ACSM'S

Resources for the Exercise Physiologist

A Practical Guide for the Health Fitness Professional

Third Edition

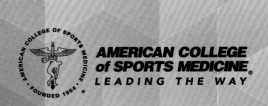

ACSM'S

Resources for the Exercise Physiologist

A Practical Guide for the Health Fitness Professional

Third Edition

SENIOR EDITOR

Benjamin T. Gordon, PhD, ACSM-EP
University of Florida
Gainesville, Florida

ASSOCIATE EDITORS

Heather Chambliss, PhD, FACSM
St. Jude Children's Research Hospital
Memphis, Tennessee

J. Larry Durstine, PhD, FACSM
University of South Carolina
Columbia, South Carolina

David M. Jett, MS, ACSM-EP
University of Louisville
Louisville, Kentucky

Leanna M. Ross, PhD
Duke University
Durham, North Carolina

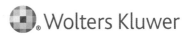. Wolters Kluwer

Philadelphia • Baltimore • New York • London
Buenos Aires • Hong Kong • Sydney • Tokyo

Acquisitions Editor: Lindsey Parambo
Senior Development Editor: Amy Millholen
Senior Editorial Coordinator: Lindsay Ries
Marketing Manager: Phyllis Hitner
Production Project Manager: Kirstin Johnson
Design Coordinator: Stephen Druding
Manufacturing Coordinator: Margie Orzech
Prepress Vendor: Absolute Service, Inc.

ACSM Committee on Certification and Registry Boards Chair: Christie Ward-Ritacco, PhD, ACSM-EP, EIM2
ACSM Publications Committee Chair: Jeffrey Potteiger, PhD, FACSM
ACSM Certification-Related Content Advisory Committee Chair: Dierdra Bycura, EdD, ACSM-CPT, ACSM-EP
ACSM Chief Operating Officer: Katie Feltman
ACSM Development Editor: Angie Chastain

Third edition

9 8 7 6 5 4 3 2 1

Printed in China

Library of Congress Cataloging-in-Publication Data

Names: Gordon, Benjamin Thomas, editor. | Chambliss, Heather, editor. |
  Durstine, J. Larry, editor. | Jett, David M., editor. | Ross, Leanna M., editor. |
  American College of Sports Medicine, issuing body.
Title: ACSM's resources for the exercise physiologist : a practical guide
  for the health fitness professional / senior editor, Benjamin T. Gordon;
  associate editors, Heather Chambliss, J. Larry Durstine, David M.
  Jett, Leanna M. Ross.
Other titles: American College of Sports Medicine's resources for the
  exercise physiologist
Description: Third edition. | Philadelphia : Wolters Kluwer, [2022] |
  Includes bibliographical references and index.
Identifiers: LCCN 2021011604 (print) | LCCN 2021011605 (ebook) | ISBN
  9781975153168 (hardcover) | ISBN 9781975153182 (epub)
Subjects: MESH: Exercise Therapy | Exercise--physiology | Physical Fitness |
  Sports Medicine | Practice Guideline | BISAC: MEDICAL / Sports Medicine
Classification: LCC RM725 (print) | LCC RM725 (ebook) | NLM WB 541 | DDC
  615.8/2—dc23
LC record available at https://lccn.loc.gov/2021011604
LC ebook record available at https://lccn.loc.gov/2021011605

Preface

The purpose of this text is to serve as the key resource for certified exercise physiologists, with particular regard to the American College of Sports Medicine (ACSM) Certified Exercise Physiologist® (ACSM-EP®). To accomplish this, *ACSM's Resources for the Exercise Physiologist* provides information about the theory and practice that forms the basis of the ACSM-EP scope of practice. This book is able to stand alone as a classroom text or serve as a supplement to many existing texts. The array and strength of the chapter contributors, many of whom are renowned experts in their fields, is a key aspect that adds to the value of this text.

The primary audience for *ACSM's Resources for the Exercise Physiologist* is the student or professional studying for the ACSM-EP certification exam. Secondary markets include ACSM-EP and personal trainers who wish to broaden their knowledge base. Other health care providers (nurses, physical therapists, etc.) looking to expand their understanding of exercise, exercise prescription, and best practices related to exercise also will find valuable information here.

Organization

This book is organized around the scope of practice domains identified for the ACSM-EP. We begin with an introductory section focused on understanding exercise and physical activity along with preexercise screening. Part II includes assessment and programming for healthy populations. Part III covers a similar underlying theme but focuses on special populations, including those with metabolic disorders, pregnant women, children, and the elderly. Part IV includes counseling and behavioral strategies for encouraging and sustaining exercise, a critical need for all exercise professionals. The final section, Part V, covers legal, management, and professional issues relevant to all exercise professionals, especially those interested in owning a business or ascending the leadership ladder. The information within this text is based on *ACSM's Guidelines for Exercise Testing and Prescription*, eleventh edition.

Features

Each of the chapters begins with **objectives** and ends with **open-ended questions** directly related to the objectives. Chapters contain **How To boxes**, which provide step-by-step instructions for different types of assessments an ACSM-EP regularly encounters, and an **Exercise is Medicine Connection**, which describes research about the role of exercise in improving health. **Case Studies** are also a key feature as they detail real-life situations ACSM-EP's face, with suggestions on how to best address them. **Icons** highlight relevant video clips that are available on Lippincott Connect.

Additional Resources

ACSM's Resources for the Exercise Physiologist includes additional resources for students and instructors.

Students

- Video clips available on Lippincott Connect

Instructors

Approved adopting instructors will be given access to the following additional resources on thePoint:

- Test bank
- Lesson plans
- PowerPoint presentations
- Image bank
- Case study answers

See the inside front cover of this text for more details, including the passcode you will need to gain access to the Web site.

Updates for the book can be found at https://www.acsm.org/get-stay-certified/get-certified /prepare-for-exams/acsm-book-updates.

Acknowledgments

Thank you to my associate editors, Larry Durstine, Mike Jett, Heather Chambliss, and Leanna Ross. Without their work, this project wouldn't have been possible. I also need to give a huge thank you to Angie Chastain who was able to masterfully organize this project despite the unprecedented times and circumstances. Thank you to all the staff at ACSM and Wolters Kluwer for their support and assistance. The staff work tirelessly to make projects like this happen. In addition, I want to thank the first two editors of this book Gary Ligouri and Peter Magyari. Without their encouragement and fantastic work, this book wouldn't be the excellent resource it has become. Furthermore, without the mentorship of Larry Durstine and Peter Magyari, I would not have the opportunity or the knowledge to complete a project of this magnitude. Lastly, thank you to my parents (Rick and Linda), brother (Matt), and longtime friend (Brandon) who have always helped and supported me regardless of the situation.

Ben Gordon, Senior Editor

Contributors

Elizabeth Anderson, MS
University of South Carolina
Columbia, South Carolina
Chapter 8

Diane Babbitt, PhD
Cedar Crest College
Allentown, Pennsylvania
Chapter 2

Bryan Blissmer, PhD
University of Rhode Island
Kingston, Rhode Island
Chapter 12

Katie Brown, PhD
Texas Tech University
Lubbock, Texas
Chapter 14

Keith J. Burns, PhD, ACSM-EP
Walsh University
North Canton, Ohio
Chapter 8

Katrina D. DuBose, PhD, FACSM
East Carolina University
Greenville, North Carolina
Chapter 7

J. Larry Durstine, PhD, FACSM
University of South Carolina
Columbia, South Carolina
Chapter 8

Gregory B. Dwyer, PhD, FACSM, ACSM-CEP, PD, EIM3
East Stroudsburg University
East Stroudsburg, Pennsylvania
Chapter 2

Avery D. Faigenbaum, EdD, FACSM, ACSM-EP
The College of New Jersey
Ewing, New Jersey
Chapter 4

Charles James Fountaine, PhD, FACSM
University of Minnesota Duluth
Duluth, Minnesota
Chapter 3

Benjamin T. Gordon, PhD, ACSM-EP
University of Florida
Gainesville, Florida
Chapter 8

Kristi King, PhD
University of Louisville
Louisville, Kentucky
Chapter 1

Matt R. Kutz, PhD
Bowling Green State University
Bowling Green, Ohio
Chapter 15

Beth Lewis, PhD
University of Minnesota
Minneapolis, Minnesota
Chapter 11

Randi S. Lite, MA, FACSM, ACSM-CEP, EIM3
Simmons University
Boston, Massachusetts
Chapter 18

Meir Magal, PhD, FACSM, ACSM-CEP
North Carolina Wesleyan College
Rocky Mount, North Carolina
Chapter 5

Peter Magyari, PhD, FACSM, ACSM-EP
University of North Florida
Jacksonville, Florida
Chapter 2

David X. Marquez, PhD, FACSM
University of Illinois at Chicago
Chicago, Illinois
Chapter 11

Michelle Y. Martin, PhD, FACSM
University of Tennessee
Memphis, Tennessee
Chapter 12

Linda E. May, PhD, FACSM
East Carolina University
Greenville, North Carolina
Chapter 10

Jessica R. Meendering, PhD, FACSM, ACSM-EP
South Dakota State University
Brookings, South Dakota
Chapter 3

A. Lynn Millar, PhD, FACSM
Winston-Salem State University
Winston-Salem, North Carolina
Chapter 9

Laurie A. Milliken, PhD, FACSM
University of Massachusetts Boston
Boston, Massachusetts
Chapter 10

Mario A. Muñoz, PhD, FACSM
Sam Houston State University
Huntsville, Texas
Chapter 10

Nicole Nelson, MHS, LMT, ACSM-EP
University of North Florida
Jacksonville, Florida
Chapter 6

Deborah A. Riebe, PhD, FACSM, ACSM-EP
University of Rhode Island
Kingston, Rhode Island
Chapter 7

James Schoffstall, EdD, FACSM, ACSM-CEP, ACSM-EP, ACSM/NCHPAD-CIFT, ACSM/NPAS-PAPHS, EIM3
Liberty University
Lynchburg, Virginia
Chapter 17

Katie J. Schuver, PhD
University of Minnesota
Minneapolis, Minnesota
Chapter 11

Matthew A. Stults-Kolehmainen, PhD, FACSM, ACSM-EP
Teachers College, Columbia University
New York, New York
Chapter 13

Stephen J. Tharrett, MS
ClubIntel
Lewisville, Texas
Chapter 16

Kathleen Sherry Thomas, PhD, ATC, ACSM-EP
Norfolk State University
Virginia Beach, Virginia
Chapter 5

Reviewers

William Boyer II, PhD
California Baptist University
Riverside, California

Matt Clark, BS
Orangetheory Fitness
Indianapolis, Indiana

Steven Gaskill, PhD
University of Montana
Missoula, Montana

Ann L. Gibson, PhD, FACSM
The University of New Mexico
Albuquerque, New Mexico

**Trevor Gillum, PhD, ACSM-EP,
EIM2**
California Baptist University
Riverside, California

Brandon Grubbs, PhD, ACSM-EP
Middle Tennessee State University
Murfreesboro, Tennessee

**Lisa Leininger, ACSM-EP, ACSM/
NPAS-PAPHS, EIM2**
California State University, Monterey Bay
Marina, California

Lydia R. Malcolm, PhD
Authentic Behavioral Health, LLC
Fort Lauderdale, Florida

Kelly P. Massey, PhD, ACSM-EP
Georgia College
Eatonton, Georgia

Amy D. Miller, DrPH
California Baptist University
Riverside, California

Jason Ng, PhD, EIM1
California State University,
San Bernardino
San Bernardino, California

Katie Potter, PhD
University of Massachusetts Amherst
Amherst, Massachusetts

Erica Rauff, PhD
Seattle University
Seattle, Washington

John R. Sirard, PhD, FACSM
University of Massachusetts Amherst
Amherst, Massachusetts

Erica M. Taylor, PhD, FACSM
Columbus State University
Columbus, Georgia

Katie J. Thralls, PhD
Seattle Pacific University
Seattle, Washington

Contents

Preface   *v*

Acknowledgments   *vii*

Contributors   *viii*

Reviewers   *x*

PART I: Overview   1

1   Understanding Physical Activity and Exercise   2

Defining Physical Activity, Exercise, and Physical Fitness   3

Historic Trends in Physical Activity   7

Ancient Times and the Rise of Exercise Physiology   7

T.K. Cureton and the Physical Fitness Movement   7

Historical Evolution of Physical Activity Epidemiology   8

Development of Physical Activity Guidelines and Recommendations   9

Relationship between Physical Activity/Exercise and Health across the Lifespan   12

Physical Activity and Health in Children and Adolescents   13

Physical Activity and Health in Adults   15

Physical Activity and Health in Older Adults   18

Physical Activity and Health in Women during Pregnancy and during the Postpartum Period   18

Physical Activity and Health in Adults with Chronic Conditions and Adults with Disabilities   18

General Risks Associated with Physical Activity/Exercise   19

Risks of Sudden Cardiac Death   20

The Risk of Cardiac Events during Exercise Testing   20

Musculoskeletal Injury Associated with Exercise   20

2   Preparticipation Physical Activity Screening Guidelines   29

Importance of Preparticipation Physical Activity Screening   30

History of Preparticipation Physical Activity Screening   31

Levels of Screening   31

Self-Guided Screening   32

  • PHYSICAL ACTIVITY READINESS QUESTIONNAIRE FOR EVERYONE   32

  • EPARMED-X+PHYSICIAN CLEARANCE FOLLOW-UP QUESTIONNAIRE   32

Professionally Supervised Screening   37

  • INFORMED CONSENT   37

  • HEALTH HISTORY QUESTIONNAIRE   39

  • MEDICAL EXAMINATION/CLEARANCE   39

  • PREPARTICIPATION PHYSICAL ACTIVITY SCREENING PROCESS   39

    Physical Activity (or Exercise) History   46

    Known Cardiovascular, Metabolic, and/or Renal Disease   46

    ACSM Major Signs or Symptoms Suggestive of Cardiovascular Disease   46

    When Should You Seek Medical Clearance?   48

American Association of Cardiovascular and Pulmonary Rehabilitation Risk Stratification   49

Challenges of ACSM Preparticipation Physical Activity Screening   49

Recommendations versus Requirements   50

Contraindications to Exercise Testing   51

What Does Contraindication Really Mean?   52

Absolute versus Relative   52

Repurposing Risk Factor Assessment and Management   52

ACSM Atherosclerotic Cardiovascular Disease Risk Factor Assessment and Defining Criteria   52

PART II: Assessments and Exercise Programming for Apparently Healthy Participants   59

---

3   Cardiorespiratory Fitness Assessments and Exercise Programming for Apparently Healthy Participants   60

Basic Anatomy and Physiology of the Cardiovascular and Pulmonary Systems as They Relate to Cardiorespiratory Fitness   61

Goal of the Cardiovascular and Respiratory Systems   61

Anatomy and Physiology of the Cardiovascular and Respiratory Systems   61

Adenosine Triphosphate Production   62

Overview of Cardiorespiratory Responses to Acute Graded Exercise of Conditioned and Unconditioned Participants   64

Oxygen Uptake Kinetics during Submaximal Single-Intensity Exercise   64

Oxygen Uptake Kinetics during Graded Intensity Exercise   65

Arteriovenous Oxygen Difference Response to Graded Intensity Exercise   66

Heart Rate, Stroke Volume, and Cardiac Output Responses to Graded Intensity Exercise   66

Pulmonary Ventilation Response to Graded Intensity Exercise   67

Blood Pressure Response to Graded Intensity Exercise   67

Measuring Blood Pressure and Heart Rate before, during, and after Graded Exercise   68

Blood Pressure and Heart Rate Assessment   68

Rate Pressure Product   69

Selecting Appropriate Cardiorespiratory Fitness Assessments for Healthy Populations   70

Cardiorespiratory Fitness Assessments Benefits   70

Types of Cardiorespiratory Fitness Assessments   70

Selecting the Appropriate Cardiorespiratory Fitness Assessment   71

Interpreting Results of Cardiorespiratory Fitness Assessments, Including Determination of $\dot{V}O_2$ and $\dot{V}O_{2max}$ 76

Metabolic Calculations as They Relate to Cardiorespiratory Exercise Programming   77

Energy Units and Conversion Factors   77

ACSM Metabolic Formula   82

• EXAMPLES   83

FITT Framework for the Development of Cardiorespiratory Fitness in Apparently Healthy People   84

Frequency   85

Intensity   85

Time   85

Type   86

Additional Variables   86

Volume   86

Progression   86

• PROGRESSIVE OVERLOAD   86

• REVERSIBILITY   86

• INDIVIDUAL DIFFERENCES   87

• SPECIFICITY OF TRAINING   87

Safe and Effective Exercises Designed to Enhance Cardiorespiratory Fitness   87

Interval Training   89

Determining Exercise Intensity   89

  Heart Rate Reserve Method   90

  Peak Heart Rate Method   90

  Peak $\dot{V}O_2$ Method   90

  Peak Metabolic Equivalent Method   91

  $\dot{V}O_2$ Reserve Method   91

  Talk Test Method   91

  Perceived Exertion Method   92

Abnormal Responses to Exercise   92

Contraindications to Cardiovascular Training Exercises   93

Effect of Common Medications on Cardiorespiratory Exercise   93

Signs and Symptoms of Common Musculoskeletal Injuries Associated with Cardiorespiratory Exercise   93

Effects of Heat, Cold, or High Altitude on the Physiological Response to Exercise   94

  Heat Stress   95

  Cold Stress   95

  Altitude   95

Acclimatization When Exercising in a Hot, Cold, or High-Altitude Environment   96

4   Muscular Strength and Muscular Endurance Assessments and Exercise Programming for Apparently Healthy Participants   103

Basic Structure and Function   105

  Muscle Fiber Types and Recruitment   105

  Types of Muscle Action   106

Assessment Protocols   108

  Assessing Muscular Strength   109

  Assessing Muscular Endurance   110

Fundamental Principles of Resistance Training   111

  Principle of Progression   111

  Principle of Regularity   112

  Principle of Overload   113

  Principle of Creativity   113

  Principle of Enjoyment   113

  Principle of Specificity   114

  Principle of Supervision   115

Program Design Considerations   115

  Types of Resistance Training   116

  • DYNAMIC CONSTANT EXTERNAL RESISTANCE TRAINING   116

  • ISOKINETICS   117

  • PLYOMETRIC TRAINING   118

  Modes of Resistance Training   119

  Safety Concerns   121

Resistance Training Program Variables   123

  Type of Exercise   124

  Order of Exercise   125

  Training Intensity   125

  Training Volume   126

  Rest Intervals between Sets   127

  Repetition Velocity   127

  Training Frequency   127

  Periodization   128

General Recommendations   129

5   Flexibility Assessments and Exercise Programming for Apparently Healthy
     Participants   136
     Basic Principles of Flexibility   137
       Factors Affecting Flexibility   137
     Modes of Flexibility Training   139
       Static Flexibility   139
       Ballistic Flexibility   140
       Proprioceptive Neuromuscular Facilitation   140
       Dynamic Flexibility   142
     Muscle and Tendon Proprioceptors   144
     Flexibility Assessment Protocols   145
       Goniometers and Inclinometers   145
     Flexibility Program Design   153
     Overall Range of Motion Recommendations   154

6   Functional Movement Assessments and Exercise Programming for Apparently
     Healthy Participants   175
     Sensorimotor Control   176
       Motor Learning   176
       Proprioception   176
       Stability and Mobility   177
     Mediators of the Proprioception, Mobility, and Stability   180
       Overweight and Obesity and Physical Inactivity   180
       Propensity for Inhibition of Stabilizing Muscles   180
       Previous Injury and Pain   180
       Everyday Posture and Limited Variety of Movement   181
       Joint Structure   181
       Age   182
     What Is Neutral Position and Why Is It so Important?   182
     Assessment and Prescription   183
       Establishing a Movement Baseline   183
         • ASSESSMENT OF STATIC NEUTRAL POSTURE   183
           Plumb Line Assessment   183
           Wall Test   183
           Progressive Approach to Developing Postural Awareness   183
         • INTEGRATIVE ASSESSMENTS AND CORRECTIONS   185
           Wall Plank-and-Roll   185
           Teaching How to Brace   185
           Diaphragmatic Breathing Assessment and Corrective Methods   186
           Rolling Patterns: Assessment and Correction   187
         • ADDRESSING ALIGNMENT ISSUES   191
           Instability Training   193
     Self-Myofascial Release and Stretching   194
     Lifestyle Recommendations   197

7   Body Composition and Weight Management   200
     Anthropometric Measurements   201
       Height and Weight   202
       Body Mass Index   202
         • CIRCUMFERENCE MEASURES   204

Measuring Body Composition   206
- *SKINFOLD MEASUREMENTS*   207
- *BIOELECTRICAL IMPEDANCE*   209
- *LABORATORY METHODS FOR MEASURING BODY COMPOSITION*   211

Weight Management   213
Energy Balance   213
Preventing Weight Gain   217
Treatment of Obesity   217
FITT Recommendations   217
Training Considerations   218
Weight Loss Goals   219
Metabolic Equations   219
Weight Management Myths   219
- *MYTH 1: FAT TURNS INTO MUSCLE*   219
- *MYTH 2: SPOT REDUCING WORKS*   220
- *MYTH 3: GAINING WEIGHT AT THE START OF AN EXERCISE PROGRAM IS FROM INCREASED MUSCLE*   220

Treatment of Obesity through Nutrition   221
Treatment of Obesity through Other Methods   223
Behavioral Strategies   224
Weight Loss Supplements   224
Dieting   225
Medications   225

PART III: Exercise Programming for Special Populations   **231**

8   Exercise for Individuals with Controlled Cardiovascular, Metabolic, Pulmonary, and Chronic Kidney Disease   232
Pathophysiology   233
Cardiovascular Disease   233
- *CORONARY HEART DISEASE*   233
- *HYPERTENSION*   234
- *PERIPHERAL ARTERY DISEASE*   235

Metabolic Diseases   235
- *DIABETES*   236
- *DYSLIPIDEMIA*   236
- *OBESITY*   236
- *METABOLIC SYNDROME*   237

Pulmonary Diseases   237
- *CHRONIC OBSTRUCTIVE PULMONARY DISEASE*   237
- *CHRONIC RESTRICTIVE PULMONARY DISEASE*   238

Chronic Kidney Disease   238
Role of Exercise Training   238
Cardiovascular Diseases   238
Metabolic Diseases   240
Pulmonary Diseases   240
Chronic Kidney Disease   240
The Art and Science of Exercise Prescription and Programming in Controlled Disease Populations   241
Special FITT Considerations for Persons with Chronic Diseases   241
- *HIGH-INTENSITY INTERVAL TRAINING*   241
- *CARDIOVASCULAR DISEASE*   244

- METABOLIC DISEASE 244
- PULMONARY DISEASE 245
- CHRONIC KIDNEY DISEASE 246

Effects of Myocardial Ischemia, Myocardial Infarction, and Hypertension on Cardiorespiratory Responses during Exercise 246

Myocardial Ischemia 246

Myocardial Infarction 247

- HYPERTENSION 247

Exercise Concerns, Precautions, and Contraindications 247

Cardiovascular Disease 247

Metabolic Disease 250

Pulmonary Disease 251

Chronic Kidney Disease 252

Effect of Common Medications on Exercise Capacity and Tolerance 253

Over-the-Counter Drugs 253

Prescription Drugs 255

Teaching and Demonstrating Safe and Effective Exercise 256

9 Exercise Programming for Individuals with Musculoskeletal Limitations 265

Traumatic Movement–Related Injuries 266

Fractures 266

Strains 267

Sprains 268

Contusions 268

- IMMEDIATE CARE 269
- MEDICATIONS FOR MUSCULOSKELETAL PAIN AND INFLAMMATION 269
- EXERCISE TO REDUCE RISK OF STRAINS AND SPRAINS 270

Overuse Injuries 271

Tendinopathy 271

- CLINICAL PRESENTATION/ASSESSMENT 271
- SAFE AND EFFECTIVE EXERCISE 272
- EXERCISE CONSIDERATIONS FOR TENDINOPATHIES 272

Bursitis 273

- CLINICAL PRESENTATION/ASSESSMENT 273
- SAFE AND EFFECTIVE EXERCISE 273

Plantar Fasciitis 273

- CLINICAL PRESENTATION/ASSESSMENT 273
- SAFE AND EFFECTIVE EXERCISE 274

Examples of Safe and Effective Exercises for Overuse Injuries 274

Low Back Pain 275

- CLINICAL PRESENTATION/ASSESSMENT 276
- SAFE AND EFFECTIVE EXERCISE 277

Chronic Conditions 281

Arthritis 281

- RHEUMATOID ARTHRITIS 281

Clinical Presentation/Assessment 281

Safe and Effective Exercise 282

- OSTEOARTHRITIS 283

Obesity and Osteoarthritis 283

Clinical Presentation/Assessment 283

Safe and Effective Exercise 283

- *MEDICATION EFFECTS FOR RHEUMATOID ARTHRITIS AND OSTEOARTHRITIS 284*
- *EXERCISE GUIDELINES FOR RHEUMATOID ARTHRITIS AND OSTEOARTHRITIS 284*

Osteoporosis 285
- *RISK FACTORS FOR OSTEOPOROSIS 285*
- *CLINICAL PRESENTATION/ASSESSMENT 287*
- *DIETARY AND PHARMACOLOGICAL SUPPORT FOR BONE HEALTH 287*
- *SAFE AND EFFECTIVE EXERCISE 288*

10 Exercise Programming across the Lifespan: Children and Adolescents, Pregnant Women, and Older Adults 299

Children and Adolescents 300

Physical and Physiological Changes 300
- *BODY SIZE AND COMPOSITION 300*
- *CARDIORESPIRATORY FUNCTION 301*
- *MUSCULAR STRENGTH, FLEXIBILITY, AND MOTOR PERFORMANCE 301*
- *RATING OF PERCEIVED EXERTION 302*
- *THERMOREGULATION 302*

Motor Skills and Physical Activity 302

The Impact of Chronic Exercise 302

Exercise Programming and Specific Exercise Considerations 303
- *CHILDREN 304*
- *ADOLESCENTS 304*

Pregnant Women 305

Physical and Physiological Changes 305

The Impact of Chronic Exercise 306

Exercise Programming and Specific Exercise Considerations 308

Special Considerations during Pregnancy 310

Older Adults 310

Physical and Physiological Changes 311
- *BODY COMPOSITION AND MUSCULOSKELETAL FUNCTION 311*
- *CARDIORESPIRATORY FUNCTION AND THERMOREGULATION 312*

The Impact of Chronic Exercise 313

Exercise Programming and Specific Exercise Considerations 313
- *AEROBIC ACTIVITY 315*
- *MUSCLE-STRENGTHENING ACTIVITY 315*
- *FLEXIBILITY ACTIVITY AND NEUROMOTOR EXERCISES 316*
- *THERMOREGULATION 316*

PART IV: Behavior Change 325

11 Theories of Behavior Change 326

Importance of Theories and Models 327

Transtheoretical Model 327

Social Cognitive Theory 328

Self-Efficacy 329

Relapse Prevention 333

Social Ecological Model 334

Theory of Planned Behavior 337

Self-Determination Theory 338

Hedonic Theory 339

12   Facilitating Health Behavior Change   347

Practical Strategies for Behavior Change   348

Identifying Benefits of Physical Activity   348

Setting Goals   349

Using Self-Monitoring Tools   349
- SELF-MONITORING RECOMMENDATIONS   350
- PHYSICAL ACTIVITY MONITORS   351

Increasing Social Support   351

Regulating Emotions   351

Enhancing Self-Efficacy   353

Problem-Solving Barriers to Physical Activity   354

Increasing Options for Physical Activity   356

Preventing Relapse   356

Facilitating Behavior Change: The Role of the Exercise Physiologist   357

Incorporating Behavior Change into Practice   357

Improving Communication   359

Using Motivational Interviewing   360

Working with Diverse Populations   366
- OLDER ADULTS   366
- RACE/ETHNICITY   367

13   Healthy Stress Management   371

The Stress Response   372

Sources of Stress   372

Appraisal of Stress   373

Coping   373
- PROBLEM-FOCUSED COPING   374
- EMOTION-FOCUSED COPING   374

The Physiological and Psychological Response to Stress   374

General Adaptation Syndrome and Allostasis   374

The Effects of Stress on Health   376
- DIGESTIVE ISSUES   376
- HEADACHES   377
- CARDIOVASCULAR AND METABOLIC DISEASES AND THE ROLE OF CORTISOL   378
- IMMUNE SUPPRESSION, CANCER, AND MULTIPLE SCLEROSIS   378

Stress and Psychological Functioning   378
- PSYCHOLOGICAL DISTRESS, ANXIETY, AND DEPRESSION   378
- FATIGUE AND BURNOUT   379
- COGNITIVE DEFICITS   379

Healthy Stress Management   379

Exercise   379

Enhancing Social Support   380

Improving Personal Control and Self-Efficacy   382

Mind–Body Techniques for Reducing Stress   383
- DIAPHRAGMATIC BREATHING AND BODY SCANS   384
- PROGRESSIVE MUSCLE RELAXATION   384
- BIOFEEDBACK   384
- MASSAGE   385
- MEDITATION AND PRAYER   385
- MINDFULNESS   385
- YOGA AND MARTIAL ARTS   386
- REFERRING A CLIENT OR PATIENT TO A PSYCHOLOGIST   386

PART V: Business   **395**

14 Legal Structure and Terminology 396
The Law and Legal System 397
Primary Sources of Law 397
  Tort Law 399
  Negligence 399
  Insurance Coverage 402
Federal Laws 403
  Sexual Harassment 403
  Occupational Safety and Health Administration Guidelines 404
  Health Insurance Portability and Accountability Act Guidelines and Recommendations 404
Client Rights and Responsibilities 405
  Client Rights 405
  Client Responsibilities 406
  Contract Law 406
  Employer and Employee Rights and Responsibilities 406
  Federal Employment Laws 407
  Hiring and Prehiring Statutes 407
  Facility Policies and Procedures 410

15 Leadership and Management 415
Defining Leadership and Management 416
  Operational Definitions 416
  Evidence-Based Management 418
Leadership: Past, Present, and Future 419
  Transactional Model 419
  Visionary Model 419
  Organic Model 420
  Leadership Theory and Model 420
Leadership Behaviors and Theories 421
  Trait Theory 421
  Situational Leadership Theory 421
  Path–Goal Leadership Theory 422
  Transformational and Transactional Leadership 422
  Lewin's Leadership Styles 423
  Servant Leadership 423
  Leader–Member Exchange Theory 424
  Emotional Intelligence 424
  Contextual Intelligence and Three-Dimensional Thinking 425
Management Techniques 427
  Management Grid (Blake and Mouton) 427
  Scientific Management (Frederick W. Taylor) 427
  Bureaucratic Model of Management (Max Weber) 428
  Total Quality Management (W. Edwards Deming) 428
  Management by Objective (Peter Drucker) 429
  Motivator-Hygiene Theory (Fredrick Herzberg) 429
  Theory X and Y (Douglas McGregor) 430
  Behavioral Approach (Mary Parker Follet) 430
Organizational Behavior 431
  Strategic Planning 431

16 General Health Fitness Management   436

Human Resource Management   437

Organizational Culture and Teamwork   437

Staffing   438

- TYPES OF POSITIONS   438
- EMPLOYEE VERSUS INDEPENDENT CONTRACTOR   439
- EXEMPT VERSUS NONEXEMPT   441
- FULL-TIME VERSUS PART-TIME   441
- JOB DESCRIPTIONS   442

Recruiting and Selection   442

- RECRUITING STRATEGIES   442
- SELECTION PROCESS   444
- INTERVIEW PROCESS   445

Compensation   445

Employee Orientation, Development, and Training   446

Performance Management and Employee Retention   447

- SETTING GOALS   447
- PERFORMANCE APPRAISALS   448
- EMPLOYEE RETENTION   449

Section Summary   449

Risk Management   449

Standards and Guidelines for Risk Management and Emergency Procedures   449

Types of Business Liability Insurance   452

Risk Management Summary   453

Facility Management and Operations   453

Clinical and Nonclinical Health/Fitness Facility Settings   453

- CLINICAL FITNESS SETTING   454
- NONCLINICAL FITNESS SETTINGS   454

Operations   455

Equipment   455

Financial Management   457

Accrual and Cash Accounting   458

Financial Statements   458

- BALANCE SHEET   458
- PROFIT AND LOSS STATEMENT   460

Budgeting   461

- TYPES OF BUDGETS   461
- CREATING A BUDGET   461

Income Management   462

Expense Management   462

Section Summary   463

Marketing and Sales   463

Marketing   463

- MARKETING TOOLS   464

Sales   465

Section Summary   465

Programming   466

Programs in Demand   466

Steps to Successful Programming   466

Section Summary   467

17 Marketing 469

Marketing Basics 470

People 470

Product 472

Place 472

Price 474

Promotion 475

- BRANDING 476
- ADVERTISING 476
- REFERRAL 476
- DIRECT MAIL/E-MAIL 477
- INTERNET 477
- BUSINESS TO BUSINESS 477
- SPONSORSHIP 477
- PERSONAL SALES 478

  Finding Leads 478

  Qualifying Prospects 479

  The Art of the Deal 479

- PUBLIC RELATIONS 479

18 Professional Behaviors and Ethics 484

History 485

Accreditation 485

Committee on the Certification and Registry Board 489

ACSM Code of Ethics 489

Scope of Practice 489

Scenario 1 491

Scenario 2 492

Scenario 3 493

Conflict of Interest 495

Providing Evidence-Based Information 495

Step 1: Develop a Question 495

Step 2: Search for Evidence 496

- PERSONAL EXPERIENCE 496
- ACADEMIC PREPARATION 496
- RESEARCH KNOWLEDGE 496

Step 3: Evaluate the Evidence 496

Step 4: Incorporate Evidence into Practice 496

Maintaining Certification 498

Ways to Earn Continuing Education Credits 499

Personal Characteristics 499

Appendix A Editors from the Previous Two Editions of *ACSM's Resources for the Exercise Physiologist* 507

Appendix B Contributors from the Previous Two Editions of *ACSM's Resources for the Exercise Physiologist* 508

Index 511

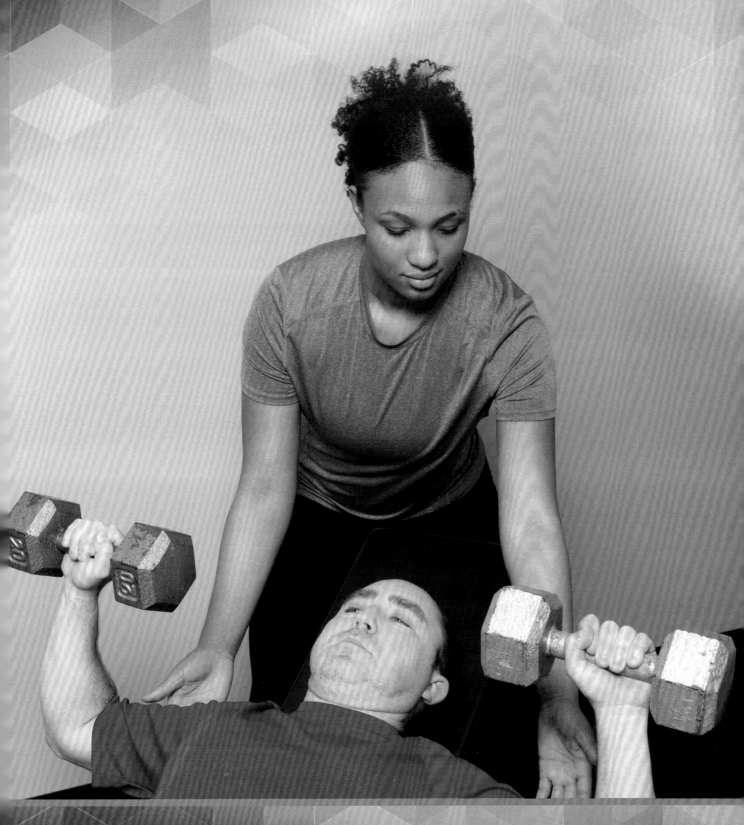

Overview

1

Understanding Physical Activity and Exercise

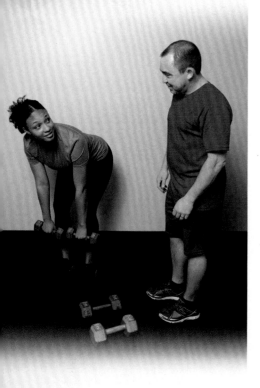

OBJECTIVES

- To define physical activity, exercise, and physical fitness.
- To identify several key historical individuals and landmark research that were instrumental in building the current knowledge base regarding the health benefits of physical activity, exercise, and physical fitness.
- To know how physical activity and exercise can positively impact health across the lifespan.
- To understand the general health risks associated with physical activity and exercise at different intensities and volumes.

INTRODUCTION

In addition to conducting exercise testing and prescription, an American College of Sports Medicine Certified Exercise Physiologist® (ACSM-EP®) should demonstrate competency in developing and implementing basic health behavior and physical activity (PA) interventions for individuals with chronic diseases or conditions as well as providing primary and secondary prevention strategies designed to improve, maintain, or attenuate declines in fitness and health in populations ranging from children to older adults (1). A practicing ACSM-EP should be able to distinguish between PA, exercise, health-related fitness, and skill-related fitness. Although the terms *PA*, *exercise*, and *physical fitness* are closely intertwined, they each have distinguishing features to make them unique. This chapter discusses some of these unique features, along with a review of important historical individuals and the landmarks in research in the evolution of PA, exercise, and physical fitness, leading to today's understanding of the health benefits as well as potential risks of PA and exercise. Finally, there is an overview of current guidelines and recommendations for using PA and exercise to promote better health.

Defining Physical Activity, Exercise, and Physical Fitness

The terms *PA*, *exercise*, and *physical fitness* are often used interchangeably; however, there are distinct characteristics that differentiate them from one another. PA and exercise are behaviors, whereas physical fitness can be an outcome of PA and exercise behaviors. Further, health- and skill-related fitness can further describe physical fitness as they are potential outcomes of PA and exercise as well.

To begin, *PA* is the broadest and most encompassing term and is defined as "any bodily movement produced by skeletal muscles that results in energy expenditure. The energy expenditure can be measured in kilocalories" (2). The total amount of caloric expenditure associated with PA is determined by the amount of muscle mass producing bodily movements and the intensity, duration, and frequency of muscular contractions. PA can be a blend of aerobic (oxygen dependent, *i.e.*, walking to the store, jogging) and anaerobic (oxygen independent, *i.e.*, moving furniture, lifting weights) activities, depending on the intensity. Within any one given activity, both aerobic and anaerobic processes may be present, as can both static and dynamic muscle contractions. Examples of PA can include walking, gardening, or riding a bicycle.

PA can be categorized by its situational context outside of competitive level sport. Typically, four PA domains include recreation, transport, occupation, and household (Fig. 1.1). "Active living"

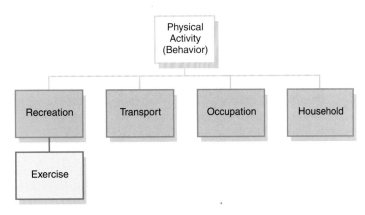

FIGURE 1.1. Domains of PA.

incorporates exercise, recreational activities, household and occupational activities, and active transportation (3). The purpose of any given bout of PA can vary by environment and can also change from day to day. For instance, transportation for some might mean using public transport and walking to and from the bus station and workplace. This type of PA is likely to provide some health-related benefits. Others might cycle vigorously to and from work at a more challenging pace. Both activities are transportation-related PA but are for a different purpose and with different outcomes.

One of the largest components of PA-related energy expenditure is occupational PA. A substantial portion of many Americans' waking day is spent working, with recent estimates indicating that employed individuals work an average of 8.5 h $\cdot$ d^{-1} (4). However, during the past 50 years, there has been a dramatic reduction in the percentage of Americans working in occupations requiring moderate-intensity PA, as the nature of work has become less physically demanding (5). Moreover, it has been estimated that occupational energy expenditure has declined by more than 100 calories $\cdot$ d^{-1} over the past five decades. The increase in obesity prevalence among American adults may be partly related to this overall decrease in occupational PA. Similar to occupational PA, observational evidence indicates that household PA in some population groups has also decreased over the past five decades (6). Gardening, home repairs, food preparation, cleaning (house and vehicle), and childcare are just some means of accumulating household PA throughout the day, and many have been made "easier" by technology.

Next, exercise is a specific subset of PA (and is typically considered within the recreational domain of PA) and, although exercise is certainly a form of PA, PA does not always include exercise. Exercise is a planned, structured, and repetitive behavior that is performed for the purpose of improving or maintaining physical fitness (2). Physical fitness is an outcome of exercise and is an attained set of attributes that relates to the ability to perform PA. Physical fitness is an outcome that directly relates to the quantity and type of PA an individual can perform. Physical fitness includes subcomponents of health- and skill-related fitness (Fig. 1.2), and although they share certain attributes, they tend to appeal to individuals with very different interests and needs.

Health-related fitness is confined to cardiorespiratory fitness, muscular endurance, muscular strength, flexibility, and body composition. Skill-related fitness can also be thought of as performance-related fitness. Skill-related fitness comprises agility, balance, coordination, power, reaction time, and speed and can result in an increased desire to participate in physical activities. Overall, skill-related fitness contributes to one's ability to function in a more skilled and efficient manner (7).

Given that most adults are not sufficiently active, promoting PA may be more conducive to engaging sedentary populations prior to recommending exercise. Although exercise may produce more health benefits, engaging in PA as opposed to exercise may be a practical first step for most physically inactive people (8). It is recommended that less fit individuals begin with lesser intense PA prior to engaging in more intense activity (9). Further, it is of great importance that an ACSM-EP works with individuals to limit long bouts of physical inactivity and sedentary behaviors (10). Sedentary behavior can be defined as sitting or reclining while engaging in minimal energy expenditure (less than 1.5 metabolic equivalents [METs]) (11,12). Physical inactivity can be defined as not meeting the recommended 30 minutes of moderate-intensity PA on at least 5 d $\cdot$ wk^{-1}, 30 minutes of vigorous-intensity PA on at least 3 d $\cdot$ wk^{-1} over at 3 or more months, or an equivalent combination achieving 600 MET-min $\cdot$ wk^{-1} (13,14). Table 1.1 shows the MET values of common physical activities.

Although there are numerous ways of accumulating PA and exercise, barriers exist for engaging in regular activity. Many adults find it difficult to acquire the necessary knowledge, attitudes, and

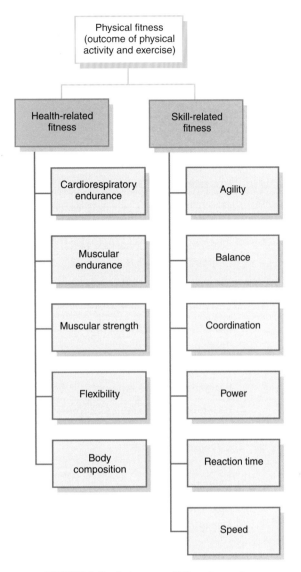

FIGURE 1.2. Outcomes of PA and exercise.

skills to reap the inherent benefits as well as the necessary social, family, financial, and geographic support and access to engage in PA regularly (Table 1.2). PA behavior may be positively or negatively influenced by differences in sex, race/ethnicity, age, educational attainment, family income, family type, country of birth, disability status, geographic location, health insurance status, sexual orientation, and marital status. An ACSM-EP should always consider these interpersonal (biological, psychological), interpersonal/cultural, organizational, physical environment (built, natural), and policy (laws, rules, regulations, codes) factors when prescribing PA and exercise (15). As an example, not having access to affordable gyms that provide childcare or sidewalks in a neighborhood so that families can exercise together may negatively impact a person's ability to be physically active. Chapters 11–13 further address behavioral strategies and examples of ways to help initiate, accumulate, and sustain meaningful PA.

Table 1.1	Metabolic Equivalents (METs) Values of Common Physical Activities Classified as Light, Moderate, or Vigorous Intensity	
Very Light/Light (<3.0 METs)	**Moderate (3.0–5.9 METs)**	**Vigorous (≥6.0 METs)**
Walking	**Walking**	**Walking, Jogging, and Running**
Walking slowly around home, store, or office = 2.0[a]	Walking 3.0 mi · h^{-1} = 3.0[a]	Walking at very, very brisk pace (4.5 mi · h^{-1}) = 6.3[a]
Household and Occupation	Walking at very brisk pace (4 mi · h^{-1}) = 5.0[a]	Walking/hiking at moderate pace and grade with no or light pack (<10 lb) = 7.0
Standing performing light work, such as making bed, washing dishes, ironing, preparing food, or store clerk = 2.0–2.5	**Household and Occupation**	Hiking at steep grades and pack 10–42 lb = 7.5–9.0
Leisure Time and Sports	Cleaning, heavy — washing windows, car, clean garage = 3.0	Jogging at 5 mi · h^{-1} = 8.0[a]
Arts and crafts, playing cards = 1.5	Sweeping floors or carpet, vacuuming, mopping = 3.0–3.5	Jogging at 6 mi · h^{-1} = 10.0[a]
Billiards = 2.5	Carpentry — general = 3.6	Running at 7 mi · h^{-1} = 11.5[a]
Boating — power = 2.5	Carrying and stacking wood = 5.5	**Household and Occupation**
Croquet = 2.5	Mowing lawn — walk power mower = 5.5	Shoveling sand, coal, etc. = 7.0
Darts = 2.5	**Leisure Time and Sports**	Carrying heavy loads, such as bricks = 7.5
Fishing — sitting = 2.5	Badminton — recreational = 4.5	Heavy farming, such as bailing hay = 8.0
Playing most musical instruments = 2.0–2.5	Basketball — shooting a round = 4.5	Shoveling, digging ditches = 8.5
	Dancing — ballroom slow = 3.0; ballroom fast = 4.5	**Leisure Time and Sports**
	Fishing from riverbank and walking = 4.0	Bicycling on flat — light effort (10–12 mi · h^{-1}) = 6.0
	Golf — walking pulling clubs = 4.3	Basketball game = 8.0
	Sailing boat, wind surfing = 3.0	Bicycling on flat — moderate effort (12–14 mi · h^{-1}) = 8; fast (14–16 mi · h^{-1}) = 10
	Table tennis = 4.0	Skiing cross-country — slow (2.5 mi · h^{-1}) = 7.0; fast (5.0–7.9 mi · h^{-1}) = 9.0
	Tennis doubles = 5.0	Soccer — casual = 7.0; competitive = 10.0
	Volleyball — noncompetitive = 3.0–4.0	Swimming leisurely = 6.0[b]
		Swimming — moderate/hard = 8–11[b]
		Tennis singles = 8.0
		Volleyball — competitive at gym or beach = 8.0

[a]On flat, hard surface.

[b]MET values can vary substantially from individual to individual during swimming as a result of different strokes and skill levels.

Adapted from Ainsworth BE, Haskell WL, Whitt MC, et al. Compendium of physical activities: an update of activity codes and MET intensities. *Med Sci Sports Exerc.* 2000;32(9 Suppl):S498–504.

Table 1.2	Popular Physical Activities and Common Barriers to Physical Activity	
Popular Physical Activities	**Common Barriers to Physical Activity**
Walking	Lack of time/inconvenience
Gardening	Lack of motivation
Calisthenics	Not enjoyable/boring
Strength training	Fear of injury
Swimming	Lack of support/access
Yoga	Lack of self-esteem/self-conscious
Dancing	Lack of coordination
Jogging	Lack of encouragement

Historic Trends in Physical Activity

Ancient Times and the Rise of Exercise Physiology

The importance of PA as a means to promote health and well-being is not a new concept. In ancient China, records of exercise for health promotion date back to approximately 2500 BC (16). Following this, teachings of the Greek physician Hippocrates (17) of the fifth and fourth centuries BC detailed the importance of exercise for health and well-being. An understanding of the pathways and mechanisms through which PA influences health and well-being remained poorly understood until recent times. Much of our current understanding in these areas evolved out of advancements in human physiology, in particular, exercise physiology.

Moving forward from ancient times to the early 20th century, pioneers such as A.V. Hill and D.B. Dill, among many others, contributed vastly to the field of exercise physiology. Hill is perhaps best known for his work studying muscle mechanics and physiology, whereas Dill and numerous colleagues at the Harvard Fatigue Laboratory extensively studied exercise responses in varying environmental conditions. Collectively, developments in exercise physiology during this period laid the groundwork for our understanding of how PA and conditioning influences physical fitness.

T.K. Cureton and the Physical Fitness Movement

Building on earlier advancements in the field of exercise physiology, T.K. Cureton's work during the 1940s focused on assessing physical fitness and the importance of physical conditioning. Cureton acted as a driving force behind the physical fitness movement in the United States while developing strong research and service programs at the University of Illinois. As a result, Cureton drew significant academic attention to the topics of physical fitness and physical conditioning (18). The cumulative contributions from Cureton and his graduate students provided much of the scientific basis for modern exercise prescription.

In addition to his scientific accomplishments, Cureton made a number of service contributions pertinent to the physical fitness movement. Several of his notable contributions included, but were not limited to, fitness training and testing of soldiers during World War II, assistance in the design of physical fitness training programs for Federal Bureau of Investigation trainees, and instrumental support in the development of the President's Council on Physical Fitness (18). Moreover, Cureton was one of the original 54 charter members of the ACSM at the time of its founding in 1954.

One of Cureton's many distinguished students who made substantial contributions to exercise physiology and the physical fitness movement was the late Michael Pollock. Pollock is perhaps most remembered as a prominent researcher who made notable contributions in the areas of exercise prescription and cardiac rehabilitation. Pollock was the lead author of the ACSM's first position statement regarding the mode and quantity of exercise necessary to elicit fitness improvements (19). In addition, Pollock was instrumental in legitimizing the role of cardiac rehabilitation as an integral part of medical treatment for patients with heart disease. Many of Pollock's significant contributions were made during his tenure at the well-known Cooper Institute for Aerobics Research in the mid-1970s.

Historical Evolution of Physical Activity Epidemiology

Although research developments in exercise physiology during the early to mid-20th century led to an improved understanding of how physical fitness could be impacted by PA, the relationships between PA and certain chronic conditions (*e.g.*, cardiovascular disease [CVD] and obesity) remained largely unknown. This was especially problematic considering the dramatic increase in CVD-related mortality that occurred during the first half of the 20th century. In an attempt to identify and understand the underlying causes of heart disease and other chronic conditions, a number of large-scale epidemiological studies (*e.g.*, Framingham Heart Study and Harvard Alumni Health Study) were initiated during the middle decades of the century. For example, the Framingham Heart Study started as a large cohort study in 1948 with the purpose of identifying and examining the effects of various risk factors on the development of CVD. Over the past 70 years, it has expanded into a multigenerational study with several cohorts and a purpose to explore the effects of cardiovascular risk factors, including physical inactivity, on various physiological diseases and conditions (20).

The first epidemiological evidence indicating that greater amounts of PA were associated with reduced risks of CVD was presented by Morris and colleagues (21) after studying double-decker bus workers in London, England. The major finding from this line of research was that physically active bus conductors suffered roughly half the coronary events than did less active bus drivers. Further illustrating the potential health benefits of being physically active, later work by Paffenbarger and coworkers (22) demonstrated that work-related caloric expenditure and the risk of death from coronary heart disease were inversely related among longshoremen in San Francisco, California.

A number of subsequent large-scale epidemiological investigations demonstrated an inverse relationship between PA and CVD incidence and mortality (23–27). In general, these investigations showed a dose-response relationship as greater levels of PA were associated with reduced risks of developing CVD (Fig. 1.3).

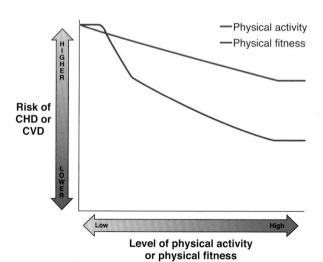

FIGURE 1.3. General relationships between PA or physical fitness level and relative risk of coronary heart disease (CHD) and CVD. (Adapted with permission from Williams PT. Physical fitness and activity as separate heart disease risk factors: a meta-analysis. *Med Sci Sports Exerc*. 2001;33[5]:754–61.)

Besides PA, research has shown that physical fitness is also inversely related to CVD incidence and mortality (see Fig. 1.3) (28–31). An important project related to this research area is the ongoing Aerobics Center Longitudinal Study (ACLS) conducted at the Cooper Clinic in Dallas, Texas. Men and women who visited the preventive medicine clinic completed a maximal treadmill test and were rated as having low, moderate, or high physical fitness based on their gender, age, and treadmill exercise time. Blair and colleagues (28) published one of the landmark papers in this research area using data from the ACLS, which demonstrated that higher levels of objectively measured physical fitness from the maximal treadmill test were associated with reduced risks of CVD mortality.

Development of Physical Activity Guidelines and Recommendations

The eventual accumulation of evidence pointing to the beneficial and protective role of PA on health-related outcomes resulted in the publication of a joint position statement by the ACSM and Centers for Disease Control and Prevention (CDC) in 1995 regarding PA and public health (32). Based on the current literature at the time, the joint position statement from the ACSM/CDC recommended that every adult accumulate 30 minutes or more of moderate-intensity PA on most, preferably all, days of the week. Soon to follow the ACSM/CDC joint position statement, the U.S. Department of Health and Human Services published the Surgeon General's report on PA and health in 1996 (33). This report presented a thorough review of the available evidence regarding PA and its relation to numerous health outcomes while restating the aerobic PA guidelines put forth by the joint ACSM/CDC position statement. Figure 1.4 shows the trend of U.S. adults reporting no leisure-time PA, which has remained steady to slightly declining, since the release of the Surgeon General's report on PA and health in 1996.

Twelve years after the joint position statement by the ACSM/CDC, an update regarding PA and public health was issued in 2007 by the ACSM and the American Heart Association (AHA) (9). The updated position statement further clarified the recommendations made in 1995. One of the main changes was the more specific frequency recommendation for moderate-intensity PA as the "most, preferably all, days of the week" qualification was changed to "five days each week." In addition, the

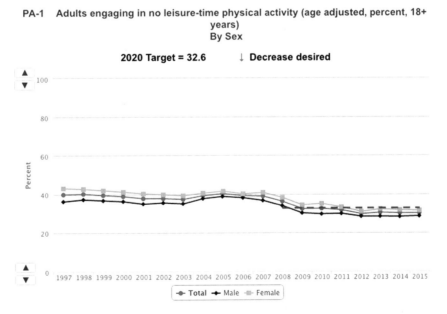

PA-1   Adults engaging in no leisure-time physical activity (age adjusted, percent, 18+ years)
By Sex

2020 Target = 32.6   ↓ Decrease desired

FIGURE 1.4. Trend line showing percentage of Americans completing no leisure-time PA. (Adapted from U.S. Department of Health and Human Services. Physical activity. Washington [DC]: U.S. Department of Health and Human Services. Available from: https://www.healthypeople.gov/2020/topics-objectives/topic/physical-activity/national-snapshot.)

update incorporated guidelines for meeting the recommendation with vigorous PA and indicated that bouts of PA should last for at least 10 minutes in duration to be counted toward the 30-minute daily goal. Specifics relating to muscle strengthening were also incorporated into the updated recommendation.

One year after the updated ACSM/AHA PA recommendations, the U.S. Department of Health and Human Services assembled a committee of PA and public health experts to review the scientific evidence on PA and health and present a detailed report, the *Physical Activity Guidelines Advisory Committee Report* (34). This report served as the foundation for the government to develop the *2008 Physical Activity Guidelines for Americans* (*2008 PAG*) (35), a practically applied set of comprehensive PA guidelines that are user-friendly for the lay community. These guidelines presented recommendations for three different age groups (children and adolescents, adults, and older adults) and incorporated specifics regarding aerobic, muscle-strengthening, and flexibility activities. Unlike the 2007 ACSM/AHA guidelines, the *2008 PAG* did not specify a weekly frequency for aerobic activity (*e.g.*, $\geq$5 d · wk^{-1}). Instead, the guidelines simply called for an accumulation of 150 minutes of moderate-intensity PA on a weekly basis and suggested that the cumulative duration be spread throughout the week.

Given the continued evidence supporting PA and health in the scientific literature throughout recent years, in 2016, the U.S. Department of Health and Human Services again assembled a committee of PA and public health experts (of which 14 of the 17 members were ACSM fellows/members) to review the latest scientific literature published since the *2008 PAG* (36). The results of these scientific reviews can be found at *ACSM's Scientific Pronouncements: Physical Activity Guidelines for Americans* (Table 1.3; https://www.acsm.org/acsm-positions-policy/physical-activity-guidelines-for-americans) (37–51). These scientific reviews were presented as the *2018 Physical Activity Guidelines Advisory Committee Scientific Report* (52), which was then used to develop the *Physical Activity Guidelines for Americans*, second edition (*2018 PAG*) (Table 1.4; https://www.health.gov/PAGuidelines/) (53).

Table 1.3	ACSM Scientific Pronouncements: *Physical Activity Guidelines for Americans, Second Edition*

Name of Article

"The US PA Guidelines Advisory Committee Report — Introduction" (37)

"Daily Step Counts for Measuring Physical Activity Exposure and Its Relation to Health" (38)

"Association between Bout Duration of Physical Activity and Health: Systematic Review" (39)

"High-Intensity Interval Training for Cardiometabolic Disease Prevention" (40)

"Sedentary Behavior and Health: Update from the 2018 Physical Activity Guidelines Advisory Committee" (41)

"Physical Activity, Cognition, and Brain Outcomes: A Review of the 2018 Physical Activity Guidelines" (42)

"Physical Activity in Cancer Prevention and Survival: A Systematic Review" (43)

"Physical Activity and the Prevention of Weight Gain in Adults: A Systematic Review" (44)

"Physical Activity, All-Cause and Cardiovascular Mortality, and Cardiovascular Disease" (45)

"Physical Activity and Health in Children Younger than 6 Years: A Systematic Review" (46)

"Benefits of Physical Activity during Pregnancy and Postpartum: An Umbrella Review" (47)

"Physical Activity, Injurious Falls, and Physical Function in Aging: An Umbrella Review" (48)

"Physical Activity to Prevent and Treat Hypertension: A Systematic Review" (49)

"Effects of Physical Activity in Knee and Hip Osteoarthritis: A Systematic Umbrella Review" (50)

"Physical Activity Promotion: Highlights from the 2018 Physical Activity Guidelines Advisory Committee Systematic Review" (51)

Table 1.4	Guidelines from the *Physical Activity Guidelines for Americans, Second Edition*
Life Stage	**Physical Activity Guidelines**
Preschool-age children	■ Preschool-age children (ages 3–5 yr) should be physically active throughout the day to enhance growth and development. ■ Adult caregivers of preschool-age children should encourage active play that includes a variety of activity types.

Children and adolescents	■ It is important to provide young people opportunities and encouragement to participate in physical activities that are appropriate for their age, that are enjoyable, and that offer variety.
	 ■ Children and adolescents ages 6–17 yr should do 60 min (1 h) or more of moderate to vigorous PA daily:
	   ■ Aerobic: Most of the 60 min or more per day should be either moderate- or vigorous-intensity aerobic PA and should include vigorous-intensity PA on at least $3 \text{ d} \cdot \text{wk}^{-1}$.
	   ■ Muscle-strengthening: as part of their 60 min or more of daily PA, children and adolescent should include muscle-strengthening PA on at least $3 \text{ d} \cdot \text{wk}^{-1}$.
	   ■ Bone-strengthening: as part of their 60 min or more of daily PA, children and adolescent should include bone-strengthening PA on at least $3 \text{ d} \cdot \text{wk}^{-1}$.

Adults	■ Adults should move more and sit less throughout the day. Some PA is better than none. Adults who sit less and do any amount of moderate to vigorous PA gain some health benefits. ■ For substantial health benefits, adults should do at least 150 (2 h and 30 min) to 300 min (5 h) a week of moderate intensity, 75 (1 h and 15 min) to 150 min (2 h and 30 min) a week of vigorous-intensity aerobic PA, or an equivalent combination of moderate- and vigorous-intensity aerobic activity. Preferably, aerobic activity should be spread throughout the week. ■ Additional health benefits are gained by engaging in PA beyond the equivalent of 300 min (5 h) of moderate-intensity PA a week. ■ Adults should also do muscle-strengthening activities of moderate or greater intensity and that involve all major muscle groups on 2 or more days a week because these activities provide additional health benefits.

Older adults	■ The key guidelines for adults also apply to older adults. In addition, the following key guidelines are just for older adults:
	   ■ As part of their weekly PA, older adults should do multicomponent PA that include balance training as well as aerobic and muscle-strengthening activities.
	   ■ Older adults should determine their level of effort for PA relative to their level of fitness.
	   ■ Older adults with chronic conditions should understand whether and how their conditions affect their ability to engage in regular PA safely.
	   ■ When older adults cannot do 150 min of moderate-intensity aerobic activity a week because of chronic conditions, they should be as physically active as their abilities and conditions allow.

Continued

Table 1.4	Guidelines from the *Physical Activity Guidelines for Americans, Second Edition* (continued)
Life Stage	**Physical Activity Guidelines**
Women during pregnancy and the postpartum period	■ Women should do at least 150 min (2 h and 30 min) of moderate-intensity aerobic activity a week during pregnancy and the postpartum period. Preferably, aerobic activity should be spread throughout the week. ■ Women who habitually engaged in vigorous-intensity aerobic activity or who were physically active before pregnancy can continue these activities during pregnancy and the postpartum period. ■ Women who are pregnant should be under the care of a health care provider who can monitor the progress of the pregnancy. Women who are pregnant can consult their health care provider about whether or how to adjust their PA during pregnancy and after the baby is born. ■ Women should gradually increase to at least 150 min (2 h and 30 min) of moderate-intensity aerobic activity spread throughout the week during pregnancy and the postpartum period once medically cleared for PA.
Adults with chronic health conditions and adults with disabilities	■ Adults with chronic conditions or disabilities, who are able, should do at least 150 (2 h and 30 min) to 300 min (5 h) a week of moderate-intensity, 75 (1 h and 15 min) to 150 min (2 h and 30 min) a week of vigorous-intensity aerobic PA, or an equivalent combination of moderate- and vigorous-intensity aerobic activity. Preferably, aerobic activity should be spread throughout the week. ■ Adults with chronic conditions or disabilities, who are able, should also do muscle-strengthening activities of moderate or greater intensity and that involve all major muscle groups on 2 or more days a week, as these activities provide additional health benefits. ■ When adults with chronic conditions or disabilities are not able to meet the above key guidelines, they should engage in regular PA according to their abilities and should avoid inactivity. ■ Adults with chronic conditions or symptoms should be under the care of a health care provider. People with chronic conditions can consult a health care professional or PA specialist about the types and amounts of activity appropriate for their abilities and chronic conditions.

In addition to updating the guidelines for children and adolescents, adults, and older adults, the *2018 PAG* clearly identify key guidelines for additional groups: preschool-age children, women during pregnancy and the postpartum period, adults with chronic health conditions, and adults with disabilities (53). Further, important updates in the *2018 PAG* included the scientific evidence to support additional health benefits related to brain health, additional cancer sites, and fall-related injuries; immediate and longer term benefits for how people feel, function, and sleep; further benefits among older adults and people with additional chronic conditions; risks of sedentary behavior and their relationship with PA; guidance for preschool children (ages 3–5 yr); elimination of the requirement for PA of adults to occur in bouts of at least 10 minutes; and tested strategies that can be used to get the population more active.

Relationship between Physical Activity/Exercise and Health across the Lifespan

Until recently, attempts to quantify daily durations of PA in free-living conditions often relied on subjective self-report methods (*e.g.*, PA questionnaires and PA logs). The best estimates for county-by-county leisure-time PA were based on CDC self-report data and give a clear picture of

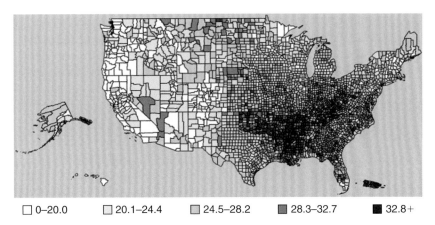

☐ 0–20.0   ☐ 20.1–24.4   ☐ 24.5–28.2   ■ 28.3–32.7   ■ 32.8+

FIGURE 1.5. 2013 Estimates of leisure-time physical inactivity among adults 20 years of age or older. (Adapted from Centers for Disease Control and Prevention. Diabetes data and statistics [Internet]. Atlanta [GA]: Centers for Disease Control and Prevention. Available from: https://www.cdc.gov/diabetes/data/county.html.)

which regions of the United States are least and most physically active (Fig. 1.5). In 2008, however, Troiano and colleagues (54) published a landmark paper detailing the first objective assessment of PA among a nationally representative sample of Americans during the 2003–2004 National Health and Nutrition Examination Survey (NHANES). This objective assessment was conducted using specialized PA accelerometers, which can measure the duration and intensity of accumulated PA. Alarming among the findings from this assessment were the extremely low daily durations of moderate to vigorous PA (≥3 METs) across all ranges as less than 4% of American adults 20 years of age and older were meeting public health recommendations for PA (*i.e.*, a minimum of 30 min of moderate PA 5 or more days per week). Concurrent estimates of self-reported PA collected during the CDC's 2003 Behavioral Risk Factor Surveillance System indicated that 47.4% of American adults were meeting current PA recommendations (55). It is difficult to explain the discrepancy between the self-report and objective measures of PA; yet, this provokes concern that most Americans are not as active as they might think.

The low levels of PA demonstrated among the majority of Americans are particularly problematic, especially when considering the numerous health benefits associated with regular PA. Across the age continuum, PA can have positive impacts in biological, psychological, and social domains. Moreover, the therapeutic and prophylactic benefits of PA can often be obtained at little to no cost and in nearly any environment. Recent scientific evidence supports an inverse relationship between daily step counts and all-cause mortality, cardiovascular events, and Type 2 diabetes (38). Daily monitoring of step counts with wearable activity monitors, coupled with appropriate behavior change strategies such as goal setting and enlisting social support, are excellent strategies to facilitate PA promotion (51).

Physical Activity and Health in Children and Adolescents

In addition to healthy eating habits, incorporating regular PA into the lives of children and adolescents (17 yr of age and younger) provides an early starting point to aid in the prevention of numerous chronic diseases. Chapters 11–13 discuss the importance of establishing positive health behaviors early in life as a means of lifelong healthy living. The *2008 PAG* included a PA recommendation for children and adolescents aged 6–17 years (35). That guideline was based on strong evidence demonstrating that in children and adolescents, higher levels of PA are associated with multiple beneficial health outcomes, including cardiorespiratory and muscular fitness, bone health, and maintenance of healthy weight status (34).

Recommendations state that school-age children and adolescents (aged 6–17 yr) should engage in at least 60 minutes of a variety of age-appropriate, enjoyable, physical activities daily. Further, in at least 3 days of the week a portion of their 60 minutes should incorporate activities that enhance aerobic, bone-, and muscle-strengthening health. Recent estimates indicate that less than one-quarter (24%) of children 6–17 years of age met these guidelines (56). In addition to continuing to support the *2008 PAG*, the updated *2018 PAG* also set out to specifically review the science behind early childhood development and further expanded the recommendations for younger children (53). The current *2018 PAG* recommend that preschool-age children (ages 3–5 yr) should be encouraged and supported in engaging in PA throughout the day (53).

An increasingly prevalent chronic disease among America's youth is obesity. Data from the early 1970s indicated that 5.0% of 2- to 5-year-olds, 4.0% of 6- to 11-year-olds, and 6.1% of 12- to 19-year-olds were obese (57). Results from the 2015–2016 NHANES estimated 16.6% of children and adolescents aged 2–19 years were overweight, 18.5% were obese, and 5.6% classified with severe obesity (58,59). Obesity prevalence among children aged 2–5 years was 13.9% in 2015–2016, with 1.9% being severely obese. Among children aged 6–11 years, 18.4% were obese and 5.2% were extremely obese. Among adolescents aged 12–19 years, 20.6% were obese and 7.7% were extremely obese (Fig. 1.6). Obesity has become a major health concern, as childhood obesity increases the risk for a host of other chronic diseases such as diabetes, hyperlipidemia, and hypertension (60). In addition, childhood obesity may result in detrimental behavioral, social, and economic effects (61,62). In fact, a 2015 U.S. Surgeon General public health report outlined the positive effects of enhancing both the physical and emotional health of adolescents in order to encourage the chances of a successful and healthy adulthood (63). The report noted that excessive consumption of sugary beverages (84% of adolescents), along with >7 hours of daily screen time (which displaces PA), are likely to lead to negative social, behavioral, and economic outcomes. The authors of the *2018 PAG* scientific report concluded from the findings of 14 scientific studies that for children 3–6 years, higher levels of PA are associated with reduced risk for excessive increases in body weight and adiposity (52).

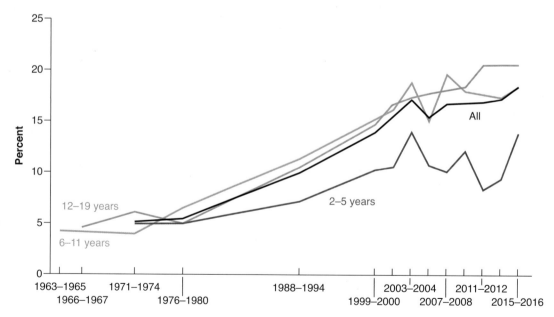

FIGURE 1.6. Prevalence of Overweight, Obesity, and Severe Obesity Among Children and Adolescents Aged 2–19 Years: United States, 1963–1965 Through 2015–2016 by Cheryl D. Fryar, M.S.P.H., Margaret D. Carroll, M.S.P.H., and Cynthia L. Ogden, Ph.D., Division of Health and Nutrition Examination Surveys, NATIONAL CENTER FOR HEALTH STATISTICS Health E-Stats, 2018. https://www.cdc.gov/nchs/data/hestat/obesity-child-17-18/obesity-child.htm.

PA has been one of many modalities suggested as a means to address the rising obesity epidemic among children and adolescents (53). Among youth, lower levels of PA are associated with a greater risk of being overweight or obese (64–66). Moreover, evidence suggests that being physically active during childhood and adolescence positively influences metabolic risk factors related to Type 2 diabetes (67,68), which has become an emerging health problem among America's youth (69). Adequate PA is also important for normal musculoskeletal development during childhood. An adequate stimulus via structured exercise and/or PA can help increase bone accretion during youth and adolescence (46,70). In turn, greater peak bone mineral density in early adulthood may be attained, which reduces the risk or delays the onset of osteoporosis in later adulthood (71). There is strong evidence to support that higher amounts of PA in children 3–6 years old are also associated with improvements in bone health as well as reduced risk of excessive increases in weight and adiposity (46).

Physical Activity and Health in Adults

Adults who engage in regular PA can enjoy many health benefits from being regularly physically active. It is recommended that adults of all ages and life stages, including older adults, women who are either pregnant or in the postpartum period, adults with chronic conditions, and adults with disabilities should engage in at least 150–300 minutes of PA per week. The recent updates in the *2018 PAG* make clear that more PA, in any amount, is better than none. In fact, attention was dedicated to determining whether the previous recommendation that PA had to be accumulated in at least 10-minute bouts was required for health benefits. The current evidence obtained from a systematic review of 29 studies concluded that any PA of any bout duration is associated with improved health outcomes (39). Further, strong scientific evidence linking sedentary behavior and increased risk for all-cause and CVD mortality as well as incidence of CVD and Type 2 diabetes was found (41). Engaging in PA can offset the excess risk of all-cause mortality that is associated with a sedentary lifestyle (Fig. 1.7) (53). Further, replacing sedentary activities (*e.g.*, sitting) with light-intensity physical activities reduces the risk of all-cause mortality. The researchers concluded that given the current high levels of sitting and low levels of PA in the population, most people would benefit from both increasing moderate to vigorous PA and reducing time spent sitting (72). These updates in the *2018 PAG* may help the ACSM-EP to encourage individuals to "sit less," "take the stairs," "get up and move more," and engage in any other types of quick, short bursts of activity.

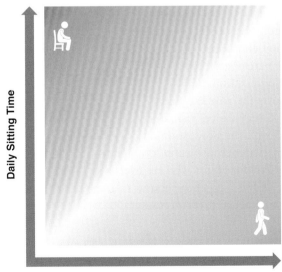

Daily Sitting Time

Moderate-to-Vigorous Physical Activity
Risk of all-cause mortality decreases as one moves from red to green.

FIGURE 1.7. Relationship among moderate-to-vigorous PA, sitting time, and risk of all-cause mortality in adults.

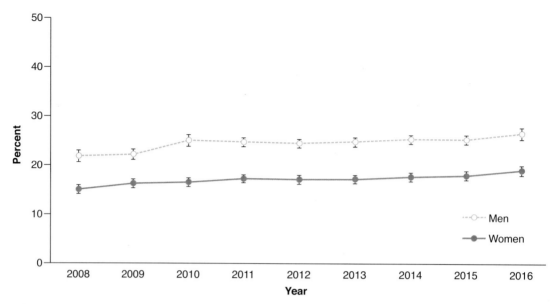

FIGURE 1.8. Estimates are age-adjusted to the 2000 U.S. standard population using five age groups: 18–24 years, 25–34 years, 35–44 years, 45–64 years, and 65+ years. National Health Interview Survey questions ask about frequency and duration of light-intensity to moderate-intensity and vigorous-intensity leisure-time PAs as well as the frequency of muscle-strengthening activities. Meeting the aerobic component of the *2008 PAG* is defined as reporting at least 150 minutes of moderate-intensity or 75 minutes of vigorous-intensity aerobic PA a week, or an equivalent combination. Meeting the muscle-strengthening component is defined as reporting muscle-strengthening activities at least 2 d · wk^{-1}. Error bars represent upper and lower bounds of the 95% confidence interval. (Data from Centers for Disease Control and Prevention, National Center for Health Statistics, National Health Interview Survey [NHIS].)

Although the scientific evidence is clear that PA improves health and well-being, almost all adults are not engaging in adequate amounts of PA (53). Only 23.6% (20.6% of women and 26.8% of men) of adults aged 18 years and older met the PA guidelines for both aerobic and muscle-strengthening activity for 2018 (at least 150 min · wk^{-1} of moderate-intensity aerobic PA, 75 min · wk^{-1} of vigorous-intensity aerobic PA, or an equivalent combination of moderate- and vigorous-intensity aerobic activity as well as muscle-strengthening activities 2 or more days a week) (Fig. 1.8) (73).

Among adults, research has shown that increases in PA can prevent or minimize weight gain (44). An increase in energy expenditure is associated with significant weight reduction (74–76). This has become especially pertinent considering 39% of men and 27% of women are overweight and 38% of men and 40% of women are obese (77,78). However, regular PA carries health benefits regardless of any changes in body composition that occur as a result of increased PA energy expenditure (79). Strong evidence supports the role PA plays in reducing breast, colon, endometrium, bladder, stomach, esophagus, and kidney cancer risk; moderate evidence in reducing lung cancer risk (43). PA has long been linked with the prevention and/or treatment of prediabetes (80) and Type 2 diabetes (81,82), and recent evidence also supports high-intensity interval training (HIIT; compared with moderate-intensity PA) for adults who are overweight or obese for the prevention of these cardiometabolic diseases, as HIIT has been found to improve insulin sensitivity, blood pressure, and body composition, but special precautions should consider musculoskeletal injury prevention (40).

Achieving the recommended amount of PA can decrease the risk of premature all-cause and cardiovascular mortality as well as the development of CVD including ischemic heart disease, ischemic stroke, and all-cause heart failure (45). CVD is the leading cause of death in the United States as well as worldwide (83). PA can prevent and treat hypertension, which is the most common, costly, and preventable CVD risk factor (49). The total direct costs attributed to hypertension are expected to rise from $130.7 billion in 2010 to $389.9 billion in 2030 and the indirect costs (*e.g.*, lost productivity) from $25.4 billion to $42.8 billion (83). Substantially increasing PA levels in the general population, and hence, the proportion of adults meeting current PA guidelines, would undoubtedly have positive effects on CVD prevalence and its associated costs. Lastly, but certainly not exhaustive of the benefits of PA, there is moderate to strong evidence to support the association between PA and improvements in cognition (*e.g.*, academic achievement, processing speed, memory, and executive function) and reduced risk for cognitive impairment (*e.g.*, Alzheimer disease) (42). For additional benefits of PA, see Table 1.5.

Table 1.5	Physical Activity-Related Health Benefits for Individuals with a Chronic Condition from the 2008 and 2018 Physical Activity Guidelines Advisory Committees (36)
Preexisting Medical Condition	
Breast cancer[a]	**Reduced risk of all-cause and breast cancer mortality**
Colorectal cancer[a]	**Reduced risk of all-cause and colorectal cancer mortality**
Prostate cancer[a]	**Reduced risk of prostate cancer mortality**
Osteoarthritis[b]	**Decreased pain**
	Improved function and quality of life
Hypertension[b]	**Reduced risk of progression of cardiovascular disease**
	Reduced risk of increased blood pressure over time
Type 2 diabetes[b]	**Reduced risk of cardiovascular mortality**
	Reduced progression of disease indicators: hemoglobin A1c, blood pressure, blood lipids, and body mass index
Recent hip fracture[c]	**Improved walking, balance, and activities of daily living**
Frailty[c]	**Improved walking, balance, and activities of daily living**
Stroke[c,d]	Improved walking, physical fitness, functional independence
	Improved cognition
Spinal cord injury[b]	Improved physical fitness
	Improved walking and wheel chair skills
Dementia[d]	**Improved cognition**
Multiple sclerosis[b,d]	Improved walking
	Improved strength and physical fitness
Parkinson's disease[c,d]	**Improved walking, balance, activities of daily living, and cognition**
Schizophrenia[d]	**Improved quality of life and cognition**
Attention deficit hyperactivity disorder[d]	**Improved cognition**

Benefits in bold are those added in 2018; benefits in normal font are those noted in the 2008 Scientific Report. Only outcomes with strong or moderate evidence of effect are included in the table. Outcomes assessed varied by chronic condition.

[a]Mortality and disease progression outcomes.

[b]Mortality, development of new chronic condition, quality of life, physical function, and progression of disease.

[c]Physical function only.

[d]Cognition.

Physical Activity and Health in Older Adults

Objectively measured evidence has shown that PA levels in America tend to decline as age increases; however, like younger adults and children, older individuals can also reap health benefits by being physically active (53,54,84). For example, in addition to the evidence supporting PA and cognition, new evidence further indicates that even single acute bouts of moderate-intensity PA produce benefits that can be seen immediately and can accumulate with more, regular PA (42). Other benefits of PA have been seen in the reduced risk of a second myocardial infarction (MI) (85). Particularly important to older adults, a physically active lifestyle can help maintain physical function during later years (84). These higher levels of functional capacity can allow older individuals to live independently and make it easier to carry out activities of daily living. Further, PA during later adulthood is associated with decreased risks of falls and osteoporotic fractures (86,87). A recent review concluded that regular PA improves (or delays) the loss of physical function and mobility while reducing the risk of fall-related injuries (48). Another recent systematic review concluded that engaging in PA (even short bouts) decreased pain, improved physical function, and improved health-related quality of life among people with hip or knee osteoarthritis (50).

Physical Activity and Health in Women during Pregnancy and during the Postpartum Period

Pregnancy is often associated with decreased levels of PA, especially during the first and third trimesters and subsequent pregnancies (88). However, there is strong evidence to support PA of moderate intensity for physical and mental health benefits during pregnancy and the postpartum period. Potential benefits of PA during this time include decreasing the risk of excessive weight gain, gestational diabetes (47), delivery of a large-for-gestational-age infant (89), and postpartum depressive symptoms (47,90). There is also building evidence to suggest that PA during this time may decrease the risk of other complications, such as preeclampsia, gestational hypertension, antenatal anxiety symptoms (47), and preterm delivery (89).

For most women, PA during pregnancy is beneficial and has minimal risks, although adjustments to the type and amount of PA during this time will likely be necessary due to the anatomical and physiological changes that occur. Current PA recommendations for women during pregnancy and the postpartum period include that women should do at least 150 minutes of aerobic PA of moderate intensity per week (53). Women who previously engaged in PA of vigorous intensity prior to pregnancy can often continue to do some vigorous PA during this time frame. All women during pregnancy and the postpartum period should be followed closely by a health care provider who can advise on needed restrictions if health complications arise. After childbirth, there is a necessary rest and healing period that varies for each person. However, once healed and medically cleared, gradually increasing PA once again is recommended (91).

Physical Activity and Health in Adults with Chronic Conditions and Adults with Disabilities

Chronic conditions are highly prevalent in the United States, with 49.8% of adults having at least one of the following chronic conditions: hypertension, coronary heart disease, stroke, diabetes, cancer, arthritis, hepatitis, kidney disease, asthma, or chronic obstructive pulmonary disease (92). Although the benefits of PA for the prevention of chronic illness are often emphasized, it is important to recognize that adults with chronic conditions or disabilities should also be encouraged to be physically active because they can obtain health benefits from PA as well. For example, among adults with hypertension, there is strong evidence to suggest that increasing PA can help to decrease blood pressure and decrease the risk of progression of CVD (49). Similarly, among adults with Type 2 diabetes, increased aerobic and strengthening PA is associated with decreased risk of disease progression, including improved management of glycolated hemoglobin, blood pressure, lipids, and body mass index (52). As such, it is recommended that, if their abilities allow, adults with chronic conditions or disabilities should meet the key PA guidelines for adults.

However, many chronic conditions and disabilities require some level of adaptation to the type or amount of PA. For example, knee or hip osteoarthritis can be a painful chronic condition that can lead to disability and limit PA. At the same time, PA among adults with hip or knee osteoarthritis is associated with decreased pain, improved physical function, and improved health-related quality of life (50). Health care providers and PA specialists, including the ACSM-EP and physical, occupational, and recreational therapists, can provide guidance and collaborate with clients to develop a plan to reach an optimal PA level that matches their abilities (53). Ultimately, the goal is for adults with chronic conditions or disability to be as physically active as possible, and avoid physical inactivity, because some benefits of PA can occur at PA levels lower than full achievement of the key PA guidelines for adults (50,53). Although adaptations may be needed, adults with chronic conditions and disabilities should be encouraged to be physically active in line with their abilities for the improvement of their current health status and to decrease the risk of additional comorbid conditions.

 ## General Risks Associated with Physical Activity/Exercise

It is the inherent responsibility of an ACSM-EP to take reasonable precautions when working with individuals who wish to become physically active or to increase their current activity level. In physically inactive, symptom-free individuals, moderate-intensity exercise does not present a risk for CVD-related events (14,92). In addition, the *2018 PAG* emphasize the importance of regular PA across all age groups, almost regardless of current health status, because the benefits are far reaching (53). Specific attention was given to assuage individual's fears from engaging PA in that the following "key guidelines" were recommended (Table 1.6).

Table 1.6	**Key Guidelines for Safe Physical Activity from the *Physical Activity Guidelines for Americans*, Second Edition (53)**

To do PA safely and reduce risk of injuries and other adverse events, people should

- Understand the risks yet be confident that PA can be safe for almost everyone.

- Choose types of PA that are appropriate for their current fitness level and health goals because some activities are safer than others.

- Increase PA gradually over time to meet key guidelines or health goals. Inactive people should "start low and go slow" by starting with lower intensity activities and gradually increasing how often and how long activities are done.

- Protect themselves by using appropriate gear and sports equipment; choosing safe environments; following rules and policies; and making sensible choices about when, where, and how to be active.

- Be under the care of a health care provider if they have chronic conditions or symptoms. People with chronic conditions and symptoms can consult a health care professional or PA specialist about the types and amounts of activity appropriate for them.

Most physically inactive or symptom-free individuals can safely begin a low- to moderate-intensity PA program without the need for baseline exercise testing or prior medical clearance (see Chapter 2 for greater detail). However, the ACSM-EP responsible for supervising vigorous-intensity exercise programs, regardless of the population, should have current training in basic and/or advanced cardiac life support and emergency procedures while also being keenly aware of the signs and symptoms of CVD.

Risks of Sudden Cardiac Death

Despite the known benefits of PA and exercise, inherent risk does exist. Sudden cardiac death associated with exercise is widely publicized, especially in children or adolescents. In truth, sudden cardiac death related to moderate exercise is extremely rare (93,94). For young individuals (younger than 30 yr), the most common causes of sudden cardiac death are congenital and hereditary abnormalities; however, there is no clear consensus on the actual rate of sudden death in young individuals (95–97). High school and college athletes are typically required to have a preparticipation screening, which is one means of detecting potential cardiac issues.

Sudden cardiac death risk increases with age and prevalence of known or unknown CVD (93,98–103). Furthermore, the rates of sudden cardiac death and acute MI are disproportionately higher in the least active individuals performing infrequent exercise (104), such as a generally inactive person shoveling heavy snow. Although the exact mechanism of sudden cardiac death or MI remains elusive, there appears to be an acute arterial insult that dislodges already present plaque, resulting in platelet aggregation or thrombosis (105–107). The ACSM-EP should have a basic understanding of this sequela and the inherent risks of sudden cardiac death or MI any one individual may carry. Appropriate screening is critical for minimizing this risk (see Chapter 2).

The Risk of Cardiac Events during Exercise Testing

A practicing ACSM-EP is likely to suggest and perform baseline and follow-up exercise tests across a wide variety of individuals. Although submaximal exercise testing is generally considered safe for most, maximal- or vigorous-intensity exercise testing does pose some risk (108–111). Similar to exercise, exercise testing is also rather safe when performed properly. Overall, the risk of cardiac events during symptom-limited exercise testing in a clinical environment is low (six cardiac events per 10,000 tests), and given proper screening and attention, most tests can be performed with a high degree of safety (112,113).

Musculoskeletal Injury Associated with Exercise

In addition to the acute risk of sudden cardiac death or MI, there is also an increased risk of musculoskeletal injury associated with exercise. The most common musculoskeletal injuries, regardless of gender, occur in the lower body, particularly at the knee or foot (114). The rate of musculoskeletal injury is highest in team and contact sports and includes injuries of all types, not just lower body injuries (106).

Walking for exercise, which is performed by approximately 30% of adults, is the most popular exercise in the United States (115). The musculoskeletal risk associated with walking is considerably lower than that with jogging (116). Compared with joggers, walkers of both genders are at 25%–30% lower risk for incurring an acute or chronic musculoskeletal injury (117). The annual rate of musculoskeletal injury associated with running revealed a higher injury incidence for novice runners (17.8%) than recreational runners (7.7%) (118). The most common injuries typically experienced by runners include medial tibial stress syndrome, Achilles tendinopathy, and plantar fasciitis (119). Although certainly not life-threatening, musculoskeletal injuries present a real and present issue.

In order to promote safety and prevent and minimize musculoskeletal injury, the ACSM-EP should consider the following safety guidelines:

- Be diligent in choosing exercise modes and prescribing exercise that are based on an individual's current fitness level and desires, along with any past exercise experiences.
- Start at a low level of intensity, frequency, and duration and progress slowly.
- Be aware and make clients aware of early signs of potential injury (*i.e.*, increasing muscle soreness, bone and joint pain, excessive fatigue, and performance decrements). When noted, take appropriate precautions, which may include temporarily ceasing the activity, more frequent rest days, or simply decreasing the frequency, intensity, or duration of exercise.
- Set realistic exercise goals to avoid overexercising (see Chapter 12 for goal setting).

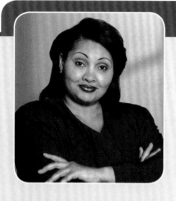

The Case of Rachel

Submitted by **Kaitlin Teser, MS, EIM Level 2 ACSM-Certified Exercise Physiologist®, Greater Boston Area, MA**

Rachel is a 43-year-old moderately active mom with no cardiovascular, metabolic, or renal disease. Rachel's initial goal of losing 10 lb shifted to wanting to incorporate more active lifestyle habits into her daily routine.

Narrative

Rachel is a 43-year-old woman who works 40 hours a week in a sedentary office job. Rachel's original goal was to lose 10 lb in 12 weeks. She was moderately active. Her two children, Zach, age 10 years, and Emily, age 8 years, are involved in karate. In addition to a walk around the local track with coworkers twice a week, Rachel also took a cardio kickboxing class on Saturday mornings.

Fitness Testing Results

The results of Rachel's fitness assessment were as follows:

Resting blood pressure	110/85 mm Hg	Good
Resting heart rate	81 bpm	Good
Body fat (%)	28.7	Fair
Body mass index	25.5	Average
Sit and reach (box)	29 cm	Fair
Muscular endurance (YMCA bench press)	16 reps	Low average
Aerobic fitness (YMCA submaximal bike test)	23.3 mL $\cdot$ kg^{-1} $\cdot$ min^{-1}	Very poor

Although Rachel's first wellness vision seemed like it related to active living, she was really focused on weight loss. I was careful to "meet her where she was" and encourage her use of the term *active living* in her wellness vision.

Rachel's First Wellness Vision

"My wellness vision is to be healthy, energetic, and vital. I am motivated by my desire to stay active with my children and continue to be active as I age. I am challenged by my demanding schedule and multiple commitments but have been a regular exerciser in the past and know the importance of active living as a way of life. I am confident that with increased social support, a regular routine and a realistic weight management plan, I will achieve success."

Rachel's program followed the FITT principle and incorporated both health- and skill-related fitness components. She added another cardio kickboxing class to her week and convinced her coworkers to walk on the track an additional day. My work with Rachel focused on increasing strength and range of motion. I introduced Rachel to a variety of modalities that could be used both at home and at the office to provide brief workouts throughout the day. The more I put myself in Rachel's shoes and developed programs that were fun, efficient, and effective, the more she seemed to be engaged in the session. I learned that Rachel often went home and tried out a modified version of our activities with her children. After 4 weeks, Rachel's attitude started to shift. When talking about food, I heard less about her examples of "willpower" and more about healthy choices. Externally, one of the first changes I noticed was how she was dressed. Rachel had begun to wear work clothes that enabled her to perform a set of "triceps dips" at her desk. Her fitness indicators were all improving, and she genuinely seemed to have more pep in her step!

On completion of the 12-week program, Rachel had lost 6 lb and increased her strength, flexibility, and aerobic fitness. What was more exciting, however, was that Rachel had gained a real appreciation of the value of daily practices of active living. She was able to restructure her work schedule to allow her to walk to school once a week with her children. She incorporated stretch breaks into the start of every meeting at work. She used the stairs instead of the elevator and always opened a door with her own strength (without assistance from an automatic door). It was only in retrospect that Rachel realized that the choices she and her family were making for recreation had shifted from inside activities, such as shopping and the movies, to hiking, cycling, and swimming. Rachel also realized that her new choices had resulted in meeting new friends who shared similar interests in being active and enjoying family activities that involved movement.

Rachel's New Wellness Vision

"My wellness vision is to move and keep moving — to move freely through a full range of motion and to move in a way that enables me to do all the things that I need to do in my life and have energy left over. I want to move with and for my children and grandchildren. I may be challenged by old habits of acting on misguided priorities, but I know that with the help of my friends and family and by incorporating brief workout breaks into my day and committing to at least one act of active living every day, I will be able to sustain and maintain my newfound joy."

Rachel was able to achieve her new goal of moving more by small choices and daily practices that reflected a new attitude about exercise. She set an achievable goal of incorporating one act of active living into every day. Rachel also became willing to meet new people who were like-minded and would support her efforts to be active. To an outside observer, Rachel's changes may seem like minor adjustments in her schedule, but to anyone who really knows her, a seismic shift took place that will enable Rachel to realize her wellness vision and goals for the future.

QUESTIONS

- What did the ACSM-EP do to support Rachel's goals?

    The ACSM-EP had a key role in actively listening to Rachel. The ACSM-EP was skilled in not only being able to identify Rachel's interest in losing weight but also wanting to incorporate active living. As a facilitator of motivation, the ACSM-EP was able to encourage Rachel to identify ways in which active living techniques could be incorporated into daily life. The ACSM-EP also provided a sound exercise program that encouraged competence, confidence, and relatedness.

- What role did social support play in Rachel's success?

    Rachel was able to establish herself as a leader and learner. She was encouraged to be creative in the completion of her goals. By including coworkers, Rachel was able to share the benefits of exercise and have support when she was challenged to work through lunch. Rachel was also able to enlist the help of her children by creating time for a walk to school morning.

- How can one act of active living a day make a difference in someone's life?

    A shift in attitude and expectations enabled Rachel to evaluate her original goals in a way that sustained her adherence to the program. By committing to one act of active living, Rachel was able to cultivate other habits of behavior around both exercise and nutrition that further aided her in reaching her weight loss and fitness goals.

References

1. Brownson RC, Eyler AA, King AC, Brown DR, Shyu Y, Sallis JF. Patterns and correlates of physical activity among US women 40 years and older. *Am J Public Health.* 2000;90(2):264–70.
2. Kerr J, Norman GJ, Sallis JF, Patrick K. Exercise aids, neighborhood safety, and physical activity in adolescents and parents. *Med Sci Sports Exerc.* 2008;40(7):1244–8.
3. Moore M, Tschannen-Moran B. *Coaching Psychology Manual.* Baltimore (MD): Lippincott Williams & Wilkins; 2009. 208 p.
4. Moustaka FC, Vlachopoulos SP, Kabitsis C, Theodorakis Y. Effects of an autonomy-supportive exercise instructing style on exercise motivation, psychological well-being, and exercise attendance in middle-age women. *J Phys Act Health.* 2012;9(1):138–50.

Case Study: Examining Misinformed Beliefs about Physical Activity

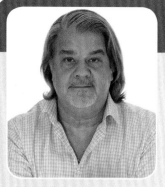

Narrative

Kevin is a 55-year-old male, who recently experienced a transient ischemic attack (TIA). At his follow-up appointment with his primary care provider, she pointed out that he needed to lose weight (current body mass index: 33) and reduce his blood pressure (current blood pressure: 165/90 mm Hg) because obesity and hypertension are risk factors for stroke. As a part of Kevin's plan, the primary care physician prescribed daily PA and recommended that Kevin should work with an ACSM-EP to develop a plan to safely incorporate increased PA into a healthy lifestyle. Kevin is currently physically inactive and has a sedentary job and is taking prescribed blood pressure medications.

See Kevin's initial comments to the ACSM-EP:

"Hi, I'm Kevin. I don't mind coming here, but I don't really know why my doctor wanted me to meet with you. I know that I'm overweight and I had a TIA, but I don't see how being more active is going to help me. Aren't the medications supposed to keep my blood pressure under control? Plus, I can eat better than I have been. That should be enough, right? I mean, I see those guys at the gym lifting weights and their faces are all red and they are straining. That doesn't look like a good idea for someone who just had a TIA. I tried running a few months ago because my friend has recently started running, and I made it a few blocks. I just couldn't do it and afterward, my knees hurt. It just seems like I missed that boat. I mean, I'm never going to be a gym goer, you know."

QUESTIONS

- What misconceptions does Kevin have about the benefits of PA given his condition?
- What misunderstandings does Kevin have about what constitutes PA?
- What information regarding PA benefits and the various types and amounts of PA do you think would be helpful for Kevin to understand at this point?

SUMMARY

As discussed earlier in this chapter, the notion that PA can improve and/or maintain health is by no means novel. However, it was not until substantial scientific advancements during the 20th century, in fields such as exercise physiology and epidemiology, that our understanding of how PA could treat and/or prevent common chronic diseases (*e.g.*, CVD, hypertension, and Type 2 diabetes mellitus) became known. Despite these advancements, there remain many unanswered questions regarding the exact pathways and mechanisms through which PA influences health. Along with that, there are also levels of uncertainty in terms of intensities and volume thresholds that can or should be performed to reap the greatest benefits without going too far.

Although there is still much to learn, the current evidence strongly indicates that regular PA and exercise can have tremendous benefits for an individual's physical, metabolic, and mental health. However, overexercising, doing too much too soon or for too long without adequate recovery methods, or exercising at an unsafe intensity can bring negative consequences, even as severe as sudden death. Although the risks associated with exercise are proportional to the amount and intensity of exercise, both acute and chronic, the benefits of habitual exercise far outweigh the risks.

This resource manual is intended to prepare the ACSM-EP with the necessary tools to assess fitness and prescribe exercise for populations able to exercise without medical supervision. Although no manual is completely comprehensive, the information within should serve as an outstanding resource for both the new and the experienced exercise professional.

STUDY QUESTIONS

1. Compare and contrast PA, exercise, health-related fitness, and skill-related fitness.
2. Describe at least two individuals and two landmark research studies that made significant contributions to the current body of knowledge regarding PA/physical fitness and associated health benefits.
3. Describe the health benefits and health risks associated with acute and chronic PA.

REFERENCES

1. American College of Sports Medicine. ACSM Certification 2018 [Internet]. Indianapolis (IN): American College of Sports Medicine; [cited 2019 Oct 9]. Available from: https://certification.acsm.org/.
2. Caspersen CJ, Powell KE, Christenson GM. Physical activity, exercise, and physical fitness: definitions and distinctions for health-related research. *Public Health Rep.* 1985;100(2):126–31.
3. Sallis JF, Linton L, Kraft MK. The first Active Living Research Conference: growth of a transdisciplinary field. *Am J Prev Med.* 2005;28(Suppl 2):93–5.
4. U.S. Bureau of Labor Statistics. American time use survey summary — 2018 results [Internet]. Washington (DC): 2019 [cited 2019 Sep 23]. Available from: https://www.bls.gov/news.release/atus.nr0.htm.
5. Church TS, Thomas DM, Tudor-Locke C, et al. Trends over 5 decades in U.S. occupation-related physical activity and their associations with obesity. *PLoS One.* 2011;6(5):e19657.
6. Archer E, Shook RP, Thomas DM, et al. 45-Year trends in women's use of time and household management energy expenditure. *PLoS One.* 2013;8(2):e56620.
7. Liguori G, Carroll-Cobb S. *FitWell: Questions and Answers.* New York (NY): McGraw-Hill; 2011. 512 p.
8. King KM. The health benefits of physical activity. In: Bayles MP, Swank AM, editors. *American College of Sports Medicine's Exercise Testing and Prescription.* Philadelphia (PA): Wolters Kluwer; 2018. p. 2–18.
9. Benefits and risks associated with physical activity. In: Riebe D, editor. *American College of Sports Medicine's Exercise Testing and Prescription.* 10th ed. Philadelphia (PA): Wolters Kluwer; 2018. p. 1–21.
10. Biswas A, Oh PI, Faulkner GE, et al. Sedentary time and its association with risk for disease incidence, mortality, and hospitalization in adults: a systematic review and meta-analysis. *Ann Intern Med.* 2015;162(2):123–32.
11. Swank AM. A first step to health: just stand up and move: could improving your health really be this easy? *ACSMs Health Fit J.* 2015;19(6):34–6.
12. Sedentary Behaviour Research Network. Standardized use of the terms "sedentary" and "sedentary behaviours" [letter]. *Appl Physiol Nutr Metab.* 2012;37(3):540–2.
13. Hallal PC, Andersen LB, Bull FC, Guthold R, Haskell W, Ekelund U. Global physical activity levels: surveillance progress, pitfalls, and prospects. *Lancet.* 2012;380(9838):247–57.
14. Riebe D, Franklin BA, Thompson PD, et al. Updating ACSM's recommendations for exercise preparticipation health screening. *Med Sci Sports Exerc.* 2015;47(11):2473–9.
15. McLeroy KR, Bibeau D, Steckler A, Glanz K. An ecological perspective on health promotion programs. *Health Educ Q.* 1988;15(4):351–77.
16. Lyons AS, Petrucelli RJ. *Medicine: An Illustrated History.* New York (NY): Abradale Press; 1978. 616 p.
17. Jones WHS, translator. *Hippocrates.* Cambridge (MA): Harvard University Press; 1952. 229 p.
18. Berryman JW. Thomas K. Cureton, Jr.: pioneer researcher, proselytizer, and proponent for physical fitness. *Res Q Exerc Sport.* 1996;67(1):1–12.
19. American College of Sports Medicine. The recommended quality and quantity of exercise for developing and maintaining fitness in healthy adults. *Med Sci Sports Exerc.* 1978;10(3):vii–x.
20. Framingham Heart Study. About the Framingham Heart Study [Internet]. Framingham (MA); 2019 [cited 2019 Oct 4]. Available from: https://www.framinghamheartstudy.org/fhs-about/.
21. Morris JN, Heady JA, Raffle PA, Roberts CG, Parks JW. Coronary heart — disease and physical activity of work. *Lancet.* 1953;265(6795):1053–7.
22. Paffenbarger RS Jr, Laughlin ME, Gima AS, Black RA. Work activity of longshoremen as related to death from coronary heart disease and stroke. *N Engl J Med.* 1970;282(20):1109–14.
23. Lee IM, Paffenbarger RS Jr. Associations of light, moderate, and vigorous intensity physical activity with longevity: the Harvard Alumni Health Study. *Am J Epidemiol.* 2000;151(3):293–9.
24. Leon AS, Connett J, Jacobs DR Jr, Rauramaa R. Leisure-time physical activity levels and risk of coronary health disease and death: the multiple risk factor intervention trial. *JAMA.* 1987;258(17):2388–95.
25. Morris JN, Everitt MG, Pollard R, Chave SP, Semmence AM. Vigorous exercise in leisure-time: protection against coronary heart disease. *Lancet.* 1980;316(8206):1207–10.
26. Sesso HD, Paffenbarger RS Jr, Lee IM. Physical activity and coronary heart disease in men: the Harvard Alumni Health Study. *Circulation.* 2000;102(9):975–80.
27. Slattery ML, Jacobs DR Jr, Nichaman MZ. Leisure time physical activity and coronary heart disease death: the US railroad study. *Circulation.* 1989;79(2):304–11.

28. Blair SN, Kohl HW III, Paffenbarger RS Jr, Clark DG, Cooper KH, Gibbons LW. Physical fitness and all-cause mortality. A prospective study of healthy men and women. *JAMA.* 1989;262(17):2395–401.

29. Ekelund LG, Haskell WL, Johnson JL, Whaley FS, Criqui MH. Physical fitness as a predictor of cardiovascular mortality in asymptomatic North American men. The Lipid Research Clinics Mortality Follow-Up Study. *N Engl J Med.* 1988;319(21):1379–84.

30. Lakka TA, Venäläinen JM, Rauramaa R, Salonen R, Tuomilehto J, Salonen JT. Relation of leisure-time physical activity and cardiorespiratory fitness to the risk of acute myocardial infarction in men. *N Eng J Med.* 1994;330(22):1549–54.

31. Sandvik L, Erikssen J, Thaulow E, Erikssen G, Mundal R, Rodahl K. Physical fitness as a predictor of mortality among healthy, middle-aged Norwegian men. *N Engl J Med.* 1993;328(8):533–7.

32. Pate RR, Pratt M, Blair SN, et al. Physical activity and public health. A recommendation for the Centers for Disease Control and Prevention and the American College of Sports Medicine. *JAMA.* 1995;273(5):402–7.

33. U.S. Department of Health and Human Services. *Physical Activity and Health: A Report of the Surgeon General.* Atlanta (GA): U.S. Department of Health and Human Services, Centers for Disease Control and Prevention, National Center for Chronic Disease Prevention and Health Promotion; 1996. 300 p.

34. Physical Activity Guidelines Advisory Committee. *2008 Physical Activity Guidelines Advisory Committee Report.* Washington (DC): U.S. Department of Health and Human Services; 2008. 683 p.

35. U.S. Department of Health and Human Services. *2008 Physical Activity Guidelines for Americans.* Washington (DC): U.S. Department of Health and Human Services; 2008. 76 p.

36. Powell KE, King AC, Buchner DM, et al. The Scientific Foundation for the Physical Activity Guidelines for Americans, 2nd edition. *J Phys Act Health.* 2018;16(1):1–11.

37. King AC, Powell KE, Kraus WE. The US Physical Activity Guidelines Advisory Committee Report — introduction. *Med Sci Sports Exerc.* 2019;51(6):1203–5.

38. Kraus WE, Janz KF, Powell KE, et al. Daily step counts for measuring physical activity exposure and its relation to health. *Med Sci Sports Exerc.* 2019;51(6):1206–12.

39. Jakicic JM, Kraus WE, Powell KE, et al. Association between bout duration of physical activity and health: systematic review. *Med Sci Sports Exerc.* 2019;51(6):1213–9.

40. Campbell WW, Kraus WE, Powell KE, et al. High-intensity interval training for cardiometabolic disease prevention. *Med Sci Sports Exerc.* 2019;51(6):1220–6.

41. Katzmarzyk PT, Powell KE, Jakicic JM, Troiano RP, Piercy K, Tennant B. Sedentary behavior and health: update from the 2018 Physical Activity Guidelines Advisory Committee. *Med Sci Sports Exerc.* 2019;51(6):1227–41.

42. Erickson KI, Hillman C, Stillman CM, et al. Physical activity, cognition, and brain outcomes: a review of the 2018 Physical Activity Guidelines. *Med Sci Sports Exerc.* 2019;51(6):1242–51.

43. McTiernan A, Friedenreich CM, Katzmarzyk PT, et al. Physical activity in cancer prevention and survival: a systematic review. *Med Sci Sports Exerc.* 2019;51(6):1252–61.

44. Jakicic JM, Powell KE, Campbell WW, et al. Physical activity and the prevention of weight gain in adults: a systematic review. *Med Sci Sports Exerc.* 2019;51(6):1262–9.

45. Kraus WE, Powell KE, Haskell WL, et al. Physical activity, all-cause and cardiovascular mortality, and cardiovascular disease. *Med Sci Sports Exerc.* 2019;51(6):1270–81.

46. Pate RR, Hillman CH, Janz KF, et al. Physical activity and health in children younger than 6 years: a systematic review. *Med Sci Sports Exerc.* 2019;51(6):1282–91.

47. Dipietro L, Evenson KR, Bloodgood B, et al. Benefits of physical activity during pregnancy and postpartum: an umbrella review. *Med Sci Sports Exerc.* 2019;51(6):1292–302.

48. Dipietro L, Campbell WW, Buchner DM, et al. Physical activity, injurious falls, and physical function in aging: an umbrella review. *Med Sci Sports Exerc.* 2019;51(6):1303–13.

49. Pescatello LS, Buchner DM, Jakicic JM, et al. Physical activity to prevent and treat hypertension: a systematic review. *Med Sci Sports Exerc.* 2019;51(6):1314–23.

50. Kraus VB, Sprow K, Powell KE, et al. Effects of physical activity in knee and hip osteoarthritis: a systematic umbrella review. *Med Sci Sports Exerc.* 2019;51(6):1324–39.

51. King AC, Whitt-Glover MC, Marquez DX, et al. Physical activity promotion: highlights from the 2018 Physical Activity Guidelines Advisory Committee Systematic Review. *Med Sci Sports Exerc.* 2019;51(6):1340–53.

52. 2018 Physical Activity Guidelines Advisory Committee. *2018 Physical Activity Guidelines Advisory Committee Scientific Report.* Washington (DC): U.S. Department of Health and Human Services; 2018. 779 p.

53. U.S. Department of Health and Human Services. *2018 Physical Activity Guidelines for Americans.* 2nd ed. Washington (DC): U.S. Department of Health and Human Services; 2018. 118 p.

54. Troiano RP, Berrigan D, Dodd KW, Mâsse LC, Tilert T, McDowell M. Physical activity in the United States measured by accelerometer. *Med Sci Sports Exerc.* 2008;40(1):181–8.

55. Centers for Disease Control and Prevention. BRFSS prevalence and trends data [Internet]. Atlanta (GA): Centers for Disease Control and Prevention; [cited 2015 Oct 3]. Available from: https://wwwn.cdc.gov/Niosh-whc/source/brfss.

56. Child and Adolescent Health Measurement Initiative, Data Resource Center for Child and Adolescent Health. *2016 National Survey of Children's Health.* Washington (DC): Data Resource Center for Child and Adolescent Health; 2016. 402 p.

57. Ogden CL, Carroll MD. *Prevalence of Obesity Among Children and Adolescents: United States Trends 1963–1965 Through 2007–2008.* Hyattsville (MD): Centers for Disease Control and Prevention, National Center for Health Statistics; 2010. 5 p.

58. Ogden CL, Carroll MD, Lawman HG, et al. Trends in obesity prevalence among children and adolescents in the United States, 1988–1994 through 2013–2014. *JAMA.* 2016;315(21):2292–9.

59. Hales CM, Fryar CD, Carroll MD, Freedman DS, Ogden CL. Trends in obesity and severe obesity prevalence in US youth and adults by sex and age, 2007–2008 to 2015–2016. *JAMA*. 2018;319(16):1723–5.

60. Must A, Anderson SE. Effects of obesity on morbidity in children and adolescents. *Nutr Clin Care*. 2003;6(1):4–12.

61. Gortmaker SL, Must A, Perrin JM, Sobol AM, Dietz WH. Social and economic consequences of overweight in adolescence and young adulthood. *N Engl J Med*. 1993;329(14):1008–12.

62. Schwimmer JB, Burwinkle TM, Varni JW. Health-related quality of life of severely obese children and adolescents. *JAMA*. 2003;289(14):1813–9.

63. Murthy VH. Surgeon general's perspectives. *Public Health Rep*. 2015;130(3):193–5.

64. Pate RR, O'Neill JR, Liese AD, et al. Factors associated with development of excessive fatness in children and adolescents: a review of prospective studies. *Obes Rev*. 2013;14(8):645–58.

65. Janssen I, Katzmarzyk PT, Boyce WF, Vereecken C, Mulvihill C, Roberts C, et al. Comparison of overweight and obesity prevalence in school-aged youth from 34 countries and their relationships with physical activity and dietary patterns. *Obes Rev*. 2005;6(2):123–32.

66. Singh GK, Kogan MD, Van Dyck PC, Siahpush M. Racial/ethnic, socioeconomic, and behavioral determinants of childhood and adolescent obesity in the United States: analyzing independent and joint associations. *Ann Epidemiol*. 2008;18(9):682–95.

67. Ku CY, Gower BA, Hunter GR, Goran MI. Racial differences in insulin secretion and sensitivity in prepubertal children: role of physical fitness and physical activity. *Obes Res*. 2000;8(7):506–15.

68. Raitakari OT, Porkka KV, Taimela S, Telama R, Räsänen L, Viikari JS. Effects of persistent physical activity and inactivity on coronary risk factors in children and young adults. The Cardiovascular Risk in Young Finns Study. *Am J Epidemiol*. 1994;140(3):195–205.

69. Amed S, Daneman D, Mahmud FH, Hamilton J. Type 2 diabetes in children and adolescents. *Expert Rev Cardiovasc Ther*. 2010;8(3):393–406.

70. Janz KF, Letuchy EM, Burns TL, Eichenberger Gilmore JM, Torner JC, Levy SM. Objectively measured physical activity trajectories predict adolescent bone strength: Iowa Bone Development Study. *Br J Sports Med*. 2014;48(13):1032–6.

71. Hernandez CJ, Beaupré GS, Carter DR. A theoretical analysis of the relative influences of peak BMD, age-related bone loss and menopause on the development of osteoporosis. *Osteoporos Int*. 2003;14(10):843–7.

72. Ekelund U, Steene-Johannessen J, Brown WJ, et al. Does physical activity attenuate, or even eliminate, the detrimental association of sitting time with mortality? A harmonised meta-analysis of data from more than 1 million men and women. *Lancet*. 2016;388(10051):1302–10.

73. National Center for Health Statistics. Early release of selected estimates based on data from the 2017 National Health Interview Survey; Atlanta (GA): Centers for Disease Control and Prevention; [cited 2019 May 22]. Available from: https://www.cdc.gov/nchs/nhis/releases /released201806.htm#7A.

74. Racette SB, Weiss EP, Villareal DT, et al. One year of caloric restriction in humans: feasibility and effects on body composition and abdominal adipose tissue. *J Gerontol A Biol Sci Med Sci*. 2006;61(9):943–50.

75. Ross R, Janssen I, Dawson J, et al. Exercise-induced reduction in obesity and insulin resistance in women: a randomized controlled trial. *Obes Res*. 2004;12(5):789–98.

76. Ross R, Dagnone D, Jones PJ, et al. Reduction in obesity and related comorbid conditions after diet-induced weight loss or exercise-induced weight loss in men. A randomized, controlled trial. *Ann Intern Med*. 2000;133(2): 92–103.

77. Fryar CD, Carroll MD, Ogden CL. *Prevalence of Overweight, Obesity, and Severe Obesity Among Adults Aged 20 and Over: United States, 1960–1962 Through 2013–2014*. Hyattsville (MD): National Center for Health Statistics; 2016. 6 p.

78. Hales CM, Carroll MD, Fryar CD, Ogden CL. *Prevalence of Obesity Among Adults and Youth: United States, 2015–2016*. Hyattsville (MD): National Center for Health Statistics;2017. 8 p.

79. Janiszewski PM, Ross R. Physical activity in the treatment of obesity: beyond body weight reduction. *Appl Physiol Nutr Metab*. 2007;32(3):512–22.

80. Jadhav RA, Hazari A, Monterio A, Kumar S, Maiya AG. Effect of physical activity intervention in prediabetes: a systematic review with meta-analysis. *J Phys Act Health*. 2017;14(9):745–55.

81. Hu FB, Sigal RJ, Rich-Edwards JW, et al. Walking compared with vigorous physical activity and risk of type 2 diabetes in women: a prospective study. *JAMA*. 1999;282(15):1433–9.

82. Aune D, Norat T, Leitzmann M, Tonstad S, Vatten LJ. Physical activity and the risk of type 2 diabetes: a systematic review and dose-response meta-analysis. *Eur J Epidemiol*. 2015;30(7):529–42.

83. Benjamin EJ, Blaha MJ, Chiuve SE, Cushman M, Das SR, Deo R, et al. Heart disease and stroke statistics — 2017 update: a report from the American Heart Association. *Circulation*. 2017;135(10):e146–603.

84. Chodzko-Zajko WJ, Proctor DN, Fiatarone Singh MA, et al. American College of Sports Medicine position stand. Exercise and physical activity for older adults. *Med Sci Sports Exerc*. 2009;41(7):1510–30.

85. Steffen-Batey L, Nichaman MZ, Goff DC Jr, et al. Change in level of physical activity and risk of all-cause mortality or reinfarction: the Corpus Christi Heart Project. *Circulation*. 2000;102(18):2204–9.

86. Feskanich D, Willett W, Colditz G. Walking and leisure-time activity and risk of hip fracture in postmenopausal women. *JAMA*. 2002;288(18):2300–6.

87. Heesch KC, Byles JE, Brown WJ. Prospective association between physical activity and falls in community-dwelling older women. *J Epidemiol Community Health*. 2008;62(5):421–6.

88. Nascimento SL, Surita FG, Godoy AC, Kasawara KT, Morais SS. Physical activity patterns and factors related to exercise during pregnancy: a cross sectional study. *PloS One*. 2015;10(6):e0128953.

89. da Silva SG, Ricardo LI, Evenson KR, Hallal PC. Leisure-time physical activity in pregnancy and maternal-child health: a systematic review and meta-analysis of randomized controlled trials and cohort studies. *Sports Med.* 2017;47(2):295–317.

90. McCurdy AP, Boulé NG, Sivak A, Davenport MH. Effects of exercise on mild-to-moderate depressive symptoms in the postpartum period: a meta-analysis. *Obstet Gynecol.* 2017;129(6):1087–97.

91. ACOG Committee Opinion No. 650: physical activity and exercise during pregnancy and the postpartum period. *Obstet Gynecol.* 2015;126(6):e135–42.

92. Ward BW, Schiller JS, Goodman RA. Multiple chronic conditions among US adults: a 2012 update. *Prev Chronic Dis.* 2014;11:E62.

93. Siscovick DS, Weiss NS, Fletcher RH, Lasky T. The incidence of primary cardiac arrest during vigorous exercise. *N Engl J Med.* 1984;311(14):874–7.

94. Goodman JM, Burr JF, Banks L, Thomas SG. The acute risks of exercise in apparently healthy adults and relevance for prevention of cardiovascular events. *Can J Cardiol.* 2016;32(4):523–32.

95. Drezner JA, Chun JS, Harmon KG, Derminer L. Survival trends in the United States following exercise-related sudden cardiac arrest in the youth: 2000-2006. *Heart Rhythm.* 2008;5(6):794–9.

96. Maron BJ, Doerer JJ, Haas TS, Tierney DM, Mueller FO. Sudden deaths in young competitive athletes: analysis of 1866 deaths in the United States, 1980–2006. *Circulation.* 2009;119(8):1085–92.

97. Van Camp SP, Bloor CM, Mueller FO, Cantu RC, Olson HG. Nontraumatic sports death in high school and college athletes. *Med Sci Sports Exerc.* 1995;27(5):641–7.

98. Giri S, Thompson PD, Kiernan FJ, et al. Clinical and angiographic characteristics of exertion-related acute myocardial infarction. *JAMA.* 1999;282(18):1731–6.

99. Hammoudeh AJ, Haft JI. Coronary-plaque rupture in acute coronary syndromes triggered by snow shoveling. *N Engl J Med.* 1996;335(26):2001.

100. Mittleman MA, Maclure M, Tofler GH, Sherwood JB, Goldberg RJ, Muller JE. Triggering of acute myocardial infarction by heavy physical exertion. Protection against triggering by regular exertion. Determinants of Myocardial Infarction Onset Study Investigators. *N Engl J Med.* 1993;329(23):1677–83.

101. Talbot LA, Morrell CH, Metter EJ, Fleg JL. Comparison of cardiorespiratory fitness versus leisure time physical activity as predictors of coronary events in men aged < or = 65 years and > 65 years. *Am J Cardiol.* 2002;89(10):1187–92.

102. Vuori I. The cardiovascular risks of physical activity. *Acta Med Scan.* 1986;200(Suppl 711):205–14.

103. Willich SN, Lewis M, Löwel H, Arntz HR, Schubert F, Schröder R. Physical exertion as a trigger of acute myocardial infarction. Triggers and Mechanisms of Myocardial Infarction Study Group. *N Engl J Med.* 1993;329(23):1684–90.

104. American College of Sports Medicine, American Heart Association. Exercise and acute cardiovascular events: placing the risks into perspective. *Med Sci Sports Exerc.* 2007;39(5):886–97.

105. Black A, Black MM, Gensini G. Exertion and acute coronary artery injury. *Angiology.* 1975;26(11):759–83.

106. Centers for Disease Control and Prevention. Nonfatal sports- and recreation-related injuries treated in emergency departments — United States, July 2000–June 2001. *MMWR Morb Mortal Wkly Rep.* 2002;51(33):736–40.

107. Ciampricotti R, Deckers JW, Taverne R, el Gamal M, Relik-van Wely L, Pool J. Characteristics of conditioned and sedentary men with acute coronary syndromes. *Am J Cardiol.* 1994;73(4):219–22.

108. Gibbons L, Blair SN, Kohl HW, Cooper K. The safety of maximal exercise testing. *Circulation.* 1989;80(4):846–52.

109. Knight JA, Laubach CA Jr, Butcher RJ, Menapace FJ. Supervision of clinical exercise testing by exercise physiologists. *Am J Cardiol.* 1995;75(5):390–1.

110. McHenry PL. Risks of graded exercise testing. *Am J Cardiol.* 1977;39(6):935–7.

111. Stuart RJ Jr, Ellestad MH. National survey of exercise stress testing facilities. *Chest.* 1980;77(1):94–7.

112. Myers J, Prakash M, Froelicher V, Do D, Partington S, Atwood JE. Exercise capacity and mortality among men referred for exercise testing. *N Engl J Med.* 2002;346(11):793–801.

113. Myers J, Voodi L, Umann T, Froelicher VF. A survey of exercise testing: methods, utilization, interpretation, and safety in the VAHCS. *J Cardiopulm Rehabil.* 2000;20(4):251–8.

114. Hootman JM, Macera CA, Ainsworth BE, Addy CL, Martin M, Blair SN. Epidemiology of musculoskeletal injuries among sedentary and physically active adults. *Med Sci Sports Exerc.* 2002;34(5):838–44.

115. U.S. Bureau of Labor Statistics. *Spotlight on Statistics: Sports and Exercise.* Washington (DC): U.S. Bureau of Labor Statistics; 2019. 14 p.

116. Powell KE, Heath GW, Kresnow MJ, Sacks JJ, Branche CM. Injury rates from walking, gardening, weightlifting, outdoor bicycling, and aerobics. *Med Sci Sports Exerc.* 1998;30(8):1246–9.

117. Colbert LH, Hootman JM, Macera CA. Physical activity-related injuries in walkers and runners in the aerobics center longitudinal study. *Clin J Sport Med.* 2000;10(4):259–63.

118. Videbæk S, Bueno AM, Nielsen RO, Rasmussen S. Incidence of running-related injuries per 1000 h of running in different types of runners: a systematic review and meta-analysis. *Sports Med.* 2015;45(7):1017–26.

119. Lopes AD, Hespanhol LC Jr, Yeung SS, Costa LO. What are the main running-related musculoskeletal injuries? A systematic review. *Sports Med.* 2012;42(10):891–905.

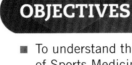

Preparticipation Physical Activity Screening Guidelines

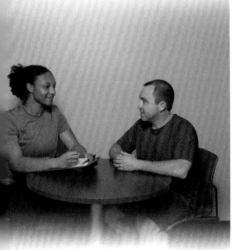

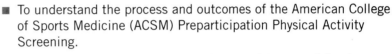

OBJECTIVES

- To understand the process and outcomes of the American College of Sports Medicine (ACSM) Preparticipation Physical Activity Screening.
- To explore the importance of and issues with preparticipation physical activity screening as well as to investigate the various tools that may be used including the Physical Activity Readiness Questionnaire for Everyone (PAR-Q+) and a health history questionnaire.
- To determine course of action with a client once his or her risk has been established.
- To discuss the concept of absolute and relative contraindications to exercise testing.

INTRODUCTION

Ever since the increased promotion of physical activity in modern times, there has been an emphasis on preparticipation physical activity screening to ensure that the risks of increased physical activity do not outweigh the benefits of this healthy behavior (1). The process of preparticipation physical activity screening has been increasingly professionalized over the years since its introduction. The American College of Sports Medicine (ACSM) is perhaps the best known organization in the area of preparticipation physical activity screening in the United States. The ACSM formally titled this process *risk stratification* in the 1990s in *ACSM's Guidelines for Exercise Testing and Prescription* (*GETP*), fourth edition, publication. This process was retitled *risk classification* in 2013 (2). With the release of the tenth edition of *GETP* in 2017, there were some substantial changes to the preparticipation physical activity screening process including the elimination of the *risk stratification/classification* terminology (including low-, moderate-, and high-risk strata) and the nonuse of adding/subtracting ACSM risk factor thresholds for overall risk classification. These changes were continued into the latest edition of *GETP* (3). This is discussed further in this chapter.

The preparticipation physical activity screening process is also intimately tied to the contraindications for graded exercise testing discussed later in this chapter. This chapter explores the preparticipation physical activity screening concept, so the ACSM Certified Exercise Physiologist® (ACSM-EP®) can make informed decisions about the readiness of an individual to undertake a physically active lifestyle.

 ## Importance of Preparticipation Physical Activity Screening

In order to reduce the likelihood of occurrence of any untoward or unwanted event(s) during a physical activity program, it is prudent to conduct some form of preparticipation physical activity screening on a client (4). Preparticipation physical activity screening, along with cardiovascular risk factor assessment discussed later in this chapter, may also be the first step in a health-related physical fitness assessment. Preparticipation physical activity screening involves gathering and analyzing demographic and health-related information on a client along with some medical/health assessments such as the presence of signs and symptoms in order to aid decision making on a client's physical activity future (3). The preparticipation physical activity screening is a dynamic process in that it may vary in its scope and components depending on the client's needs from a medical/health standpoint (*e.g.*, the client has some form of cardiovascular, metabolic, and/or renal [CMR] disease) as well as the presence of signs and symptoms suggestive of CMR disease (*e.g.*, chest pain of an ischemic nature) and his or her physical activity program status (he or she currently participates in moderate physical activity for the past 3 mo).

The following is a partial list of the reasons why it is important to first screen clients for participation in physical activity programs (3,5):

- To identify those with medical contraindications (exclusion criteria) for performing physical activity
- To identify those who should receive a medical/physical evaluation/exam and clearance prior to performing a physical activity program
- To identify those who should participate in a medically supervised physical activity program
- To identify those with other health/medical concerns (*i.e.*, orthopedic injuries, etc.)

History of Preparticipation Physical Activity Screening

There are several national and international organizations that have made suggestions about what these preparticipation physical activity screening guidelines should be including the ACSM (1,2,6,7). However, it is helpful to remember that these are just guidelines or suggestions. The prudent ACSM-EP should devise a preparticipation physical activity screening scheme that best meets the needs of his or her client(s) and environment(s).

For instance, the U.S. Surgeon General in the 1996 report on *Physical Activity and Health* stated that (4)

> Previously inactive men over age 40, women over age 50, and people at high risk for CVD [CVD is an abbreviation for cardiovascular disease] should first consult a physician before embarking on a program of vigorous physical activity to which they are unaccustomed. People with disease should be evaluated by a physician first. . . .

In addition, a summary of the "cautions" listed on many pieces of exercise equipment as well as in exercise books and videos is to

- "First consult your physician before starting an exercise program."
- "This is especially important for
    - Men ≥45 years old; women ≥55 years old
    - Those who are going to perform vigorous physical activity
    - And for those who are new to exercise or are unaccustomed to exercise"

There is one major set of formal screening guidelines for individuals who wish to embark on a physical activity program. This set comes from the ACSM. The ACSM has published this set in their popular and often revised text, *GETP*, starting with their fourth edition in 1991. Several other professional organizations including the American Heart Association (AHA) have also published and revised their own set of preparticipation physical activity screening guidelines. The AHA guidelines were published most recently in their journal *Circulation* in 2001 (2,8).

As stated earlier, the ACSM, through its *GETP* text, has addressed preparticipation physical activity screening (4). In the past, the ACSM has listed these preparticipation physical activity screening guidelines often under the moniker, "Risk Stratification." Through the first eight editions (although risk stratification did not appear formally in the first three editions) of the *GETP*, there have been several revisions made to this risk stratification section. The ninth edition of the *GETP* terms this process as *risk classification*. The tenth edition of *GETP* has put forth major changes to the preparticipation physical activity screening process (2). We would categorize the revisions made to the *GETP* preparticipation screening process as mostly an elimination of the "strata" or levels used as well as the elimination of the use of the ACSM risk factor thresholds for this process. In the place of the ACSM risk factor thresholds is the dependence on the physical activity history of the participant as well as the presence of CMR disease and the presence of signs and symptoms suggestive of CMR disease (3).

Levels of Screening

According to the ACSM, there are two basic approaches to preparticipation physical activity screening (3). One of these approaches can be performed by the individual wishing to become more physically active without direct input from an exercise professional (self-guided screening). The other approach involves interaction with an exercise professional such as an ACSM-EP (professionally supervised screening). These two levels of screening are not mutually exclusive; for instance, an individual may first use the self-guided method before seeking an ACSM-EP for professional guidance in preparticipation physical activity screening.

Self-Guided Screening

Self-guided approaches to preparticipation physical activity screening have been suggested by many organizations from the ACSM to the AHA as a minimum or starting point for the individual who wishes to increase his or her physical activity (2). The Physical Activity Readiness Questionnaire for Everyone (PAR-Q+) has been suggested for use in self-guided screening and is discussed next.

Physical Activity Readiness Questionnaire for Everyone

The Health History Questionnaire (HHQ) is generally thought of as being a comprehensive assessment of a client's medical and health history. Because the HHQ can be more information than is needed in some situations, the original Physical Activity Readiness Questionnaire, or PAR-Q, was developed in Canada to be simpler in both scope and use (9). The original PAR-Q contains seven YES/NO questions that have been found to be both readable and understandable for an individual to answer. The PAR-Q was designed to screen out those clients from not participating in physical activities that may be too strenuous for them. The PAR-Q has been recommended as a minimal standard for entry into moderate-intensity exercise programs. Thus, the PAR-Q may be considered a useful tool for individuals to gauge their own "medical" readiness to participate in physical activity programs (3). However, because the PAR-Q may be best used to screen those who are at high risk for exercise complications and thus may need a medical exam, it may not be as effective in screening low- to moderate-risk individuals (7). Thus, the PAR-Q has recently morphed into the PAR-Q+ with some word changes among the seven YES/NO questions to better classify all individuals (Fig. 2.1) (3).

Thus, at the minimum, a prudent ACSM-EP should consider suggesting to his or her clients that they fill out a PAR-Q+ (Figs. 2.1 and 2.2) prior to participation in any self-guided physical activity program (3,10).

The PAR-Q has been found to be a useful tool (6). In one article by de Oliveira Luz and colleagues (6), the PAR-Q was found to have a high (89%) sensitivity (producing many true positives) for picking up potential medical conditions that might impact an individual's exercise responses in older subjects. However, it should be noted that the specificity (or true negatives) of the PAR-Q in this subject pool was estimated at 42% (6). Thus, the PAR-Q may be quite good at detecting potential problems in clients before they occur in an exercise setting, but the form may also wrongly identify clients as having a potential problem when on further evaluation, there is no need for concern. This may not be a bad situation as the form errors of the side of caution. The prudent ACSM-EP may therefore need to intervene in such cases as well as involve further health care professionals.

Because there are some potential problems noted with the PAR-Q as far as its ability to discern if an individual's potential adverse medical condition might impact his or her exercise response, the PAR-Q+ was developed. However, the PAR-Q+ is updated annually and thus statistics related to the PAR-Q+ effectiveness are not yet available. It has been suggested by Jamnik and colleagues (5) that a qualified health/fitness professional (ACSM-EP) may, using ACSM preparticipation physical activity screening process, perform a thorough screening process.

ePARmed-X+Physician Clearance Follow-Up Questionnaire

The ePARmed-X+Physician Clearance Follow-Up Questionnaire was developed also in Canada as a tool that a physician can use to refer individuals to a professionally supervised physical activity program and make recommendations for that program. This form was designed to be used in those cases where a YES answer on one of the seven questions in the PAR-Q+ necessitates further medical clearance using the self-guided method. It is also worth noting that although not required, the ePARmed-X+Physician Clearance Follow-Up Questionnaire (see http://www.eparmedx.com) could be used for medical clearance in a professionally supervised preparticipation physical activity screening.

2021 PAR-Q+

The Physical Activity Readiness Questionnaire for Everyone

The health benefits of regular physical activity are clear; more people should engage in physical activity every day of the week. Participating in physical activity is very safe for MOST people. This questionnaire will tell you whether it is necessary for you to seek further advice from your doctor OR a qualified exercise professional before becoming more physically active.

GENERAL HEALTH QUESTIONS

Please read the 7 questions below carefully and answer each one honestly: check YES or NO.	YES	NO
1) Has your doctor ever said that you have a heart condition ☐ OR high blood pressure☐ ?	☐	☐
2) Do you feel pain in your chest at rest, during your daily activities of living, OR when you do physical activity?	☐	☐
3) Do you lose balance because of dizziness OR have you lost consciousness in the last 12 months? Please answer NO if your dizziness was associated with over-breathing (including during vigorous exercise).	☐	☐
4) Have you ever been diagnosed with another chronic medical condition (other than heart disease or high blood pressure)? PLEASE LIST CONDITION(S) HERE: _____	☐	☐
5) Are you currently taking prescribed medications for a chronic medical condition? PLEASE LIST CONDITION(S) AND MEDICATIONS HERE: _____	☐	☐
6) Do you currently have (or have had within the past 12 months) a bone, joint, or soft tissue (muscle, ligament, or tendon) problem that could be made worse by becoming more physically active? Please answer NO if you had a problem in the past, but it does not limit your current ability to be physically active. PLEASE LIST CONDITION(S) HERE: _____	☐	☐
7) Has your doctor ever said that you should only do medically supervised physical activity?	☐	☐

☑ **If you answered NO to all of the questions above, you are cleared for physical activity.**
Please sign the PARTICIPANT DECLARATION. You do not need to complete Pages 2 and 3.

- ▶ Start becoming much more physically active – start slowly and build up gradually.
- ▶ Follow Global Physical Activity Guidelines for your age (https://www.who.int/publications/i/item/9789240015128).
- ▶ You may take part in a health and fitness appraisal.
- ▶ If you are over the age of 45 yr and NOT accustomed to regular vigorous to maximal effort exercise, consult a qualified exercise professional before engaging in this intensity of exercise.
- ▶ If you have any further questions, contact a qualified exercise professional.

PARTICIPANT DECLARATION
If you are less than the legal age required for consent or require the assent of a care provider, your parent, guardian or care provider must also sign this form.

I, the undersigned, have read, understood to my full satisfaction and completed this questionnaire. I acknowledge that this physical activity clearance is valid for a maximum of 12 months from the date it is completed and becomes invalid if my condition changes. I also acknowledge that the community/fitness center may retain a copy of this form for its records. In these instances, it will maintain the confidentiality of the same, complying with applicable law.

NAME _____ DATE _____

SIGNATURE _____ WITNESS _____

SIGNATURE OF PARENT/GUARDIAN/CARE PROVIDER _____

⬤ **If you answered YES to one or more of the questions above, COMPLETE PAGES 2 AND 3.**

⚠ **Delay becoming more active if:**

- ✓ You have a temporary illness such as a cold or fever; it is best to wait until you feel better.
- ✓ You are pregnant - talk to your health care practitioner, your physician, a qualified exercise professional, and/or complete the ePARmed-X+ at www.eparmedx.com before becoming more physically active.
- ✓ Your health changes - answer the questions on Pages 2 and 3 of this document and/or talk to your doctor or a qualified exercise professional before continuing with any physical activity program.

FIGURE 2.1. First page of the PAR-Q+. (Reprinted with permission from the PAR-Q+ Collaboration and the authors of the PAR-Q+. See http://eparmedx.com for the most current annual update of the PAR-Q+.)

2021 PAR-Q+
FOLLOW-UP QUESTIONS ABOUT YOUR MEDICAL CONDITION(S)

1.   Do you have Arthritis, Osteoporosis, or Back Problems?

If the above condition(s) is/are present, answer questions 1a-1c   If **NO** ☐ go to question 2

1a.	Do you have difficulty controlling your condition with medications or other physician-prescribed therapies? (Answer **NO** if you are not currently taking medications or other treatments)	YES☐ NO☐
1b.	Do you have joint problems causing pain, a recent fracture or fracture caused by osteoporosis or cancer, displaced vertebra (e.g., spondylolisthesis), and/or spondylolysis/pars defect (a crack in the bony ring on the back of the spinal column)?	YES☐ NO☐
1c.	Have you had steroid injections or taken steroid tablets regularly for more than 3 months?	YES☐ NO☐

2.   Do you currently have Cancer of any kind?

If the above condition(s) is/are present, answer questions 2a-2b   If **NO** ☐ go to question 3

2a.	Does your cancer diagnosis include any of the following types: lung/bronchogenic, multiple myeloma (cancer of plasma cells), head, and/or neck?	YES☐ NO☐
2b.	Are you currently receiving cancer therapy (such as chemotheraphy or radiotherapy)?	YES☐ NO☐

3.   Do you have a Heart or Cardiovascular Condition? This includes Coronary Artery Disease, Heart Failure, Diagnosed Abnormality of Heart Rhythm

If the above condition(s) is/are present, answer questions 3a-3d   If **NO** ☐ go to question 4

3a.	Do you have difficulty controlling your condition with medications or other physician-prescribed therapies? (Answer **NO** if you are not currently taking medications or other treatments)	YES☐ NO☐
3b.	Do you have an irregular heart beat that requires medical management? (e.g., atrial fibrillation, premature ventricular contraction)	YES☐ NO☐
3c.	Do you have chronic heart failure?	YES☐ NO☐
3d.	Do you have diagnosed coronary artery (cardiovascular) disease and have not participated in regular physical activity in the last 2 months?	YES☐ NO☐

4.   Do you currently have High Blood Pressure?

If the above condition(s) is/are present, answer questions 4a-4b   If **NO** ☐ go to question 5

4a.	Do you have difficulty controlling your condition with medications or other physician-prescribed therapies? (Answer **NO** if you are not currently taking medications or other treatments)	YES☐ NO☐
4b.	Do you have a resting blood pressure equal to or greater than 160/90 mmHg with or without medication? (Answer **YES** if you do not know your resting blood pressure)	YES☐ NO☐

5.   Do you have any Metabolic Conditions? This includes Type 1 Diabetes, Type 2 Diabetes, Pre-Diabetes

If the above condition(s) is/are present, answer questions 5a-5e   If **NO** ☐ go to question 6

5a.	Do you often have difficulty controlling your blood sugar levels with foods, medications, or other physician-prescribed therapies?	YES☐ NO☐
5b.	Do you often suffer from signs and symptoms of low blood sugar (hypoglycemia) following exercise and/or during activities of daily living? Signs of hypoglycemia may include shakiness, nervousness, unusual irritability, abnormal sweating, dizziness or light-headedness, mental confusion, difficulty speaking, weakness, or sleepiness.	YES☐ NO☐
5c.	Do you have any signs or symptoms of diabetes complications such as heart or vascular disease and/or complications affecting your eyes, kidneys, **OR** the sensation in your toes and feet?	YES☐ NO☐
5d.	Do you have other metabolic conditions (such as current pregnancy-related diabetes, chronic kidney disease, or liver problems)?	YES☐ NO☐
5e.	Are you planning to engage in what for you is unusually high (or vigorous) intensity exercise in the near future?	YES☐ NO☐

FIGURE 2.2. The PAR-Q+ follow-up questions about medical conditions.

2021 PAR-Q+

6.   **Do you have any Mental Health Problems or Learning Difficulties?** This includes Alzheimer's, Dementia, Depression, Anxiety Disorder, Eating Disorder, Psychotic Disorder, Intellectual Disability, Down Syndrome

If the above condition(s) is/are present, answer questions 6a-6b   If **NO** ☐ go to question 7

6a.	Do you have difficulty controlling your condition with medications or other physician-prescribed therapies? (Answer **NO** if you are not currently taking medications or other treatments)	YES☐ NO☐
6b.	Do you have Down Syndrome **AND** back problems affecting nerves or muscles?	YES☐ NO☐

7.   **Do you have a Respiratory Disease?** This includes Chronic Obstructive Pulmonary Disease, Asthma, Pulmonary High Blood Pressure

If the above condition(s) is/are present, answer questions 7a-7d   If **NO** ☐ go to question 8

7a.	Do you have difficulty controlling your condition with medications or other physician-prescribed therapies? (Answer **NO** if you are not currently taking medications or other treatments)	YES☐ NO☐
7b.	Has your doctor ever said your blood oxygen level is low at rest or during exercise and/or that you require supplemental oxygen therapy?	YES☐ NO☐
7c.	If asthmatic, do you currently have symptoms of chest tightness, wheezing, laboured breathing, consistent cough (more than 2 days/week), or have you used your rescue medication more than twice in the last week?	YES☐ NO☐
7d.	Has your doctor ever said you have high blood pressure in the blood vessels of your lungs?	YES☐ NO☐

8.   **Do you have a Spinal Cord Injury?** This includes Tetraplegia and Paraplegia

If the above condition(s) is/are present, answer questions 8a-8c   If **NO** ☐ go to question 9

8a.	Do you have difficulty controlling your condition with medications or other physician-prescribed therapies? (Answer **NO** if you are not currently taking medications or other treatments)	YES☐ NO☐
8b.	Do you commonly exhibit low resting blood pressure significant enough to cause dizziness, light-headedness, and/or fainting?	YES☐ NO☐
8c.	Has your physician indicated that you exhibit sudden bouts of high blood pressure (known as Autonomic Dysreflexia)?	YES☐ NO☐

9.   **Have you had a Stroke?** This includes Transient Ischemic Attack (TIA) or Cerebrovascular Event

If the above condition(s) is/are present, answer questions 9a-9c   If **NO** ☐ go to question 10

9a.	Do you have difficulty controlling your condition with medications or other physician-prescribed therapies? (Answer **NO** if you are not currently taking medications or other treatments)	YES☐ NO☐
9b.	Do you have any impairment in walking or mobility?	YES☐ NO☐
9c.	Have you experienced a stroke or impairment in nerves or muscles in the past 6 months?	YES☐ NO☐

10.   **Do you have any other medical condition not listed above or do you have two or more medical conditions?**

If you have other medical conditions, answer questions 10a-10c   If **NO** ☐ read the Page 4 recommendations

10a.	Have you experienced a blackout, fainted, or lost consciousness as a result of a head injury within the last 12 months **OR** have you had a diagnosed concussion within the last 12 months?	YES☐ NO☐
10b.	Do you have a medical condition that is not listed (such as epilepsy, neurological conditions, kidney problems)?	YES☐ NO☐
10c.	Do you currently live with two or more medical conditions?	YES☐ NO☐

PLEASE LIST YOUR MEDICAL CONDITION(S) AND ANY RELATED MEDICATIONS HERE: _____

_____

> ## GO to Page 4 for recommendations about your current medical condition(s) and sign the PARTICIPANT DECLARATION.

FIGURE 2.2. (continued)

2021 PAR-Q+

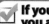 **If you answered NO to all of the FOLLOW-UP questions (pgs. 2-3) about your medical condition, you are ready to become more physically active - sign the PARTICIPANT DECLARATION below:**

▶ It is advised that you consult a qualified exercise professional to help you develop a safe and effective physical activity plan to meet your health needs.

▶ You are encouraged to start slowly and build up gradually - 20 to 60 minutes of low to moderate intensity exercise, 3-5 days per week including aerobic and muscle strengthening exercises.

▶ As you progress, you should aim to accumulate 150 minutes or more of moderate intensity physical activity per week.

▶ If you are over the age of 45 yr and **NOT** accustomed to regular vigorous to maximal effort exercise, consult a qualified exercise professional before engaging in this intensity of exercise.

 If you answered YES to one or more of the follow-up questions about your medical condition:

You should seek further information before becoming more physically active or engaging in a fitness appraisal. You should complete the specially designed online screening and exercise recommendations program - the **ePARmed-X+ at www.eparmedx.com** and/or visit a qualified exercise professional to work through the ePARmed-X+ and for further information.

⚠ **Delay becoming more active if:**

 You have a temporary illness such as a cold or fever; it is best to wait until you feel better.

 You are pregnant - talk to your health care practitioner, your physician, a qualified exercise professional, and/or complete the ePARmed-X+ **at www.eparmedx.com** before becoming more physically active.

 Your health changes - talk to your doctor or qualified exercise professional before continuing with any physical activity program.

● You are encouraged to photocopy the PAR-Q+. You must use the entire questionnaire and NO changes are permitted.
● The authors, the PAR-Q+ Collaboration, partner organizations, and their agents assume no liability for persons who undertake physical activity and/or make use of the PAR-Q+ or ePARmed-X+. If in doubt after completing the questionnaire, consult your doctor prior to physical activity.

PARTICIPANT DECLARATION

● All persons who have completed the PAR-Q+ please read and sign the declaration below.

● If you are less than the legal age required for consent or require the assent of a care provider, your parent, guardian or care provider must also sign this form.

I, the undersigned, have read, understood to my full satisfaction and completed this questionnaire. I acknowledge that this physical activity clearance is valid for a maximum of 12 months from the date it is completed and becomes invalid if my condition changes. I also acknowledge that the community/fitness center may retain a copy of this form for records. In these instances, it will maintain the confidentiality of the same, complying with applicable law.

NAME _____   DATE _____

SIGNATURE _____   WITNESS _____

SIGNATURE OF PARENT/GUARDIAN/CARE PROVIDER _____

———— **For more information, please contact** ————
www.eparmedx.com
Email: eparmedx@gmail.com

Citation for PAR-Q+
Warburton DER, Jamnik VK, Bredin SSD, and Gledhill N on behalf of the PAR-Q+ Collaboration. The Physical Activity Readiness Questionnaire for Everyone (PAR-Q+) and Electronic Physical Activity Readiness Medical Examination (ePARmed-X+). Health & Fitness Journal of Canada 4(2):3-23, 2011.

The PAR-Q+ was created using the evidence-based AGREE process (1) by the PAR-Q+ Collaboration chaired by Dr. Darren E. R. Warburton with Dr. Norman Gledhill, Dr. Veronica Jamnik, and Dr. Donald C. McKenzie (2). Production of this document has been made possible through financial contributions from the Public Health Agency of Canada and the BC Ministry of Health Services. The views expressed herein do not necessarily represent the views of the Public Health Agency of Canada or the BC Ministry of Health Services.

Key References
1. Jamnik VK, Warburton DER, Makarski J, McKenzie DC, Shephard RJ, Stone J, and Gledhill N. Enhancing the effectiveness of clearance for physical activity participation; background and overall process. APNM 36(S1):S3-S13, 2011.
2. Warburton DER, Gledhill N, Jamnik VK, Bredin SSD, McKenzie DC, Stone J, Charlesworth S, and Shephard RJ. Evidence-based risk assessment and recommendations for physical activity clearance; Consensus Document. APNM 36(S1):S266-s298, 2011.
3. Chisholm DM, Collis ML, Kulak LL, Davenport W, and Gruber N. Physical activity readiness. British Columbia Medical Journal. 1975;17:375-378.
4. Thomas S, Reading J, and Shephard RJ. Revision of the Physical Activity Readiness Questionnaire (PAR-Q). Canadian Journal of Sport Science 1992;17:4 338-345.

FIGURE 2.2. *(continued)*

Professionally Supervised Screening

Self-analysis of risk for physical activity is important with the large number of individuals who are currently not physically active but hopefully will become more active soon perhaps by self-guidance. Thus, they will need to, or should, use some means to determine their physical readiness, such as the PAR-Q+. However, many individuals will seek the knowledge and guidance of an ACSM-EP for this service. Professionally supervised screening, under the guidance of an ACSM-EP, should include the following components: (a) informed consent process, (b) preparticipation physical activity screening, (c) health history, and (d) cardiovascular risk factor analysis (and possibly medical clearance, if warranted) while following the ACSM preexercise evaluation process (3). The ACSM-EP may be involved in professional screening at the "lower" levels of risk (*i.e.*, general nonclinical population who does not meet any of the ACSM risk factor thresholds), whereas professionals such as the ACSM Certified Clinical Exercise Physiologist® (ACSM-CEP®) will be more likely involved with individuals at higher risk levels (who meet more than one ACSM risk factor threshold). In the following section, we discuss the informed consent process, HHQ, and the medical evaluation/clearance.

Informed Consent

The informed consent process is the first step when working with a new patient or client and must be completed prior to the collection of (a) any personal and confidential information, (b) any form of fitness testing, or (c) exercise participation. The informed consent should be written to "inform" the participant of any personal and confidential information that will be collected and how it will be stored as well as the purpose(s) of, and risks involved with, any of the exercise testing and exercise program participation. Remember, it is equally as important to present the benefits of exercise (as well as the risks) so that the participant can make an informed decision about participation.

Although the consent form is a legal document, its contents should be verbally explained to the participant and should include a statement indicating the individual has been given an opportunity to ask questions about the preparticipation physical activity, exercise testing or fitness assessment, or the exercise program and has been given sufficient information to provide an informed "consent." Any questions asked by the participant and the response provided by the ACSM-EP should be included on the signed informed consent document. The consent form must indicate the participant is free to withdraw at any time. Also, all reasonable efforts must be made to protect the privacy of individual's health information (*e.g.*, medical history, test results) as described in the Health Insurance Portability and Accountability Act (HIPAA) (3,11). The participant's signature on the informed consent document indicates that the participant has been adequately "informed" of the risks and benefits involved and have given his or her "consent" to proceed. A sample consent form for exercise testing is provided in Figure 2.3. However, it is advisable to check with those responsible for legal decisions in your facility to determine the most appropriate informed consent process for your needs. Sample forms should not be adopted unless approved by legal counsel and/ or the appropriate institutional review board.

When any participant information is being used in a research setting, this should be indicated during the consent process and reflected on the informed consent form, and applicable policies for the testing of human subjects must be implemented. Health care professionals and research scientists should obtain approval from the participant and the institutional review board when conducting an exercise test for research purposes.

It is imperative that personnel are properly trained and authorized to carry out any emergency procedure and use any equipment identified in the informed consent. Written emergency policies and procedures should be in place, and emergency drills should be practiced at least once every 3 months or more frequently when there is a change in staff (11).

Informed Consent for an Exercise Test

1. **Purpose and Explanation of the Test**

   You will perform an exercise test on a cycle ergometer or a motor-driven treadmill. The exercise intensity will begin at a low level and will be advanced in stages depending on your fitness level. We may stop the test at any time because of signs of fatigue or changes in your heart rate, electrocardiogram, or blood pressure, or symptoms you may experience. It is important for you to realize that you may stop when you wish because of feelings of fatigue or any other discomfort.

2. **Attendant Risks and Discomforts**

   There exists the possibility of certain changes occurring during the test that increase risk. These include abnormal blood pressure; fainting; irregular, fast, or slow heart rhythm; and, in rare instances, heart attack, stroke, or death. Every effort will be made to minimize these risks by evaluation of preliminary information relating to your health and fitness and by careful observations during testing. Emergency equipment and trained personnel are available to deal with unusual situations that may arise.

3. **Responsibilities of the Participant**

   Information you possess about your health status or previous experiences of heart-related symptoms (*e.g.*, shortness of breath with low-level activity; pain; pressure; tightness; heaviness in the chest, neck, jaw, back and/or arms) with physical effort may affect the safety of your exercise test. Your prompt reporting of these and any other unusual feelings with effort during the exercise test itself is very important. You are responsible for fully disclosing your medical history as well as symptoms that may occur during the test. You are also expected to report all medications (including nonprescription) taken recently and, in particular, those taken today to the testing staff.

4. **Benefits to be Expected**

   The results obtained from the exercise test may assist in the diagnosis of your illness, in evaluating the effect of your medications, or in evaluating what type of physical activities you might do with low risk.

5. **Inquiries**

   Any questions about the procedures used in the exercise test or the results of your test are encouraged. If you have any concerns or questions, please ask us for further explanations.

6. **Use of Medical Records**

   The information that is obtained during exercise testing will be treated as privileged and confidential as described in the Health Insurance Portability and Accountability Act of 1996. It is not to be released or revealed to any individual except your referring physician without your written consent. However, the information obtained may be used for statistical analysis or scientific purposes with your right to privacy retained.

7. **Freedom of Consent**

   I hereby consent to voluntarily engage in an exercise test to determine my exercise capacity and state of cardiovascular health. My permission to perform this exercise test is given voluntarily. I understand that I am free to stop the test at any point if I so desire.

   I have read this form, and I understand the test procedures that I will perform and the attendant risks and discomforts. Knowing these risks and discomforts, and having had an opportunity to ask questions that have been answered to my satisfaction, I consent to participate in this test.

Date	Signature of Patient
Date	Signature of Witness
Date	Signature of Physician or Authorized Delegate

FIGURE 2.3. Sample of informed consent form for a symptom-limited exercise test. (Reprinted from American College of Sports Medicine. *ACSM's Guidelines for Exercise Testing and Prescription.* 11th ed. Philadelphia [PA]: Wolters Kluwer; 2022. 548 p., Figure 2.1).

Health History Questionnaire

Some form of an HHQ is necessary to use with a client to establish his or her medical/health risks for participation in a physical activity program (7,12). The HHQ, along with other medical/health data, is also used in the process of exercise preparticipation physical activity screening. The HHQ should be tailored to fit the needs of the program as far as asking for the specific information needed from a client. In general, the HHQ should minimally assess a client's (3)

- Family history of CMR disease
- Personal history of various diseases and illnesses including CMR disease
- Surgical history
- Past and present health behaviors/habits (such as history of cigarette smoking and physical activity)
- Current use of various drugs/medications
- Specific history of various signs and symptoms suggested of CMR disease among other things

The current edition of the *GETP* contains a more detailed list of the specifics of the health and medical evaluations (including desirable laboratory tests) (3). Again, the prudent ACSM-EP should tailor the HHQ to his or her client's specific needs. A sample HHQ is included in this chapter (Fig. 2.4).

Medical Examination/Clearance

A medical examination led by a physician (or other qualified health care professional) may also be necessary or desirable to help evaluate the health and/or medical status of your client prior to a physical activity program. The suggested components of this medical examination can be found in the most current edition of the *GETP* (3). In addition to a medical examination, it may be desirable to perform some routine laboratory assessments (*i.e.*, fasting blood cholesterol and/or resting blood pressure) on your client prior to physical activity programming (7). Clients who are at a higher risk for exercise complications (those who show signs or symptoms suggestive of CMR disease) may need (it is recommended) a medical clearance prior to participation in a physical activity program.

Preparticipation Physical Activity Screening Process

The process for screening prior to participation in a physical activity program had been altered significantly with the publication of *GETP* (2). Essentially, only three items need to be considered to complete the process, as is displayed in Figure 2.5. In addition, the ACSM preparticipation physical activity screening algorithm can be found in Figure 2.6. The first item to consider in the process is the individual's past physical activity history. The individual can be queried about his or her physical activity history using the HHQ and/or by questioning. Next, the individual should be evaluated for the presence of known CMR disease. This, too, can be assessed using the HHQ and/or by questioning. Last in the process is the assessment of the individual's presence of signs and symptoms that can be suggestive of CMR disease. The ACSM in its recent *GETP* provides a form for the assessment of all three of these components of the process. This form can be found in Figure 2.7 (3).

It is important to note that the process of ACSM preparticipation physical activity screening has been divorced from the concept of the need for and supervisory qualifications of a graded exercise test and other health-related physical fitness assessments. Recent professional society opinions and research have devalued the use of graded exercise testing for many adults as part of the diagnostic workup for cardiovascular disease (3). Thus, preparticipation physical activity screening is about participating in a physical activity program not about exercise testing. We discuss all three components of the preparticipation physical activity screening process in the following section.

HEALTH HISTORY QUESTIONNAIRE

NAME_____AGE_____DATE_____DATE OF BIRTH_____
     First   M.I.   Last   day/month/yr   day/month/yr

ADDRESS_____
        Street   City/State/Zip

TELEPHONE (home)_____(business)_____(cell)_____

OCCUPATION_____PLACE OF EMPLOYMENT_____

MARITAL STATUS: (circle one)   SINGLE   MARRIED   DIVORCED   WIDOWED

SPOUSE:_____

EDUCATION: (check highest level)   ELEMENTARY_____   HIGH SCHOOL_____   COLLEGE_____

GRADUATE_____

ETHNICITY:_____ PERSONAL PHYSICIAN_____

LOCATION_____

Reason for last doctor visit?_____ Date of last physician exam_____

Have you previously been tested for an exercise Program?   YES _____   NO _____   YEAR(s) _____

LOCATION OF TEST_____

Person to contact in case of an emergency_____ Phone #_____

(relationship)_____

PLEASE CHECK YES or NO

PAST (Have you ever had?)	YES	NO
High blood pressure	☐	☐
Heart problems	☐	☐
Disease of the arteries	☐	☐
Varicose veins	☐	☐
Lung disease	☐	☐
Asthma	☐	☐
Kidney disease	☐	☐
Hepatitis	☐	☐
Diabetes	☐	☐
Orthopedic problems	☐	☐
Arthritis	☐	☐

FAMILY (Have any immediate family or grandparents had?)	YES	NO
Heart attacks	☐	☐
High blood pressure	☐	☐
High cholesterol	☐	☐
Stroke	☐	☐
Diabetes	☐	☐
Congenital heart defect	☐	☐
Heart operations	☐	☐
Early death	☐	☐
Other family illness _____		
_____		
_____		

PRESENT SYMPTOMS (Have you recently had?)	YES	NO
Chest pain/discomfort	☐	☐
Shortness of breath	☐	☐
Dizzy spells	☐	☐
Skipped heart beats	☐	☐
Trouble sleeping	☐	☐
Ankle swelling	☐	☐
Leg pain/cramping	☐	☐
Frequent headaches	☐	☐
Frequent colds	☐	☐
Back pain	☐	☐
Orthopedic problems	☐	☐

(FOR STAFF COMMENTS)

_____
_____
_____

FIGURE 2.4. HHQ used at East Stroudsburg University.

HEALTH HISTORY QUESTIONNAIRE

HOSPITALIZATIONS: Please list recent hospitalizations (Women: do not list normal pregnancies)

Year   Location   Reason

_____

_____

Any other medical problems/concerns not already identified? Yes_____ No_____ (Please list below)

_____

_____

Have you ever had your cholesterol measures? Yes_____ No_____; If yes, (value)_____ (Date)_____

Are you taking any Prescription or Non-Prescription medications? Yes_____ No_____ (include birth control pills)

Medication   Reason for Taking   For How Long?

_____

_____

Do you currently smoke? Yes_____ No_____ If so, what? Cigarettes_____ Cigars_____ Pipe_____

How much per day: < .5 pack_____   0.5 to 1pack_____   1.5 to 2 packs_____   > 2 packs_____

Have you ever quit smoking? Yes_____ No_____ When?_____ How many years and how

much did you smoke?_____

Do you drink any alcoholic beverages? Yes_____ No_____ If Yes, how much in 1 week?

Beer_____(cans)   Wine_____(glasses)   Hard liquor_____(drinks)

Do you drink any caffeinated beverages? Yes_____ No_____ If Yes, how much in 1 week?

Coffee_____(cups)   Tea_____(glasses)   Soft drinks_____(cans)

ACTIVITY LEVEL EVALUATION

What is your occupational activity level?   sedentary_____; light_____; moderate_____; heavy_____

Do you currently engage in vigorous physical activity on a regular basis? Yes_____ No_____

If so, what type?_____ How many days per week?_____

How much time per day? (check one)   < 15 min_____   15–30 min_____   30–45 min_____   > 60 min_____

Do you ever have an uncomfortable shortness of breath during exercise? Yes_____ No_____

Do you ever have chest discomfort during exercise? Yes_____ No_____ If so, does it go away with rest?_____

Do you engage in any recreational or leisure-time physical activities on a regular basis? Yes_____ No_____

If so, what activities?_____

On average: How often?_____times/week;   For how long?_____time/session

FIGURE 2.4. (*continued*)

HEALTH HISTORY QUESTIONNAIRE

Are you currently following a weight reduction diet plan? Yes_____ No_____ Name:_____

If so, how long have you been dieting? _____months   Is the plan prescribed by your doctor? Yes_____ No_____

Have you used weight reduction diets in the past? Yes_____ No_____;   If yes, how often and which type(s)?

_____

_____

Please indicate the reasons why you want to join the exercise program.

To lose weight _____ Doctor's recommendation_____ For good health _____ Enjoyment_____

Release of tension_____ Improve physical appearance _____ Other _____

FOR STAFF USE:

_____

_____

FIGURE 2.4. (*continued*)

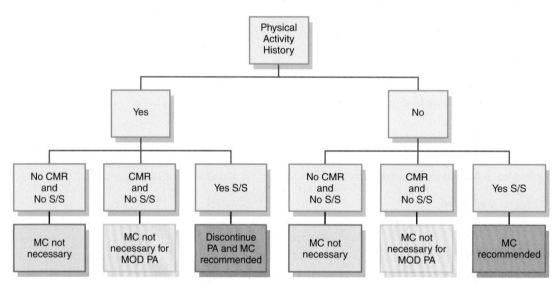

Physical Activity History: 30 min of MOD PA on 3 d · wk⁻¹ for at least last 3 mo
CMR: cardiovascular, metabolic, or renal disease
S/S: signs and symptoms suggestive of CMR
MC: medical clearance
MOD PA: moderate physical activity or exercise

FIGURE 2.5. Decision tree for preparticipation screening; simplified algorithm.

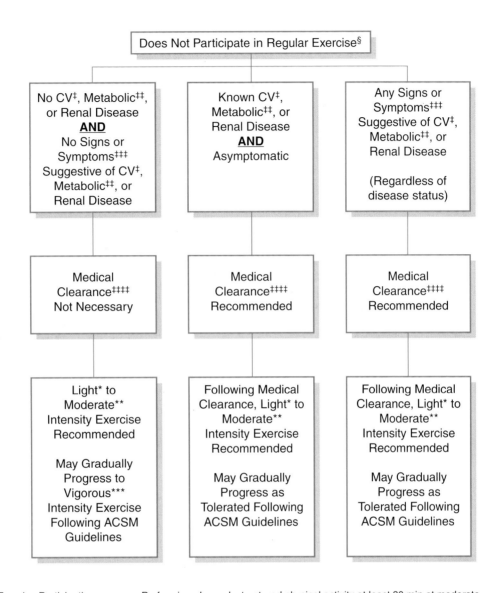

§Exercise Participation	Performing planned, structured physical activity at least 30 min at moderate intensity on at least 3 d · wk⁻¹ for at least the last 3 mo	
*Light Intensity Exercise	30%–39% HRR or V̇O₂R, 2–2.9 METs, RPE 9–11, an intensity that causes slight increases in HR and breathing	
**Moderate Intensity Exercise	40%–59% HRR or V̇O₂R, 3–5.9 METs, RPE 12–13, an intensity that causes noticeable increases in HR and breathing	
***Vigorous Intensity Exercise	60% HRR or V̇O₂R, 6 METs, RPE 14, an intensity that causes substantial increases in HR and breathing	
‡Cardiovascular (CV) Disease	Cardiac, peripheral vascular, or cerebrovascular disease	
‡‡Metabolic Disease	Type 1 and 2 diabetes mellitus	
‡‡‡Signs and Symptoms	At rest or during activity. Includes pain, discomfort in the chest, neck, jaw, arms, or other areas that may result from ischemia; shortness of breath at rest or with mild exertion; dizziness or syncope; orthopnea or paroxysmal nocturnal dyspnea; ankle edema; palpitations or tachycardia; intermittent claudication; known heart murmur; unusual fatigue or shortness of breath with usual activities.	
‡‡‡‡Medical Clearance	Approval from a health care professional to engage in exercise	
ACSM Guidelines	See the most current edition of *ACSM's Guidelines for Exercise Testing and Prescription*	

FIGURE 2.6. The ACSM preparticipation screening algorithm. HR, heart rate; HRR, heart rate reserve. (Reprinted from Riebe D, Franklin BA, Thompson PD, et al. Updating ACSM's recommendations for exercise preparticipation health screening. *Med Sci Sports Exerc.* 2015;47[11]:2473–9.) (*continued*)

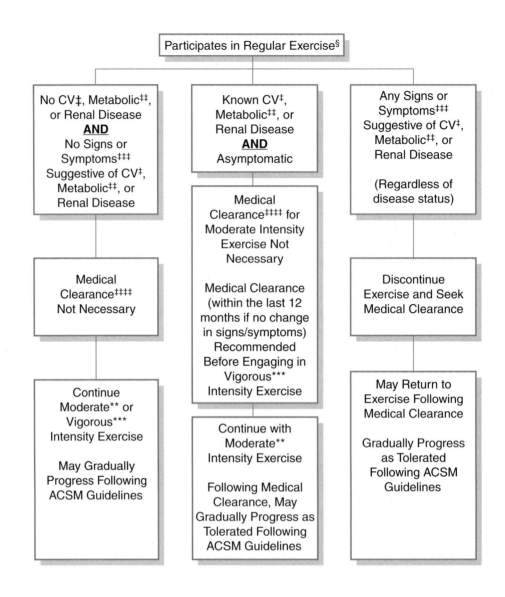

§Exercise Participation — Performing planned, structured physical activity at least 30 min at moderate intensity on at least 3 d · wk^{-1} for at least the last 3 mo

*Light Intensity Exercise — 30%–39% HRR or $\dot{V}O_2R$, 2–2.9 METs, RPE 9–11, an intensity that causes slight increases in HR and breathing

**Moderate Intensity Exercise — 40%–59% HRR or $\dot{V}O_2R$, 3–5.9 METs, RPE 12–13, an intensity that causes noticeable increases in HR and breathing

***Vigorous Intensity Exercise — 60% HRR or $\dot{V}O_2R$, 6 METs, RPE 14, an intensity that causes substantial increases in HR and breathing

‡Cardiovascular (CV) Disease — Cardiac, peripheral vascular, or cerebrovascular disease

‡‡Metabolic Disease — Type 1 and 2 diabetes mellitus

‡‡‡Signs and Symptoms — At rest or during activity. Includes pain, discomfort in the chest, neck, jaw, arms, or other areas that may result from ischemia; shortness of breath at rest or with mild exertion; dizziness or syncope; orthopnea or paroxysmal nocturnal dyspnea; ankle edema; palpitations or tachycardia; intermittent claudication; known heart murmur; unusual fatigue or shortness of breath with usual activities.

‡‡‡‡Medical Clearance — Approval from a health care professional to engage in exercise

ACSM Guidelines — See the most current edition of *ACSM's Guidelines for Exercise Testing and Prescription*

FIGURE 2.6. (*continued*)

Exercise Preparticipation Health Screening Questionnaire for Exercise Professionals

Assess your client's health needs by marking all *true* statements.

Step 1

SIGNS AND SYMPTOMS
Does your client experience:
____ chest discomfort with exertion
____ unreasonable breathlessness
____ dizziness, fainting, blackouts
____ ankle swelling
____ unpleasant awareness of a forceful, rapid or irregular heart rate
____ burning or cramping sensations in your lower legs when walking short distance
____ known heart murmur

If you **did** mark any of these statements under the symptoms, **STOP**, your client should seek medical clearance before engaging in or resuming exercise. Your client may need to use a facility with a **medically qualified staff**.

If you **did not** mark any symptoms, continue to steps 2 and 3.

Step 2

CURRENT ACTIVITY
Has your client performed planned, structured physical activity for at least 30 min at moderate intensity on at least 3 days per week for at least the last 3 months?

Yes ☐ No ☐

Continue to Step 3.

Step 3

MEDICAL CONDITIONS
Has your client had or do they currently have:
____ a heart attack
____ heart surgery, cardiac catheterization, or coronary angioplasty
____ pacemaker/implantable cardiac defibrillator/rhythm disturbance
____ heart valve disease
____ heart failure
____ heart transplantation
____ congenital heart disease
____ diabetes
____ renal disease

Evaluating Steps 2 and 3:

- If you **did not mark any of the statements in Step 3**, medical clearance is not necessary.
- If you marked Step 2 "**yes**" and **marked any of the statements in Step 3**, your client may continue to exercise at light to moderate intensity without medical clearance. However, medical clearance is recommended before engaging in vigorous exercise.
- If you marked Step 2 "**no**" and **marked any of the statements in Step 3**, medical clearance is recommended. Your client may need to use a facility with a **medically qualified staff**.

FIGURE 2.7. Preparticipation physical activity screening questionnaire for exercise professionals. (Reprinted from Magal M, Riebe D. New preparticipation health screening recommendations: what exercise professionals need to know. *ACSMs Health Fit J*. 2016;20[3]:22–7.)

Physical Activity (or Exercise) History

An individual who currently engages in physical activity is considered to be at lower risk for a cardio-vascular event during exercise than one who is sedentary. An individual is considered to be currently engaged in physical activity if he or she has been performing planned, structured physical activity of at least 30 minutes at a moderate intensity, at least 3 d · wk^{-1}, for the last 3 months. These criteria are based on the dose of physical activity that is necessary to lower one's risk, according to the ACSM. Moderate-intensity physical activity has several descriptors associated with it including exercise at a level that is between 40% and 59% of the individual's heart rate reserve or maximal oxygen uptake reserve. Moderate-intensity physical activity or exercise is further described as between 3 and 5.9 metabolic equivalents (METs) and at a rating of perceived exertion (RPE) of around 12–13 on the traditional 6–20 scale. Also, moderate intensity causes noticeable increases in heart rate and breathing (3).

Known Cardiovascular, Metabolic, and/or Renal Disease

Clients with any of the CMR diseases are at a higher risk for an untoward event during exercise. Thus, the presence of a CMR disease will influence the level of preparticipation physical activity screening. The specific diseases and/or conditions covered are as follows:

- Heart attack
- Heart surgery, cardiac catheterization, or coronary angioplasty
- Pacemaker/implantable cardiac defibrillator/rhythm disturbance
- Heart valve disease
- Heart failure
- Heart transplantation
- Congenital heart disease (Congenital refers to birth.)
- Diabetes, Types 1 and 2
- Renal disease such as renal failure

Note the absence of pulmonary diseases from this list of diseases and/or conditions. Pulmonary disease has been shown to be less likely to cause untoward events during exercise than CMR disease and thus has been removed from the list (3).

ACSM Major Signs or Symptoms Suggestive of Cardiovascular Disease

There are several outward signs or symptoms that may indicate a client has current CMR disease. These signs and symptoms can be found in the following sections along with further discussion of these signs or symptoms. If a client has any of these signs or symptoms, then he or she is considered at a higher risk, and it is recommended that the individual seek medical clearance before participation in a physical activity program. It is important to remember that these signs or symptoms must be interpreted within the clinical context in which they appear because they are not all specific for CMR disease (3).

Discussion of ACSM signs or symptoms

There are nine signs and symptoms suggestive of CMR disease, which include the following:

- Pain or discomfort in the chest, neck, jaw, arms, or other areas that may be due to ischemia or lack of oxygenated blood flow to the tissue, such as the heart (13). Remember that chest pain or angina is not always located in the chest area of a client. Women in particular may experience low back pain or feelings of indigestion as opposed to chest pain. Some key features of this pain that favors an ischemic origin include the following:
  - Character: The pain is felt as constricting, squeezing, burning, "heaviness," or "heavy feeling."
  - Location: The pain is substernal, across the midthorax, anteriorly; in one or both arms or shoulders; in neck, cheeks, or teeth; or in forearms, fingers, and/or in the interscapular region.
  - Provoking factors: The pain comes on with exercise or exertion, excitement, other forms of stress, cold weather, or after meals (3).

- *Dyspnea* is the medical term for shortness of breath (13). Dyspnea is expected in most individuals during moderate to severe exertion such as stair climbing. However, shortness of breath at rest or with mild exertion may indicate cardiac and/or pulmonary disease and should be examined by a physician. Dyspnea (defined as an abnormally uncomfortable awareness of breathing) is one of the principal symptoms of cardiac and pulmonary disease. It commonly occurs during strenuous exertion in healthy, well-trained individuals and during moderate exertion in healthy, untrained individuals. However, it should be regarded as abnormal when it occurs at a level of exertion that is not expected to evoke this symptom in a given individual. Abnormal exertional dyspnea suggests the presence of cardiopulmonary disorders, in particular, left ventricular dysfunction or chronic obstructive pulmonary disease (3).

- Syncope, or fainting, and dizziness during exercise may indicate poor blood flow to the brain due to inadequate cardiac output from a number of cardiac disorders (13). However, syncope and dizziness upon sudden cessation of exercise is relatively common even among healthy individuals due to a sudden decrease in venous return and consequent reduction in blood flow to the brain. Cardiac disorders that are associated with syncope and dizziness are potentially life-threatening and include severe coronary artery disease, hypertrophic cardiomyopathy, aortic stenosis, and malignant ventricular dysrhythmias. Although dizziness or syncope shortly after cessation of exercise should not be ignored, these symptoms may occur even in healthy individuals as a result of a reduction in venous return to the heart (3).

- Orthopnea refers to trouble breathing while lying down. Paroxysmal nocturnal dyspnea refers to difficulty breathing while asleep, beginning usually 2–5 hours after the onset of sleep, which may be relieved by sitting on the side of the bed or getting out of bed (13). Both are indicative of poor left ventricular function. Patients with these conditions often report sleeping in recliners to lessen the symptoms of this disorder. Orthopnea is relieved promptly by sitting upright or standing. Although nocturnal dyspnea may occur in individuals with chronic obstructive pulmonary disease, it differs in that it is usually relieved following a bowel movement rather than specifically by sitting up (3).

- Ankle edema, or swelling, that is not due to injury is suggestive of heart failure, a blood clot, insufficiency of the veins, or a lymph system blockage (13). Generalized edema (known as anasarca) occurs in individuals with the nephrotic (from the kidneys) syndrome, severe heart failure, or hepatic (from the liver) cirrhosis. Bilateral ankle edema that is most evident at night is a characteristic sign of heart failure or bilateral chronic venous insufficiency. Unilateral edema of a limb often results from venous thrombosis or lymphatic blockage in the limb (3).

- Palpitations and tachycardia both refer to rapid beating or fluttering of the heart (13). The client may report a feeling of unpleasantness associated with the unusual heart rhythm. Palpitations (defined as an unpleasant awareness of the forceful or rapid beating of the heart) may be induced by various disorders of cardiac rhythm. These include tachycardia, bradycardia of sudden onset, ectopic beats, compensatory pauses, and accentuated stroke volume resulting from valvular regurgitation. Palpitations also often result from anxiety states and high cardiac output (or hyperkinetic) states, such as anemia, fever, thyrotoxicosis, arteriovenous fistula, and the so-called idiopathic hyperkinetic heart syndrome (3).

- Intermittent claudication refers to severe calf pain when walking (13). This pain indicates a lack of oxygenated blood flow to the working muscles similar in origin to chest pain. The pain does not occur with standing or sitting, is reproducible from day to day, is more severe when walking upstairs or up a hill, and is often described as a cramp, which disappears within 1–2 minutes after stopping exercise. Coronary artery disease is more prevalent in individuals with intermittent claudication. Patients with diabetes are at increased risk for this condition (3).

- Heart murmurs are unusual sounds caused by blood flowing through the heart (13). Although some murmurs may be innocent, heart murmurs may indicate valvular or other cardiovascular disease. From an exercise safety standpoint, it is especially important to exclude hypertrophic cardiomyopathy and aortic stenosis as underlying causes because these are among the more common causes of exertion-related sudden cardiac death. Unless previously diagnosed and determined to be safe, all murmurs should be evaluated by a physician (3).

■ Unusual fatigue or shortness of breath that occurs during light exertion or normal activity and not during strenuous activity (13). Although there may be benign origins for these symptoms, they also may signal the onset of or change in the status of cardiovascular and/or metabolic disease (3).

When Should You Seek Medical Clearance?

Figure 2.5 illustrates an attempt to simplify and clarify some of the decisions aided by the ACSM preparticipation physical activity screening process. The ACSM-EP should always keep in mind that the ACSM preparticipation physical activity screening process is a guideline and may need to be modified based on several issues such as local medical practice or custom.

Essentially, Figure 2.5 represents a paradigm shift in preparticipation screening from previous ACSM screening paradigms, and we have chosen to simplify and colorize the figure to aid the ACSM-EP with this decision tree. Medical clearance, which may include a medical examination by a health care professional including a physician, is suggested and recommended to be a part of the preparticipation physical activity screening workup if your client has signs and symptoms suggestive of CMR disease. We have denoted this outcome using the color red in Figure 2.5. In fact, individuals who meet these criteria (signs and symptoms suggestive of CMR disease) should only participate after getting medical clearance to do so. Individuals who may be free of signs and symptoms but have the presence of CMR disease may benefit from medical clearance, and thus, we have used the color yellow for caution in Figure 2.5. This is appropriate for clients who currently do not participate in a physical activity program. However, in most "apparently healthy" clients (free of CMR disease and signs and symptoms suggestive of CMR disease), it is acceptable to get them started in a moderate-intensity physical activity program without the need for previous medical clearance. We have used the color green for this outcome in Figure 2.5.

As you can see in Figure 2.5, the current physical activity history of a client does influence these decisions. For instance, if your client has not been physically active in the recent past (last 3 mo), then you are more likely to recommend medical clearance to start a low to moderate physical activity program, whereas the previously physically active client may be able to proceed to a more moderate to vigorous physical activity program.

The prudent ACSM-EP would always err on the side of caution when there are uncertainties and request full medical clearance. The ePARmed-X+Physician Clearance Follow-Up Questionnaire may be used for medical clearance.

Vigorous exercise is often defined as greater than or equal to 60% of your client's functional capacity (≥ 6 METs, ≥ 14 on a 6–20 RPE scale, and cause substantial increases in heart rate and breathing), whereas low to moderate exercise programs would be less than 60% of functional capacity (14–17).

Two previous features of the ACSM risk stratification/classification process were the use and supervision of graded exercise testing. Nondiagnostic exercise testing is generally performed for exercise prescriptive and/or functional capacity purposes, whereas diagnostic exercise testing may be performed to assess the presence or impact of cardiovascular disease (18). Submaximal exercise testing may also be useful in individualizing your client's exercise prescription as well as gaining functional capacity information as is discussed in other chapters of this textbook. Research and expert opinion has recently questioned the value of the diagnostic exercise test (15,19).

The supervision criterion of exercise testing has also undergone much revision in recent years. Training in exercise testing administration is required and includes certification in emergency care (*i.e.*, AHA Advanced Cardiac Life Support Certification) as well as experience in exercise testing interpretation and emergency plan practice (15,19,20).

Thus, a competent ACSM-EP may oversee the judicious use of the preparticipation physical activity screening and graded exercise test for exercise prescription purposes in his or her lower risk clients. However, other personnel may need to become involved if the preparticipation physical activity screening suggests the need for medical clearance (3,20).

American Association of Cardiovascular and Pulmonary Rehabilitation Risk Stratification

Other professional organizations have also published guidelines that address risk stratification and preparticipation physical activity screening (3,11,16,21–23). Most prominently among these are AHA and American Association of Cardiovascular and Pulmonary Rehabilitation (AACVPR). Similar to the recent changes in ACSM preparticipation exercise screening, other guidelines have been modified to reduce impediments to begin or continue safe and effective exercise programming.

The AACVPR has contributed to the field of preparticipation physical activity screening and risk stratification with guidelines revised most recently in 2012 (3,4,11,18). The AACVPR risk stratification scheme continues to use Low, Moderate, and High risk categories to identify level of risk of physical activity triggering an untoward event.

Overall health risk exists as a continuum from apparently healthy to known disease. The AACVPR risk stratification scheme thus may serve as a nice bridge to ACSM preparticipation by offering services and programming to more "risky" or diseased clients as might be found in clinical exercise programs such as cardiac rehabilitation or medical fitness facilities, perhaps supervised by an ACSM Certified Clinical Exercise Physiologist®. The AACVPR risk stratification guidelines are listed in Box 2.1 (3,23).

Challenges of ACSM Preparticipation Physical Activity Screening

Perhaps the greatest challenge of ACSM preparticipation physical activity screening is overlooking a sign or symptom of ongoing cardiovascular disease, potentially leading to the client experiencing a cardiac event during a supervised exercise session. Although the incidence of such events is rare (see "Exercise is Medicine" box), the prudent ACSM-EP should exercise caution in minimizing such risk (24–27). To reduce the risk of such an event, the ACSM-EP should obtain as much medical history information as possible through the HHQ and client interviews. When in doubt, particularly in a general, nonclinical client who may be a higher risk client, the ACSM recommends consulting with a health care professional for advice on how to proceed. Remember, it is better to be conservative and prudent than to endanger the client's health (15).

Of course, the conservative approach to preparticipation physical activity screening must be balanced by the public health argument of putting up too many obstacles or barriers to participation in front of the client, potentially resulting in driving the client away from adopting a physically active and healthy lifestyle. Thus, the client might be encouraged to begin a low- to moderate-intensity program, where the overall risks of untoward events are minimal, before he or she undergoes further medical evaluation and clearance (3). It is perhaps important for all individuals beginning a physical activity program that the initial intensity be low to moderate and increase gradually in a progressive overload fashion as discussed in other chapters in this text and the *GETP* (2,3,28).

Box 2.1	**American Association of Cardiovascular and Pulmonary Rehabilitation Risk Stratification Algorithm for Risk of Event**

Patient is at **HIGH RISK** if ANY ONE OR MORE of the following factors are present:

- Left ventricular ejection fraction <40%
- Survivor of cardiac arrest or sudden death
- Complex ventricular dysrhythmias (ventricular tachycardia, frequent [>6 beats $\cdot$ min^{-1}] multiform PVCs) at rest or with exercise
- MI or cardiac surgery complicated by cardiogenic shock, CHF, and/or signs/symptoms of postprocedure ischemia
- Abnormal hemodynamics with exercise, especially flat or decreasing systolic blood pressure or chronotropic incompetence with increasing workload
- Significant silent ischemia (ST depression 2 mm or greater without symptoms) with exercise or in recovery
- Signs/symptoms including angina pectoris, dizziness, light-headedness or dyspnea at low levels of exercise (<5.0 METs) or in recovery
- Maximal functional capacity of less than 5.0 METs
  - If measured functional capacity is not available, this factor can be excluded.
- Clinically significant depression or depressive symptoms

Patient is at **MODERATE RISK** if they meet neither high-risk nor low-risk standards:

- Left ventricular ejection fraction = 40%–50%
- Signs/symptoms including angina at "moderate" levels of exercise (60%–75% of maximal functional capacity) or in recovery
- Mild to moderate silent ischemia (ST depression less than 2 mm) with exercise or in recovery

Patient is at **LOW RISK** if ALL of the following factors are present:

- Left ventricular ejection fraction >50%
- No resting or exercise-induced complex dysrhythmias
- Uncomplicated MI, CABG, angioplasty, atherectomy, or stent:
  - Absence of CHF or signs/symptoms indicating postevent ischemia
- Normal hemodynamic and ECG responses with exercise and in recovery
- Asymptomatic with exercise or in recovery, including absence of angina
- Maximal functional capacity at least 7.0 METs
  - If measured functional capacity is not available, this factor can be excluded.
- Absence of clinical depression or depressive symptoms

CABG, coronary artery bypass graft; CHF, congestive heart failure; ECG, electrocardiogram; METs, metabolic equivalents; MI, myocardial infarction; PVCs, premature ventricular contractions.

Reprinted with permission from American Association of Cardiovascular and Pulmonary Rehabilitation. *AACVPR Stratification Algorithm for Risk of Event* [Internet]. Chicago (IL): American Association of Cardiovascular and Pulmonary Rehabilitation; 2012 [cited 2018 Aug 24]. Available from: https://www.aacvpr.org/Portals/0/Registry/Cardiac%20Registry/Cardiac%20Registry%20User%20Resources/AACVPR%20Risk%20Stratification%20Algorithm.pdf.

Recommendations versus Requirements

It is important to remember that the goal of *GETP* is to provide direction on how to screen participants and proceed with physical activity programming. In all cases, the ACSM-EP should exercise caution and use his or her best judgment when handling an individual client. When in doubt, referring a client for a medical evaluation and clearance is always in good judgment.

The ACSM prepaticipation health screening protocol was assessed in a recent article by Price and colleagues (29) and demonstrated a reduction in medical clearances versus the previously used system presented in the ninth edition of *GETP* in a younger population. To date, there are no published reports on the effectiveness of the AACVPR risk classification scheme. Thus, although it is prudent to recommend that the ACSM-EP follow the prepaticipation screening scheme, it may be difficult to suggest this as a requirement to follow for a quality exercise program because it is lacking an evidence base (5).

Contraindications to Exercise Testing

The process of evaluating risk (through a medical exam/health history and the ACSM prepatici-pation physical activity screening) may identify clinical characteristics of an individual that make physical activity risky and, thus, contraindicated. There are a host of clinical characteristics that have been identified and published by ACSM (as well as other organizations, such as the AHA) that are termed *contraindications*. These contraindications generally refer to exercise testing. This list can be found in Box 2.2 (3). As you can see, many of these contraindications are cardiovascular disease–related and only revealed by consultation with a physician and likely sophisticated medical testing. However, the resting blood pressure relative contraindication criterion (>200 mm Hg systolic blood pressure or 110 mm Hg diastolic blood pressure) is likely to be known by the ACSM-EP during basic health-related physical fitness testing.

Box 2.2	Contraindications to Symptom-Limited Maximal Exercise Testing

Absolute Contraindications
- Acute myocardial infarction within 2 d
- Ongoing unstable angina
- Uncontrolled cardiac arrhythmia with hemodynamic compromise
- Active endocarditis
- Symptomatic severe aortic stenosis
- Decompensated heart failure
- Acute pulmonary embolism, pulmonary infarction, or deep venous thrombosis
- Acute myocarditis or pericarditis
- Acute aortic dissection
- Physical disability that precludes safe and adequate testing

Relative Contraindications
- Known obstructive left main coronary artery stenosis
- Moderate to severe aortic stenosis with uncertain relationship to symptoms
- Tachyarrhythmias with uncontrolled ventricular rates
- Acquired advanced or complete heart block
- Recent stroke or transient ischemia attack
- Mental impairment with limited ability to cooperate
- Resting hypertension with systolic >200 mm Hg or diastolic >110 mm Hg
- Uncorrected medical conditions, such as significant anemia, important electrolyte imbalance, and hyperthyroidism

Reprinted with permission from (3).

What Does Contraindication Really Mean?

A contraindication is a clinical characteristic that may increase the risk associated with the participation in physical activity and/or exercise testing. For example, if an individual has unstable angina, or chest pain (unstable angina refers to chest pain that is not well controlled or predictable), then he or she may experience ischemia during exercise that could lead to a myocardial infarction, or heart attack. Although it is important to note that the incidence of cardiovascular complications is rare during exercise, a prudent ACSM-EP would be advised to follow the contraindications listed to minimize this incidence (3,4,28). As previously discussed, many of the contraindications listed are uncommon, but the ACSM-EP should protect the individual from all known and likely risks.

Absolute versus Relative

The list of contraindications is often divided between those that are as either absolute or relative. Absolute refers to those criteria that are absolute contraindications; individuals with these biomarkers should not be allowed to participate in any form of physical activity program and/or exercise test. However, those individuals with clinical contraindications that are listed as relative may be accepted or allowed into a physical activity assessment and/or program if it is deemed that the benefits for the individual outweigh the risks to the individual (4,28). For instance, if a client has a resting blood pressure of 210/105 mm Hg, it may be decided by a medical director and/or physician to allow the client to enter into the physical activity program because the benefits to the individual may outweigh the risks of exercising with this particular relative contraindication.

Repurposing Risk Factor Assessment and Management

As mentioned previously, the ACSM CVD risk assessment is no longer a mandatory component for determining if medical clearance is warranted before individuals begin an exercise program. However, identifying and controlling CVD risk factors remains an important objective of disease prevention and management. Therefore, under the current recommendations, the ACSM-EP is encouraged to complete a CVD risk factor analysis with his or her patients and clients. The goal has simply shifted from using the ACSM CVD risk factor assessment as a tool for preparticipation health screening and risk stratification to identifying and managing CVD risk in patients and clients. As addressed later in this textbook, CVD risk factors may significantly impact exercise prescription.

Another important reason to provide CVD risk assessment is to help educate and inform the client about his or her need to make lifestyle modifications such as increasing physical activity and incorporating more healthful food choices in his or her diets.

ACSM Atherosclerotic Cardiovascular Disease Risk Factor Assessment and Defining Criteria

Using the client's health history (and basic health evaluation data such as resting blood pressure), simply compare your client's information to the list of the ACSM CVD risk factor criteria to determine which ones the client meets. Meeting one or none of these indicates a low risk of future cardiovascular disease, whereas the presence of two or more risk factors indicates an increased risk of disease. Note that only one positive factor is assigned per ACSM CVD risk factor criteria. For example, in obesity, a body mass index (BMI) greater than $30\,\mathrm{kg} \cdot \mathrm{m}^{-2}$ and a waist circumference of 105 cm (for men) would count as only one positive risk factor. Likewise, having both high systolic and high diastolic resting blood pressure readings would result in only one positive factor. If a client is taking a medication for hypertension or high cholesterol, he or she is considered positive for the associated risk factor regardless of his or her actual resting blood pressure or blood cholesterol measurements. There is also one negative factor (having a high high-density lipoprotein cholesterol [HDL-C]) that would offset one positive risk factor. The following is a detailed list of the ACSM atherosclerotic CVD risk factors and defining criteria (3):

- Client's age of 45 years or older for males and 55 years or older for females (4)
- Family history of specific cardiovascular events including myocardial infarction (heart attack), coronary revascularization (bypass surgery or angioplasty), or sudden cardiac death. This applies to first-degree relatives only. First-degree relatives are biological parents, siblings, and children. The risk factor criteria are met when at least one male relative has had one of the three specific events prior to age 55 years or before age 65 years in a female relative (30).
- If the client currently smokes cigarettes, quit smoking within the last 6 months, or if he or she is exposed to environmental tobacco smoke; secondhand smoke exposure can be assessed by the presence of cotinine in your client's urine (8,31).
- A sedentary lifestyle is defined as not participating in a regular exercise program or not meeting the minimal recommendations of 30 minutes or more of moderate-intensity physical activity (40%–59% oxygen uptake reserve [$\dot{V}O_2R$]) on at least 3 d $\cdot$ wk^{-1} for at least 3 months (32).
- Obesity is defined as a BMI $\geq$30 kg $\cdot$ m^{-2} or a waist circumference of greater than 102 cm (~40 in) for men and greater than 88 cm (~35 in) for women. If available, body fat percentage values could also be used with appropriate judgment of the ACSM-EP (8).
- Hypertension refers to having a resting blood pressure $\geq$130 mm Hg systolic or $\geq$80 mm Hg diastolic, or if the client is currently taking any antihypertensive medication. Importantly, these resting blood pressures must have been assessed on at least two separate occasions (18,33,34).
- Dyslipidemia refers to having a low-density lipoprotein cholesterol (LDL-C) $\geq$130 mg $\cdot$ dL^{-1} (3.37 mmol $\cdot$ L^{-1}), an HDL-C of <40 mg $\cdot$ dL^{-1} (1.04 mmol $\cdot$ L^{-1}), or if the client is taking a lipid-lowering medication. Use $\geq$200 mg $\cdot$ dL^{-1} (5.18 mmol $\cdot$ L^{-1}) only if the total serum cholesterol measurement is available (35). Also, LDL-C is typically not measured but rather estimated from HDL-C, total cholesterol (TC), and triglycerides (35).
- Diabetes is defined as having a fasting blood glucose $\geq$126 mg $\cdot$ dL^{-1} (7.0 mmol $\cdot$ L^{-1}) or 2-hour plasma glucose values in oral glucose tolerance test (OGTT) $\geq$200 mg $\cdot$ dL^{-1} (11.1 mmol $\cdot$ L^{-1}) or glycolated hemoglobin (HbA1C) $\geq$6.5% (21).
- HDL-C has a cardioprotective effect so is considered a negative risk factor if $\geq$60 mg $\cdot$ dL^{-1} (1.55 mmol $\cdot$ L^{-1}). HDL-C participates in reverse cholesterol transport and thus may lower the risk of cardiovascular disease.

Comparing the client's personal data to the ACSM atherosclerotic CVD risk factor criteria outlined previously will help the ACSM-EP to educate the client about his or her current health risk and evaluate the effectiveness of the exercise protocol at managing and/or attenuating this risk.

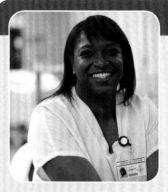

The Case of Hollie

In the following text is a case study using one individual (Hollie Lankford) for the purpose of exploring further the processes of ACSM preparticipation physical activity screening and ACSM atherosclerotic CVD risk factor assessment. Refer to the preparticipation screening simplified algorithm (see Fig. 2.5) for guidance while reviewing this case study.

ACSM Preparticipation Physical Activity Screening Case Study

Hollie Lankford, a 42-year-old female, decides she wants to begin exercising in your program. As the ACSM-EP, you administer your ACSM preparticipation physical activity screening protocol. She is 5 ft 6 in tall and weighs 188 lb. Ms. Lankford provides you with the following information: Her father died of a heart attack at the age of 56 years. Her mother was put on medication for hypertension 10 years ago at the age of 62 years. She presents with no signs or symptoms of CMR disease. After 24 years of smoking one pack of cigarettes per day, she quit smoking 3 years ago. Her percentage body fat was measured at 34% via skinfolds. Fasting blood chemistries revealed a TC of 190 mg · dL^{-1}, an HDL-C of 72 mg · dL^{-1}, and a resting blood glucose of 84 mg · dL^{-1}. Her resting heart rate was measured at 70 bpm, and resting blood pressure was measured at 142/82 mm Hg and 144/84 mm Hg on two separate occasions. She reports that she works in a sedentary office job and sits at her desk all day. She complains that being in a high management position is stressful and doesn't have time to exercise during her workday. She reports routinely walking her dogs approximately 0.5 mi each morning and 0.25 mi each evening. Hollie states that she drinks one glass of wine most evenings before bed. Ms. Lankford has been diagnosed with rheumatoid arthritis, which she reports is not made worse by exercise. In addition, Hollie sustained a musculoskeletal injury to her low back last year that forced her to miss 1 week of work; however, she reports that her low back area has been problem free for the last 7 months.

Follow the ACSM preparticipation physical activity screening algorithm (see Fig. 2.6) for the individual in this case study to determine the need for a medical evaluation and for prescribed exercise intensity before beginning an exercise program.

Physical Activity History

She walks her dogs daily for a total of approximately 0.75 mi and thus is not considered physically active as defined by the ACSM.

Presence of Cardiovascular, Metabolic, and/or Renal Disease

None noted.

Major Symptoms or Signs Suggestive of Cardiovascular, Metabolic, and/or Renal Disease

None noted.

ACSM Preparticipation Physical Activity Screening Status

Medical clearance is not necessary prior to starting a physical activity program of light to moderate intensity. She may progress to more vigorous intensity exercise following *GETP* (3,28). As an ACSM-EP, you may want to conduct exercise tests for prescriptive purposes while being careful not to exacerbate Hollie's previous back injury. A physical activity program should be recommended that incorporates strengthening her core and lower back muscles.

ACSM CVD Risk Factors and Defining Criteria

	ACSM Risk Factors	Comment
	Age	42 yr old (below criteria of 55 yr old)
	Family history	Father had heart attack (myocardial infarction) at 56 yr old (was not before 55 yr old); mother with hypertension doesn't count.
	Cigarette smoking	Quit smoking more than 6 mo ago so not a risk factor.
+	Sedentary lifestyle	Walking dogs 0.75 mi each day is not considered physically active.
+	Obesity	BMI = 30.34 kg $\cdot$ m^{-2} (above 30 kg $\cdot$ m^{-2} is obese)
+	Hypertension	Systolic blood pressure = 142/82 mm Hg and 144/84 mm Hg (considered hypertensive)
	Dyslipidemia	TC = 190 mg $\cdot$ dL^{-1} (below criteria level of 200 mg $\cdot$ dL^{-1})
	Diabetes	Fasting blood glucose = 82 mg $\cdot$ dL^{-1} (below criteria level of 126 mg $\cdot$ dL^{-1})
−	High HDL-C	HDL-C = 72 mg $\cdot$ dL^{-1} (60 mg $\cdot$ dL^{-1} and above is considered a negative risk factor)
2	(+) Risk factors	3 positive risk factors − 1 negative risk factor = 2

ACSM Risk Factor Analysis

Hollie has a risk factor profile that includes hypertension, obesity, and a sedentary lifestyle. Her high HDL-C decreases her overall risk for CVD. Thus, a prudent ACSM-EP should stress to this client the importance of adopting a physically active lifestyle with an initial moderate-intensity exercise program. In addition, Ms. Lankford should consult with appropriate health care professionals regarding her diet and possible medical intervention for hypertension.

EXERCISE IS MEDICINE

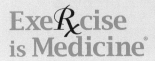

"Don't exercise too much, you may have a heart attack." How often have you heard that before? Dr. Paul Thompson and his colleagues from around the world have conducted many studies over the years to help refute that claim. In one particular study published back in 1996 in the *Archives of Internal Medicine*, Dr. Thompson studied the complications that may occur from participation in exercise (29). That study found that only 6 per 100,000 men die of exertion each year. In this article, Dr. Thompson suggested that the routine use of cardiovascular exercise tests has little diagnostic value for cardiovascular disease because of the rarity of sudden cardiac death in the population. In a scientific statement from the AHA published in *Circulation* in 2007, the writing team (Dr. Thompson and his colleagues) further suggested that the risk of sudden death from exercise is greatest in those least accustomed to physical activity (27). This lends further support to the concepts of performing diagnostic exercise tests only on those at high risk for cardiovascular disease as well as using the principle of progressive overload in exercise training by starting those who are unaccustomed to exercise at a lower exercise load (intensity and duration) and gradually increasing the exercise load as they become more accustomed to exercise. Thus, the incidence of sudden cardiac death is lessened in the client. From this study and others, you can see the influence on the current ACSM preparticipation physical activity screening guidelines (3,28).

SUMMARY

Preparticipation physical activity screening is a process that may include health/medical history and informed consent of an individual client. The process is one where the client is prepared for the upcoming physical activity program. Although there are several examples or models that can be followed for the preparticipation physical activity screening process, the bottom line is the need to evaluate a client's medical readiness to undertake the physical activity program planned for his or her. Thus, the preparticipation physical activity screening gives the relative assurance that the client is ready and able (based on national guidelines, such as from ACSM) to participate in the rigors of the physical activity training process. It is thus important that the ACSM-EP perform the preparticipation physical activity screening on his or her client.

STUDY QUESTIONS

1. Discuss each individual ACSM risk factor threshold. Specifically, how do the individual ACSM risk factor thresholds match up with the modifiable and nonmodifiable risk factors for coronary heart disease listed by the AHA?
2. Given the 2013 scientific statement from the AHA as well as the *2018 Physical Activity Guidelines for Americans*, does the ACSM preparticipation physical activity screening guidelines aid or hinder the concept of increasing physical activity behavior of all Americans?
3. Diabetes is relatively stressed in the ACSM preparticipation physical activity screening guidelines. (Diabetes is a CMR disease.) What are some of the complications of diabetes that justifies its inclusion in the preparticipation guidelines?

REFERENCES

1. Buchner DM. Physical activity to prevent or reverse disability in sedentary older adults. *Am J Prev Med*. 2003; 25(3 Suppl 2):214–5.
2. American College of Sports Medicine. *ACSM's Guidelines for Exercise Testing and Prescription*. 10th ed. Philadelphia (PA): Wolters Kluwer; 2018. 480 p.
3. American College of Sports Medicine. *ACSM's Guidelines for Exercise Testing and Prescription*. 11th ed. Philadelphia (PA): Wolters Kluwer; 2022. 548 p.
4. *Physical Activity and Health: A Report of the Surgeon General*. Atlanta (GA): U.S. Department of Health and Human Services, Centers for Disease Control and Prevention, National Center for Chronic Disease Prevention and Health Promotion; 1996. 278 p.
5. Jamnik VK, Gledhill N, Shephard RJ. Revised clearance for participation in physical activity: greater screening responsibility for qualified university-educated fitness professionals. *Appl Physiol Nutr Metab*. 2007;32(6):1191–7.
6. de Oliveira Luz LG, de Albuquerque Maranhao Neto G, de Tarso Veras Farinatti P. Validity of the Physical Activity Readiness Questionnaire (PAR-Q) in elder subjects. *Rer Brasileira de Cine Desempenho Hun*. 2007; 9(4):366–71.
7. Swain DP. *ACSM's Resource Manual for Guidelines for Exercise Testing and Prescription*. 7th ed. Philadelphia (PA): Lippincott Williams & Wilkins; 2013. 896 p.
8. Fletcher GF, Ades PA, Kligfield P, et al. Exercise standards for testing and training: a scientific statement from the American Heart Association. *Circulation*. 2013;128(8):873–934.
9. Shephard RJ, Thomas S, Weller I. The Canadian Home Fitness Test. 1991 update. *Sports Med*. 1991;11(6):358–66.
10. 2018 Physical Activity Guidelines Advisory Committee. *2018 Physical Activity Guidelines Advisory Committee Scientific Report*. Washington (DC): U.S. Department of Health and Human Services; 2018. 779 p.
11. American Association of Cardiovascular and Pulmonary Rehabilitation. *Guidelines for Cardiac Rehabilitation and Secondary Prevention Programs*. 4th ed. Champaign (IL): Human Kinetics; 2004. 288 p.
12. Gibbons RJ, Balady GJ, Bricker JT, et al. ACC/AHA 2002 guideline update for exercise testing: summary article. A report of the American College of Cardiology/American Heart Association Task Force on Practice Guidelines (committee to update the 1997 exercise testing guidelines). *J Am Coll Cardiol*. 2002;40(8):1531–40.

13. Stedman, editor. *Stedman's Medical Dictionary for the Health Professions and Nursing.* 5th ed. Baltimore (MD): Lippincott Williams & Wilkins; 2005. 2154 p.

14. Brawner CA, Vanzant MA, Ehrman JK, et al. Guiding exercise using the talk test among patients with coronary artery disease. *J Cardiopulm Rehabil.* 2006;26(2):72–7.

15. Garber CE, Blissmer B, Deschenes MR, et al. American College of Sports Medicine position stand. Quantity and quality of exercise for developing and maintaining cardio-respiratory, musculoskeletal, and neuromotor fitness in apparently healthy adults: guidance for prescribing exercise. *Med Sci Sports Exer.* 2011;43(7):1334–59.

16. Haskell WL, Lee IM, Pate RR, et al. Physical activity and public health: updated recommendation for adults from the American College of Sports Medicine and the American Heart Association. *Circulation.* 2007;116(9):1081–93.

17. Persinger R, Foster C, Gibson M, Fater DC, Porcari JP. Consistency of the talk test for exercise prescription. *Med Sci Sports Exerc.* 2004;36(9):1632–6.

18. James PA, Oparil S, Carter BL, et al. 2014 Evidence-based guideline for the management of high blood pressure in adults: report from the panel members appointed to the Eighth Joint National Committee (JNC 8). *JAMA.* 2014;311(5):507–20.

19. Lahav D, Leshno M, Brezis M. Is an exercise tolerance test indicated before beginning regular exercise? A decision analysis. *J Gen Intern Med.* 2009;24(8):934–8.

20. American College of Sports Medicine. *ACSM's Health-Related Physical Fitness Assessment Manual.* 5th ed. Philadelphia (PA): Wolters Kluwer; 2017. 192 p.

21. American Diabetes Association. Diagnosis and classification of diabetes mellitus. *Diabetes Care.* 2007;30(Suppl 1):S42–7.

22. Executive summary of the clinical guidelines on the identification, evaluation, and treatment of overweight and obesity in adults. *Arch Intern Med.* 1998;158(17):1855–67.

23. Williams MA. Exercise testing in cardiac rehabilitation. Exercise prescription and beyond. *Cardiol Clin.* 2001;19(3):415–31.

24. Giri S, Thompson PD, Kiernan FJ, et al. Clinical and angiographic characteristics of exertion-related acute myocardial infarction. *JAMA.* 1999;282(18):1731–6.

25. Thompson PD. The cardiovascular complications of vigorous physical activity. *Arch Intern Med.* 1996;156(20):2297–302.

26. Thompson PD, Buchner D, Pina IL, et al. Exercise and physical activity in the prevention and treatment of atherosclerotic cardiovascular disease: a statement from the Council on Clinical Cardiology (Subcommittee on Exercise, Rehabilitation, and Prevention) and the Council on Nutrition, Physical Activity, and Metabolism (Subcommittee on Physical Activity). *Circulation.* 2003;107(24):3109–16.

27. Thompson PD, Franklin BA, Balady GJ, et al. Exercise and acute cardiovascular events placing the risks into perspective: a scientific statement from the American Heart Association Council on Nutrition, Physical Activity, and Metabolism and the Council on Clinical Cardiology. *Circulation.* 2007;115(17):2358–68.

28. Riebe D, Franklin BA, Thompson PD, et al. Updating ACSM's recommendations for exercise preparticipation health screening. *Med Sci Sports Exerc.* 2015;47(11):2473–9.

29. Price O, Tsakirides C, Gray M. Stavropoulos-Kalinoglou A. ACSM preparticipation health screening guidelines: a UK university cohort perspective. *Med Sci Sports Exerc.* 2019;51(5):1047–54.

30. U.S. Preventive Services Task Force. Screening for coronary heart disease: recommendation statement. *Ann Intern Med.* 2004;140(7):569–72.

31. Maron BJ, Araújo CG, Thompson PD, et al. Recommendations for preparticipation screening and the assessment of cardiovascular disease in masters athletes: an advisory for healthcare professionals from the working groups of the World Heart Federation, the International Federation of Sports Medicine, and the American Heart Association Committee on Exercise, Cardiac Rehabilitation, and Prevention. *Circulation.* 2001;103(2):327–34.

32. Pate RR, Pratt M, Blair SN, et al. Physical activity and public health. A recommendation from the Centers for Disease Control and Prevention and the American College of Sports Medicine. *JAMA.* 1995;273(5):402–7.

33. Arnett DK, Blumenthal RS, Albert MA, et al. 2019 ACC/AHA guideline on the primary prevention of cardiovascular disease: executive summary: a report of the American College of Cardiology/American Heart Association Task Force on Clinical Practice Guidelines. *Circulation.* 2019;140:e563–95.

34. Whelton PK, Carey RM, Aronow WS, et al. 2017 ACC/AHA/AAPA/ABC/ACPM/AGS/APhA/ASH/ASPC/NMA/PCNA guideline for the prevention, detection, evaluation, and management of high blood pressure in adults: a report of the American College of Cardiology/American Heart Association Task Force on Clinical Practice Guidelines. *Hypertension.* 2018;71(6):e13–115.

35. Stone NJ, Robinson J, Lichtenstein AH, et al. 2013 ACC/AHA guideline on the treatment of blood cholesterol to reduce atherosclerotic cardiovascular risk in adults: a report of the American College of Cardiology/American Heart Association Task Force on Practice Guidelines. *J Am Coll Cardiol.* 2013;129(5):1047–54.

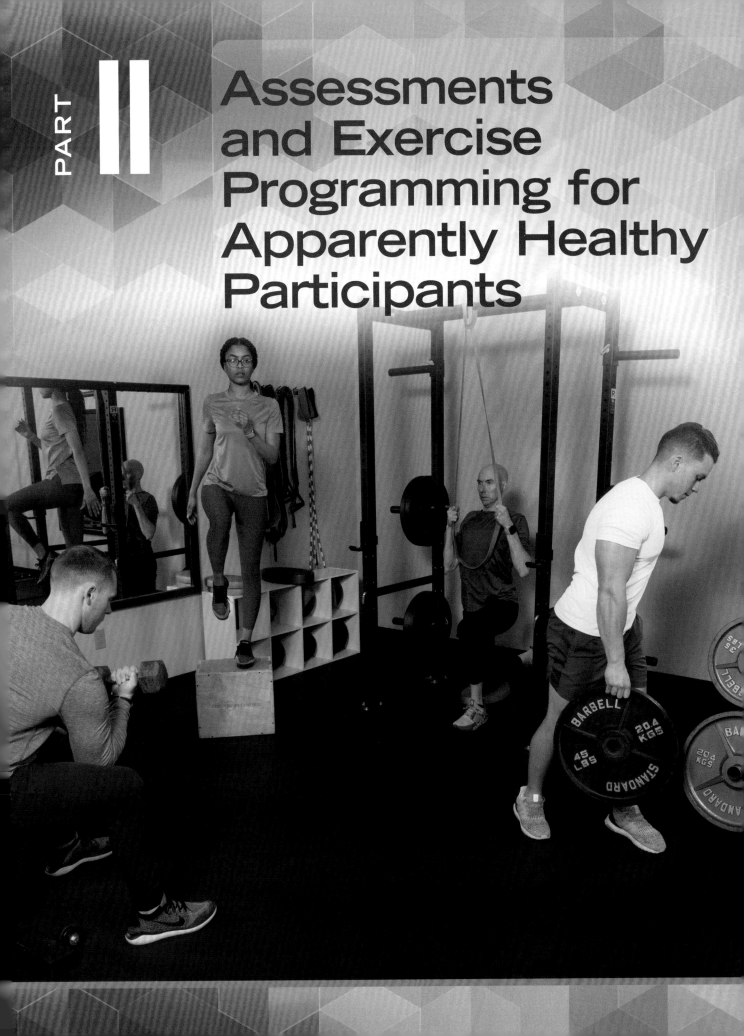

Assessments and Exercise Programming for Apparently Healthy Participants

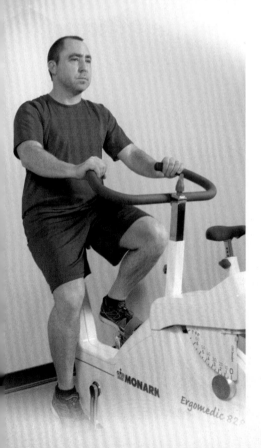

Cardiorespiratory Fitness Assessments and Exercise Programming for Apparently Healthy Participants

OBJECTIVES

- To understand basic anatomy and physiology of the cardiovascular and pulmonary systems as they relate to cardiorespiratory fitness.
- To select appropriate cardiorespiratory fitness assessments.
- To use the FITT framework to develop cardiorespiratory fitness.

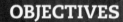

INTRODUCTION

Cardiorespiratory fitness (CRF) may be defined as the ability of the circulatory and respiratory systems to supply oxygen to the muscles to perform dynamic physical activity (1,2). High CRF is associated with increase health benefits (1), and it has been well established that individuals who do moderate- or vigorous-intensity aerobic physical activity have significantly lower risk of cardiovascular disease than inactive people (2). A dose-response relationship exists between aerobic fitness and health outcomes, as increased levels of CRF are associated with numerous positive health outcomes and reductions in chronic disease and all-cause mortality (1).

Therefore, the principal role of the American College of Sports Medicine (ACSM) Certified Exercise Physiologist® (ACSM-EP®) is to provide the development and maintenance of CRF to clientele. To provide safe, evidence-based instruction, the ACSM-EP needs a firm science foundation in the physiology of the cardiovascular and pulmonary systems. Once this groundwork has been established, the ACSM-EP can then begin the art of individualized exercise prescription.

 ## Basic Anatomy and Physiology of the Cardiovascular and Pulmonary Systems as They Relate to Cardiorespiratory Fitness

Goal of the Cardiovascular and Respiratory Systems

The cardiovascular and respiratory systems work in synchrony to provide oxygen and remove waste from the body. The respiratory system supports gas exchange, promoting the movement of oxygen and carbon dioxide from the environment into the blood and from the blood back into the environment. The cardiovascular system is responsible for the delivery of oxygenated blood and nutrients to the cell to make energy in the form of adenosine triphosphate (ATP). The cardiovascular system is also responsible for the removal of "waste" from the cell, so it can be transported to its appropriate destination for elimination or recycling (Fig. 3.1).

Anatomy and Physiology of the Cardiovascular and Respiratory Systems

The main components of the cardiovascular system are the heart and vasculature. The heart is a four-chambered muscular pump composed of the right and left atria (upper chambers) and the right and left ventricles (lower chambers). Specifically, the right ventricle is responsible for pumping deoxygenated blood to the lungs for oxygen loading and carbon dioxide unloading. After gas exchange occurs in the pulmonary circulation, blood returns to the left atrium. The left ventricle is then responsible for generating the force necessary to drive the blood out of its chamber and through the vasculature. The right and left atria act to provide support to their respective ventricles, serving as a reservoir of blood that eventually moves into the ventricles. The vasculature consists of arteries, arterioles, capillaries, venules, and veins; they can be thought of as a series of tubes that branch and become smaller in diameter as they move away from the heart (see Fig. 3.1).

The cardiovascular system is composed of two circulatory paths: the pulmonary circulation and the systemic circulation. The pulmonary circulation (pulmonary artery to pulmonary vein) is responsible for moving blood between the heart and lungs to oxygenate the blood, and the systemic circulation is responsible for moving blood from the heart to the rest of the body to deliver oxygen to tissues that need it for aerobic energy production. As the vasculature extends distal from the heart, arteries branch into smaller arterioles, which in turn branch and merge with the capillaries. The capillary is the smallest and most numerous of the blood vessels and is the location of gas and nutrient exchange. Deoxygenated blood and metabolic byproducts move out of capillaries into venules, which

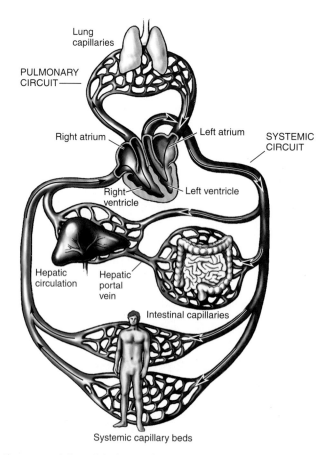

Lung
capillaries

PULMONARY
CIRCUIT——

Right atrium

Left atrium

SYSTEMIC
CIRCUIT

Right
ventricle

Left ventricle

Hepatic
circulation

Hepatic
portal
vein

Intestinal capillaries

Systemic capillary beds

FIGURE 3.1. Schematic representation of the integration between the cardiovascular system and the respiratory system. (Reprinted from American College of Sports Medicine. *ACSM's Resource Manual for Guidelines for Exercise Testing and Prescription.* 7th ed. Philadelphia [PA]: Lippincott Williams & Wilkins; 2014. 896 p.)

consolidate into veins as they move closer to the heart. Veins are responsible for delivering the deoxygenated blood back to the right side of the heart, where the cycle then repeats endlessly. In overview, blood moves through the major components of the heart and circulatory system in the following order: right atrium, right ventricle, pulmonary artery, lungs, pulmonary vein, left atrium, left ventricle, aorta, organs and tissues, and finally the vena cava, before returning back to the right atrium.

Adenosine Triphosphate Production

ATP is an energy-bearing molecule composed of carbon, hydrogen, nitrogen, oxygen, and phosphorus atoms and is found in all living cells. Nervous transmission, muscle contractions, formation of nucleic acids, and many other energy-consuming reactions of metabolism are possible because of the energy in ATP molecules.

Cells break down the food we eat with the ultimate goal of producing ATP, which is the cellular form of energy used within the body to fuel work. Muscle cells are very limited in the amount of ATP they can store. To support muscle contraction during continuous exercise, cells must continuously create ATP at a rate equal to ATP use through a combination of three primary metabolic systems: creatine phosphate (CP), anaerobic glycolysis, and the oxidative system.

The most immediate source of ATP is the CP system. Small amounts of CP are stored within each cell, and one CP donates a phosphate group to adenosine diphosphate (ADP) to create one ATP, or a simple one-to-one trade-off. This simplicity allows for the rapid production of ATP within the cell; however, this production is short-lived. Because of this, the CP system can provide

ATP to fuel work only during short intense bouts of exercise, owing to the limited storage capacity of CP within each cell. Therefore, the CP system is the primary source of ATP during very short, intense movements, such as discus throw, shot put, and high jump, and any maximal-intensity exercise lasting less than approximately 10 seconds.

Anaerobic glycolysis is the next most immediate energy source and consists of a metabolic pathway that breaks down carbohydrates (glucose or glycogen) into pyruvate. The bond energy produced from the breakdown of glucose and glycogen is used to phosphorylate ADP and create ATP. The net energy yield for anaerobic glycolysis, without further oxidation through the subsequent oxidative systems, is two ATPs if glucose is the substrate and three ATPs if glycogen is the substrate. When oxygen is available in the mitochondria of the cell, pyruvate continues to be broken down to acetyl-coenzyme A (acetyl-CoA) and enters the aerobic energy system. Alternatively, in the absence of adequate oxygen supply, pyruvate is converted to lactic acid, which gradually builds up in muscle cells and the blood. Anaerobic glycolysis is the primary source of ATP during medium-duration, intense exercise, such as the 200- and 400-m sprint events or any exercise of an intensity that cannot be continued for more than approximately 90 seconds.

Anaerobic energy systems can produce ATP quickly, but they are limited in the duration for which they can continue to produce ATP. For longer duration exercise or low-intensity exercise regardless of duration, the body relies most heavily on the oxidative metabolic energy systems. The aerobic or oxidative energy system does not contribute much energy at the onset of exercise but is able to sustain energy production for a longer duration. As exercise intensity decreases, allowing for longer exercise duration, the relative contribution of the anaerobic energy systems decreases and the relative contribution of the aerobic energy systems increases (Fig. 3.2).

The oxidative system includes two metabolic pathways: the Krebs cycle (aerobic glycolysis) and the electron transport chain. Unlike the anaerobic energy systems mentioned earlier, the oxidative systems require the presence of oxygen to produce ATP, which takes place in the mitochondria of the cell. This is why the mitochondria are known as the "powerhouse of the cell" because that is where the majority of ATP is generated.

The Krebs cycle requires the presence of carbohydrates, proteins, or fats. These macronutrients are broken down through a series of chemical reactions with their subsequent energy collected and

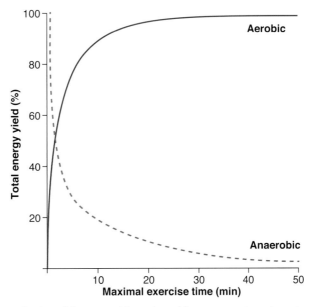

FIGURE 3.2. Relative contribution of the anaerobic and aerobic energy systems based on duration of exercise. (Reprinted from American College of Sports Medicine. *ACSM's Resource Manual for Guidelines for Exercise Testing and Prescription.* 7th ed. Philadelphia [PA]: Lippincott Williams & Wilkins; 2014. 896 p.)

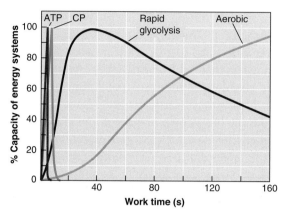

FIGURE 3.3. Relative contribution of the CP system, glycolysis, and the aerobic oxidative system to total energy production based on duration of exercise. (Reprinted from American College of Sports Medicine. *ACSM's Resource Manual for Guidelines for Exercise Testing and Prescription.* 7th ed. Philadelphia [PA]: Lippincott Williams & Wilkins; 2014. 896 p.)

used to create ATP independently and within the electron transport chain. This oxidative system is the primary source of ATP used during low- to moderate-intensity aerobic exercise lasting longer than 1–2 minutes all the way up to long-distance endurance events.

The anaerobic and aerobic energy systems work together to create ATP to fuel exercise. The ATP stored within the muscle cell will be used during the first few seconds of exercise onset. As stored ATP decreases, the contribution of ATP production via the CP system increases. Subsequently, as the stores of CP are reduced, anaerobic glycolysis becomes the primary contributing energy system to ATP creation. Aerobic ATP production becomes the primary fuel source in exercise lasting more than approximately 1–2 minutes. Figure 3.3 depicts the relative contribution of each source for exercise lasting between 1 and 160 seconds. Although the contribution of energy production differs on the basis of intensity and duration of exercise within the CP system, anaerobic glycolysis, and the oxidative systems, all of these primary metabolic pathways work in synchrony to produce the energy required to sustain the biological work of the human body.

The ACSM-EP should be familiar with the metabolic pathways used to create energy in the body and the link between the oxidative metabolic pathways, the cardiovascular system, and the respiratory system. Within this context, anaerobic metabolism can be called on even during long-duration exercise, particularly when using interval training consisting of intermittent high-intensity bouts.

Overview of Cardiorespiratory Responses to Acute Graded Exercise of Conditioned and Unconditioned Participants

Oxygen Uptake Kinetics during Submaximal Single-Intensity Exercise

As discussed in the previous section, oxygen is required to create ATP via the oxidative energy system. As workload increases, so does the energy requirement, and more oxygen is required to make ATP. Therefore, the volume of oxygen the body consumes per unit time ($\dot{V}O_2$) is proportional to workload. Upon the transition from rest to submaximal exercise, $\dot{V}O_2$ increases and reaches a steady state in 1–4 minutes (3). Steady state is the point at which $\dot{V}O_2$ plateaus during submaximal aerobic exercise and energy production via the aerobic energy systems is equal to the energy required to perform the set intensity of work. Prior to steady state, $\dot{V}O_2$ is lower than required to create adequate energy for the given task primarily via the oxidative energy systems. This period of inadequate oxygen consumption has been termed *the oxygen deficit* (4).

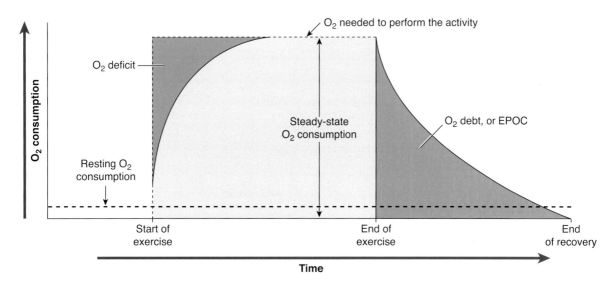

FIGURE 3.4. Oxygen uptake kinetics upon transition from rest to exercise, during submaximal single-intensity exercise, and upon transition from exercise back to a resting condition. (From Kraemer W, Fleck S, Deschenes M. *Exercise Physiology: Integrating Theory and Application.* Philadelphia [PA]: Lippincott Williams & Wilkins; 2012. 512 p.)

During this period, the anaerobic energy systems are responsible for providing the energy to make up for the difference between the energy produced via the aerobic energy systems and the energy required to perform the work required (5). The time required to reach steady state is influenced by the training state and the magnitude of the increase in exercise intensity (6,7). Aerobic exercise training decreases the time required to reach steady state, thus reducing the oxygen deficit. This is beneficial because less ATP production will be required and therefore less anaerobic byproducts from the anaerobic energy systems at the start of exercise and upon transition to a higher workload of exercise (6,7).

After cessation of exercise, $\dot{V}O_2$ remains elevated because of the increased work associated with the resynthesis of ATP and CP within muscle cells; lactate removal; and elevated body temperature, hormones, heart rate (HR), and respiratory rate (8). This elevation after exercise was first called *oxygen debt* (9) but is now commonly referred to as *excess postexercise oxygen consumption* (EPOC). Figure 3.4 provides a visual representation of the oxygen uptake kinetics upon transition from rest to exercise and depicts oxygen deficit, steady state, and EPOC.

Oxygen Uptake Kinetics during Graded Intensity Exercise

Graded exercise testing is used in many settings to determine baseline fitness and relevant health risks. Typically, the ACSM-EP will use either maximal or submaximal graded exercise testing to determine baseline fitness, which can be compared at future time points for assessing fitness improvements. It is important for the ACSM-EP conducting graded exercise tests to be well aware of the normal and abnormal hemodynamic response to incremental exercise, as described in the sections that follow.

During incremental exercise, $\dot{V}O_2$ increases slowly within the first few minutes of exercise and eventually reaches a steady state at each submaximal exercise intensity. Steady-state $\dot{V}O_2$ continues to increase linearly as workload increases (Fig. 3.5) until maximal $\dot{V}O_2$ ($\dot{V}O_{2max}$) is reached. $\dot{V}O_{2max}$ is the highest volume of oxygen the body can consume. It is often used as an indicator of aerobic fitness and endurance exercise performance because a higher $\dot{V}O_{2max}$ indicates a greater capacity to create ATP via oxidative energy production and a greater ability to supply the energy required to support higher intensity exercise workloads.

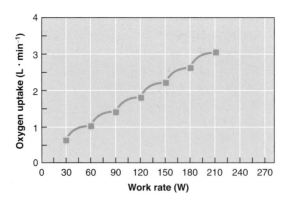

FIGURE 3.5. Relationship between oxygen uptake and workload during graded intensity exercise. (Reprinted from American College of Sports Medicine. *ACSM's Resource Manual for Guidelines for Exercise Testing and Prescription.* 7th ed. Philadelphia [PA]: Lippincott Williams & Wilkins; 2014. 896 p.)

The Fick equation can be used to determine $\dot{V}O_{2max}$. The Fick principle states that $\dot{V}O_{2max} = HR_{max} \times SV_{max} \times$ a-$\dot{V}O_2$ difference max, where $\dot{V}O_2$ = oxygen consumption ($mL \cdot kg^{-1} \cdot min^{-1}$), HR = heart rate (bpm), SV = stroke volume (mL per beat), and a-$\dot{V}O_2$ difference = arteriovenous oxygen difference. This equation demonstrates that $\dot{V}O_{2max}$ is dictated by maximal cardiac output ($SV_{max} \times HR_{max}$) and maximal a-$\dot{V}O_2$ difference.

Arteriovenous Oxygen Difference Response to Graded Intensity Exercise

The a-$\dot{V}O_2$ difference reflects the difference in oxygen content between the arterial and the venous blood. The a-$\dot{V}O_2$ difference provides a measure of the amount of oxygen taken up by the working muscles from the arterial blood. Resting oxygen content is approximately 20 $mL \cdot dL^{-1}$ in arterial blood and 15 $mL \cdot dL^{-1}$ in venous blood, yielding an a-$\dot{V}O_2$ of about 5 $mL \cdot dL^{-1}$. During exercise, venous oxygen content decreases as a result of the increased consumption of oxygen by the working muscles, thus resulting in an increase in a-$\dot{V}O_2$ difference with increasing exercise intensity.

Heart Rate, Stroke Volume, and Cardiac Output Responses to Graded Intensity Exercise

HR increases linearly with increasing workload until HR maximum is reached, which is also typically the point of exercise maximum. Although maximal HR (HR_{max}) declines with age (10), trained athletes have lower resting HRs throughout the lifespan. Training itself has little impact on HR_{max}. However, training can decrease an individual's HR at a given submaximal workload from pre- to postaerobic exercise training as a sign of increased fitness. SV is the volume of blood the heart ejects with each beat. Similar to HR, SV increases with workload but only up to approximately 40%–60% of $\dot{V}O_{2max}$ in the general population (11,12). Beyond 40%–60% of $\dot{V}O_{2max}$, SV has been shown to decrease slightly in sedentary individuals (13,14) while continuing to increase beyond 40%–60% of $\dot{V}O_{2max}$ in highly trained individuals (15,16). As SV increases with training, resting HR tends to decrease because more blood being pumped per beat allows the heart to beat less often at rest.

Cardiac output is the product of SV and HR and is also a measure of blood pumped per minute. Cardiac output increases steadily during graded intensity exercise because of the linear rise in HR and curvilinear rise in SV. Increases in cardiac output beyond ~50% of $\dot{V}O_{2max}$ are primarily mediated by increases in HR in untrained individuals. Trained individuals also have the capacity to increase cardiac output via increases in HR, but because they can see continued increase in SV past that of an untrained individual, they have a greater capacity to increase cardiac output (10).

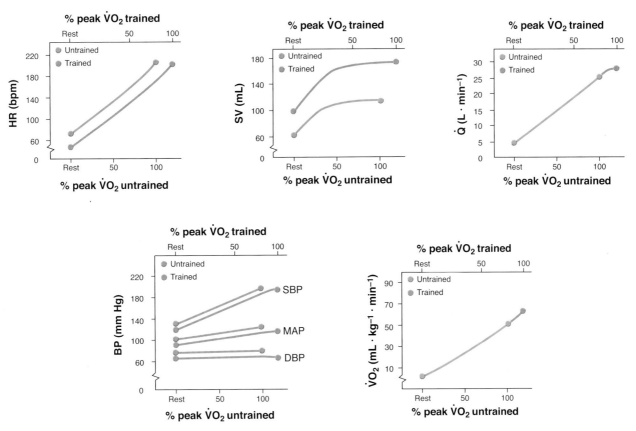

FIGURE 3.6. Cardiovascular responses to graded intensity exercise in trained and untrained individuals. (From Kraemer W, Fleck S, Deschenes M. *Exercise Physiology: Integrating Theory and Application.* Philadelphia [PA]: Lippincott Williams & Wilkins; 2012. 512 p.)

See Figure 3.6 for a visual comparison of HR, SV, and cardiac output responses to graded exercise intensity between trained and untrained individuals.

Pulmonary Ventilation Response to Graded Intensity Exercise

Pulmonary ventilation is the volume of air inhaled and exhaled per minute. It is calculated by multiplying the frequency of breathing by the volume of air moved per breath (tidal volume). Pulmonary ventilation increases linearly with work rate until 50%–80% of $\dot{V}O_{2max}$, at which point it reaches the ventilatory threshold and ventilation begins to increase exponentially (17). Ventilatory threshold has been used as an indicator of performance and training intensity; trained subjects can reach higher workloads than untrained subjects before reaching their ventilatory threshold (18).

Blood Pressure Response to Graded Intensity Exercise

Blood pressure (BP) is proportional to the product of cardiac output and total peripheral resistance (TPR) (the overall resistance to blood flow by the blood vessels). Systolic blood pressure (SBP) is the pressure in the arteries during ventricular contraction, or systole, and is heavily influenced by changes in cardiac output. Thus, just as cardiac output increases linearly with increasing workload, so does SBP. Diastolic blood pressure (DBP) is the pressure in the arteries when the heart is relaxed, or diastole, and is heavily influenced by TPR. During dynamic, large muscle mass exercise, vascular beds within active muscle vasodilate, decreasing resistance within these blood vessels. In contrast, blood vessels in less metabolically active tissues constrict, increasing resistance within these blood vessels. TPR is determined by the systemic resistance throughout the entire vasculature and is thus determined by the relative proportion of the vasculature that has undergone vasodilation versus vasoconstriction during exercise. During graded exercise, TPR may drop slightly because of the large muscle vasodilation. As a result of this and the contrasting increase in cardiac output, DBP remains relatively stable (19).

Mean arterial pressure (MAP) is the average BP in the arterial system over one complete cardiac cycle (MAP = DBP + 0.33 [SBP − DBP]). MAP is not a critical value to assess during regular exercise and instead is more commonly used in a clinical or diagnostic setting. However, it is worth noting that as a result of training, SBP, DBP, and MAP are all reduced slightly at submaximal workloads (20). See Figure 3.6 for a visual comparison of the BP responses to graded exercise intensity between trained and untrained individuals.

In summary, the ACSM-EP should understand that HR, pulmonary ventilation, a-$\dot{V}O_2$ difference, SV, cardiac output, SBP, and mean arterial BP increase during graded intensity exercise, whereas DBP remains stable or decreases slightly during aerobic type exercise. These cardiovascular and pulmonary responses support greater oxygen uptake to allow for the increase in aerobic energy production required during exercise.

Measuring Blood Pressure and Heart Rate before, during, and after Graded Exercise

Blood Pressure and Heart Rate Assessment

To determine whether clients have an appropriate cardiovascular response to graded exercise, the ACSM-EP should assess BP and HR before, during, and after exercise. (See previous section for a description of the expected HR and BP response to graded intensity exercise.) Prior to exercise, BP and HR should be assessed while resting in the exercise position that will subsequently be used for exercise testing. HR can be accessed via multiple techniques, such as radial and carotid pulse palpation, auscultation with a stethoscope, or the use of a reliable HR monitor. If using pulse palpation, the pulse should be counted for a minimum of 15 seconds and multiplied by 4 to calculate HR in units of beats per minute (bpm). Counting HR for less than 15 seconds reduces the accuracy and reliability of this technique. If the pulse palpation technique is to be used during and after exercise to assess HR, palpation of the radial artery may be a superior choice to the carotid artery because of the possibility of activating the carotid baroreceptors and inducing a reduction in HR, SV, TPR, and MAP (21). BP is typically assessed via brachial artery auscultation. To obtain accurate and reliable BP readings, the ACSM-EP should practice standard BP assessment techniques as specified in the box entitled "How to Assess Resting Blood Pressure" (22,23).

> Visit ⊙ Lippincott® Connect to watch video 3.1 about blood pressure measurement.

During graded exercise testing, BP and HR should be assessed at each exercise intensity. For some tests, it is important for HR to reach a steady state before advancing, and therefore, HR should be assessed at least two times at each stage to ensure that it is appropriate to move to the next workload. Generally, this is done at the end of each of the last 2 minutes of each exercise stage. BP should also be assessed during the last minute of each exercise stage. Taking accurate HR and BP assessments during exercise is a skill that requires significant practice by the ACSM-EP in order to be completed accurately and in a timely manner while the client continues to exercise.

| **HOW TO** | **Assess Resting Blood Pressure** |

1. Patients should be seated quietly for at least 5 min in a chair with back support (rather than on an examination table) with their feet on the floor and their arm supported at heart level. Patients should refrain from smoking cigarettes or ingesting caffeine for at least 30 min preceding the measurement.

2. Measuring supine and standing values may be indicated under special circumstances.

3. Wrap cuff firmly around upper arm at heart level; align cuff with brachial artery.

4. The appropriate cuff size must be used to ensure accurate measurement. The bladder within the cuff should encircle at least 80% of the upper arm. Many adults require a large adult cuff.

5. Place stethoscope chest piece below the antecubital space over the brachial artery. Bell and diaphragm side of chest piece seem to be equally effective in assessing BP (24). Avoid using the thumb to secure the stethoscope against the arm as this may allow the evaluators pulse to be detected through the stethoscope.

6. Quickly inflate cuff pressure to 20 mm Hg above first Korotkoff sound.

7. Slowly release pressure at rate equal to 2–5 mm Hg $\cdot$ s^{-1}.

8. SBP is the point at which the first of two or more Korotkoff sounds is heard (phase 1), and DBP is the point before the disappearance of Korotkoff sounds (phase 5).

9. At least two measurements should be made (minimum of 1 min apart), and the average should be taken.

10. BP should be measured in both arms during the first examination. Higher pressure should be used when there is consistent interarm difference.

11. Provide to patients, verbally and in writing, their specific BP numbers and BP goals.

Modified from American College of Sports Medicine. *ACSM's Health-Related Physical Fitness Assessment Manual.* 5th ed. Philadelphia (PA): Wolters Kluwer; 2018. 177 p.

When performing exercise HR and BP assessments, the ACSM-EP needs to ensure that the client's arm is relaxed, at heart level, and not touching any exercise equipment. After completion of exercise, BP and HR should be assessed for a minimum of 5 minutes of recovery or until each become stable (21).

Rate Pressure Product

In addition to checking for appropriate cardiovascular responses, the ACSM-EP can use these data to calculate an individual's "rate pressure product" (RPP). RPP, also referred to as double product, is the product of HR and SBP that occurs concomitantly and serves as an estimate of myocardial oxygen demand (M$\dot{V}O_2$) (RPP = HR × SBP). At rest, the heart consumes approximately 70% of the oxygen delivered to the cardiac muscle. During exercise, the cardiac muscle performs more work because of increased HR and increased contractility, and thus, M$\dot{V}O_2$ increases during exercise in direct proportion to exercise intensity (25). Therefore, if HR and SBP are lower at a given submaximal exercise intensity, the M$\dot{V}O_2$ will be lower, indicating increased fitness. The RPP can be useful to the ACSM-EP when performing exercise testing or prescribing exercise to clients with cardiovascular disease who have been medically cleared for exercise (24).

Selecting Appropriate Cardiorespiratory Fitness Assessments for Healthy Populations

Cardiorespiratory Fitness Assessments Benefits

CRF is an umbrella term that serves as an indicator of the functional capacity of the heart, lungs, blood vessels, and muscles to work in synchrony to support dynamic, large muscle mass exercise (24). CRF assessment is regularly performed in both healthy and clinical populations. In clinical populations, CRF testing is used for screening, diagnosis, and prognosis of medical conditions. CRF testing is also used in both clinical and healthy populations to gain insight into the most appropriate frequency, intensity, duration, and mode of exercise to prescribe when creating individualized exercise programs and as a motivational tool to help track progress and continually set obtainable, short-term goals (25).

Types of Cardiorespiratory Fitness Assessments

CRF can be assessed through a variety of step tests, field tests, and submaximal $\dot{V}O_2$ prediction tests. The wide variety of well-respected and widely used CRF tests allows the ACSM-EP the opportunity to select an assessment that provides the desired physiological informational while adhering to the needs of the client and the resources available. Table 3.1 provides an organizational chart of the most popular CRF tests for your reference. A detailed description of the most popular cardiorespiratory testing protocols can be found in the *ACSM's Health-Related Physical Fitness Assessment Manual* (24), and additional references are listed in Table 3.1.

The gold standard used to measure CRF is the assessment of $\dot{V}O_{2max}$ via open-circuit spirometry during maximal-intensity aerobic exercise. Open-circuit spirometry requires the collection of expired air from the client during a graded intensity exercise test to maximal exertion. The volume and content of oxygen and carbon dioxide in the expired air is analyzed with a highly specific gas analyzer. These data allow for the calculation of oxygen consumption at each workload of a graded

Table 3.1	Cardiorespiratory Fitness Assessment Techniques		
Type of Test	**Intensity**	**Specific Test Protocols**	**Major Equipment Needed**
Maximal oxygen uptake $\dot{V}O_{2max}$	Maximal	Open-circuit spirometry during graded exercise test to volitional fatigue (26)	Treadmill, cycle ergometer, arm ergometer, etc.
Submaximal oxygen uptake	Submaximal	Astrand-Rhyming Cycle Ergometer Test (27)	Cycle ergometer
		YMCA Cycle Ergometer Test (28)	Cycle ergometer
Step tests	Maximal or submaximal	Queens College/McArdle Step Test (29)	Aerobic step or specific height bench, metronome
		Harvard Step Test (30)	
		Astrand-Rhyming Step Test (27)	
Field tests	Maximal or submaximal	Rockport walk (31)	Level walking/running surface
		12-min walk/run test (32,33)	
		1.5-mile run test (24)	

exercise test. As discussed previously, $\dot{V}O_2$ will increase linearly as workload increases until $\dot{V}O_2$ plateaus and $\dot{V}O_{2max}$ is reached. Although assessment of $\dot{V}O_{2max}$ with gas analysis is the gold standard of CRF assessment, it requires expensive equipment, technical expertise, and maximal intensity exercise performance by the client. These requirements limit the use of $\dot{V}O_{2max}$ testing using open-circuit spirometry to primarily clinical laboratory and research settings (21).

Submaximal $\dot{V}O_2$ estimates $\dot{V}O_{2max}$ from the HR response to submaximal single-stage or graded exercise. Therefore, precise assessment of HR is a critical factor in determining $\dot{V}O_{2max}$ and should be a well-developed skill by the ACSM-EP. HR can easily be affected by environmental, dietary, and behavioral factors, and the ACSM-EP should do his or her best to control these factors during submaximal $\dot{V}O_2$ testing. Because submaximal testing relies on predictions, there is an increased chance of error because of a variety of factors, such as estimations on resting and maximum HR. To minimize the error of prediction, the following assumptions must be met during submaximal exercise testing: (a) Steady-state HR is achieved within 3–4 minutes at each workload, (b) HR increases linearly with work rate, (c) a consistent work rate should be maintained throughout each stage of testing, and (d) estimation/prediction of should be accurate (24). Unfortunately, estimation/prediction of HR_{max} is not an exact science and is highly variable. If true HR_{max} differs significantly from predicted HR_{max}, this assumption may introduce a source of error into the prediction of $\dot{V}O_{2max}$ via submaximal $\dot{V}O_2$ testing (34).

Step tests are a widely used form of CRF assessment because of the practicality of this technique. They are short in duration, require little equipment yet are easily portable, and allow for assessment of large groups. Various step test protocols range from submaximal to maximal, giving the ACSM-EP a wide range of choices that he or she should critically assess before determining which is most appropriate for the client. Intensity is determined by step height and step cadence. Most step tests predict $\dot{V}O_{2max}$ from recovery HR (27,29,30), whereas some step tests use steady-state exercise HR to estimate CRF (35). The lower the exercise HR and the greater the rate of recovery, the higher the estimated $\dot{V}O_{2max}$.

Field tests are also widely used to assess CRF. The most common forms of field tests include assessment of the amount of time required to cover a set distance or assessment of the distance covered in a set amount of time. Field tests are versatile, in that they can use many modes of exercise, such as walking, running, cycling, and swimming. Field tests have many of the same benefits as step tests, in that they are short in duration, require little equipment, can be used for large groups, and can be performed wherever a safe, flat, known distance is available. However, field tests can be more subjective in nature, largely because of the dependency on client effort and therefore are not as reliable as laboratory tests for assessing CRF.

Selecting the Appropriate Cardiorespiratory Fitness Assessment

When choosing which cardiorespiratory assessment to use, the ACSM-EP should consider intensity, length, and expense of the test; type and number of personnel needed; equipment and facilities needed; physician supervision needs and safety concerns; information required as a result of the assessment; required accuracy of results; appropriateness of mode of exercise; and the willingness of the participant to perform the test (24). The ACSM-EP should review the Physical Activity Readiness Questionnaire, health history, and risk assessment documents collected during the prescreening visit to help determine which assessment will be best (see Chapter 2 on prescreening and risk classification). On the basis of the client's risk classification category, the intent of the exercise test, and the other considerations, the ACSM-EP should think critically to determine whether a submaximal or maximal test is most appropriate on a case-by-case basis and to avoid a "one-size-fits-all" approach. Although maximal testing may be quite precise, it has many drawbacks, including first and foremost the increased risk of exercising to exhaustion, especially in clients presenting with any level of risk other than "low" (21). Other drawbacks to maximal testing include increased costs and time, specialized personnel and supplies, and the discomfort of asking the client to exercise to complete exhaustion. Submaximal tests may therefore be more appropriate for many individuals and, when conducted appropriately, result in a reasonable estimate of $\dot{V}O_{2max}$ (36).

HOW TO — Assess Cardiorespiratory Fitness: The Rockport Walking Test

Equipment Needed

1. Track or level surface
2. Stopwatch
3. HR monitor (optional)
4. Scale to measure body weight
5. Clipboard, recording sheet, and pencil
6. Calculator

Procedure

1. Locate a level surface, preferably a track, and determine the distance or lap that is equivalent to 1 mile.

2. After a proper warm-up, instruct the client to walk 1 mi as fast as possible, without jogging or running.

3. Immediately after 1 mi has been completed, record the walk time in minutes.

4. If the individual is wearing an HR monitor, record the HR achieved immediately upon reaching the 1-mi mark. If an HR monitor is not available, upon completion of the mile, take the client's pulse for 15 s and multiply by 4 to determine peak HR.

5. Data may now be entered into the following formula:

   $\dot{V}O_{2max}$ (mL $\cdot$ kg^{-1} $\cdot$ min^{-1}) 5 = 132.853 − (0.0769 × body weight in lb) − (0.3877 × age in yr) + (6.315 × gender [1 for men, 0 for women]) − (3.2649 × 1-mi walk time in minutes) − (0.1565 × HR)

Example

1. What is the predicted maximal aerobic capacity for a 64-yr-old woman who weighs 155 lb and who completes the Rockport test in 16 min with an HR of 142 bpm?

   $\dot{V}O_{2max}$ = 132.853 − (0.0769 × 155) − (0.3877 × 64) + (6.315 × 0) − (3.2649 × 16)
   − (0.1565 × 142) = 21.7 mL $\cdot$ kg^{-1} $\cdot$ min^{-1}

2. Normative data suggest that this individual would be rated as "low average" for her age.

Reference

Kline GM, Porcari JP, Hintermeister R, et al. Estimation of $\dot{V}O_{2max}$ from a one-mile track walk, gender, age, and body weight. *Med Sci Sports Exerc.* 1987;19(3):253–9.

HOW TO	**Assess Cardiorespiratory Fitness: Queens College Step Test**

Equipment Needed

1. Step/bleacher
2. Metronome
3. Stopwatch
4. HR monitor (optional)
5. Clipboard, recording sheet, and pencil
6. Calculator

Protocol

1. The step test requires that the individual step up and down on a standardized step height of 16.25 in (41.25 cm) for 3 min. (Many gymnasium bleachers have a riser height of 16.25 in.)

2. Men step at a rate (cadence) of 24 per minute, whereas women step at a rate of 22 per minute. This cadence should be closely monitored and set with the use of an electronic metronome. A 24-steps-per-minute cadence means that the complete cycle of step up with one leg, step up with the other, step down with the first leg, and finally step down with the last leg is performed 24 times in a minute. Commonly, the metronome is set at a cadence of four times the step rate, in this case, 96 bpm for men, to coordinate each leg's movement with a beat of the metronome. The women's step cadence would be 88 bpm. Although it may be possible to test more than one client at a time, the group would need to be of the same gender.

3. At the conclusion of 3 min, the client stops and palpates the pulse (typically at the radial site) while standing, within the first 5 s. A 15-s pulse count is then taken and multiplied by 4 to determine HR in bpm. This recovery HR should occur within the first 30 s of immediate recovery from the end of the step test. The subject's $\dot{V}O_{2max}$ is determined from the recovery HR by the following formulas:

$$\text{For men: } \dot{V}O_{2max} \text{ (mL} \cdot \text{kg}^{-1} \cdot \text{min}^{-1}) = 111.33 - (0.42 \times HR)$$

$$\text{For women: } \dot{V}O_{2max} \text{ (mL} \cdot \text{kg}^{-1} \cdot \text{min}^{-1}) = 65.81 - (0.1847 \times HR)$$

> Visit ⊙ Lippincott® Connect to watch video 3.2 demonstrating the Queens College Step Test.

Example

For example, if a man finished the test with a recovery HR = 144 bpm (36 beats in 15 s), then

$$\dot{V}O_{2max} \text{ (mL} \cdot \text{kg}^{-1} \cdot \text{min}^{-1}) = 111.33 - (0.42 \times 144) = 50.85 \text{ mL} \cdot \text{kg}^{-1} \cdot \text{min}^{-1}$$

Reference

American College of Sports Medicine. *ACSM's Health-Related Physical Fitness Assessment Manual.* 5th ed. Philadelphia (PA): Wolters Kluwer; 2018. 177 p.

HOW TO: Assess Cardiorespiratory Fitness: Ebbeling Single-Stage Submaximal Treadmill Walking Test

Equipment Needed

1. Treadmill
2. Stopwatch
3. HR monitor (optional)
4. Clipboard, recording sheet, and pencil
5. Calculator

Protocol

1. Warm up for 4 min at a 0% grade and a walking speed between 2.0 and 4.5 mph that elicits a HR between 50% and 70% of age-predicted HR_{max}, adjusting speed after first minute as needed.

2. Following the warm-up, elevate treadmill to a 5% grade and continue walking for an additional 4 min at a speed of 2.0, 3.0, 4.0, or 4.5 mph. Record the steady-state HR (SS HR) from the average of the final 30 s of the last 2 min at the 5% grade. If HR differs by more than 5 bpm, extend the test by an additional minute and record the SS HR from the new final 2 min.

3. Enter the SS HR into the equation below to estimate $\dot{V}O_{2max}$.

$$\dot{V}O_{2max}\ (mL \cdot kg^{-1} \cdot min^{-1}) = 15.1 + (21.8 \times \text{speed in mph}) - (0.327 \times \text{SS HR in bpm}) - (0.263 \times \text{speed in mph} \times \text{age in yr}) + (0.00504 \times \text{SS HR in bpm} \times \text{age in yr}) + (5.98 \times \text{gender: female} = 0,\ \text{male} = 1)$$

Visit ◉ Lippincott® Connect to watch video 3.3 demonstrating the Ebbeling Single-Stage Submaximal Treadmill Walking Test.

Example

A 42-yr-old female walked at 4 mph (5% grade) with an SS HR of 160 bpm.

$$\dot{V}O_{2max}\ (mL \cdot kg^{-1} \cdot min^{-1}) = 15.1 + (21.8 \times 4.0) - (0.327 \times 160) - (0.263 \times 4.0 \times 42) + (0.00504 \times 160 \times 42) + (5.98 \times 0) = 39.7\ mL \cdot kg^{-1} \cdot min^{-1}$$

Adapted from Ebbeling CB, Ward A, Puleo EM, Widrick J, Rippe JM. Development of a single-stage submaximal treadmill walking test. *Med Sci Sports Exerc.* 1991;23(8):966–73.

HOW TO	**Assess Cardiorespiratory Fitness in Adults: The Astrand-Rhyming Cycle Ergometer Test**

Equipment Needed

1. Cycle ergometer
2. Stopwatch
3. HR monitor (optional)
4. Clipboard, recording sheet, and pencil
5. Calculator

Protocol

1. Position the seat on the cycle ergometer per ACSM guidelines.
2. Select the work rate for your client based on sex and self-reported fitness level.
   - Men, unconditioned: 300 or 600 kg-m $\cdot$ min^{-1} (50 or 100 W)
   - Men, conditioned: 600 or 900 kg-m $\cdot$ min^{-1} (100 or 150 W)
   - Women, unconditioned: 300 or 450 kg-m $\cdot$ min^{-1} (50 or 75 W)
   - Women, conditioned: 450 or 600 kg-m $\cdot$ min^{-1} (75 or 100 W)
3. After proper warm-up, instruct your client to pedal at 50 rpm for 6 min at the work rate selected above.
4. Assess HR two times during minute 5–6 and average the values.
5. Estimate $\dot{V}O_{2max}$ from a nomogram (Fig. 3.7).
6. Because HR$_{max}$ decreases with age, the value from the nomogram must be adjusted for age by multiplying $\dot{V}O_{2max}$ value by the following correction factors.

AGE	CORRECTION FACTOR
15	1.10
25	1.00
35	0.87
40	0.83
45	0.78
50	0.75
55	0.71
60	0.68
65	0.65

Visit ⬤ Lippincott® Connect to watch video 3.4 demonstrating the Astrand-Rhyming Cycle Ergometer Test and video 3.5 on determining the correct seat height.

Example

1. What is the predicted maximal aerobic capacity for a 35-yr-old man who has an average HR of 146 bpm during the last minute of the test at a work rate of 900 kgm $\cdot$ min^{-1}?
2. Based on the nomogram, the predicted $\dot{V}O_{2max}$ is 3.2 L $\cdot$ min^{-1}. After adjusting for age, the predicted $\dot{V}O_{2max}$ is 2.784 L $\cdot$ min^{-1}.

Reference

Astrand PO, Rhyming I. A nomogram for calculation of aerobic capacity (physical fitness) from pulse rate during sub-maximal work. *J Appl Physiol.* 1954;7(2):218–21.

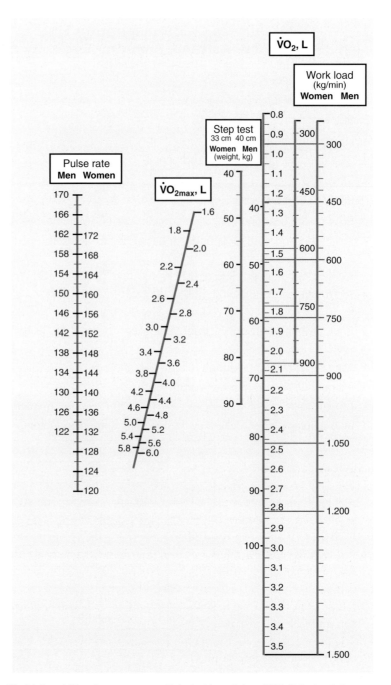

FIGURE 3.7. Modified Astrand-Rhyming nomogram. (Adapted from Astrand PO, Ryhming I. A nomogram for calculation of aerobic capacity [physical fitness] from pulse rate during sub-maximal work. *J Appl Physiol.* 1954;7[2]:218–21.)

Interpreting Results of Cardiorespiratory Fitness Assessments, Including Determination of $\dot{V}O_2$ and $\dot{V}O_{2max}$

After completing cardiopulmonary exercise assessment, the ACSM-EP should interpret the results of the assessment and share the information with his or her client. To maximize client understanding of CRF testing, individual $\dot{V}O_{2max}$ data are often compared with established criterion-referenced and normative standards. Criterion-referenced standards classify individuals into categories or groups, such as "excellent" or "needs improvement," on the basis of external criteria.

In contrast, normative standards provide percentiles from data collected within a specific population. The ACSM-EP can use either type of standard when interpreting data and may find it helpful to present data to clients using both types of standards, as one may have more impact with a client on the basis of his or her perspective. Care should be taken when using normative standards to ensure that the client population and the normative standard population are similar. If there is discrepancy within the populations, normative data are not appropriate for comparisons (25). Table 3.2 provides both normative and criterion-referenced $\dot{V}O_{2max}$ data specific to age and sex.

Low CRF levels have been shown to be an independent predictor of cardiovascular disease and all-cause mortality (37,38). The ACSM-EP should discuss this relationship with clients, as it may bring added meaning to the test results and help motivate clients to improve their CRF. Both maximal and submaximal tests can be used to evaluate CRF at a given point in time as well as changes in CRF that result from physical activity participation (21). A higher $\dot{V}O_{2max}$, a lower HR at a given intensity of submaximal exercise, or a lower recovery HR indicates an overall improvement in CRF.

Metabolic Calculations as They Relate to Cardiorespiratory Exercise Programming

Metabolic calculations can be a tremendous asset to the ACSM-EP. An ACSM-EP can use these calculations to determine calorie expenditure for clients interested in weight control, along with helping other clients reach daily and weekly goals for exercise.

Energy Units and Conversion Factors

Energy can be presented using many different terms in the field of exercise physiology, such as absolute oxygen consumption ($L \cdot min^{-1}$ or $mL \cdot min^{-1}$), relative oxygen consumption ($mL \cdot kg^{-1} \cdot min^{-1}$), metabolic equivalents (METs), and kilocalories. The ACSM-EP should possess a firm understanding of the different terms used to express energy expenditure to allow for easy conversion of data from one term to another.

Oxygen consumption refers to the rate at which oxygen is consumed by the body. It can be expressed in absolute ($L \cdot min^{-1}$) or relative ($mL \cdot kg^{-1} \cdot min^{-1}$) terms. Absolute oxygen consumption is the raw volume of oxygen consumed by the body, whereas relative oxygen consumption is the volume of oxygen consumed relative to body weight and can serve as a useful measure of fitness between individuals.

METs present the energy cost of exercise in a simple format that can be easily used by the general public to gauge exercise intensity. One MET is equal to the relative oxygen consumption at rest, which is approximately $3.5 \ mL \cdot kg^{-1} \cdot min^{-1}$. Using METs as energy cost units allows for the energy cost of exercise to be presented in multiples of rest. For example, if an individual is working at an energy cost of 10 METs, he or she is completing approximately 10 times the amount of work and using 10 times the amount of energy of that at rest. The Compendium of Physical Activities provides a list of the energy cost for different forms of physical activity using METs (39–41). In addition, METs can be used to calculate energy expenditure over time ([MET $\times$ kg $\times$ 3.5] / 200 = $kcal \cdot min^{-1}$).

Kilocalorie is an estimate of energy cost that can be related directly to physical activity and exercise, and the ACSM-EP can calculate the number of kilocalories expended during an exercise bout if oxygen consumption is measured or estimated using previously mentioned methods. As an ACSM-EP, understanding the conversion of energy between units is crucial. The flowchart in Figure 3.8 provides a visual tool to help the ACSM-EP understand the link between energy units and serves as a helpful guide when practicing unit conversions.

Table 3.2	Treadmill-Based Cardiorespiratory Fitness Classifications ($\dot{V}O_{2max}$) by Age and Sex

$\dot{V}O_{2max}$ (mL $O_2 \cdot kg^{-1} \cdot min^{-1}$)

MEN

		Age Group (yr)				
Percentile		20–29	30–39	40–49	50–59	60–69
95	Superior	66.3	59.8	55.6	50.7	43.0
90	Excellent	61.8	56.5	52.1	45.6	40.3
85		59.3	54.2	49.3	43.2	38.2
80		57.1	51.6	46.7	41.2	36.1
75	Good	55.2	49.2	45.0	39.7	34.5
70		53.7	48.0	43.9	38.2	32.9
65		52.1	46.6	42.1	36.3	31.6
60		50.2	45.2	40.3	35.1	30.5
55	Fair	49.0	43.8	38.9	33.8	29.1
50		48.0	42.4	37.8	32.6	28.2
45		46.5	41.3	36.7	31.6	27.2
40		44.9	39.6	35.7	30.7	26.6
35	Poor	43.5	38.5	34.6	29.5	25.7
30		41.9	37.4	33.3	28.4	24.6
25		40.1	35.9	31.9	27.1	23.7
20		38.1	34.1	30.5	26.1	22.4
15	Very poor	35.4	32.7	29.0	24.4	21.2
10		32.1	30.2	26.8	22.8	19.8
5		29.0	27.2	24.2	20.9	17.4

WOMEN

		Age Group (yr)				
Percentile		20–29	30–39	40–49	50–59	60–69
95	Superior	56.0	45.8	41.7	35.9	29.4
90	Excellent	51.3	41.4	38.4	32.0	27.0
85		48.3	39.3	36.0	30.2	25.6
80		46.5	37.5	34.0	28.6	24.6
75	Good	44.7	36.1	32.4	27.6	23.8
70		43.2	34.6	31.1	26.8	23.1
65		41.6	33.5	30.0	26.0	22.0
60		40.6	32.2	28.7	25.2	21.2
55	Fair	38.9	31.2	27.7	24.4	20.5
50		37.6	30.2	26.7	23.4	20.0
45		35.9	29.3	25.9	22.7	19.6
40		34.6	28.2	24.9	21.8	18.9

| Table 3.2 | Treadmill-Based Cardiorespiratory Fitness Classifications ($\dot{V}O_{2max}$) by Age and Sex (continued) | | | | |

WOMEN

		Age Group (yr)				
Percentile		20–29	30–39	40–49	50–59	60–69
35	Poor	33.6	27.4	24.1	21.2	18.4
30		32.0	26.4	23.3	20.6	17.9
25		30.5	25.3	22.1	19.9	17.2
20		28.6	24.1	21.3	19.1	16.5
15	Very poor	26.2	22.5	20.0	18.3	15.6
10		23.9	20.9	18.8	17.3	14.6
5		21.7	19.0	17.0	16.0	13.4
		(n = 410)	(n = 608)	(n = 843)	(n = 805)	(n = 408)

Percentiles from cardiopulmonary exercise testing on a treadmill with measured $\dot{V}O_{2max}$ (mL $O_2 \cdot kg^{-1} \cdot min^{-1}$). Data obtained from the Fitness Registry and the Importance of Exercise National Database (FRIEND) Registry for men and women who were considered free from known cardiovascular disease.

Adapted with permission from Kaminsky LA, Imboden MT, Arena R, Myers J. Reference standards for cardiorespiratory fitness measured with cardiopulmonary exercise testing using cycle ergometry: data from the Fitness Registry and the Importance of Exercise National Database (FRIEND) Registry. *Mayo Clin Proc.* 2017;92(2):228–33.

HOW TO   Sample Cross-Training Program

The following is an example of a typical mix of activities which may be available at a health club. An overall scheme of a 6-mo training progression is shown for an apparently healthy client. Use of the terms *beginner*, *intermediate*, and *established* to describe the fitness level of the client is somewhat subjective. For some individuals, even the beginner stage may present too much of a challenge. If so, starting out with only 5–10 min of exercise may be more appropriate. The progression should not be overly aggressive. Do not focus on achieving target goals quickly but rather to gradually increase the overall workload to establish compliance and promote adherence. Progression should be individualized on the basis of the client's initial fitness level, health status, age, and individual goals.

For each stage, a range rather than a single number is included for frequency, intensity, and duration. Assist the client with the appropriate balance based on individual responses. Frequency of exercise progresses gradually over the 6-month period outlined from 3 d $\cdot$ wk^{-1} up to a target of 3–5 d $\cdot$ wk^{-1}. Intensity increases from relatively low to a target of 70%–85% HRR. By slowly increasing the intensity, the client is able to adapt to the higher levels of exercise without becoming discouraged or experiencing retrogression (*i.e.*, a reversal of gains due to excessive overload). The duration of the exercise session also increases in small steps to allow for appropriate adaptations. Finally, consider changing the mode of exercise to provide more variety in the program.

Recall that the activities are classified by group. Walking is a group A activity and is appropriate for anyone. For each activity, the sequence in time, intensity, and frequency as well as progression of the different types

Continued

of activities should be noted. When designing a program, occasionally including new modes of exercise can provide much-appreciated variety but should be introduced gradually so that appropriate adjustments can be made (*i.e.*, appropriate overload). Most importantly, remember that the overall training program must match the goals of the client.

Sample Cross-Training Program at a Health Club

Status	Time Point	Warm-Up	Workout[a]	Cool-Down
Beginner	First week	Slow, easy walking pace for a couple of minutes	Pick one activity each day at a light level of exertion (level 3 or 4) for 10 min at least twice a day for a total of 20 min each day (3 d · wk^{-1}). Select from walking on the treadmill or stationary biking. Your weekly total should be 60 min.	Slow, easy walking pace for a couple of minutes
	Progression, part 1	Slow, easy walking pace for 5 min	Each week, add 15 min to your weekly total until you reach 120 min of activity (*e.g.*, 30 min 4 d · wk^{-1}). Potential activities include treadmill walking, stationary biking, and using a stair climber. Stay at this duration and increase your intensity over the next couple of weeks from light (level 3 or 4) to moderate (level 5 or 6). Once you are comfortable with this time and intensity for a couple of weeks, continue to add 10–15 min · wk^{-1} until you reach 150 min.	Slow, easy walking pace for 5 min
	Progression, part 2	Easy walking pace for 5–10 min	Exercise at an intensity that gives a moderate level of exertion (level 5 or 6); continue to add 10–15 min each week to progress from 150 min · wk^{-1} to a total of 200 min.	Easy walking pace for 5–10 min
	Final week	Easy walking pace for 5–10 min	Exercise at an intensity that gives a moderate level of exertion (level 5 or 6) for 30–60 min (3–5 d · wk^{-1}); activities may include treadmill walking; stationary biking; or using a stair climber, elliptical trainer, rowing machine, or Nordic ski machine. Your weekly total should be 200 min.	Easy walking pace for 5–10 min
Intermediate	Initial week	Easy walking pace for 5–10 min	Exercise at a level that feels moderate (level 5 or 6) for 30–60 min (3–5 d · wk^{-1}) using a treadmill, stationary bike, stair climber, elliptical trainer, or Nordic ski machine; your weekly total should be 200 min.	Easy walking pace for 5–10 min

Status	Time Point	Warm-Up	Workout[a]	Cool-Down
	Progression	Easy walking pace for 5–10 min	Continue to increase exercise duration by 10–15 min d · wk^{-1} to approach 300 min of moderate activity accumulated on a weekly basis. Another option is to introduce more vigorous activity a couple of days per week, such as jogging on the treadmill, taking a spinning class, or taking a step aerobics class, realizing that the time needed will be less (typically, 2 min of moderate activity equals 1 min of vigorous activity).	Easy walking pace for 5–10 min
	Final week	Easy walking pace for 5–10 min	Exercise at a level that feels moderate (level 5 or 6) for 45–90 min (3–5 d · wk^{-1}); your weekly total should be 300 min (moderate intensity). OR Combine moderate and vigorous walking on alternate days. Your weekly total should be equivalent amounts of moderate and vigorous activity (*e.g.*, 200 min of moderate plus 50 min of vigorous).	Easy walking pace for 5–10 min
Established	Continue/ maintain	Easy walking pace for 5–10 min	Exercise at an intensity that feels moderate (level 5 or 6); your weekly total should be a minimum of 300 min (moderate intensity). OR Exercise at a higher intensity (level 7 or 8); your weekly total should be a minimum of 150 min (vigorous intensity). OR Combine moderate and vigorous walking on alternate days. Your weekly total should be equivalent amounts of moderate and vigorous activity (*e.g.*, 200 min of moderate plus 50 min of vigorous).	Easy walking pace for 5–10 min

[a]Level of exertion is on a scale of 0–10 (sitting at rest is 0 and your highest effort level is 10).

Adapted with permission from American College of Sports Medicine. *ACSM's Complete Guide to Fitness and Health.* Champaign (IL): Human Kinetics; 2011. 408 p.

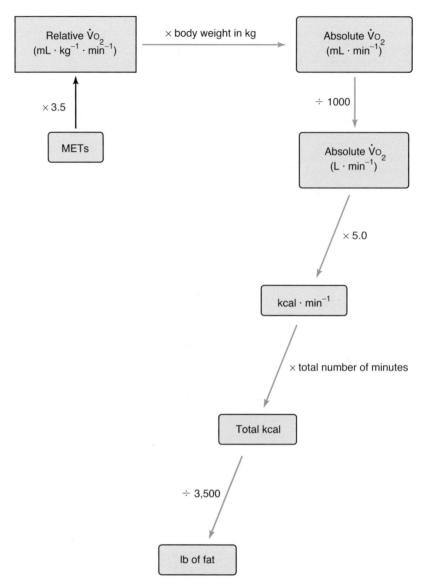

FIGURE 3.8. The energy equivalency chart: the seven energy expressions. (From American College of Sports Medicine. *ACSM's Certification Review*. 3rd ed. Philadelphia [PA]: Lippincott Williams & Wilkins; 2010. 308 p.)

ACSM Metabolic Formula

Although open-circuit spirometry is the gold standard technique used to assess oxygen consumption and estimate energy cost during exercise, it is not accessible and/or feasible in all applications. The ACSM provides metabolic formulas (21) to allow the ACSM-EP an alternative method of energy cost estimation for popular modes of physical activity. The metabolic formula calculates gross energy expenditure, which refers to the sum of energy used at rest and during exercise (Table 3.3). In contrast, net energy expenditure refers to the energy cost of exercise that exceeds the energy required to support the body at rest. Thus, the energy costs calculated from the metabolic formula will represent the amount of energy required to complete the exercise task, including the energy required to support resting energy requirements. After energy cost is estimated, the conversion factors discussed earlier can be used to convert into the appropriate energy expression required for application purposes, such as weight loss or weight gain goals.

Table 3.3	Metabolic Calculations for the Estimation of Energy Expenditure ($\dot{V}O_2$ [mL $\cdot$ kg^{-1} $\cdot$ min^{-1}]) during Common Physical Activities			
	Sum These Components			
Activity	**Resting Component**	**Horizontal Component**	**Vertical Component/ Resistance Component**	**Limitations**
Walking	3.5	0.1 $\times$ speed[a]	1.8 $\times$ speed[a] $\times$ grade[b]	Most accurate for speeds of 1.9–3.7 min $\cdot$ h^{-1} (50–100 m $\cdot$ min^{-1})
Running	3.5	0.2 $\times$ speed[a]	0.9 $\times$ speed[a] $\times$ grade[b]	Most accurate for speeds >5 min $\cdot$ h^{-1} (134 m $\cdot$ min^{-1})
Stepping	3.5	0.2 $\times$ steps $\cdot$ min^{-1}	1.33 $\times$ (1.8 $\times$ step height[c] $\times$ steps $\cdot$ min^{-1})	Most accurate for stepping rates of 12–30 steps $\cdot$ min^{-1}
Leg cycling	3.5	3.5	(1.8 $\times$ work rate[d]) / body mass[e]	Most accurate for work rates of 300–1,200 kg $\cdot$ m $\cdot$ min^{-1} (50–200 W)
Arm cycling	3.5		(3 $\times$ work rate[d]) / body mass[e]	Most accurate for work rates between 150 and 750 kg $\cdot$ m $\cdot$ min^{-1} (25 and 125 W)

[a]Speed in m $\cdot$ min^{-1}.

[b]Grade is percentage grade expressed in decimal format (*e.g.*, 10% = 0.10).

[c]Step height in meter. *Multiply by the following conversion factors:* lb to kg: 0.454; in to cm: 2.54; ft to m: 0.3048; m to km: 1.609; min $\cdot$ h^{-1} to m $\cdot$ min^{-1}: 26.8; kg-m $\cdot$ min^{-1} to W: 0.164; W to kg-m $\cdot$ min^{-1}: 6.12; $\dot{V}O_{2max}$ L $\cdot$ min^{-1} to kcal $\cdot$ min^{-1}: 4.9; $\dot{V}O_{2max}$ mL $\cdot$ kg^{-1} $\cdot$ min^{-1} to MET: 3.5.

[d]Work rate in kilogram meters per minute (kg-m $\cdot$ min^{-1}) is calculated as resistance (kg) $\times$ distance per revolution of flywheel $\times$ pedal frequency per minute. Note: Distance per revolution is 6 m for Monark leg ergometer, 3 m for the Tunturi and BodyGuard ergometers, and 2.4 m for Monark arm ergometer.

[e]Body mass in kilogram.

Adapted from Table D.1, American College of Sports Medicine. *ACSM's Guidelines for Exercise Testing and Prescription.* 11th ed. Philadelphia (PA): Wolters Kluwer; 2022. 548 p.

Examples

Tracy, a 58-kg woman, would like to begin an exercise program.

1. You advise Tracy to walk at 3 mph on a treadmill at 10% grade. What is her $\dot{V}O_2$?
   Walking $\dot{V}O_2$ mL $\cdot$ kg^{-1} $\cdot$ min^{-1} = (0.1 $\times$ speed) + (1.8 $\times$ speed $\times$ fractional grade) + 3.5 mL $\cdot$ kg^{-1} $\cdot$ min^{-1}
   3.0 mph $\times$ 26.8 = 80.4 m $\cdot$ min^{-1}
   10% grade = 0.10
   Walking $\dot{V}O_2$ mL $\cdot$ kg^{-1} $\cdot$ min^{-1} = (0.1 $\times$ 80.4) + (1.8 $\times$ 80.4 $\times$ 0.10) + 3.5 mL $\cdot$ kg^{-1} $\cdot$ min^{-1}
   Walking $\dot{V}O_2$ mL $\cdot$ kg^{-1} $\cdot$ min^{-1} = 26 mL $\cdot$ kg^{-1} $\cdot$ min^{-1}

2. How many METs is this exercise intensity?
   METs = $\dot{V}O_2$ mL $\cdot$ kg^{-1} $\cdot$ min^{-1} / 3.5
   METs = 26 mL $\cdot$ kg^{-1} $\cdot$ min^{-1} / 3.5
   METs = 7.43

3. Tracy decides that she would rather ride a stationary bicycle. What would be the equivalent work rate on the cycle ergometer?
   Leg cycling $\dot{V}O_{2max}$ mL $\cdot$ kg^{-1} $\cdot$ min^{-1} = (1.8 $\times$ work rate / body weight) + (3.5) + (3.5 mL $\cdot$ kg $\cdot$ min^{-1})
   26 mL $\cdot$ kg^{-1} $\cdot$ min^{-1} = (1.8 $\times$ work rate / 58) + (3.5) + (3.5 mL $\cdot$ kg^{-1} $\cdot$ min^{-1})

EXERCISE IS MEDICINE CONNECTION

Exe**R**cise is Medicine®

Morris JN, Heady JA, Raffle PAB, Roberts CG, Parks JW. Coronary heart disease and physical activity of work. *Lancet.* 1953;265(6795):1053–7.

Famed British epidemiologist Dr. Jeremy Morris was one of the pioneers in helping establish a link between physical activity and coronary heart disease (CHD). In his landmark 1953 study, Morris and colleagues (42) compared the incidence of CHD between conductors and drivers in London transport employees. Morris et al.'s main findings showed that the physically active conductors, whose job duties required climbing the stairs of London's fabled double-decker buses, had a different pattern of CHD from that of the bus drivers, who were sedentary for the majority of their workday. The physically active conductors had lower rates of CHD than the bus drivers; displayed symptoms of CHD at a much later age than the drivers, which were less severe; and had a substantially lower mortality rate of fatal myocardial infarction. Morris et al.'s findings that physical activity was protective against CHD were met with heavy skepticism from the prevailing conventional wisdom of the day, yet Morris pressed on, replicating his findings in future studies of postal workers and civil servants, consistently demonstrating the protective effects of regular physical activity and exercise in work and/or recreational pursuits. Dr. Morris's work also lends credence to the hazards of sedentary behavior, which have come under increased focus with the advent of inactivity physiology research. Thanks to the efforts of Dr. Morris, the ACSM-EP can enthusiastically educate clients that Exercise is Medicine.

$19 \text{ mL} \cdot \text{kg}^{-1} \cdot \text{min}^{-1} = (1.8 \times \text{work rate} / 58)$

$612 \text{ kg} \cdot \text{m} \cdot \text{min}^{-1} = \text{work rate}$

4. If Tracy exercises as prescribed for 30 minutes, 5 d · wk^{-1}, for 5 weeks, how many kilocalories will Tracy expend during her exercise sessions? (Assume that her caloric intake stays consistent.)

$30 \text{ min} \cdot \text{d}^{-1} \times 5 \text{ d} \cdot \text{wk}^{-1} = 150 \text{ min} \cdot \text{wk}^{-1}$

$150 \text{ min} \cdot \text{wk}^{-1} \times 5 \text{ weeks} = 750 \text{ total minutes}$

$\dot{V}O_2 = 26 \text{ mL} \cdot \text{kg}^{-1} \cdot \text{min}^{-1}$

$26 \text{ mL} \cdot \text{kg}^{-1} \cdot \text{min}^{-1} \times 58 \text{ kg} = 1{,}508 \text{ mL} \cdot \text{min}^{-1}$

$1{,}508 \text{ mL} \cdot \text{min}^{-1} / 1{,}000 = 1.508 \text{ L} \cdot \text{min}^{-1}$

$1.508 \text{ L} \cdot \text{min}^{-1} \times 5 \text{ kcal} = 7.54 \text{ kcal} \cdot \text{min}^{-1}$

$7.54 \text{ kcal} \cdot \text{min}^{-1} \times 750 \text{ minutes} = 5{,}655 \text{ kcal}$

$5{,}655 / 3{,}500 = 1.62 \text{ lb of fat}$

FITT Framework for the Development of Cardiorespiratory Fitness in Apparently Healthy People

The acronym FITT (F = frequency, I = intensity, T = time or duration, T = type or mode) provides the framework to establish an exercise prescription in healthy individuals (Table 3.4). Given the wide array of fitness levels the ACSM-EP may encounter, the FITT principle may be customized to meet the unique goals and needs of the individual. To optimize CRF, the FITT principle of exercise prescription is presented as F-Frequency (d · wk^{-1}), I-Intensity (percentage of heart rate

Table 3.4	Aerobic (Cardiovascular Endurance) Exercise Recommendations
FITT	**Recommendation**
Frequency	▪ At least 3 d $\cdot$ wk^{-1}
	▪ For most adults, spreading the exercise sessions across 3–5 d $\cdot$ wk^{-1} may be the most conducive strategy to reach the recommended amounts of physical activity.
Intensity	▪ Moderate (40%–59% HRR) and/or vigorous (60%–89% HRR) intensity is recommended for most adults.
Time	▪ Most adults should accumulate 30–60 min $\cdot$ d^{-1} ($\geq$150 min $\cdot$ wk^{-1}) of moderate-intensity exercise, 20–60 min $\cdot$ d^{-1} ($\geq$75 min $\cdot$ wk^{-1}) of vigorous-intensity exercise, or a combination of moderate- and vigorous-intensity exercise daily to attain the recommended targeted volumes of exercise.
Type	▪ Aerobic exercise performed in a continuous or intermittent manner that involves major muscle groups is recommended for most adults.

From American College of Sports Medicine. *ACSM's Guidelines for Exercise Testing and Prescription.* 11th ed. Philadelphia (PA): Wolters Kluwer; 2022. 548 p.

reserve [HRR], $\dot{V}O_{2max}$), T-Time (duration per session), and T-Type (mode of physical activity), with additional recommendations for quantifying volume (product of training frequency, exercise intensity, and exercise duration), and the implementation of progressive overload. The FITT principle of exercise prescription for CRF is summarized in Table 3.4.

The CRF components of the FITT principle have been adopted from the most recent recommendations from ACSM and the *2018 Physical Activity Guidelines for Americans.*

The recommendations for CRF using the FITT framework for exercise prescription are as follows (1,2,21):

Frequency

According to the *2018 Physical Activity Guidelines*, aerobic exercise is recommended to be performed on at least 3 d $\cdot$ wk^{-1} (2). For most adults, spreading the exercise sessions across 3–5 d $\cdot$ wk^{-1} while incorporating both moderate- and vigorous-intensity exercise options may be best to reach the recommended amount of physical activity.

Intensity

A combination of moderate- (40%–59% HRR) and/or vigorous-intensity (60%–84% HRR) exercise is recommended for most healthy individuals. Intensity may be prescribed using multiple methods such as, but not limited to, HRR, rating of perceived exertion (RPE), percentage $\dot{V}O_{2max}$, and percentage of age-predicted HR$_{max}$.

Time

Most adults are recommended to accumulate 30–60 min $\cdot$ d^{-1} of moderate-intensity exercise, 20–60 min $\cdot$ d^{-1} of vigorous-intensity exercise, or a combination of moderate- and vigorous-intensity exercise per day (1,2,21). A general guideline for aerobic exercise prescription is that 2 minutes of moderate-intensity aerobic exercise is equivalent to 1 minute of vigorous-intensity aerobic exercise (2).

Type

All types of physical activity are beneficial as long as they are of sufficient intensity and duration. Rhythmic, continuous exercise that involves major muscle groups is the most typical choice; however, for more advanced individuals, intermittent exercise such as interval training or stop-and-go sports may be used to accumulate the recommended frequency, intensity, and time needed for CRF.

 Additional Variables

Volume

Exercise volume is the product of training frequency, exercise intensity, and the duration of the exercise session. A dose-response relationship exists between physical activity and health outcomes, in which greater amounts of physical activity are associated with greater health benefits. For substantial health benefits, adults are recommended to accumulate 150 min $\cdot$ wk^{-1} of moderate-intensity aerobic exercise, or 75 min $\cdot$ wk^{-1} of vigorous-intensity aerobic exercise, or an equivalent combination of moderate and vigorous-intensity aerobic exercise per week to attain the volume of recommended physical activity (2). For additional and more extensive health benefits, adults should increase their aerobic physical activity to 300 min $\cdot$ wk^{-1} of moderate-intensity aerobic exercise, or 150 min $\cdot$ wk^{-1} of vigorous-intensity aerobic exercise, or an equivalent combination of moderate- and vigorous-intensity aerobic exercise (2).

Progression

The recommended rate of progression of an exercise program is dependent on the individual's health status, physical fitness, training responses, and exercise program goals. Therefore, progression may consist of increasing any of the components of the FITT principles as tolerated by the individual. Any progression should be made gradually, avoiding large increases in any of the FITT components to minimize risks. The progression of exercise may be from a single session per day or in multiple sessions.

Inherent within the FITT framework are the following principles of training that the ACSM-EP must consider when prescribing cardiorespiratory exercise:

Progressive Overload

The overload principle is at the foundation of all exercise prescription. To improve CRF, the individual must exercise at a level greater than accustomed to induce adaptation. The ACSM-EP can implement the overload principle by manipulating the frequency, intensity, or time of the exercise prescription. For example, if an ACSM-EP is working with a client who typically runs on a treadmill at 75% HR$_{max}$, for 30 minutes, 3 d $\cdot$ wk^{-1}, the overload principle may be adhered to by increasing the intensity of the run to 80% of HR$_{max}$, increasing the time spent running to 40 minutes, or increasing running to 4 d $\cdot$ wk^{-1}. It is important for the ACSM-EP to understand that all variables should not be increased simultaneously, as small incremental progression allows the body to adapt, which is key to reducing the risk of overuse injuries (2).

Reversibility

The principle of reversibility can be viewed as the opposite of the overload principle. Commonly referred to as the "use it or lose it" principle, the reversibility principle dictates that once cardiorespiratory training is decreased or stopped for a significant period (2–4 wk), previous improvements will reverse and decrease, and the body will readjust to the demands of the reduced physiological stimuli (3). Hard-earned gains in CRF can be lost if the training stimulus is removed, and the ACSM-EP should be aware that prior gains made with clients who have taken long breaks from training will necessitate readjusting previous exercise prescriptions.

Individual Differences

The principle of individual differences states that all individuals will not respond similarly to a given training stimulus (29). The ACSM-EP will encounter a wide range of individuals of varying age and fitness levels, each of whom will demonstrate varied responses to a given exercise stimulus. Within an exercise prescription for CRF, the ACSM-EP will encounter high and low responders because of the large genetic component that affects the degree of potential change in $\dot{V}O_{2max}$ (43). The variation in fitness levels necessitates a personalized exercise prescription based on the unique needs of the individual.

Specificity of Training

The specificity principle, also known as the SAID (specific adaptations to imposed demands) principle, is dependent on the type and mode of exercise. The specificity principle states that specific exercise elicits specific adaptations, creating specific training effects (29). For example, if an ACSM-EP is working with a client who wishes to improve his or her time in an upcoming half-marathon, the principle of specificity dictates that, in order to improve, the ACSM-EP needs to select a training stimulus specific to the activity in question. Thus, running would be the appropriate mode to select because activities such as cycling or swimming do not train the specific muscles and movement patterns needed to complete a half-marathon.

Safe and Effective Exercises Designed to Enhance Cardiorespiratory Fitness

As discussed in the introduction to the FITT framework, when designing an exercise program to develop CRF, the type of exercise that is generally prescribed to improve health and fitness is rhythmic and continuous and uses large muscle groups (21). Given the nearly unlimited number of ways to be physically active, there is no shortage of exercise options for the ACSM-EP to choose from when prescribing physical activity to enhance CRF. Exercise options can be viewed on a continuum, ranging from the relatively simple, such as brisk walking, to much more complex and vigorous, such as repeat 400-m interval sprints approaching 100% $\dot{V}O_{2max}$. Although the options to improve CRF may seem overwhelming at times, the ACSM has created a classification scheme to help the ACSM-EP make an appropriate exercise selection that matches the fitness level and unique interests of the clientele an ACSM-EP may be serving (21). Cardiovascular endurance exercises may be divided into four categories (Table 3.5):

Type A: endurance exercises requiring minimal skill or physical fitness to perform, such as walking or water aerobics

Type B: vigorous-intensity endurance exercises requiring minimal skill, such as running or spinning

Type C: endurance activities requiring skill to perform, such as cross-country skiing or in-line skating

Type D: recreational sports, such as tennis or basketball

Subsequently, the ACSM-EP can modify any activity from the four categories to best accommodate the skill level, physical fitness stage, and personal preferences of the individual or groups the ACSM-EP may be serving.

Table 3.5	Modes of Aerobic (Cardiorespiratory Endurance) Exercises to Improve Physical Fitness		
Exercise Group	**Exercise Description**	**Recommended for**	**Examples**
A	Endurance activities requiring minimal skill or physical fitness to perform	All adults	Walking, leisurely cycling, aqua-aerobics, slow dancing
B	Vigorous-intensity endurance activities requiring minimal skill	Adults (as per the preparticipation screening guidelines in Chapter 2) who are habitually physically active and/or at least average physical fitness	Jogging, running, rowing, aerobics, spinning, elliptical exercise, stepping exercise, fast dancing
C	Endurance activities requiring skill to perform	Adults with acquired skill and/or at least average physical fitness levels	Swimming, cross-country skiing, skating
D	Recreational sports	Adults with a regular exercise program and at least average physical fitness	Racquet sports, basketball, soccer, downhill skiing, hiking

Reprinted from Table D.1, American College of Sports Medicine. *ACSM's Guidelines for Exercise Testing and Prescription.* 11th ed. Philadelphia (PA): Wolters Kluwer; 2022. 548 p.

An additional method of classifying cardiorespiratory exercise that may be useful to the ACSM-EP is by weight-bearing or non–weight-bearing activities. Weight-bearing activities cause muscles and bones to work against gravity, such as jogging or aerobic dance, versus non–weight-bearing activities in which the stress on the bones, joints, and muscles is lessened, such as in cycling or swimming. Although some weight-bearing physical activity is important for bone health (2), many individuals may have orthopedic limitations that may necessitate the need to choose more nonimpact physical activity options. In addition, low-impact physical activity has a third or less of the injury risk of higher impact activities (2). Table 3.6 highlights popular exercise modalities and the advantages and disadvantages of each.

Table 3.6	Advantages and Disadvantages of Different Exercises	
Exercise	**Advantages**	**Disadvantages**
Walking	Does not require expensive equipment, special skill, or special facilities; can be done indoors or outdoors	Potential safety concerns of walking environment
Jogging/running	Easily accessible and large caloric expenditure; promotes bone health	Increased injury risk because of higher impact, environmental concerns
Bicycling	Reduced impact on bones and joints	Cost of bicycle, weather, safety of cycling environment
Swimming	Buoyancy provides great alternative for individuals with joint pain; warm moist air may benefit asthmatics	Skill level needed; chlorinated pool may aggravate respiratory conditions.
Aerobic machines	Multiple options allowing exercise, regardless of weather; many provide low-impact workout option.	Ownership and maintenance costs of home aerobic machines; use of aerobic machines may necessitate membership at fitness facility.

Interval Training

The implementation of interval training to improve CRF and/or metabolic health is an additional method of exercise prescription that the ACSM-EP may wish to consider. Interval training, broadly defined as intermittent periods of intense exercise separated by periods of recovery (44), typically consists of alternating bouts of vigorous-to-supramaximal intensity exercise (20–240 s) followed by equal or longer bouts of light-to-moderate intensity exercise (60–360 s).

Interval training has long been used in the conditioning of athletes for energy system development and performance enhancement purposes (45). However, the use of interval training within sedentary or recreationally active populations has been growing in popularity among fitness professionals (46). From an exercise efficiency standpoint, the lower exercise volume and subsequent time commitment needed for interval training could be very appealing to individuals with limited time, a common barrier to exercise participation (47).

Previous research has found that interval training elicits physiological adaptations similar to traditional endurance training despite a lower total workload, and superior physiological adaptations when total exercise dose is matched (44,48–51). When prescribing interval training, the ACSM-EP is encouraged to consider the interval training nomenclature first proposed by Weston et al. (52) that differentiate high-intensity interval training (HIIT) from sprint interval training (SIT). HIIT is traditionally performed at an intensity that is greater than the anaerobic threshold and is often performed at an intensity close to that which elicits ≥80–100% peak HR, whereas SIT is characterized by an all-out, supramaximal effort equal to or greater than the pace that elicits ≥100% $\dot{V}O_{2peak}$ (44,52). Of potential great interest to the ACSM-EP is a recent systematic review and meta-analysis of HIIT of patients with lifestyle-induced chronic diseases, which recommended that a 4 × 4 protocol (work = four intervals at 4 min at 85%–95% peak HR; rest = three intervals at 3 min at 70% peak HR, 3 d · wk^{-1}) demonstrated the biggest changes in $\dot{V}O_{2peak}$, was well tolerated, and had excellent adherence (52). Furthermore, there is emerging research for the ACSM-EP to consider as to the value of low-volume interval training (LVIT), in which a total exercise time commitment of >15 minutes can provide a potent stimulus to physiological adaptations associated with improved health (49). LVIT protocols range from the extraordinarily demanding (eight bouts of all-out 20 s efforts with 10 s rest in between; 4 d · wk^{-1}) (53–55) to much less severe protocols (two to three bouts of all-out 20 s efforts with 2–3 min rest in between; 3 d · wk^{-1}), all of which yielded significant changes in indices of metabolic health and aerobic capacity (56–59).

When prescribing interval training, the ACSM-EP can manipulate at least nine different variables that could impact the desired metabolic, cardiopulmonary, or neuromuscular responses (60,61); however, the primary factors of interest concern (a) the intensity and duration of the exercise and recovery interval and (b) the total number of intervals performed (60,61). Consistent with the principles of exercise prescription and FITT framework, the decision for the ACSM-EP to implement interval training will be dependent on initial CRF assessments, the specific goals of the clientele, and selecting the exercise modality that will best lead to exercise adherence and self-efficacy (62).

Determining Exercise Intensity

The ACSM-EP has multiple options to determine the appropriate exercise intensity when prescribing physical activity to improve CRF. Options range from direct measurements in clinical or laboratory settings to more subjective ratings based on feelings of exertion or fatigue. The precision needed to determine exercise intensity will be dependent on the unique conditions, needs, and preferences of the clientele the ACSM-EP may be serving. The ACSM-EP may consider using any of the following methods to determine exercise intensity.

Heart Rate Reserve Method

HRR, or Karvonen, method requires the ACSM-EP to determine the resting HR and maximum HR of the client. Resting HR is optimally measured in the morning while the client is in bed before rising (29), whereas maximum HR is best measured during a progressive maximal exercise test but can also be estimated via age-predicted formulas (21). The HRR is the difference between maximum HR and resting HR. Target HR will be determined by considering the habitual physical activity, exercise level, and goals of the client (21). To assign a target HR, use the following formula:

$$\text{Target HR} = [(\text{Maximum HR} - \text{Resting HR}) \times \% \text{ intensity desired}] + \text{Resting HR}$$

For example, if your client has a maximum HR of 200 bpm and a resting HR of 60 bpm and wishes to exercise at 65%–75% of HRR, the HR range would be 151–165 bpm:

$[(200 - 60) \times 65\%] + 60 = \text{Target HR of 151 bpm}$
$[(200 - 60) \times 75\%] + 60 = \text{Target HR of 165 bpm}$

Peak Heart Rate Method

The peak HR method requires the ACSM-EP to determine the client's HR_{max}. This may be accomplished from direct measurement, such as a $\dot{V}O_{2max}$ treadmill test, or maximum HR may be estimated from age-predicted formulas. Common estimation equations that the ACSM-EP may consider include the following:

- Maximum HR = 207 − (0.7 × age in yr) (63) for men and women participants in an adult fitness program with broad range of age and fitness levels
- Maximum HR = 208 − (0.7 × age in yr) (64) for healthy men and women

The ACSM-EP should be aware that each of the earlier equations might overestimate maximum HR in certain populations, whereas underestimating in others (21). The ACSM-EP is advised to use HR_{max} estimations only as a guide and to realize that estimates may not be accurate for certain individuals. Once HR_{max} has been determined, the ACSM-EP may assign a target HR by following the formula:

$$\text{Target HR} = \text{Maximum HR} \times \% \text{ intensity desired}$$

For example, if a client is 40 years old and has a selected workload of 85% of maximum HR, and the ACSM-EP chooses the equation, Maximum HR = 208 − (0.7 × age) to estimate maximum HR, the calculations would be as follows:

$$208 - (0.7 \times 40) = \text{Estimated maximum HR of 180 bpm}$$
$$180 \times 85\% = \text{Target HR of 153 bpm}$$

Peak $\dot{V}O_2$ Method

The peak $\dot{V}O_2$ method may be used if the ACSM-EP has measured or estimated the $\dot{V}O_{2max}$ of the client in a laboratory or field setting. However, one should be cautious when assigning workload on the basis of estimates because of the expected error in extrapolating HR (*e.g.*, 220 − age = standard deviation of 12–15 bpm) (21). Once the $\dot{V}O_{2max}$ has been determined, the following formula may be followed:

$$\text{Target } \dot{V}O_2 = \dot{V}O_{2max} \times \% \text{ intensity desired}$$

For example, an ACSM-EP working with an individual with a measured $\dot{V}O_{2max}$ of 60 mL · kg^{-1} · min^{-1}, with an exercise prescription of 90% maximum, would calculate the target $\dot{V}O_2$ as follows:

$$60 \times 90\% = \text{Target } \dot{V}O_{2max} \text{ of } 54 \text{ mL} \cdot kg^{-1} \cdot min^{-1}$$

Peak Metabolic Equivalent Method

In some instances, the ACSM-EP may choose the peak MET method to guide intensity. Whereas $\dot{V}O_{2max}$ is a relative measure of intensity, METs provide an absolute measure, allowing the intensity of various physical activity options to be compared with each other. Resources such as the Compendium of Physical Activities (39–41) feature extensive MET listings for a wide array physical activity options. Because 1 MET is equivalent to 3.5 mL · kg^{-1} · min^{-1}, an individual's peak MET level can be determined simply by dividing one's measured or estimated $\dot{V}O_{2max}$ by 3.5. For example, an individual with a $\dot{V}O_{2max}$ of 35 would have a peak MET level of 10 METs. Once an individual's peak MET has been determined, the ACSM-EP can prescribe exercise at an appropriate workload by using a target MET level. The formula for determining target METs is as follows (25):

$$\text{Target METs} = (\% \text{ intensity desired}) \, [(\dot{V}O_{2max} \text{ in METs}) - 1] + 1$$

For example, for an individual with a $\dot{V}O_{2max}$ of 35 mL · kg^{-1} · min^{-1} and who wants to exercise at an intensity of 70% the target METs can be calculated as follows:

Step 1: $\dot{V}O_{2max}$ in METs = 35 mL · kg^{-1} · min^{-1} / 3.5 mL · kg^{-1} · min^{-1} = 10 METs
Step 2: Target METs = (0.70) (10 − 1) + 1
Step 3: Target METs = (0.70) (9) + 1
Step 4: Target METs = 6.3 + 1 = 7.3 METs

Thus, the ACSM-EP could select activities from the Compendium of Physical Activities that correspond with a MET level between 7.0 and 7.5.

$\dot{V}O_2$ Reserve Method

The $\dot{V}O_2$ reserve ($\dot{V}O_2R$) method may be used when the ACSM-EP has directly measured or estimated the client's $\dot{V}O_{2max}$ and resting $\dot{V}O_2$ in a laboratory setting. The $\dot{V}O_2R$ is the difference between $\dot{V}O_{2max}$ and resting $\dot{V}O_2$. Target $\dot{V}O_2R$ will be dependent on the goals of the client:

$$\text{Target } \dot{V}O_2R = [(\dot{V}O_{2max} - \dot{V}O_{2rest}) \times \text{intensity desired}] + \dot{V}O_{2rest}$$

For example, for a client with a $\dot{V}O_{2max}$ of 35 mL · kg^{-1} · min^{-1}, a resting $\dot{V}O_2$ of 3.5 mL · kg^{-1} · min^{-1}, and a selected workload of 60% $\dot{V}O_2R$, the calculation would be as follows:

$$[(35 - 3.5) \times 60\%] + 3.5 = \text{Target } \dot{V}O_2R \text{ of } 22.4 \text{ mL} \cdot kg^{-1} \cdot min^{-1}$$

Talk Test Method

The talk test is a simple and convenient method to determine exercise intensity, especially for individuals who may be unaccustomed to physical activity. The talk test is a subjective measure of relative intensity, which helps differentiate between moderate and vigorous physical activity. If an individual is able to talk, but not sing, the physical activity is considered moderate. However, once the intensity of the activity increases to a point at which an individual is not able to say more than a few words without pausing for breath, the intensity would be considered vigorous (65). Once comfortable speech is no longer possible, the vigorousness of the exercise may be outside the range for the individual to sustain, and the ACSM-EP can instruct the client to stop or reduce the level of effort.

Perceived Exertion Method

The perceived exertion method is another subjective rating of how hard one may be working. Perceived exertion is most commonly measured through Borg's RPE Scale, which ranges from 6 to 20, 6 meaning no exertion at all and 20 meaning maximal exertion. An RPE range from 10 to 16 should be safe and health promoting for most adults (66).

An additional perceived exertion scale for the ACSM-EP to be familiar with is Borg's Category Ratio Scale, commonly abbreviated as CR-10. The CR-10 uses a scale of 0–10, in which sitting is 0 and the highest level of effort possible is 10. A CR-10 range of 5–8 corresponds with moderate- (CR 5–6) and vigorous-intensity (CR 7–8) physical activity (2).

 Abnormal Responses to Exercise

Increases in HR, SBP, and ventilation, from rest, are normal responses to cardiorespiratory exercise in healthy individuals. Although the benefits and overall safety of cardiorespiratory exercise have been well established (1,21), the ACSM-EP should be aware of potential abnormal responses to exercise that may necessitate the termination of exercise session and possibly require medical assistance. The "How to Read the Signs: Stopping an Exercise Test" box provides general indications for stopping an exercise session (21). The ACSM-EP should consider that individuals who are detrained, returning from injury, or unaccustomed to physical activity may have a very low tolerance and capacity for exercise, and thus, in addition to the general indications highlighted in the box, the ACSM-EP should be judicious in the design of initial exercise prescriptions and communicate with his or her clients at all times.

HOW TO   Read the Signs: Stopping an Exercise Test

The following lists general indications the ACSM-EP should watch for when giving an exercise test; being able to recognize these will avoid injury or problems.

- Onset of angina or angina-like symptoms
- Drop in SBP of ≥10 mm Hg with an increase in work rate, or if SBP decreases below the value obtained in the same position before testing
- Excessive rise in BP: SBP >250 mm Hg and/or DBP >115 mm Hg
- Shortness of breath, wheezing, leg cramps, or claudication
- Signs of poor perfusion: light-headedness, confusion, ataxia, pallor, cyanosis, nausea, or cold and clammy skin
- Failure of HR to increase with increased exercise intensity
- Noticeable change in heart rhythm by palpation or auscultation
- Participant requests to stop
- Physical or verbal manifestations of severe fatigue
- Failure of the testing equipment

Contraindications to Cardiovascular Training Exercises

The ACSM-EP will undoubtedly encounter individuals with physical or clinical limitations in which the risks of exercise testing and subsequent prescription may outweigh any potential benefits (21). Individuals with cardiac, respiratory, metabolic, or musculoskeletal disorders should be supervised by clinically trained personnel when beginning an exercise program (see Chapter 8 for more details on these populations). A thorough preexercise screening, obtaining informed consent, and review of medical history are necessary for the ACSM-EP to identify potential contraindications and to ensure the safety of the client (21). However, it is inevitable that the ACSM-EP will encounter apparently healthy clients who develop chest pain, breathing difficulty, musculoskeletal distress, or other worrisome symptoms during an exercise session. The ACSM-EP should immediately stop exercise, ensure client safety, and then refer the client to the appropriate health care professional. Please refer to Chapter 2 for greater detail on properly assessing risk factors.

Effect of Common Medications on Cardiorespiratory Exercise

It is not uncommon for the ACSM-EP to work with clients who may be taking prescribed and over-the-counter (OTC) medications. Although it is never the role of the ACSM-EP to administer, prescribe, or educate clients on the use or effects of medications, it is important for the ACSM-EP to understand the potential complex interactions of medication and exercise. Medications may alter HR, BP, and/or exercise capacity (21), and therefore, clients taking medication should be strongly encouraged to communicate any changes in medication routines to the ACSM-EP. Please refer to Chapter 8 for the effect common OTC and prescription medications have on exercise.

Signs and Symptoms of Common Musculoskeletal Injuries Associated with Cardiorespiratory Exercise

Although a properly designed CRF prescription results in minimal risk (2), the ACSM-EP should be aware of the signs and symptoms of common musculoskeletal injuries associated with exercise (67).

- Exquisite point tenderness
- Pain that persists even when the body part is at rest
- Joint pain
- Pain that does not go away after warming up
- Swelling or discoloration
- Increased pain with weight-bearing activities or with active movements
- Changes in normal bodily functions

Previous research suggests the risk of injury is directly related to the increase in the amount of physical activity performed (2), and thus, the chance for musculoskeletal injury increases as the individual performs exercise at greater levels of frequency and intensity (67). The individuals with whom the ACSM-EP may work will come from varied backgrounds, presenting a wide array of potential intrinsic and extrinsic risk factors that may predispose clients to injury. Common risk factors that the ACSM-EP may encounter are listed as follows (modified from 68):

Intrinsic Risk Factors

History of previous injury
Inadequate fitness or conditioning

Body composition
Bony alignment abnormalities
Strength or flexibility imbalances
Joint or ligamentous laxity
Predisposing musculoskeletal disease

Extrinsic Risk Factors

Excessive load on the body
Type of movement
Speed of movement
Number of repetitions
Footwear
Surface
Training errors
Excessive distances
Fast progression
High intensity
Running on hills
Poor technique
Fatigue
Adverse environmental conditions
Air quality
Darkness
Heat or cold
High humidity
Altitude
Wind
Worn or faulty equipment

Once the ACSM-EP has addressed potential risks, strategies to minimize injury may be employed, especially in at-risk individuals. The ACSM-EP should consider the age, level of fitness, and prior experience of potential clients when individualizing exercise prescriptions (2). It is recommended that the ACSM-EP use an intensity relative to a client's fitness level to usher in a desired level of effort while slowly increasing the duration and frequency of physical activity before increasing intensity (2). Previous research suggests that the injury risk is increased in individuals who run, participate in sports, and engage in more than $1.25\,\text{h} \cdot \text{wk}^{-1}$ of physical activity (69). Therefore, when working with clients who may fit this profile, the ACSM-EP should take steps to minimize potential risk via proper assessment, client education, and exercise program design. In addition, the ACSM-EP should closely monitor increases in physical activity, especially in previously sedentary individuals, as the larger the overload to one's baseline physical activity, the greater the chance of injury (2).

Effects of Heat, Cold, or High Altitude on the Physiological Response to Exercise

Hot, cold, and high-altitude environments alter the typical physiological response to exercise. These extreme environments have the ability to stress our physiological systems to their maximal capacity and may negatively impact exercise performance before acclimatization (70). The ACSM-EP should be aware of the major challenges of exercise in hot, cold, and/or high-altitude environments and the impact of these environments on the physiological response to exercise.

Heat Stress

Hot environments reduce the body's ability to dissipate heat and thus promote an increase in core body temperature. In an effort to maintain a neutral body temperature when exposed to a hot environment, sweat rate and skin blood flow increase to promote heat loss (71). Although critical for heat dissipation, increased sweat rates and skin blood flow challenge the capacity of the cardiovascular system and may be the primary performance-limiting factors during exercise in a hot environment (72). Increased sweat rates can cause a reduction in plasma volume and increase the risk of dehydration (73). Furthermore, increased sweat rates may lead to a decrease in SV, which then prompts an increase in HR to maintain cardiac output at submaximal workloads. This "HR drift," or elevated HR at submaximal loads, can decrease performance dramatically in a hot environment. Increased blood flow to the skin circulation comes at the expense of reduced blood flow to the working muscle (19). In addition to these primary cardiovascular limiting factors, other physiological changes occur during exercise in the heat that may contribute to reduced performance capacity, such as diminished central nervous system function and increased muscle glycogen utilization (72). The ACSM-EP should expect higher HR values at a given workload during exercise in the heat compared with exercise in a thermoneutral environment. HR may not reach a steady state during prolonged, submaximal intensity exercise because of the increased sweat rate, leading to cardiovascular drift. During cardiovascular drift, HR climbs over time, thereby decreasing overall performance (74,75). Staying well hydrated during exercise may help attenuate cardiovascular drift.

Cold Stress

Exercise in a cold environment facilitates heat loss produced during exercise. However, long duration exercise events in a cold environment increase the risk of hypothermia. If core temperature is challenged, the body attempts to increase heat production and limit heat loss via shivering and vasoconstriction of blood vessels in the skin (72). Individuals with greater subcutaneous fat mass have an advantage at limiting heat loss in cold environments, as their thicker subcutaneous fat layer acts as form of insulation or barrier between the warm blood and the cold environment (76). The HR and cardiac output responses to exercise in a cold environment are similar to those of a thermoneutral environment (77); however, respiratory rate is higher at a given submaximal intensity and $\dot{V}O_{2max}$ may be slightly lower. The primary barrier to maximal performance in a cold environment may simply be the extra work associated with wearing bulky clothing during exercise. Bulky clothing increases the energy cost of exercise because of the extra weight of the clothing, alterations in movement resulting in augmented extraneous work, and increased friction as layers of clothing slide against each other during exercise (78,79). Overall, the effect on $\dot{V}O_{2max}$ in a cold environment is negligible compared with that in a hot environment.

Altitude

Barometric pressure decreases with ascent to altitude. The partial pressure of oxygen (PO_2) is equal to the product of barometric pressure and the percentage of oxygen in the air. For example, the partial pressure at sea level is 760 mm Hg and the percentage of oxygen in dry air is 20.93%. Thus, the PO_2 at sea level is approximately 159 mm Hg ($PO_2 = 760 \times 0.2093$). If, however, you are at an altitude at which barometric pressure is only 550 mm Hg, the PO_2 now decreases to 115 mm Hg ($PO_2 = 760 \times 0.2093$). It is a common misconception that the "thin air" at altitude has less oxygen than the air at sea level; the percentage of oxygen in the air remains the same at all elevations in the stratosphere. It is the change in barometric pressure that causes the PO_2 to decrease at altitude and reduces our ability to provide oxygen to working muscles. In response to lower PO_2

at altitude, pulmonary ventilation increases. During the initial days of high-altitude exposure, SV decreases (80,81), yet HR increases (82) to a greater extent, causing an increase in cardiac output at a given submaximal exercise intensity (83). There is typically no change noted in BP (81). Other changes that could affect performance when transferring to altitude include weight loss (84) and sleep disturbances (83). To stay at the same relative intensity of exercise (*e.g.*, submaximal HR), unacclimatized individuals will have to reduce the absolute intensity of exercise at a higher altitude because of the greater difficulty of doing exercise at the higher altitude. The time it takes to become acclimatized to altitude varies greatly between individuals and also depends on the local altitude. It is best for the ACSM-EP to assume that there will need to be a significant reduction in intensity and duration of exercise during the initial days of altitude adjustment, but that over time, exercise should become more comfortable.

Acclimatization When Exercising in a Hot, Cold, or High-Altitude Environment

Acclimatization is the process of physiological adaptation that occurs in response to changes in the natural environment. *Acclimation* is a related term but refers to the process of physiological adaptation that occurs in response to experimentally induced changes in climate, such as an environmental chamber in a research laboratory (72). Both acclimatization and acclimation can improve exercise performance in extreme environments.

Heat acclimatization has been shown to elicit many favorable physiological responses that may improve exercise performance in a hot environment (85–87), such as lower core body temperature, lower skin temperature, higher sweat rate, higher plasma volume, lower HR at a specific workload, lower perception of effort, and improved conservation of sodium. As a whole, these physiological adaptations improve heat dissipation from the body to the environment and limit cardiovascular strain.

In general, heat acclimatization requires gradual exposure to exercise in the heat on consecutive days. In order for complete adaptation to occur, 2–4 hours of moderate- to high-intensity exercise in a hot environment for 10 consecutive days is suggested (88). Partial acclimation to the heat can also be completed by training athletes wearing additional layers of clothing in a cool environment (89). Although the acclimation benefits of this technique will never reach the magnitude of true acclimatization, it may serve a purpose when the alternative choice is no acclimation. The first few days of exercise in a hot or humid environment should be light in intensity with frequent rest periods provided. The intensity of exercise should gradually build to the length and intensity desired for performance. The benefits of acclimation decrease after only days of exposure to another climate (90) and completely dissipate after approximately 2–3 weeks (86). Thus, acclimatization to the heat occurs annually in individuals living in areas where there is a wide variation in climate across the course of the year.

Cold acclimatization causes the shivering threshold to be reset to a lower mean skin temperature. This is a positive adaptation as it suggests cold acclimatization enhances the ability to maintain heat production through means besides shivering (91). In addition, cold acclimatization has also been shown to improve maintenance of hand and feet temperatures (92), potentially attenuating the loss of dexterity that normally accompanies cold extremities.

Altitude acclimatization requires adjusting to the lower PO_2. The lower PO_2 at altitude stimulates the production of additional red blood cells (erythropoiesis) to increase the oxygen-carrying capacity of the blood. Within hours of ascent to altitude, the kidneys increase the release of the hormone erythropoietin to stimulate erythropoiesis, but this process takes time, and the full benefits of erythropoiesis may not take effect for 4 or more weeks (72). After the oxygen-carrying capacity of the blood is restored via erythropoiesis, the HR, SV, cardiac output, and pulmonary ventilation responses to exercise revert back to more typical conditions. Today, many endurance athletes use altitude training to improve their athletic performance by practicing the "live high, train low" strategy (93), which is a unique strategy of gaining the benefits of high-altitude acclimatization ("live high") and the maintenance of high-intensity training at sea level ("train low") to occur in synchrony. After returning to sea level, the benefits of altitude acclimatization have been shown to last up to 3 weeks (93).

The Case of Lakisha

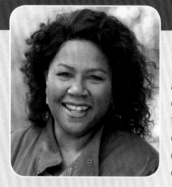

Lakisha is a 45-year-old stay-at-home mother of three who has had sporadic adherence to an exercise program since her youngest child was born. Lakisha enjoys being outside and prefers outdoor settings to indoors when she has the time to exercise, but recently, it has been a challenge to accumulate 75 minutes a week of structured walking around the neighborhood. Lakisha is not a big fan of running or similar high-impact activities but does enjoy walking as her primary mode of exercise. Lakisha is planning a family vacation to the Grand Canyon in 3 months and wants to make sure she improves her fitness so she and her husband can hike some of the more challenging trails at the park. A sample program using the FITT framework with considerations for volume and progression follows.

Physical Data

Resting BP: 119/77 mm Hg
Resting HR: 58 bpm
Weight: 155 lb
Height: 65 in
Body mass index: 25.8 kg $\cdot$ m^{-2}
Body fat percentage measured by calipers: 27.5
CRF measured by Ebbeling Single-Stage Submaximal Treadmill Walking Test: $\dot{V}O_{2max}$: 35.2 mL $\cdot$ kg^{-1} $\cdot$ min^{-1}

Lakisha's 12-Week Walking Program for Cardiorespiratory Fitness

Weeks 1–4

Frequency (F): 3 d $\cdot$ wk^{-1}
Intensity (I): perceived exertion method, CR-5; ~50% HRR
Time (T): week 1: 25 minutes; week 2: 30 minutes; week 3: 35 minutes; week 4: 40 minutes
Type (T): walking
Volume (V): week 1: 75 minutes; week 2; 90 minutes; week 3: 105 minutes; week 4: 120 minutes

Weeks 5–8

F: 4 d $\cdot$ wk^{-1}
I: walking: 3 d $\cdot$ wk^{-1} at CR-5, ~50% HRR
  Interval walking: 1 d $\cdot$ wk^{-1} of interval walking at CR-7, ~70% HRR for 1 minute, 1-minute regular pace at CR-5
T: walking: week 5: 40 minutes; week 6: 45 minutes; week 7: 50 minutes; week 8: 55 minutes
  Interval walking: week 5: 15 minutes; week 6: 15 minutes; week 7: 15 minutes; week 8: 15 minutes
T: walking, interval walking
V: week 5: 135 minutes; week 6: 150 minutes; week 7: 165 minutes; week 8: 180 minutes

Weeks 9–12

F: 5 d $\cdot$ wk^{-1}
I: walking: 3 d $\cdot$ wk^{-1} at CR-6, ~55% HRR
  Interval walking: 1 d $\cdot$ wk^{-1} of interval walking at CR-8, ~75% HRR for 1 minute, 1-minute regular pace at CR-5
  Hill climbing: 1 d $\cdot$ wk^{-1} at CR-7, ~70% HRR
T: walking: week 9: 55 minutes; week 10: 60 minutes; week 11: 60 minutes; week 12: 65 minutes
  Interval walking: week 9: 20 minutes; week 10: 20 minutes; week 11: 30 minutes; week 12: 30 minutes
Hill climbing: week 9: 10 minutes; week 10: 10 minutes; week 11: 15 minutes; week 12: 15 minutes
T: walking, interval walking, hill climbing
V: week 9: 195 minutes; week 10: 210 minutes; week 11: 225 minutes; week 12: 240 minutes

SUMMARY

Assessing and prescribing exercise is both an art and a science; it should be taken as a serious responsibility by the ACSM-EP. There are numerous means of assessing CRF so that the ACSM-EP can accommodate a wide range of clientele safely. Also, the FITT principle provides a framework of prescribing exercise that also allows for tremendous individual variation.

Properly assessing and prescribing exercise can play a significant role in helping individuals initiate an enjoyable exercise program. Using the most appropriate assessment and prescription techniques limits all types of risk and provides the individual with a solid foundation to begin his or her lifetime of physical activity.

STUDY QUESTIONS

1. $\dot{V}O_{2max}$ is commonly used as a marker of aerobic exercise capacity. Explain the science behind this concept. In other words, how is oxygen used in the body and why does a greater maximal oxygen uptake equate to greater aerobic exercise capacity?
2. Write out the Fick equation. Define each term within the Fick equation and discuss how each component of the equation changes with exercise training.
3. A 165-lb woman is walking on the treadmill at 3 mph at 2% grade for 30 minutes. Calculate the $\dot{V}O_2$, MET, and estimated caloric expenditure of this activity.
4. Using the HRR method, what is the target HR range for a 55-year-old man with a resting HR of 72 bpm, with an exercise prescription of 60%–70% of HRR?

REFERENCES

1. Garber CE, Blissmer B, Deschenes MR, et al. American College of Sports Medicine position stand. Quantity and quality of exercise for developing and maintaining cardiorespiratory, musculoskeletal, and neuromotor fitness in apparently healthy adults: guidance for prescribing exercise. *Med Sci Sports Exerc.* 2011;43(7):1334–59.
2. U.S. Department of Health and Human Services. *2018 Physical Activity Guidelines for Americans.* 2nd ed. [Internet]. Washington (DC): U.S. Department of Health and Human Services. Available from: https://health.gov/paguidelines/secondedition/pdf/Physical_Activity_Guidelines_2nd_edition.pdf.
3. Plowman SA, Smith DL. *Exercise Physiology for Health, Fitness, and Performance.* 3rd ed. Philadelphia (PA): Lippincott Williams & Wilkins; 2011. 744 p.
4. Medbø JI, Mohn AC, Tabata I, Bahr R, Vaage O, Sejersted OM. Anaerobic capacity determined maximal accumulated O_2 deficit. *J Appl Physiol.* 1988;64(1):50–60.
5. Di Prampero P, Boutellier U, Pietsch P. Oxygen deficit and stores at onset of muscular exercise in humans. *J Appl Physiol.* 1983;55(1 Pt 1):146–53.
6. Hickson RC, Bomze HA, Holloszy JO. Faster adjustment of O2 update to the energy requirement of exercise in the trained state. *J Appl Physiol.* 1978;44(6):877–81.
7. Powers S, Dodd S, Beadle R. Oxygen uptake kinetics in trained athletes differing in VO_{2max}. *Eur J Appl Physiol.* 1985;54(3):306–8.
8. Gaesser G, Brooks G. Metabolic bases of excess post exercise oxygen consumption: a review. *Med Sci Sports Exerc.* 1984;16(1):29–43.
9. Hill A. The oxidative removal of lactic acid. *J Physiol.* 1914;48:x–xi.
10. Astrand PO, Rodahl K, Dahl HA, Stromme SB. *Textbook of Work Physiology: Physiological Bases of Exercise.* 4th ed. Champaign (IL): Human Kinetics; 2003. 656 p.
11. Astrand PO, Cuddy TE, Saltin B, Stenberg J. Cardiac output during submaximal and maximal work. *J Appl Physiol.* 1964;19:268–74.
12. Holmgren A, Johnson B, Sjostrand T. Circulatory data in normal subjects at rest and during exercise in recumbent position, with special reference to the stroke volume at different work intensities. *Acta Physiol Scand.* 1960;49:343–63.
13. Christie J, Sheldahl LM, Tristani FE, Sagar KB, Ptacin JJ, Wann S. Determination of stroke volume and cardiac output during exercise: comparison of two-dimensional and Doppler echocardiography, Fick oximetry, and thermodilution. *Circulation.* 1987;76:539–47.

14. Higginbotham MB, Morris KG, Williams RS, McHale PA, Coleman RE, Cobb FR. Regulation of stroke volume during submaximal and maximal upright exercise in normal man. *Circ Res*. 1986;58(2):281–91.

15. Gledhill N, Cox D, Jamnik V. Endurance athletes' stroke volume does not plateau: major advantage is diastolic function. *Med Sci Sports Exerc*. 1994;26(9):1116–21.

16. Zhou B, Conlee RK, Jensen R, Fellingham GW, George JD, Fisher AG. Stroke volume does not plateau during graded exercise in elite male distance runners. *Med Sci Sports Exerc*. 2001;33:1849–54.

17. Wasserman K, Whipp BJ, Koyal SN, Beaver WL. Anaerobic threshold and respiratory gas exchange during exercise. *J Appl Physiol*. 1973;35(2):236–43.

18. Dawson B. Exercise training in sweat clothing in cool conditions to improve heat tolerance. *Sports Med*. 1994;17(4):233–44.

19. Rowell LB. *Human Cardiovascular Control*. New York (NY): Oxford University Press; 1993. 500 p.

20. Kraemer, WJ, Fleck SJ, Deschenes MR. *Exercise Physiology: Integrating Theory and Application*. Philadelphia (PA): Lippincott Williams & Wilkins; 2012. 512 p.

21. American College of Sports Medicine. *ACSM's Guidelines for Exercise Testing and Prescription*. 11th ed. Philadelphia (PA): Wolters Kluwer; 2022. 548 p.

22. Pickering TG, Hall JE, Appel LJ, et al. Recommendations for blood pressure measurement in humans and experimental animals: part 1: blood pressure measurement in humans: a statement for professionals from the Subcommittee of Professional and Public Education of the American Heart Association Council on High Blood Pressure Research. *Hypertension*. 2005;45:142–61.

23. U.S. Department of Health and Human Services. *The Seventh Report of the Joint National Committee on Prevention, Detection, Evaluation, and Treatment of High Blood Pressure — Complete Report*. Bethesda (MD): National Heart, Lung, and Blood Institute; 2004. 104 p.

24. American College of Sports Medicine. *ACSM's Health-Related Physical Fitness Assessment Manual*. 5th ed. Philadelphia (PA): Wolters Kluwer; 2018. 177 p.

25. American College of Sports Medicine. *ACSM's Resource Manual for Guidelines for Exercise Testing and Prescription*. 6th ed. Philadelphia (PA): Lippincott Williams & Wilkins; 2010. 868 p.

26. Adams GM, Beam WC. *Exercise Physiology: Laboratory Manual*. 5th ed. New York (NY): McGraw-Hill; 2008. 320 p.

27. Astrand PO, Rhyming I. A nomogram for calculation of aerobic capacity (physical fitness) from pulse rate during submaximal work. *J Appl Physiol*. 1954;7(2):218–21.

28. YMCA of the USA. *YMCA Fitness Testing and Assessment Manual*. Champaign (IL): Human Kinetics; 1989. 247 p.

29. McArdle WD, Katch FI, Katch VL. *Exercise Physiology: Nutrition, Energy, and Human Performance*. 7th ed. Philadelphia (PA): Lippincott Williams & Wilkins; 2010. 1104 p.

30. Brouha L. The step test: a simple method of measuring physical fitness for muscular work in young men. *Res Quart Exerc Sport*. 1991;14:31–6.

31. Kline GM, Porcari JP, Hintermeister R, et al. Estimation of $\dot{V}O_{2max}$ from a one-mile track walk, gender, age, and body weight. *Med Sci Sports Exerc*. 1987;19(3):253–9.

32. Cooper KH. A means of assessing maximal oxygen intake. Correlation between field and treadmill testing. *JAMA*. 1968;203(3):201–4.

33. Cooper KH. Testing and developing cardiovascular fitness within the United States Air Force. *J Occup Med*. 1968;10(11):636–9.

34. Astrand PO. Aerobic work capacity in men and women with specific reference to age. *Acta Physiol Scand*. 1960;49(Suppl 169):45–60.

35. Mariz JS, Morrison JF, Peter J. A practical method of estimating an individual's maximal oxygen uptake. *Ergonomics*. 1961;4:97–122.

36. Astrand PO. Principles of ergometry and their implications in sport practice. *Int J Sports Med*. 1984;5:102–5.

37. Blair SN, Kohl HW, Barlow CE, Paffenbarger RS, Gibbons LW, Macera CA. Changes in physical fitness and all-cause mortality: a prospective study of healthy and unhealthy men. *JAMA*. 1995;273:1093–8.

38. Wei M, Kampert JB, Barlow CE, et al. Relationship between low cardiorespiratory fitness and mortality in normal-weight, overweight, and obese men. *JAMA*. 1999;282(16):1547–53.

39. Ainsworth BE, Haskell WL, Leon AS, et al. Compendium of physical activities: classification of energy costs of human physical activities. *Med Sci Sports Exerc*. 1993;25(1):71–80.

40. Ainsworth BE, Haskell WL, Whitt MC, et al. Compendium of physical activities: an update of activity codes and MET intensities. *Med Sci Sports Exerc*. 2000;32(Suppl 9):S498–516.

41. Ainsworth BE, Haskell WL, Herrmann SD, et al. 2011 Compendium of physical activities: a second update of codes and MET values. *Med Sci Sports Exerc*. 2011;43(8):1575–81.

42. Morris JN, Heady JA, Raffle PA, Roberts CG, Parks JW. Coronary heart disease and physical activity of work. *Lancet*. 1953;265(6795):1053–7.

43. Wilmore JH, Costill DL, Kenney WL. *Physiology of Sport and Exercise*. 4th ed. Champaign (IL): Human Kinetics; 2008. 592 p.

44. MacInnis MJ, Gibala MJ. Physiological adaptations to interval training and the role of exercise intensity. *J Physiol*. 2017;595(9):2915–30.

45. Laursen PB, Jenkins DG. The scientific basis for high-intensity interval training: optimising training programmes and maximising performance in highly trained endurance athletes. *Sports Med*. 2002;32(1):53–73.

46. Thompson WR. Worldwide survey of fitness trends for 2019. *ACSMs Health Fit J*. 2018;22(6):10–17.

47. Gibala MJ. High-intensity interval training: a time-efficient strategy for health promotion? *Curr Sports Med Rep*. 2007;6(4):211–3.

48. Gist NH, Fedewa MV, Dishman RK, Cureton KJ. Sprint interval training effects on aerobic capacity: a systematic review and meta-analysis. *Sports Med*. 2014;44(2):269–79.

49. Gillen JB, Gibala MJ. Is high-intensity interval training a time-efficient exercise strategy to improve health and fitness? *Appl Physiol Nutr Metab*. 2014;39(3):409–12.

50. Milanović Z, Sporiš G, Weston M. Effectiveness of high-intensity interval training (HIT) and continuous endurance training for VO$_{2max}$ improvements: a systematic review and meta-analysis of controlled trials. *Sports Med.* 2015;45(10):1469–81.

51. Batacan RB Jr, Duncan MJ, Dalbo VJ, Tucker PS, Fenning AS. Effects of high-intensity interval training on cardiometabolic health: a systematic review and meta-analysis of intervention studies. *Br J Sports Med.* 2017;51(6):494–503.

52. Weston KS, Wisløff U, Coombes JS. High-intensity interval training in patients with lifestyle-induced cardiometabolic disease: a systematic review and meta-analysis. *Br J Sports Med.* 2014;48(16):1227–34.

53. Ma JK, Scribbans TD, Edgett BA, et al. Extremely low-volume, high-intensity interval training improves exercise capacity and increases mitochondrial protein content in human skeletal muscle. *Open J Mol Integr Physiol.* 2013;3(4):202–10.

54. Tabata I, Irisawa K, Kouzaki M, Nishimura K, Ogita F, Miyachi M. Metabolic profile of high intensity intermittent exercise. *Med Sci Sports Exerc.* 1997;29(3):390–5.

55. Tabata I, Nishimura K, Kouzaki M, et al. Effects of moderate-intensity endurance and high intensity intermittent training on anaerobic capacity and VO$_{2max}$. *Med Sci Sports Exerc.* 1996;28(10):1327–30.

56. Allison MK, Baglole JH, Martin BJ, MacInnis MJ, Gurd BJ, Gibala MJ. Brief intense stair climbing improves cardiorespiratory fitness. *Med Sci Sports Exerc.* 2017;49(2):298–307.

57. Gillen JB, Martin BJ, MacInnis MJ, Skelly LE, Tarnopolsky MA, Gibala MJ. Twelve weeks of sprint interval training improves indices of cardiometabolic health similar to traditional endurance training despite a five-fold lower exercise volume and time commitment. *PLoS One.* 2016;11(4):e0154075.

58. Gillen JB, Percival ME, Skelly LE, et al. Three minutes of all-out intermittent exercise per week increases skeletal muscle oxidative capacity and improves cardiometabolic health. *PLoS One.* 2014;9(11):e111489.

59. Metcalfe RS, Babraj JA, Fawkner SG, Vollaard NBJ. Towards the minimal amount of exercise for improving metabolic health: beneficial effects of reduced-exertion high-intensity interval training. *Eur J Appl Physiol.* 2012;112(7):2767–75.

60. Buchheit M, Laursen PB. High-intensity interval training, solutions to the programming puzzle: part I: cardiopulmonary emphasis. *Sports Med.* 2013;43(5):313–38.

61. Buchheit M, Laursen PB. High-intensity interval training, solutions to the programming puzzle: part II: anaerobic energy, neuromuscular load and practical applications. *Sports Med.* 2013;43(10):927–54.

62. Trost SG, Owen N, Bauman AE, Sallis JF, Brown W. Correlates of adults' participation in physical activity: review and update. *Med Sci Sport Exerc.* 2002;34(12):1996–2001.

63. Gellish RL, Goslin BR, Olson RE, McDonald A, Russi GD, Moudgil VK. Longitudinal modeling of the relationship between age and maximal heart rate. *Med Sci Sports Exerc.* 2007;39(5):822–9.

64. Tanaka HK, Monahan KD, Seals DR. Age-predicted maximal heart rate revisited. *J Am Coll Cardiol.* 2001;37(1):153–6.

65. Reed JL, Pipe AL. The talk test: a useful tool for prescribing and monitoring exercise intensity. *Curr Opin Cardiol.* 2014;29(5):475–480.

66. Dishman RK. Prescribing exercise intensity for healthy adults using perceived exertion. *Med Sci Sports Exerc.* 1994;26(9):1087–94.

67. Howley ET, Franks BD. *Health Fitness Instructor's Handbook.* 4th ed. Champaign (IL): Human Kinetics; 2003. 573 p.

68. Renstrom P, Kannus P. Prevention of sports injuries. In: Strauss RH, editor. *Sports Medicine.* Philadelphia (PA): WB Saunders; 1992. p. 307–29.

69. Hootman JM, Macera CA, Ainsworth BE, Martin M, Addy CL, Blair SN. Association among physical activity level, cardiorespiratory fitness, and risk of musculoskeletal injury. *Am J Epidemiol.* 2001;154(3):251–8.

70. Suzuki Y. Human physical performance and cardiorespiratory responses to hot environments during submaximal upright cycling. *Ergonomics.* 1980;23(6):527–42.

71. Kenney WL, Munce T. Aging and human temperature regulation. *J Appl Physiol.* 2003;95:2598–603.

72. Cheung SS. *Advanced Environmental Exercise Physiology.* Champaign (IL): Human Kinetics; 2010. 272 p.

73. Shirreffs SM, Armstrong LE, Cheuvront SN. Fluid and electrolyte needs for preparation and recovery from training and competition. *J Sports Sci.* 2004;22:57–63.

74. Ekelund LG. Circulatory and respiratory adaptation during prolonged exercise of moderate intensity in the sitting position. *Acta Physiol Scand.* 1967;69(4):327–40.

75. Johnson JM, Rowell LB. Forearm and skin vascular responses to prolonged exercise in man. *J Appl Physiol.* 1975;39(6):920–92.

76. Smith RM, Hanna JM. Skinfolds and resting heat loss in cold air and water: temperature equivalence. *J Appl Physiol.* 1975;39:93–102.

77. Doubt TJ. Physiology of exercise in the cold. *Sports Med.* 1991;11(6):367–81.

78. Patton JF. The effects of acute cold exposure on exercise performance. *J Appl Sport Sci Res.* 1988;2:72–8.

79. Teitlebaum A, Goldman RF. Increased energy cost with multiple clothing layers. *J Appl Physiol.* 1972;32(6):743–4.

80. Alexander JK, Hartley LH, Modelski M, Grover RF. Reduction of stroke volume during exercise in man following ascent to 3,100 m altitude. *J Appl Physiol.* 1967;23(6):849–58.

81. Reeves JT, Groves BM, Sutton JR, et al. Operation Everest II: preservation of cardiac function at extreme altitude. *J Appl Physiol.* 1987;63:531–9.

82. Grover R, Reeves JT, Grover EB, Leathers JE. Muscular exercise in young men native to 3,100 m altitude. *J Appl Physiol.* 1967;22(3):555–64.

83. West JB. Physiology of extreme altitude. In: Fregly MJ, Blatteis CM, editors. *Handbook of Physiology: Section 4: Environmental Physiology.* vol 2. New York (NY): Oxford University Press; 1996. 1586 p.

84. Pugh LG. Physiological and medical aspects of the Himalayan Scientific and Mountaineering Expedition, 1960-61. *BMJ.* 1962;2:621–33.

85. Armstrong LE, Costill DL, Fink WK. Changes in body water and electrolytes during heat acclimation: effects of dietary sodium. *Aviat Space Environ Med.* 1987;58(2):143–8.

86. Armstrong LE, Maresh CM. The induction and decay of heat acclimatization in trained athletes. *Sports Med.* 1991;12(5):302–12.

87. Cheung SS, McLellan TM. Influence of heat acclimation, aerobic fitness, and hydration effects on tolerance during uncompensable heat stress. *J Appl Physiol.* 2000;84(5):1731–9.

88. Lind AR, Bass DE. Optimal exposure time for development of acclimatization to heat. *Fed Proc.* 1963;22:704–8.

89. Davis JH. Anaerobic threshold: review of the concept and directions for future research. *Med Sci Sports Exerc.* 1985;17(1):6–21.

90. Lee SM, Williams WJ, Schneider SM. Role of skin blood flow and sweating rate in exercise thermoregulation after bed rest. *J Appl Physiol.* 2002;92(5):2026–34.

91. Brück K. Basic mechanisms in longtime thermal adaptation. In: Szelenyi Z, Szekely M, editors. *Advances in Physiological Science.* vol 23. Oxford (United Kingdom): Pergamon Press; 1980. p. 263–73.

92. Stocks J, Taylor N, Tipton M, Greenleaf J. Human physiological responses to cold exposure. *Aviat Space Environ Med.* 2004;75(5):444–57.

93. Levine BD, Stray-Gundersen J. "Living high-training low": effect of moderate-altitude acclimatization with low-altitude training on performance. *J Appl Physiol.* 1997;83(1):102–12.

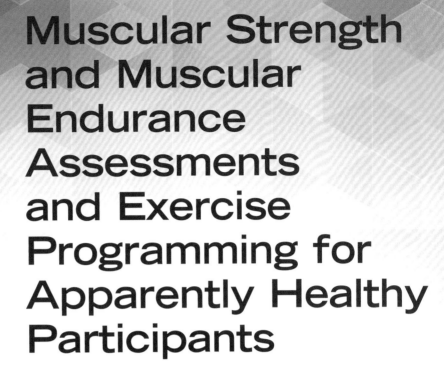

CHAPTER 4

Muscular Strength and Muscular Endurance Assessments and Exercise Programming for Apparently Healthy Participants

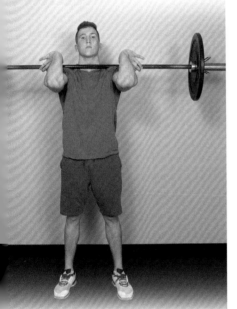

OBJECTIVES

- To understand the importance of muscular strength and muscular endurance for health and fitness.
- To describe the basic structure and function of muscle.
- To explain the fundamental principles of resistance training.
- To identify resistance training program variables.
- To compare different resistance exercise modalities.
- To design resistance training programs for apparently healthy adults and individuals with medically controlled disease.

INTRODUCTION

The development of muscular strength and muscular endurance is an essential component of health-related physical fitness. There has been a tremendous increase in the number of scientific publications on this topic, and resistance training has become a popular worldwide fitness trend (1–3). Regular participation in a training program designed to enhance muscular strength and muscular endurance can improve the health, fitness, and performance of men and women with different needs, goals, and abilities (4–8). As such, resistance exercise is often considered "medicine" due to the well-established benefits associated with this type of training (7). The American College of Sports Medicine (ACSM) recommends participating in a comprehensive fitness program that includes resistance exercise, and the *Physical Activity Guidelines for Americans* report recognizes the potential benefits of muscle-strengthening activities for adults (4,9,10).

In addition to enhancing all components of muscular fitness (*i.e.*, muscular strength, muscular endurance, and muscular power), higher levels of muscular fitness are associated with significantly better cardiometabolic risk profiles, lower risk of all-cause mortality, fewer cardiovascular disease (CVD) events, and improvements in health-related quality of life (11–16). Resistance training can improve body composition as well as selected health-related biomarkers including blood glucose levels and blood pressure in individuals with mild or moderate hypertension (7,9,17–19). Regular participation in muscle-strengthening activities can lower the risk of developing Type 2 diabetes (17,20) and can improve glycemic control and insulin sensitivity in adults with this condition (21,22). Furthermore, regular participation in a resistance training program can significantly reduce depressive symptoms and improve anxiety symptoms among adults regardless of health status (23,24).

EXERCISE IS MEDICINE CONNECTION

Exe$R$cise is Medicine®

Yang J, Christophi C, Farioli A, et al. Association between push-up exercise capacity and future cardiovascular events among active adult men. *JAMA Netw Open*. 2019;2(2):e188341.

Although increased aerobic fitness is associated with a lower risk of CVD and improved longevity, little is known about the association between field measures of muscular fitness and future cardiovascular events among adults. Yang and colleagues (25) assessed push-up performance and exercise tolerance in male firefighters. The number of push-ups performed was divided into five categories in increments of 10 push-ups for each category and exercise tolerance tests were performed on a treadmill. Participants were followed for 10 years, and the main outcome was incident CVD-related events. Significant negative associations were found between increasing push-up capacity and CVD events. Participants able to perform more than 40 push-ups had a significantly lower risk of CVD-related events compared with those completing fewer than 10 push-ups. Also, push-up capacity was more strongly associated with CVD risk than aerobic capacity. These findings suggest that push-up performance may be a simple, low-cost measure for assessing functional status and CVD risk in healthy adult men (25).

Resistance training over months or years can increase bone mass and has proven to be a valuable strategy for preventing the loss of bone mass in people with osteoporosis (26,27). Importantly, regular participation in a resistance training program can contribute to an improved health-related quality of life by enhancing physical function, building strength reserves, and enabling people to do what they enjoy while maintaining their independence (8,14,28,29). Moreover, there is growing interest in increasing patient's muscular strength with preoperative resistance training to improve physical fitness and postoperative outcomes (30,31). Concerted efforts are needed to educate adults about the unique benefits of resistance exercise and incorporate this type of training into fitness programs because a vast majority of adults do not engage in adequate muscle-strengthening activity (32,33).

This rest of this chapter provides a basic overview of muscle structure and function; highlights the fundamental principles of resistance exercise; and outlines program design considerations for developing, implementing, and progressing resistance training programs that are consistent with individual needs, goals, and abilities. In this chapter, the term *resistance training* (also known as *strength training*) refers to a specialized method of physical conditioning that involves the progressive use of a wide range of resistive loads and a variety of training modalities designed to enhance muscular fitness. The term *resistance training* should be distinguished from the terms *bodybuilding* and *powerlifting*, which are competitive sports.

Basic Structure and Function

An understanding of the basic structure and function of the muscular system is important for designing fitness programs and optimizing training adaptations. Many of the fundamental principles of resistance training discussed later in this chapter are grounded in an understanding of muscle structure and function. Although the body has more than 600 skeletal muscles that vary in shape and size, the basic purpose of skeletal muscle, especially during resistance training, is to provide force to move the joints of the body in different directions.

The smallest contractile unit within a muscle is called a sarcomere, which is made up of different proteins. A myofibril consists of many sarcomeres, and groups of myofibrils make up a single muscle fiber or muscle cell. Different types of connective tissue called fascia surround these structures and create a stable, yet flexible, environment. The connective tissue in muscle is like a rubber band that stretches and recoils to provide added force to a muscle contraction.

The muscles that are the primary movers of a joint are called the agonists, and the muscles that assist in that movement are called synergists. Antagonists are muscles that oppose a movement. For example, during the biceps curl exercise, the biceps brachii and brachialis are the agonists for that movement, the brachioradialis is the synergist, and the triceps brachii is the antagonist. Only the parts of a muscle that are used during an exercise will adapt to the training stress; furthermore, different training loads stimulate different amounts of muscle. That is why it is important to understand muscle structure and be aware that different training loads recruit different muscle fibers.

Muscle Fiber Types and Recruitment

Although skeletal muscle is made up of thousands of muscle fibers, there are generally two types of muscle fibers. Type I fibers (also called slow-twitch fibers) have a high oxidative capacity and a lower contractile force capability and are better for endurance activities. Type II fibers (also called fast-twitch fibers) have a high glycolytic capacity and a higher contractile force capability and are better for strength and power activities. Although each muscle fiber type has various subtypes

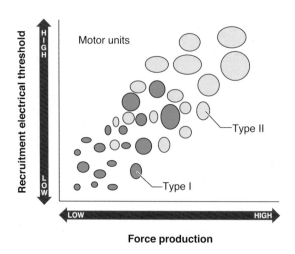

FIGURE 4.1. Size principle of motor unit recruitment. (Reproduced with permission from Haff G, Triplett N, editors. *Essentials of Strength Training and Conditioning.* 4th ed. Champaign [IL]: Human Kinetics; 2016. 752 p.)

(type IIa, IIx), the ratio of type I and II fibers in the body varies for each person and depends mainly on hereditary factors. Regular resistance training may cause a small change in fiber type composition, but these changes are primarily from one subgroup of fiber to another subgroup of fiber. Thus, resistance training will not convert type I fibers to type II fibers, but different training loads and different movement speeds can alter the involvement of different types of muscle fibers and influence exercise-induced changes in muscle metabolism (34,35).

Because muscle fibers that are not stimulated will not reap the benefits of training, it is important to understand how muscle fibers are recruited for action. Muscle fibers are innervated by a motor neuron, and this neuromuscular gathering is called a motor unit. Although each motor unit is composed of either all type I or all type II fibers, the size of a motor unit as well as the number of fibers within a motor unit varies within different muscles. The size principle of motor unit activation states that motor units are recruited from the smallest to the largest, depending on the force production demands. Smaller or low-threshold motor units (mostly type I fibers) are recruited first, and larger or high-threshold motor units (mostly type II fibers) are recruited later, depending on the demands of the exercise (Fig. 4.1) (3,34).

Training with heavy loads that can be lifted only four to six times (*e.g.*, a 4–6 repetition maximum [RM]) will activate higher threshold motor units than training with a load that can be lifted 12–15 times (34,36). However, even if heavy loads are lifted, low-threshold motor units will be recruited first, and then high-threshold motor units will be activated as needed to produce the necessary force. Although exceptions exist, to recruit high-threshold motor units, specific types of resistance exercise that involve lifting heavy loads, moving lighter loads at a fast velocity, or both are needed to achieve a training effect in these muscle fibers (3,34). The principle that different training loads and power requirements recruit different types and numbers of motor units is the rationale for the concept of training periodization or program variation discussed later in this chapter (37).

Types of Muscle Action

Muscles can perform different types of muscle actions. When a weight is lifted, the involved muscles normally shorten, and this is called a concentric muscle contraction, and when a weight is lowered, the involved muscles lengthen, and this is called an eccentric muscle action. For example, when an individual extends the hips and knees from a parallel squat position to the standing phase,

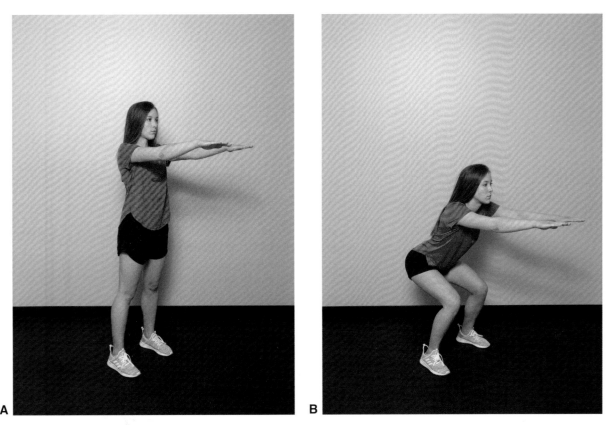

FIGURE 4.2. Squat without weights starting position **(A)** and squat position **(B)**.

the gluteus maximus and vastus lateralis perform concentric muscle contractions (Fig. 4.2). The gluteus maximus and vastus lateralis perform eccentric muscle action when the body is lowered from the standing phase to the parallel squat position. If a muscle is activated but no movement at the joint takes place, the muscle action is called isometric (or static). This type of muscle action takes place during the standing phase of the squat exercise when the weight is held stationary and no visible movement occurs. Isometric muscle actions also occur when the weight is too heavy to lift any further. This typically happens during the "sticking point" of an exercise when the force produced by the muscle equals the resistance (3).

The amount of force produced by a muscle is dependent on a number of factors, including the type of muscle action. The highest force produced occurs during an eccentric muscle action, and maximal force produced during an isometric muscle action is greater than that seen during a concentric contraction. Furthermore, as the velocity of movement increases, the amount of force that is generated decreases during a concentric muscle contraction and increases during an eccentric muscle action (Fig. 4.3) (34). This is an important consideration when designing resistance training programs because high force development during maximal eccentric muscle actions has been linked to increased delayed-onset muscle soreness (38). Although eccentric muscle actions are a potent stimulus for increases in muscle size and strength due to its unique physiological and mechanical properties (38), a gradual and progressive introduction to resistance training is warranted to reduce the risk of a muscle strain. Even resistance-trained individuals who accentuate the eccentric phase of a lift can experience muscle soreness for several days after an exercise session, albeit they are less susceptible to muscle damage than untrained adults (39,40).

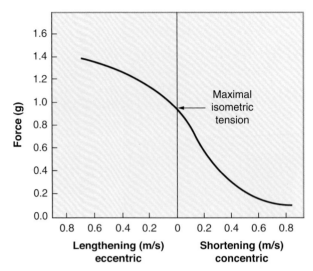

FIGURE 4.3. Force–velocity relationship. (From American College of Sports Medicine. *ACSM's Foundations of Strength Training and Conditioning*. Philadelphia [PA]: Lippincott Williams & Wilkins; 2012. 560 p.)

Assessment Protocols

Muscular fitness can be assessed by a variety of laboratory and field-based measures. Results from muscular fitness tests can provide valuable information about an individual's baseline fitness and can be used to design individualized resistance training programs that target muscle weaknesses and imbalances. Moreover, data from periodic muscular fitness assessments can be used to highlight a client's progress and provide positive feedback that can promote exercise adherence. For safety purposes, physically inactive adults with known cardiovascular, metabolic, and/or renal disease or any signs or symptoms suggestive of these diseases should seek medical clearance before beginning a resistance training program (41,42). Physically active asymptomatic adults may begin a light- to moderate-intensity resistance training program without medical clearance and progress gradually as tolerated (41). More information on exercise preparticipation health screening can be found in Chapter 2.

Muscular fitness tests are specific to the muscle groups being assessed, the velocity of movement, the joint range of motion (ROM), and the type of equipment available (3). Furthermore, no single test exists for evaluating total-body muscular fitness, so professionals need to carefully select and supervise the most appropriate muscular fitness tests for each client. Also, individuals should participate in several familiarization/practice sessions before testing and adhere to a specific protocol (including repetition duration and ROM) to obtain a reliable fitness score that can be used to track fitness changes over time. Because an acute bout of static stretching may have adverse effects on subsequent strength and power performance, large amplitude dynamic movements (also known as dynamic stretching) and test-specific activities should precede muscular fitness testing (43–45).

An initial assessment of muscular fitness and a change in muscular strength or muscular endurance over time can be based on the absolute value of the weight lifted or the total number of repetitions performed with a given resistance. Alternatively, a relative value can be determined by assessing the maximum number of repetitions performed at a percentage (*e.g.*, 70%) of the 1-RM pre- and posttesting. Although population-specific norms are available for most health-related muscular fitness tests, when strength comparisons are made between individuals, the values should be expressed as relative values (per kilogram of body weight). For example, a client who weighs 100 kg and lifts 75 kg on the chest press exercise has a relative strength score of

$0.75 \text{ kg} \cdot \text{kg}^{-1}$, whereas a client who weighs 80 kg and lifts the same amount of weight on the same exercise has a relative strength score of $0.94 \text{ kg} \cdot \text{kg}^{-1}$. Although both clients have the same absolute strength on the chest press exercise, the lighter client has a higher measure of relative upper body strength, and this is an important consideration when comparing individual strength performance between clients.

Assessing Muscular Strength

Muscular strength can be assessed in fitness facilities with different measures. For example, static or isometric strength can be measured conveniently using handgrip dynamometers. Although static or isometric strength measures are specific to the muscle group and joint angle being tested, handgrip strength has been found to be a valid marker of functional status and mortality in adults (46,47). When administering the handgrip test, it is important to consider the position of the shoulder, elbow, forearm, and wrist (48). The ACSM Certified Exercise Physiologist® (ACSM-EP®) should adjust the grip bar so the second joint of the fingers fits snugly over the handle and participants should hold the handgrip dynamometer in line with the forearm at the level of the thigh away from the body. Two trials should be allowed with each hand and the highest value attained from either hand (to the nearest kilogram) should be recorded (9).

The 1-RM, which is the heaviest weight that can be lifted only once using proper technique, is the standard muscular strength assessment (3). However, a multiple RM such as a 5-RM or a 10-RM can also be used to provide valuable information regarding an individual's resistance training program. For example, if a client was training with an 8- to 12-RM weight, the performance of a 10-RM test could provide an index of training-induced changes over time. The ACSM-EP should consider the number of warm-up sets and rest intervals between trials when performing RM testing. For example, additional warm-up sets and longer rest intervals between trials may be needed if participants are lifting heavy weights during 1-RM trials.

Procedures for administering 1-RM (or multiple-RM) strength tests after the familiarization period and an adequate warm-up are outlined in the "How to Assess One Repetition Maximum or Multiple Repetition Maximum" box (3,9). The general testing procedures for administering a 1-RM or a multiple RM are similar because both tests require maximal effort on the last trial.

HOW TO | **Assess One Repetition Maximum or Multiple Repetition Maximum**

1. Warm up for 5–10 min with low-intensity aerobic exercise and dynamic stretching.
2. Perform a warm-up with a submaximal load on the specific exercise used for testing.
3. After a brief rest, perform a second warm-up set with a moderate load (about 50%–70% of perceived capacity).
4. Attempt a 1-RM lift (or any multiple of 1-RM); if successful, rest approximately ~3 min before the next trial.
5. Increase resistance progressively depending on the effort required for the previous trial (5%–10% for upper body and 10%–20% for lower body). If lift is successful, rest ~3 min before next attempt. Continue testing until a failed attempt occurs. A 1-RM should be obtained within four trials to avoid excessive fatigue.
6. The final weight lifted successfully with proper exercise technique should be recorded as the absolute 1-RM or multiple-RM.

Notably, the prediction accuracy of multiple-RM testing improves as the RM gets closer to the 1-RM (49). A familiarization period is particularly important for individuals with no prior resistance exercise experience because they need to learn proper exercise technique and be taught how to produce maximal effort during the test. A proper familiarization period (*e.g.*, two to three practice sessions for each exercise) will likely achieve appropriate familiarization and reliability for RM strength testing (50,51). Moreover, communication between the ACSM-EP and the client can help determine a progression pattern of loading with reasonable accuracy. Properly trained spotters are needed to ensure the safety of strength testing procedures, particularly during the performance of free weight exercises such as the bench press and back squat.

Normative data for the chest press and leg press exercises are available in *ACSM's Guidelines for Exercise Testing and Prescription* (9). However, additional research is needed to provide norms for different exercises and different types of resistance training equipment because 1-RM performance is significantly greater on weight machines than free weights (49,52).

Assessing Muscular Endurance

Muscular endurance is the ability to perform repeated contractions over a period and is typically assessed with field measures such as the push-up test (Fig. 4.4). This test can be used independently or in combination with other tests of muscular endurance to screen for muscle weaknesses and aid in the exercise prescription. Procedures for administering the push-up test are described in

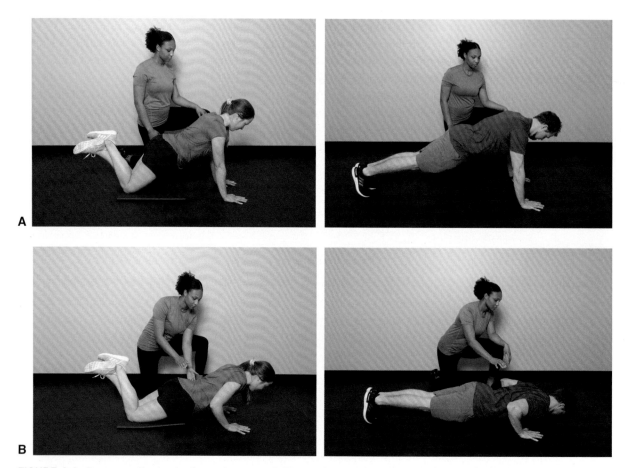

FIGURE 4.4. Proper positioning for the push-up test. **A.** The starting positions for women and men. **B.** The downward positions for women and men.

the "How to Assess Upper Body Strength and Endurance with the Push-Up Test" box. Normative data for the push-up test is available in *ACSM's Guidelines for Exercise Testing and Prescription* (9). Of note, overweight individuals may find this test difficult to perform, and poor results obtained during testing may discourage participation in an exercise program. The ACSM-EP should carefully consider which tests are appropriate for each individual and most likely to yield beneficial information. As an alternative, muscular endurance may also be evaluated using a set percentage of 1-RM, with the ACSM-EP determining how many repetitions an individual can successfully perform using, for example, 70% on an individual's 1-RM for any given exercise.

Fundamental Principles of Resistance Training

Although adults should be encouraged to incorporate resistance training into their exercise routine, unstructured and inconsistent programming does not ensure that muscular fitness gains will occur. Training programs need to be based on fundamental training principles and carefully prescribed to optimize training outcomes and maximize exercise adherence. Although factors such as initial level of fitness, resistance training experience, heredity, age, sex, nutritional status, and health habits (*e.g.*, sleep) will influence the rate and magnitude of adaptation that occurs, there are seven fundamental principles that can help determine the effectiveness of all resistance training programs. These principles are (a) *Progression*, (b) *Regularity*, (c) *Overload*, (d) *Creativity*, (e) *Enjoyment*, (f) *Specificity*, and (g) *Supervision*. These basic principles can be remembered as the PROCESS of resistance training program design (53).

Principle of Progression

The principle of progression refers to the fact that the demands placed on the body must be continually and progressively increased over time to achieve long-term gains in muscular fitness. This does not mean that heavier weights should be used every workout but rather that over time, the physical stress placed on the body should gradually become more challenging to continually stimulate adaptations and avoid accommodation or staleness resulting from the same training program (3,54). Without a more challenging exercise stimulus that is consistent with individual needs, goals, and abilities, the human body has no reason to adapt any further. This principle is related to the law of diminishing returns because the rate and magnitude of training-induced adaptations will become limited if training variables remain constant (3). Notably, after the first few months of resistance training and strength gains, the threshold for training-induced adaptations is higher (*i.e.*, harder to attain) as individuals move closer to their genetic ceiling (3).

At the start of a resistance training program, the 10-RM on the leg press might be 50 kg, which is likely an adequate stimulus to promote adaptations. But as training progresses, 10 repetitions with 50 kg would be suboptimal for stimulating gains in muscle fitness strength as 50 kg "feels easy" for 10 repetitions. If the training load is not increased at a rate that is compatible with the training-induced adaptations that are occurring, no further gains in muscular fitness will occur. A reasonable guideline for a beginner is to increase the training weight about 5%–10% a week and to decrease the repetitions by two to four when a given load can be performed for the desired number of repetitions with proper exercise technique. For example, if an adult client can perform 12 repetitions of the leg press exercise with proper exercise technique using 50 kg, the client should increase the weight to 55 kg and decrease the repetitions to 8 in order to continually make gains in muscular strength. A more conservative approach would be to follow the "2 plus 2" rule (55). That is, once this client can perform two or more additional repetitions over the assigned repetition goal on two consecutive workouts, weight should be added to the leg press exercise during the next

HOW TO   Assess Upper Body Strength and Endurance with the Push-Up Test

1. Explain the purpose of the test to the client (to determine how many push-ups can be completed as a reflection of upper body muscular endurance).

2. Inform clients of proper breathing technique (to exhale with the effort, which occurs when pushing away from the floor).

3. The push-up test usually is administered with men starting in the standard "down" position (hands pointing forward and under the shoulder, back straight, and head up, using the toes as the pivotal point). For women, the modified knee push-up position is often used, with legs together, lower leg in contact with mat, ankles plantarflexed, back straight, hands shoulder width-apart, and head up, using the knees as the pivotal point. (Note: Some men will need to use the modified position, and some women can use the full-body position. However, norms are established using the full-body position for males and the modified position for females.)

4. The subject must raise the body by straightening the elbows and return to the "down" position, until the chin touches the mat. The stomach should not touch the mat.

5. For both men and women, the subject's back must be straight at all times, and the subject must push up to a straight-arm position.

6. Demonstrate the test and allow the client to practice if desired.

7. Remind the client that the maximal number of push-ups performed consecutively without rest is counted as the score.

8. Begin the test when the client is ready. Stop the test when the client strains forcibly or is unable to maintain the appropriate exercise technique within two repetitions.

Descriptions of procedures are adapted from the American College of Sports Medicine. *ACSM's Guidelines for Exercise Testing and Prescription.* 11th ed. Philadelphia (PA): Wolters Kluwer; 2022. 548 p.

training session. Alternatively, the client could increase the number of sets, increase the number of repetitions, or add another leg exercise to the exercise routine (55).

Individuals who have achieved a desired level of muscular fitness may not need to progress the training program to maintain that level of performance. However, program variation is important for exercise adherence, and experienced exercisers may benefit from periodically changing program variables to keep the training stimulus fresh and challenging. For example, altering the mode of resistance training, changing the exercise order, or increasing the weekly set volume can limit training plateaus (37,56).

Principle of Regularity

In order to make continued gains in muscular fitness, resistance training should be performed regularly at least two times per week (10). Although the optimal training frequency may depend on training status, training volume, and training goals (57), two to three training sessions per week on nonconsecutive days are reasonable for most adults. Inconsistent training will result in only modest training adaptations, and periods of inactivity will result in a decrease in muscular strength and size (58). This concept is known as reversibility because strength gains will be lost when resistance training stops as training-induced adaptations cannot be stored. Although adequate recovery is needed between resistance training sessions, the principle of regularity states that long-term gains in muscular fitness will be realized only if the program is performed on a consistent basis.

Principle of Overload

The overload principle is a basic tenet of all resistance training programs. The overload principle simply states that to enhance muscular fitness, the body must exercise at a level beyond that at which it is normally stressed (59). For example, an adult who can easily complete 10 repetitions with 20 kg while performing a chest press exercise must increase the weight, the repetitions, or the number of sets if the individual wants to increase upper body strength. Otherwise, if the training stimulus is not increased beyond the level to which the muscles are accustomed, training adaptations will not be maximized even if other aspects of the training program are well designed. Although overload is typically manipulated by changing the exercise intensity, duration, or frequency, adding more complex exercises to a training program is another way to place greater overload on the body (60). For example, progressing from a weight machine leg press to a free weight squat can place a new training demand on the body.

Principle of Creativity

The creativity principle refers to the imagination and ingenuity that can help to optimize training-induced adaptations and enhance exercise adherence. Because an intimidating gym environment, a lack of confidence in using exercise equipment, and limited support from family friends may be a barrier to attendance (61), creative approaches for designing and implementing exercise programs are needed. For example, the provision of exercise variety and technology-based exercise interventions have been found to provide a creative means for promoting physical activity in adults (62). In order for clients to remain engaged and interested in resistance training, an ACSM-EP will need to use creative thinking to facilitate the development of training programs that are safe, effective, and enjoyable. By creatively incorporating new training equipment and corrective exercises into the training program, the ACSM-EP can help clients overcome barriers, address limitations, and maintain interest in resistance exercise (37,60,63). Depending on each client's needs, abilities, and goals, implements such as battle ropes, medicine balls, kettlebells, or suspension trainers can be incorporated into resistance training programs to optimize strength gains, increase energy expenditure, enhance adherence, promote enjoyment, and stimulate an ongoing interest in this type of exercise (64–66).

Although the quantitative aspects of resistance training and its physiological adaptations are important considerations, the qualitative aspects of exercise program design should not be overlooked (67). This is where the art and science of designing resistance training programs come into play because the principles of exercise science need to be balanced with imagination and creativity. Sharing experiences with other certified professionals can help to foster creative expression and spark an appreciation for original ideas related to the design of resistance training programs. By taking time to reflect on the design and implementation of resistance training programs, creative solutions to challenging situations can be identified. Notwithstanding the critical importance of exercise safety and proper technique, novelty and training variety are important for stimulating strength development (37,60,68).

Principle of Enjoyment

Enjoyment of physical activity is an important determinant of long-term participation in recreational fitness activities and structured exercise programs (69,70). The principle of enjoyment states that participants who genuinely enjoy exercising are more likely to adhere to the exercise program and achieve training goals. Although encouragement from the ACSM-EP and support from family and friends can influence exercise behaviors (61), the enjoyment an individual feels during and after a resistance training session can facilitate the sustainability of the desired behavior (64,71,72).

Although resistance training programs should be challenging, clients should have the competence and confidence in their physical abilities to perform the exercises or activities with energy and vigor. As such, enjoyment can be defined as a balance between skill and challenge (73). If the resistance training program is too advanced, clients will be anxious and will lose interest.

Conversely, if the training program is too easy, clients will become bored. Resistance training programs should be matched with the physical abilities of the participants in order for the training experience to be enjoyable. ACSM-certified professionals who provide immediate and meaningful feedback on challenging exercises can help clients negotiate demanding situations and therefore maintain a state of enjoyment while training.

Principle of Specificity

The principle of specificity refers to the distinct adaptations that take place as a result of the training program. For example, the adaptations to resistance training are specific to the muscle actions, velocity of movement, exercise ROM, muscle groups trained, energy systems involved, and intensity and volume of training (36,74). The principle of specificity is often referred to as the SAID principle (which stands for specific adaptations to imposed demands). In terms of designing resistance training programs, only muscle groups that are trained will make desired adaptations in selected parameters of muscular fitness. Exercises such as the squat and leg press can be used to enhance lower body strength, but these exercises will not affect upper body strength.

In addition, the adaptations that take place in a muscle or muscle group will be as simple or as complex as the stress placed on them. For example, because basketball requires multiple-joint and multiplanar movements in the sagittal (*i.e.*, left to right), frontal (*i.e.*, front to back), and transverse (*i.e.*, upper to lower) planes, it seems prudent for basketball players to include muscle actions and complex movements that closely mimic the demands of their sport. Anatomical views of the sagittal, frontal, and transverse planes of the human body are shown in Figure 4.5. An understanding of basic biomechanics and exercise movements that take place in these planes will aid in

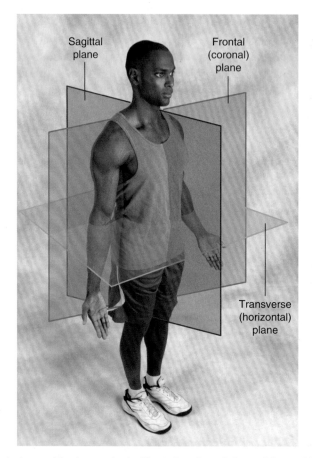

FIGURE 4.5. Anatomical planes of the human body. (From American College of Sports Medicine. *ACSM's Resources for the Personal Trainer.* 6th ed. Philadelphia [PA]: Wolters Kluwer; 2021. 650 p.)

the appropriate selection of exercises that are consistent with specific movement patterns, muscle actions, and joint angles that need to be trained.

It is also important that the exercises and joint ranges of motion in the training program are consistent with the demands of the target activity. Hence, the specificity principle also applies to the design of resistance training programs for individuals who want to enhance their abilities to perform activities of daily life such as stair climbing and yard work, which require multiple-joint and multiplanar movements. Observations of a sport or activity (with or without video analysis) can provide the ACSM-EP with information regarding the relevant movements and appropriate ranges of motion that are particularly important to train. The potential benefits of movement-specific resistance training are highlighted by the growing popularity of medicine balls, stability balls, kettlebells, and other exercise devices that are often used to enhance rotational strength, muscle power, postural control, and agility.

Principle of Supervision

The principle of supervision states that the safety and efficacy of exercise programs are maximized when qualified fitness professionals supervise activities while providing instruction and encouragement (72,75,76). There is strong evidence of a relationship between program leadership and participation in resistance training, and clients who participate in supervised resistance training programs are likely to make greater gains in muscular fitness and performance than unsupervised training (72,76–78). By providing meaningful feedback on movement skill technique during resistance training sessions, the ACSM-EP can enhance a client's resistance training self-efficacy and, in turn, improve adherence and training-induced outcomes (72,78). Moreover, a qualified supervising individual can dispel the misperceptions associated with resistance training and remind clients that heavy weights are not only for elite athletes and that well-designed training will not result in "bulky muscles" unless that is desired. Qualified supervision is a critical component of any resistance training program particularly for beginners who need education and instruction on proper exercise technique, appropriate training loads, and general resistance training guidelines.

Adults who participate in supervised resistance training programs tend to self-select higher training loads and, consequently, have higher levels of maximal strength (79). Because most men and women tend to self-select resistance training loads that are below recommended training intensities (80–82), specific instruction is needed to gradually increase the training load to optimize resistance training skill competency and strength development. Resistance training programs are most effective when they are designed and supervised by qualified fitness professionals who understand the PROCESS of resistance exercise program design (37,53,72).

 ## Program Design Considerations

Because most adults are not meeting current muscle strengthening recommendations, tailored interventions and qualified supervision and instruction are warranted (3,32,33). Resistance training programs should be based on a participant's health status, current fitness level, training experience, personal interests, and individual goals. In addition, fitness professionals should consider the number of days per week their client can resistance train. By assessing the needs of each participant and applying the fundamental principles of training to the program design, safe and effective resistance training programs can be developed for each individual. Of note, the health status of each participant should be assessed before participating in a resistance training program because it is important to identify "at-risk" individuals who may need medical clearance and a modification of their exercise prescription (41). Risk assessment procedures can be found in Chapter 2.

An important factor to consider when designing resistance training programs is the participant's current fitness status and/or previous experience resistance training. Those who have the least experience resistance training tend to have a greater capacity for improvement compared with those who have been resistance training for several years. Although any reasonable resistance training program can be used to increase the muscle strength of untrained individuals, more advanced programs are needed to produce desirable adaptations in trained individuals. As noted previously, the potential for adaptation gradually diminishes as resistance training experience increases. Thus, as individuals gain experience with resistance training, more complex programs are needed to make continual gains in muscular fitness (60,68,83).

Types of Resistance Training

Different types of resistance training have proven to be effective for enhancing muscular fitness (3,34,54). Although each type of resistance exercise has advantages and disadvantages, there are several important factors to consider when selecting one type of training over another or including multiple types within a given training program. The most common types of resistance training include dynamic constant external resistance (DCER) training, variable resistance training, isokinetics, and plyometrics.

Dynamic Constant External Resistance Training

DCER training is the most common method of resistance training for enhancing muscular fitness. DCER describes a type of training in which the weight lifted does not change during the lifting (concentric) and lowering (eccentric) phase of an exercise. Although the term *isotonic* was traditionally used to describe this type of training, this term literally means constant (*iso*) tension (*tonic*). Because tension exerted by a muscle as it shortens varies with the mechanical advantage of the joint and the length of the muscle fibers at a particular joint angle, the term *isotonic* does not accurately describe this method of resistance exercise.

Different types of training equipment, including free weights (*e.g.*, barbells and dumbbells), weight machines, and medicine balls, and endless combinations of sets and repetitions, can be used for DCER training. Weight machines generally limit the user to fixed planes of motion. However, they are easy to use and are ideal for isolating muscle groups. Free weights and medicine balls are less expensive and can be used for a wide variety of different exercises that require greater proprioception, balance, and coordination. In addition to improving health and fitness, DCER training is commonly used to enhance motor performance skills and sports performance. For example, weightlifting exercises such as the power clean (Fig. 4.6) and snatch are recognized as some of the most effective exercises for increasing muscle power because they require explosive movements and a more complex neural activation pattern than do traditional strength-building exercises such as the chest press or leg extension (68,84).

During DCER training, the weight lifted does not change throughout the ROM. Because muscle tension can vary significantly when a DCER exercise is performed, the heaviest weight that can be lifted throughout a full ROM is limited by the strength of a muscle at the weakest joint angle. As a result, DCER exercise provides enough resistance in some parts of the movement range but not enough resistance in others. For example, during the barbell bench press exercise, more weight can be lifted during the last part of the exercise than in the first part of the movement when the barbell is being pressed off the chest.

In an attempt to overcome this limitation, mechanical devices that operate through a lever arm or cam have been designed to vary the resistance throughout the exercise's ROM. These devices are known as variable resistance machines and theoretically force the muscle to contract maximally throughout the ROM by varying the resistance to match the exercise strength curve. These machines can be used to train all the major muscle groups, and by automatically changing the resistive force throughout the movement range, they provide proportionally less resistance in weaker segments of the movement and more resistance in stronger segments of the movement.

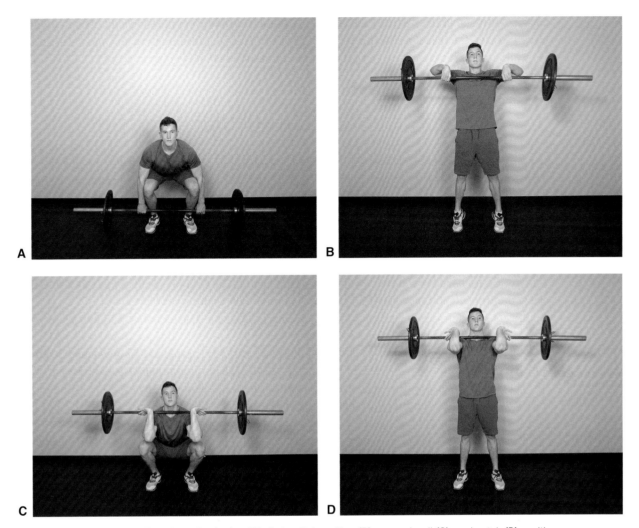

FIGURE 4.6. The clean: beginning **(A)**, first pull, transition **(B)**, second pull **(C)**, and catch **(D)** positions.

Like all weight machines, variable resistance machines provide a specific movement path that makes the exercise easier to perform. To overcome this limitation, resistance-trained individuals can use bands or chains to create variable resistance during free weight training (3). For example, if an elastic band is attached to each end of a barbell and secured to the floor during the bench press exercise, more resistance will be applied to the barbell the farther the band is stretched. Likewise, if heavy chains are attached to both ends of a barbell during the squat exercise, progressively more weight will be applied to the barbell as the chains are lifted off the floor.

Isokinetics

Isokinetic training involves dynamic muscular actions that are performed at a constant angular limb velocity. This type of muscular action requires specialized equipment, and isokinetic devices are designed to train movements around various joints (*e.g.*, knee, hip, shoulder, elbow). Isokinetic dynamometers generally are not used in fitness centers, but this type of equipment is used by clinicians for injury rehabilitation and research (85,86). Unlike other types of resistance exercise, the speed of movement — rather than the resistance — is controlled during isokinetic training. Isokinetic velocities of 60°, 180°, and 300° · s^{-1} are commonly referred to as the slow, medium, and fast velocities, respectively. If the purpose of the exercise program is to increase strength at higher velocities (*e.g.*, for enhanced sports performance), performing faster speed isokinetic training appears prudent (87,88). Because data from isokinetic studies support velocity specificity adaptations (3,34), the best approach may be to perform isokinetic training at slow, medium, and fast velocities to develop increased strength and power at different movement speeds.

Plyometric Training

Plyometric training refers to a specialized method of conditioning designed to enhance neuromuscular performance (89). Unlike traditional strength-building exercises such as the bench press and squat, plyometric training is characterized by quick, powerful movements that involve a rapid stretch of a muscle (eccentric muscle action) immediately followed by a rapid shortening of the same muscle (concentric muscle action). This type of muscle action provides a physiological advantage because the muscle force generated during the concentric muscle action is potentiated by the preceding eccentric muscle action (90). Although both concentric and eccentric muscle actions are important for plyometric training, the amount of time it takes to change direction from the eccentric to the concentric phase of the movement is a critical factor in plyometric training. This period is called the amortization phase, which should be as short as possible (<0.1 s) to maximize training adaptations. Healthy adults, including older adults over 60 years of age, can achieve significant gains in muscular fitness from a training program that includes plyometrics provided the exercises are sensibly progressed and performed with proper technique (91,92).

Exercises that involve jumping, skipping, hopping, and other explosive movements with medicine balls can be considered a type of plyometric training. Although plyometric exercises are often associated with high-intensity drills such as depth jumps (*i.e.*, jumping from a box to the ground and then immediately jumping upward; Fig. 4.7), less intense activities such as double leg hops and jumping jacks can also be considered a type of plyometric exercise because every time the feet hit the ground, the quadriceps go through a stretch-shortening cycle. Of practical importance, plyometric exercises can place a great amount of stress on the involved muscles, connective tissues, and joints. Therefore, this type of training needs to be carefully prescribed and progressed to reduce the likelihood of musculoskeletal injury. The importance of starting with basic movements (*e.g.*, jumps in place) or establishing an adequate foundation of strength before participating in a plyometric program should not be overlooked by the ACSM-EP (3).

It is reasonable for individuals to begin plyometric training with one or two sets of six to eight repetitions of lower intensity drills and gradually progress to several sets of moderate to higher

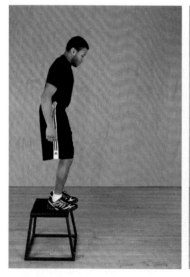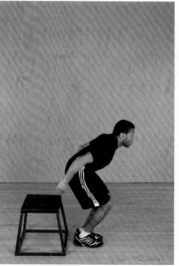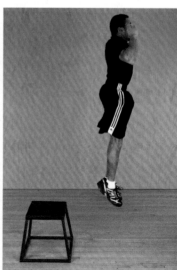

FIGURE 4.7. Depth jump. (From American College of Sports Medicine. *ACSM's Foundations of Strength Training and Conditioning.* Philadelphia [PA]: Lippincott Williams & Wilkins; 2012. 560 p.)

intensity exercises over time as technical competence improves (89). Of note, plyometrics are not a stand-alone fitness program and should be incorporated into a training session that includes other types of resistance training. Other considerations for plyometric training include proper footwear and a shock-absorbing landing surface (*e.g.*, suspended floor or grass playing field).

Modes of Resistance Training

Almost any mode of resistance training can be used to enhance muscular fitness provided that the fundamental principles of training are adhered to and the program is sensibly progressed over time. Some types of equipment are relatively easy to use, whereas others require balance, coordination, and high levels of skill. A decision to use a certain mode of resistance training should be based on an individual's health status, training experience, and personal goals. The major modes of resistance training are weight machines, free weights, body weight exercises, and a broadly defined category of balls, bands, and elastic tubing.

Single-joint exercises such as the biceps curl target a specific muscle group and require less skill to perform, whereas multiple-joint exercises such as the barbell squat involve more than one joint or major muscle group and require more balance and coordination. Although both single- and multiple-joint exercises are effective for enhancing muscular fitness, multiple-joint exercises are generally considered more effective for increasing muscle strength because they involve a greater amount of muscle mass and therefore enable a heavier weight to be lifted (37,93). Multiple-joint exercises have also been shown to have the greatest acute metabolic and anabolic hormonal response (*e.g.*, testosterone and growth hormone), which could have a favorable impact on the design of resistance training programs targeting improvements in muscle size and body composition (94,95).

Weight machines are designed to train all the major muscle groups and can be found in most fitness centers. Both single- (*e.g.*, leg extension) and multiple-joint (*e.g.*, leg press) exercises can be performed on weight machines, which are relatively easy to use because the exercise motion is controlled by the machine and typically occurs in only one anatomical plane. This may be particularly important to consider when designing resistance training programs for inactive or inexperienced individuals. Weight machines are designed to fit the average male or female, although a seat pad or back pad can be used to adjust the body position of individuals who are smaller or larger. Two examples of multiple-joint exercises performed on weight machines are shown in Figures 4.8 (lat pull-down) and 4.9 (pull-up).

Free weights are also popular in fitness centers and come in a variety of shapes and sizes. Although it typically takes longer to learn proper exercise technique when using free weights compared with weight machines, there are several advantages of free weight training. For example, free weights offer a greater variety of exercises than weight machines because they can be moved in many different directions. Another important benefit of using free weights is that they require the use of additional stabilizing and assisting muscles to hold the correct body position during an exercise. Qualified instruction, sensible starting weights, technique-driven progression, and the appropriate use of a spotter are needed to reduce the risk of an accident (96–98).

Total-body free weight exercises, including modified cleans, pulls, and presses, can be incorporated into a training program provided that qualified instruction is available and safety measures are in place (*e.g.*, a safe lifting environment and appropriate loads) (3,99,100). However, the ACSM-EP should be aware of the extra time it takes to teach advanced free weight exercises and should be knowledgeable of the progression from basic exercises (*e.g.*, front squat) to skill-transfer exercises (*e.g.*, overhead squat) and finally to weightlifting movements (*e.g.*, clean and jerk).

Visit ● Lippincott® Connect to watch videos 4.1 through 4.3, which demonstrate a curl-up, a labile push-up, and a pull-up/chin-up, respectively.

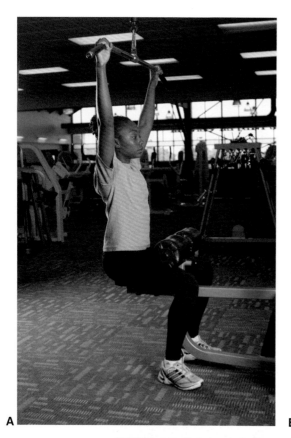
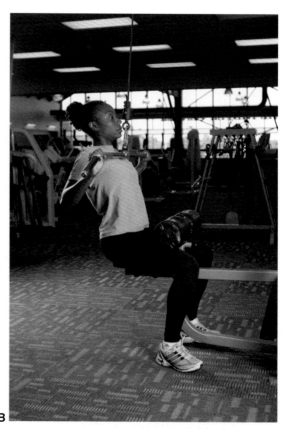

FIGURE 4.8. Pull-down: starting position **(A)** and pull-down position **(B)**.

Body weight exercises such as push-ups and pull-ups are some of the oldest modes of resistance training. Obviously, a major advantage of body weight training is that equipment is not needed and a variety of exercises can be performed. Conversely, a limitation of body weight training is the difficulty in adjusting the body weight to the individual's strength level. Inactive or overweight participants may not be strong enough to perform even one repetition of a body weight exercise.

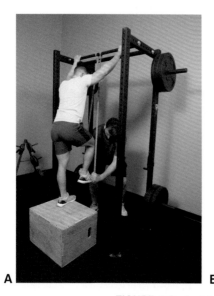
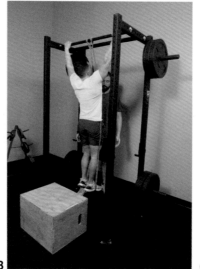
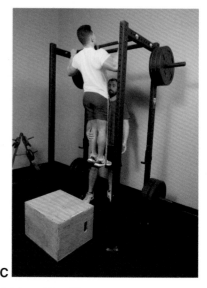

FIGURE 4.9. Assisted pull-up: set-up **(A)**, starting position **(B)**, finish position **(C)**.

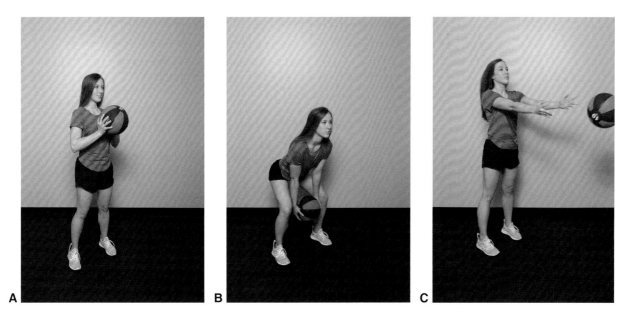

FIGURE 4.10. Underhand medicine ball toss.

In such cases, using exercise machines and training devices that allow individuals to perform body weight exercises such as pull-ups and dips by using a predetermined percentage of their body weight is desirable. This type of equipment provides an opportunity for participants of all abilities to incorporate body weight exercises into their resistance training program and feel good about their accomplishments.

Stability balls, medicine balls, and elastic tubing are effective training modes that are used by fitness professionals and therapists. Stability balls are lightweight, inflatable balls (about 45–75 cm in diameter) that add the elements of balance and coordination to any exercise while targeting selected muscle groups. Medicine balls come in different shapes and sizes (about 1–>10 kg) and are an effective alternative to free weights and weight machines; Figure 4.10 shows an underhand medicine ball toss; others include the side-to-side toss, chest pass, overhead throw, back throw, vertical throw, slams, pullover pass, side toss, and front rotation throw. Resistance training with an elastic rubber cord involves performing an exercise against the force required to stretch the cord and then returning it to its unstretched state. Stability balls, medicine balls, and elastic tubing are not only relatively inexpensive but are also being used more and more commonly as tools to enhance strength, muscular endurance, and power. In addition, exercises performed with these devices can be proprioceptively challenging, which carries added benefit. Table 4.1 summarizes the advantages and disadvantages of different modes of resistance training.

Safety Concerns

Although all resistance training activities have some degree of medical risk, the chance of injury can be reduced by following established training guidelines and safety procedures. In addition, due to interindividual variability in the response to resistance training, an ACSM-EP needs to monitor the ability of all participants to tolerate the stress of strength and conditioning programs. Without proper supervision and technique-driven progression, injuries that require medical attention can happen.

In an evaluation of resistance training–related injuries presenting to emergency departments in the United States, researchers reported that men suffered more trunk injuries than women,

Table 4.1	Comparison of Different Modes of Resistance Training			
	Weight Machines	**Free Weights**	**Body Weight**	**Balls and Cords**[a]
Cost	High	Low	None	Very low
Portability	Limited	Variable	Excellent	Excellent
Ease of use	Excellent	Variable	Variable	Variable
Muscle isolation	Excellent	Variable	Variable	Variable
Functionality	Limited	Excellent	Excellent	Excellent
Exercise variety	Limited	Excellent	Excellent	Excellent
Space requirements	High	Variable	Low	Low

[a]Medicine balls, stability balls, and elastic cords.

whereas women had more accidental injuries compared with men (97). Figure 4.11 illustrates the percentage of resistance training–related injuries at each body part for men and women between the ages of 14 and 30 years who presented to U.S. emergency departments.

Although there have not been any prospective trials that have focused specifically on measures to prevent resistance training–related injuries, an ACSM-EP who understands resistance training guidelines and acknowledges individual differences should provide supervision and instruction. This is particularly important for beginners who need to receive instruction on proper exercise technique as well as basic education on resistance training procedures (*e.g.*, weight room etiquette, appropriate spotting procedures, and the proper storage of equipment). Resistance exercises should

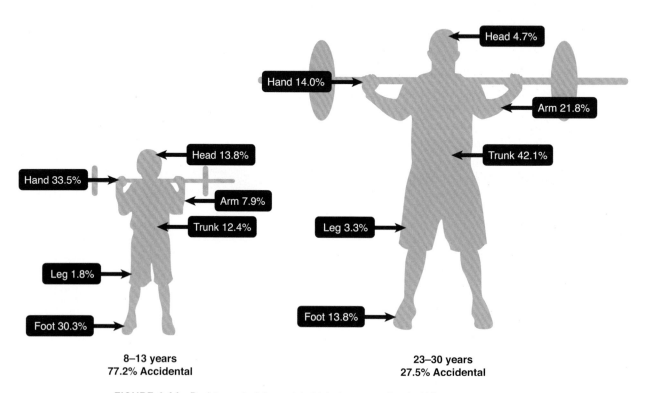

FIGURE 4.11. Resistance training–related injuries presenting to U.S. emergency rooms.

Table 4.2	Modifiable Risk Factors Associated with Resistance Training Injuries that Can Be Reduced (or Eliminated) with Qualified Supervision and Instruction	
Risk Factor	**Modification by Qualified ACSM-EP**
Health-related concern	Communicate with treating clinician and modify program
Unsafe exercise environment	Adequate training space and proper equipment layout
Improper use of equipment	Clear instruction on exercise technique and training
Excessive load and volume	Gradual progression of training program
Poor trunk control	Targeted resistance exercises for core musculature
Muscle imbalances	Include agonist and antagonist exercises for selected muscle groups
Inadequate recuperation	Modify training program and consider lifestyle factors such as proper nutrition and adequate sleep

be performed in a controlled manner using proper breathing techniques (*i.e.*, exhalation during the concentric phase and inhalation during the eccentric phase) to avoid the Valsalva maneuver and transient elevations in systolic and diastolic blood pressure (3). Individuals with orthopedic injuries or pain should use a symptom-limited ROM when performing selected resistance exercises. Furthermore, extended periods of high-intensity resistance training can result in serious complications such as rhabdomyolysis, which may harm kidney function (101). Modifiable risk factors associated with resistance training injuries that can be reduced or eliminated with qualified supervision and instruction are outlined in Table 4.2.

An ACSM-EP should be able to correctly perform the exercises they prescribe and should be able to modify exercise form and technique if necessary. When working in a fitness facility, the staff should be attentive and should try to position themselves with a clear view of the training center so that they can have quick access to individuals who need assistance. The resistance training area should be well lit and large enough to handle the number of individuals exercising in the facility at any given time. The facility should be clean, and the equipment should be well maintained. In addition, fitness professionals are responsible for enforcing safety rules (*e.g.*, proper footwear and safe storage of weights) and ensuring that individuals are training effectively.

 ## Resistance Training Program Variables

Despite various claims about the best resistance training program, there is not one *optimal* combination of sets, repetitions, and exercises that will promote long-term adaptations in muscular fitness for all individuals. Rather, many program variables need to be systematically altered over time to achieve desirable outcomes (37,102). Clearly, resistance training programs need to be individualized and based on one's health history, training experience, training goals, and training availability.

The program variables that should be considered when designing a resistance training program include (a) type of exercise, (b) order of exercise, (c) training intensity, (d) training volume (total number of sets and repetitions), (e) rest intervals between sets and exercises, (f) repetition velocity, and (g) training frequency (34). By varying one or more of these program variables, a limitless number of resistance training programs can be designed. Because individuals will respond

Table 4.3	Summary of ACSM's Guidelines for Resistance Training
Frequency	Untrained individuals should resistance train at least 2 nonconsecutive days per week.
	Trained individuals can select a frequency based on their weekly training volume.
Intensity	Untrained individuals can resistance train with 60%–70% 1-RM for 8–12 repetitions to improve muscular fitness.
	Trained individuals can resistance train with >80% 1-RM for 1- to 6-RM to optimize strength gains; a wide range of intensities can be used for other muscular fitness goals.
Volume	Untrained individuals can perform one set per muscle group per session.
	Trained individuals can perform multiple sets per muscle group per session to improve muscular fitness.
Type	Multiple-joint exercises that target agonist and antagonist muscle groups are recommended.
	Single-joint and core exercises may also be included in a resistance training program, typically after multiple-joint exercises.
	Different types of equipment and body weight exercises can be used.

Adapted with permission from American College of Sports Medicine. *ACSM's Guidelines for Exercise Testing and Prescription*. 11th ed. Philadelphia (PA): Wolters Kluwer; 2022. 548 p.

differently to the same resistance training program, sound decisions must be made on the basis of an understanding of resistance exercise, individual needs, and personal goals. Table 4.3 summarizes ACSM's principles for resistance training for apparently healthy adults (9).

Type of Exercise

A limitless number of exercises can be used to enhance muscular fitness. It is important to select exercises that are appropriate for an individual's exercise technique experience and training goals. Also, the type of exercises should promote muscle balance across joints and between opposing muscle groups (*i.e.*, agonists and antagonists) such as the quadriceps and hamstrings or the chest and upper back. Exercises generally can be classified as single-joint (*e.g.*, biceps curl and leg extension) or multiple-joint (*e.g.*, bench press and squats). Although single-joint exercises that isolate muscle groups can be incorporated into a resistance training program, it is important to include multiple-joint exercises to promote the coordinated use of multiple-joint movements (2). Additionally, it is recommended that resistance exercises include concentric, eccentric, and isometric muscle actions (9).

Exercises can also be classified as closed kinetic chain or open kinetic chain. Closed kinetic chain exercises are those in which the distal joint segment is stationary (*e.g.*, squat), whereas open chain exercises are those in which the terminal joint is free to move (*e.g.*, leg extension). Closed kinetic chain exercises more closely mimic everyday activities and include more functional movement patterns (3).

Visit ⦿ Lippincott® Connect to watch videos 4.4 through 4.8, which demonstrate a wood chop, squats, lunges, and a dumbbell bench press, respectively.

Another issue regarding the choice of exercise is the inclusion of exercises for the lumbopelvic hip complex, which is commonly referred to as the core musculature (3,9). Strengthening the abdominals, hip, and low back enhances body control and may also reduce the risk of injury during athletic events and activities of daily life (103–106). If individuals lack proper postural control during the performance of a resistance exercise, they will not be able to transfer energy efficiently to the distal segments and will be more susceptible to an injury. Thus, prehabilitation exercises for the core musculature should be included in resistance training programs. That is, exercises that may be prescribed for the rehabilitation of an injury should be prescribed beforehand as a preventive health measure.

> Visit ● Lippincott® Connect to watch videos 4.9 and 4.10, which demonstrate plank and a side bridge, respectively.

Exercises such as planks and bridges are effective for core conditioning. Multidirectional exercises that involve rotational movements and diagonal patterns performed with one's own body weight or a medicine ball can also be effective in strengthening the core musculature. In addition, research has indicated that the progressive introduction of greater instability during resistance training might have application for improving dynamic balance and functional mobility in older adults (107). Depending on the needs and goals of the individual, other prehabilitation exercises (*e.g.*, internal and external rotation for the rotator cuff musculature) can be incorporated into the training session.

Order of Exercise

There are many ways to arrange the sequence of exercises in a training session. Traditionally, beginners or clients with limited training availability perform total-body workouts that involve multiple exercises stressing all major muscle groups each session. In this type of workout, large muscle group exercises should be performed before smaller muscle group exercises and multiple-joint exercises should be performed before single-joint exercises. Following this exercise order will allow heavier weights to be used on the multiple-joint exercises because fatigue will be less of a factor. It is also helpful to perform more challenging exercises earlier in the workout when the neuromuscular system is less fatigued. Thus, power exercises such as plyometrics and weightlifting movements such as the snatch and clean and jerk lifts (or variations of these lifts) should be performed before more traditional strength exercises such as a back squat or bench press so that an individual can train for maximal power without undue fatigue (3).

Individuals with resistance training experience who have more time to train may modify their programs by performing a split routine. For example, they could perform lower body exercises only on Monday and Thursday and upper body exercises only on Tuesday and Friday. Although different training programs are effective for enhancing muscular strength and performance, individual goals, time available for training, and personal preference should determine the exercise program that is used.

Training Intensity

One of the most important variables in the design of a resistance training program is the training intensity, which refers to the magnitude of loading (*i.e.*, amount of weight lifted). Gains in muscular fitness are influenced by the amount of weight lifted, which is dependent on other program variables such as exercise order, training volume, repetition speed, and rest interval length (3,108). Depending on the goals of the resistance training program (*e.g.*, strength, hypertrophy, or local muscular endurance), the recommended training intensity can vary (37,109). Thus, fitness professionals should be aware of individual training goals in order to prescribe an appropriate resistance training intensity.

The use of RM loads is a relatively common method to prescribe resistance training intensity. RM loads of >60% are recommended for increasing muscular strength (110). A repetition range between 8 and 12 (at ~60%–80% 1-RM) is commonly used to enhance general muscular fitness (9). If the 1-RM on the leg press exercise is 100 kg, a training intensity of 60% would be 60 kg. It is reasonable for beginners or inactive individuals to use a resistance training intensity of approximately 40%–50% 1-RM because they are mostly improving motor performance at this stage, and learning how to perform each exercise properly is of paramount importance. As individuals get stronger and their resistance training skill competency improves, heavier resistances will be needed to make continual gains in muscular strength and performance (37,110). Experienced clients may resistance train at intensities greater than 80% 1-RM (*e.g.*, 1- to 6-RM) to achieve the desired gains in muscle strength (9,37,110).

If the primary goal of the resistance training program is to increase muscular hypertrophy, a wide range of training intensities may be effective. Although a resistance training intensity of 60%–80% 1-RM is typically used to increase (or preserve) muscle mass (37), less intense resistance training performed to volitional failure may also be an effective stimulus for muscle hypertrophy (110). Therefore, both light and heavy loads, with a repetition range of 6- to 20-RM, could be used to stimulate muscle hypertrophy in adults (110).

When resistance training to improve local muscular endurance, different training intensities may be effective (37,111). Lighter loads can be performed for higher repetitions (*e.g.*, 15–25) or moderate to heavy loads could be performed for fewer repetitions with a shorter rest interval between sets and exercises. Circuit training or high-intensity functional training are examples of programs that could stimulate cardiometabolic adaptations (37,111).

Because each repetition zone (*e.g.*, 3–6, 8–12, or 15–20) has its advantages, one approach may be to systematically vary the resistance training intensity to avoid training plateaus and optimize adaptations (37). Consistent training at high intensities to muscular failure on every exercise increases the risk of overtraining, which is characterized by fatigue, performance decline, and mood disturbances (112). Additionally, determining the desired resistance training intensity based on a percentage of a 1-RM requires frequent strength testing. In many cases, this is not realistic because of the time required to perform 1-RM (or multiple-RM) testing correctly on different exercises. Furthermore, maximal resistance testing for small muscle group assistance exercises is not typically performed. Thus, an ACSM-EP may also introduce clients to resistance training with lighter loads and gradually increase the weight lifted to achieve the target repetition range. Clients may benefit from resistance training at a relative percentage of their 1-RM for a predetermined number of repetitions not performed to muscular fatigue (113,114). However, fitness professionals should be aware that the number of repetitions that can be performed at a given percentage of the 1-RM varies with the amount of muscle mass required to perform the exercise. For example, research has shown that at a given percentage of the 1-RM, adults can perform more repetitions on a large muscle group exercise such as the squat compared with a smaller muscle group exercise such as the biceps curl (115). Therefore, a desired RM range (*e.g.*, 8- to 12-RM) may not be consistent with the same percentage of the 1-RM for all upper and lower body exercises.

Training Volume

The number of exercises performed per session, the repetitions performed per set, and the number of sets performed per exercise all influence the training volume (34). Although untrained individuals can respond favorably to single-set training, multiple-set training is more effective than single-set training for both muscular hypertrophy and strength enhancement in adults with resistance training experience (59,108,116). Thus, novice trainees could perform less than 5 sets per muscle group per week, whereas experienced clients could perform more than 10 sets per muscle group per week to enhance training adaptations (59,109,110).

The desired weekly volume of resistance training can be achieved with different exercises for the same muscle group (37). For example, during a given week, the leg muscles can be trained with either four sets of squats or two sets of squats and two sets of leg press. It is important to remember that every training session and every exercise does not need to be characterized by the same number of sets and repetitions. Program variation can provide needed recovery for individuals who have been participating in a high-volume training program for a prolonged period. Because recovery is an integral part of any training program, high-volume training needs to be balanced with low-volume sessions to facilitate recovery. In addition, low-volume sessions provide a learning opportunity for the ACSM-EP to reinforce proper exercise technique on specific movement patterns.

Rest Intervals between Sets

The length of the rest period between sets will influence energy recovery and the training adaptations that take place. If the primary goal of the program is to maximize gains in muscular strength, heavier weights and longer rest intervals (*e.g.*, >2 min) are desirable, whereas both short and longer rest intervals may be useful when training for muscular hypertrophy (117,118). As previously noted with other program variables, the same rest interval does not need to be used for all exercises, and short rest intervals (*e.g.*, 1 min) may be a time-efficient option for clients with limited training availability.

Repetition Velocity

The velocity or cadence at which a resistance exercise is performed can affect the adaptations to a training program because gains in muscular fitness are specific to the training velocity. For example, fast-velocity plyometric training or weightlifting exercises such as the snatch and clean and jerk lifts are more likely to enhance speed and power than slower velocity resistance exercise on a weight machine (68,84,89). In any case, beginners need to learn how to perform each exercise correctly and develop an adequate level of strength before optimal gains in power performance are realized. As individuals improve muscular strength and gain experience performing higher velocity movements, heavier loads or more complex exercises may be used to optimize training adaptations. It is likely that the performance of different training velocities and the integration of numerous training techniques may provide the most effective training stimulus (37,60,68).

Training Frequency

A resistance training frequency of two to three times per week on nonconsecutive days is recommended for beginners (9). Although a resistance training frequency of once per week may increase muscular fitness in untrained adults, more frequent training sessions may be needed to optimize adaptations (57). A training frequency of two to three times per week on nonconsecutive days will allow for more frequent motor learning of the desired movement patterns as well as adequate recovery between sessions (48–72 h) (4). However, total training volume appears to be more important than training frequency in adults with resistance training experience (119,120). Trained adults can achieve similar gains in muscular fitness with a training frequency of once, twice, or thrice weekly when training volume is equal (119,121). Although higher training frequencies may be a desirable option for some trained individuals, clients with limited training availability may benefit from less frequent sessions performed at a higher training volume. Factors including training experience, training volume, and training availability can influence the range of training frequency options for each individual.

Periodization

Periodization is a concept that refers to the systematic variation in training program design. Because it is impossible to continually improve at the same rate over long-term training, properly varying the training variables can limit training plateaus, maximize performance gains, and reduce the likelihood of overtraining (54,65). The underlying concept of periodization is based on Selye general adaptation syndrome, which proposes that after a certain period, adaptations to a new stimulus will no longer take place unless the stimulus is altered (102). In essence, periodization is a process whereby a fitness professional systematically changes the training stimulus to keep it effective and enjoyable. Although the concept of periodization has been part of athletic training programs for many years (65), our understanding of the potential benefits of periodized training programs compared with nonperiodized programs for untrained individuals and older adults continues to be explored in the literature (83,122,123).

By periodically varying program variables such as the choice of exercise, training intensity, number of sets, rest periods between sets, or any combination of these, long-term performance gains will be optimized and the risk of "overuse" injuries may be reduced (37,54). Moreover, it is reasonable to suggest that individuals who participate in periodized resistance training programs and continue to improve their health and fitness may be more likely to adhere to an exercise program for the long term. For example, if a trained individual's lower body routine typically consists of the leg press, leg extension, and leg curl exercises, performing the back squat and dumbbell lunge exercises on alternate workout days will likely increase the effectiveness of the training program and reduce the likelihood of staleness and boredom. Furthermore, varying the training weights, number of sets, and/or rest interval between sets can help prevent training plateaus, which are not uncommon among fitness enthusiasts. Many times, a strength plateau can be avoided by periodically varying the exercises or varying the training intensity and training volume to allow for ample recovery. In the long term, program variation with adequate recovery will allow an individual to make even greater gains because the body will be challenged to adapt to even greater demands (37).

The general concept of periodization is to prioritize training goals and then develop a long-term plan that varies throughout the year (54). In general, the year is divided into specific training cycles (*e.g.*, a macrocycle, a mesocycle, and a microcycle), with each cycle having a specific goal (*e.g.*, hypertrophy, strength, or power). One model of periodization is referred to as a linear model because the volume and intensity of training gradually change over time (3). For example, at the start of a macrocycle, the training volume may be high and the training intensity may be low. As the year progresses, the volume is decreased as the intensity of training increases. Although this type of training originally was designed for athletes who attempted to elicit peak performance for a specific competition, it can be modified for enhancing health and fitness goals. For example, individuals who routinely perform the same combination of sets and repetitions on all exercises will benefit from gradually increasing the weight and decreasing the number of repetitions as strength improves.

A second model of periodization is referred to as an undulating (nonlinear) model because of the daily fluctuations in training volume and intensity (3). For example, on the major exercises, a trained individual may perform two or three sets with 8- to 10-RM loads on Monday, three or four sets with 4- to 6-RM loads on Wednesday, and one or two sets with 12- to 15-RM loads on Friday. Whereas the heavy training days will maximally activate the trained musculature, selected muscle fibers may not be maximally taxed on light and moderate training days. By varying training volume and intensity, the participant can minimize the risk of overtraining and maximize the potential for achieving performance goals (3,54,65).

General Recommendations

Resistance training has the potential to offer unique benefits to men and women of all ages and abilities. Regular participation in a progressive resistance training program can enhance muscular fitness and improve an individual's health status. However, the design of resistance training programs can be complex, and program variables including the choice of exercise, order of exercise, training intensity, training volume, repetition velocity, and rest period between sets and exercises need to be systematically varied over time to optimize gains in muscle fitness and performance. In addition, resistance training programs need to be individualized and consistent with personal goals and training availability to maximize outcomes and exercise adherence. Ultimately, knowledge of muscle structure and function along with an understanding of resistance training principles will determine the effectiveness of the training program.

In addition to understanding the science of resistance exercise, an ACSM-EP needs to appreciate the art of prescribing exercise. Resistance training programs need to be individualized and consistent with personal needs, goals, and abilities. A key factor for safe and effective resistance training is proper program design that includes exercise instruction, technique-driven progression, and periodic evaluations to assess progress toward training goals. This requires effective leadership, realistic goal setting, and a solid understanding of training-induced adaptations that take place in both beginners and experienced exercisers.

Although the creation of a basic resistance training program must be individualized based on a variety of factors mentioned earlier, one simple way to gain experience writing basic and balanced resistance training programming is to use movement pattern-based exercise prescription.

Visit ⊙ Lippincott® Connect to watch videos 4.11 through 4.13, which demonstrate the one-repetition maximum bench testing procedure, the multi-rep bench press test, and the push-up test.

The Case of Jeremy

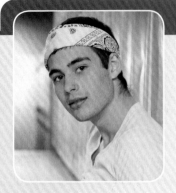

Submitted by **Benjamin Gleason, ACSM-HFS, NSCA-CSCS, US Air Force, Niceville, FL**
Jeremy is a former high school athlete, now 23 years old and apparently healthy.

Narrative

Jeremy's body composition is within normal ranges, as are his blood pressure and heart rate. He cites no family history of disease. He works out in the local gym for four sessions per week and spends 1–2 hours per session. This has been his primary mode of regular exercise since high school, and he plays recreational sports in the local city league in his free time. He wishes to continue his current exercise pattern but has come to see you to discuss some issues he's been having lately. He casually complains to you during his fitness screening that he suffers mild knee pain and low back pain during and after his workouts. On observing him in a gym session, you notice that when he performs the squat, he rounds his back and places most of his weight on the balls of his feet. He also rounds his back slightly when he performs the deadlift and hyperextends his spine at the end of the lift. During standing overhead pressing movements, he leans back to force out a few extra reps. He has been suffering from mild pain in his knees and back for some time now and says his high school sports coach used to tell him "No pain, no gain!" when he brought it up from time to time several years ago. He asks you if this pain is normal and says he doesn't want to sound like a wimp to the other guys in the gym. His typical weight program involves three or four sets of 6–12 repetitions on every exercise, and he performs at least three exercises for each body part in his program. Mondays, he does chest and triceps; Tuesdays he does legs; Thursdays he does back and biceps; and Fridays he does shoulders. He includes some light cardio on a stationary bike or a treadmill after most workouts.

Analysis

Jeremy's workout program is a typical one used by many bodybuilders, but his attention to detail on form leaves much to be desired. Apparently, he was not taught the proper exercise technique by his coach in high school or the fitness center staff, and Jeremy has developed some movement pattern disorders. To reduce the likelihood of knee and back pain during the squat and deadlift, he should keep the majority of his bodyweight on his heels as he descends and rises throughout the ROM and keep his back in the neutral position. It will take time to break old habits, and Jeremy will need to use a lighter load to learn proper technique on these free weight exercises. Jeremy should visit a medical professional to address any possible injuries beyond the minor pain he experiences during exercise. His habits of hyperextending his back at the top of the deadlift and arching his back to get more reps on overhead presses are likely contributors to his back pain and serve no practical advantage in resistance training as they are high-risk methods. A deadlift is complete when the lifter returns to the standing position only and not beyond (hyperextension). The posterior chain musculature (low back, gluteals, hamstrings) requires considerable attention in an effective training program, and the correct initiation of movement is imperative to reduce the risk of injury and produce the desired performance effects.

QUESTIONS

- Discuss Jeremy's tendency to round his back during deadlifts and how it may be causing his low back pain.
- Why is knee pain common in individuals who squat in an anterior-dominant manner?
- Provide at least three exercises to address Jeremy's apparent posterior chain deficiency.
- Suggest two core stability exercises that may help Jeremy hold spinal stability better.

References

1. Bird S, Barrington-Higgs S. Exploring the deadlift. *Strength Cond J.* 2010;32(2):46–51.
2. Chiu L. A teaching progression for squatting exercises. *Strength Cond J.* 2011;33(2):46–54.
3. Gamble P. An integrated approach to training core stability. *Strength Cond J.* 2007;29(1):58–68.
4. McGill S. *Low Back Disorders, Evidence-Based Prevention and Rehabilitation.* Champaign (IL): Human Kinetics; 2002. 295 p.

SUMMARY

In this chapter, the benefits and importance of muscular strength and endurance for health and fitness were described. An overview of the basic structure and function of the muscle was also provided. Fundamental principles relating to resistance training for health and fitness were reviewed. The primary variables of a resistance training program were described. The role of the ACSM-EP in designing a resistance training program for apparently healthy adults and individuals with controlled disease was discussed. Tools for developing an individualized resistance training program from assessment to implementation to evaluation were provided.

STUDY QUESTIONS

1. Describe the size principle of motor unit recruitment and explain its practical application to resistance exercise program design.
2. Discuss seven fundamental principles that influence the effectiveness of resistance training programs.
3. Compare and contrast three different modes of resistance training and discuss the advantages and disadvantages of each method.
4. Outline testing procedures for assessing a 1-RM leg press on a trained adult client.
5. Design a resistance training program for an untrained healthy adult and include recommendations for participant safety, program progression, and exercise adherence.

REFERENCES

1. Kercher V. International comparisons: ACSM's worldwide survey of fitness trends. *ACSMs Health Fit J.* 2018;22(6):24–9.
2. Kraemer W, Ratamess N, Flanagan S, Shurley J, Todd J, Todd T. Understanding the science of resistance training: an evolutionary perspective. *Sports Med.* 2017;47(12): 2415–35.
3. Ratamess N. *ACSM's Foundations of Strength Training and Conditioning.* Philadelphia (PA): Lippincott Williams & Wilkins; 2012. 560 p.
4. Garber C, Blissmer B, Deschenes M, et al. American College of Sports Medicine position stand. Quantity and quality of exercise for developing and maintaining cardiorespiratory, musculoskeletal, and neuromotor fitness in apparently healthy adults: guidance for prescribing exercise. *Med Sci Sports Exerc.* 2011;43(7):1334–59.
5. Squires R, Kaminsky L, Porcari J, Ruff J, Savage P, Williams M. Progression of exercise training in early outpatient cardiac rehabilitation: an official statement from the American Association of Cardiovascular and Pulmonary Rehabilitation. *J Cardiopulm Rehabil Prev.* 2018;38(3): 139–46.
6. Wolfe RR. The underappreciated role of muscle in health and disease. *Am J Clin Nutr.* 2006;84(3):475–82.
7. Westcott W. Resistance training is medicine: effects of strength training on health. *Curr Sports Med Rep.* 2012;11(4): 209–16.
8. Fragala M, Cadore E, Dorgo S, et al. Resistance training for older adults: position statement from the National Strength and Conditioning Association. *J Strength Cond Res.* 2019;33(8):2019–52.

9. American College of Sports Medicine. *ACSM's Guidelines for Exercise Testing and Prescription.* 11th ed. Philadelphia (PA): Wolters Kluwer; 2022. 548 p.

10. U.S. Department of Health and Human Services. *Physical Activity Guidelines for Americans.* 2nd ed. Washington (DC): U.S. Department of Health and Human Services; 2018. 118 p.

11. Mcleod J, Stokes T, Phillips S. Resistance exercise training as a primary countermeasure to age-related chronic disease. *Front Physiol.* 2019;10:645.

12. Saeidifard F, Medina-Inojosa J, West C, et al. The association of resistance training with mortality: a systematic review and meta-analysis. *Eur J Prev Cardiol.* 2019;26(15):1647–65.

13. Artero E, Lee D, Lavie C, et al. Effects of muscular strength on cardiovascular risk factors and prognosis. *J Cardiopulm Rehabil Prev.* 2012;32(6):351–8.

14. Hart P, Buck D. The effect of resistance training on health-related quality of life in older adults: systematic review and meta-analysis. *Health Promot Perspect.* 2019;9(1):1–12.

15. García-Hermoso A, Cavero-Redondo I, Ramírez-Vélez R, et al. Muscular strength as a predictor of all-cause mortality in an apparently healthy population: a systematic review and meta-analysis of data from approximately 2 million men and women. *Arch Phys Med Rehabil.* 2018;99(10):2100–13.e5.

16. Siahpush M, Farazi P, Wang H, Robbins R, Singh G, Su D. Muscle-strengthening physical activity is associated with cancer mortality: results from the 1998-2011 National Health Interview Surveys, National Death Index record linkage. *Cancer Causes Control.* 2019;30(6):663–70.

17. Grøntved A, Pan A, Mekary R, et al. Muscle-strengthening and conditioning activities and risk of type 2 diabetes: a prospective study in two cohorts of US women. *PLoS Med.* 2014;11(1):e1001587.

18. Figueroa A, Okamoto T, Jaime S, Fahs C. Impact of high-and low-intensity resistance training on arterial stiffness and blood pressure in adults across the lifespan: a review. *Pflügers Arch.* 2019;471(3):467–78.

19. Peterson M, Sen A, Gordon P. Influence of resistance exercise on lean body mass in aging adults: a meta-analysis. *Med Sci Sports Exerc.* 2011;43(2):249–58.

20. Ashton R, Tew G, Aning J, Gilbert S, Lewis L, Saxton J. Effects of short-term, medium-term and long-term resistance exercise training on cardiometabolic health outcomes in adults: systematic review with meta-analysis. *Br J Sports Med.* 2020;54(6):341–8.

21. Pan B, Ge L, Xun Y-Q, et al. Exercise training modalities in patients with type 2 diabetes mellitus: a systematic review and network meta-analysis. *Int J Behav Nutr Phys Act.* 2018;15(1):72.

22. Gordon BA, Benson AC, Bird SR, Fraser SF. Resistance training improves metabolic health in type 2 diabetes: a systematic review. *Diabetes Res Clin Pract.* 2009;83(2):157–75.

23. Gordon B, McDowell C, Lyons M, Herring M. The effects of resistance exercise training on anxiety: a meta-analysis and meta-regression analysis of randomized controlled trials. *Sports Med.* 2017;47(12):2521–32.

24. Gordon B, McDowell C, Hallgren M, Meyer J, Lyons M, Herring M. Association of efficacy of resistance exercise training with depressive symptoms: meta-analysis and meta-regression analysis of randomized clinical trials. *JAMA Psychiatry.* 2018;75(6):566–76.

25. Yang J, Christophi C, Farioli A, et al. Association between push-up exercise capacity and future cardiovascular events among active adult men. *JAMA Netw Open.* 2019;2(2):e188341.

26. American College of Sports Medicine position stand: physical activity and bone health. *Med Sci Sports Exerc.* 2004;36:1985–96.

27. Hong A, Kim S. Effects of resistance exercise on bone health. *Endocrinol Metab (Seoul).* 2018;33(4):435–44.

28. Kim Y, Kim K, Paik N, Kim K, Jang H, Lim J. Muscle strength: a better index of low physical performance than muscle mass in older adults. *Geriatr Gerontol Int.* 2016;16(5):577–85.

29. Ciolac E, Rodrigues-da-Silva J. Resistance training as a tool for preventing and treating musculoskeletal disorders. *Sports Med.* 2016;46(9):1239–48.

30. Carli F, Ferreira V. Prehabilitation: a new area of integration between geriatricians, anesthesiologists, and exercise therapists. *Aging Clin Exp Res.* 2018;30(3):241–4.

31. Piraux E, Caty G, Reychler G. Effects of preoperative combined aerobic and resistance exercise training in cancer patients undergoing tumour resection surgery: a systematic review of randomised trials. *Surg Oncol.* 2018;27(3):584–94.

32. Vezina J, Der Ananian C, Greenberg E, Kurka J. Sociodemographic correlates of meeting US Department of Health and Human Services muscle strengthening recommendations in middle-aged and older adults. *Prev Chronic Dis.* 2014;11:E162.

33. Bennie J, Pedisic Z, van Uffelen J, et al. Pumping iron in Australia: prevalence, trends and sociodemographic correlates of muscle strengthening activity participation from a national sample of 195,926 adults. *PLoS One.* 2016;11(4):e0153225.

34. Fleck S, Kraemer W. *Designing Resistance Training Programs.* 4th ed. Champaign (IL): Human Kinetics; 2014. 520 p.

35. Lim C, Kim H, Morton R, et al. Resistance exercise-induced changes in muscle metabolism are load-dependent. *Med Sci Sports Exerc.* 2019;51(12):2578–85.

36. Campos GE, Luecke TJ, Wendeln HK, et al. Muscular adaptations in response to three different resistance-training regimens: specificity of repetition maximum training zones. *Eur J Appl Physiol.* 2002;88(1–2):50–60.

37. Ratamess N, Alvar B, Evetoch T, et al. American College of Sports Medicine position stand. Progression models in resistance training in healthy adults. *Med Sci Sports Exerc.* 2009;41(3):687–708.

38. Hody S, Croisier J, Bury T, Rogister B, Leprince P. Eccentric muscle contractions: risks and benefits. *Front Physiol.* 2019;10:536.

39. Ye X, Beck T, Wages N. Reduced susceptibility to eccentric exercise-induced muscle damage in resistance-trained men is not linked to resistance training-related neural adaptations. *Biol Sport.* 2015;32(3):199–205.

40. Newton M, Morgan G, Sacco P, Chapman D, Nosaka K. Comparison of responses to strenuous eccentric exercise of the elbow flexors between resistance-trained and untrained men. *J Strength Cond Res.* 2008;22(2):597–607.

41. Riebe D, Franklin B, Thompson P, et al. Updating ACSM's recommendations for exercise preparticipation health screening. *Med Sci Sports Exerc.* 2015;47(11):2473–9.

42. Williams MA, Haskell WL, Ades PA, et al. Resistance exercise in individuals with and without cardiovascular disease: 2007 update: a scientific statement from the American Heart Association Council on Clinical Cardiology and Council on Nutrition, Physical Activity, and Metabolism. *Circulation.* 2007;116(5):572–84.

43. Simic L, Sarabon N, Markovic G. Does pre-exercise static stretching inhibit maximal muscular performance? A meta-analytical review. *Scand J Med Sci Sports.* 2013;23(2):131–48.

44. Behm D, Chaouachi A. A review of the acute effects of static and dynamic stretching on performance. *Eur J Appl Physiol.* 2011;111(11):2633–51.

45. Opplert J, Babault N. Acute effects of dynamic stretching on muscle flexibility and performance: an analysis of the current literature. *Sports Med.* 2018;48(2):299–325.

46. Rijk J, Roos P, Deckx L, van den Akker M, Buntinx F. Prognostic value of handgrip strength in people aged 60 years and older: a systematic review and meta-analysis. *Geriatr Gerontol Int.* 2018;16(1):5–20.

47. Celis-Morales C, Welsh P, Lyall D, et al. Associations of grip strength with cardiovascular, respiratory, and cancer outcomes and all cause mortality: prospective cohort study of half a million UK Biobank participants. *Br Med J.* 2018;361:k1651.

48. Cronin J, Lawton T, Harris N, Kilding A, McMaster D. A brief review of handgrip strength and sport performance. *J Strength Cond Res.* 2017;31(11):3187–217.

49. Reynolds J, Gordon T, Robergs R. Prediction of one repetition maximum strength from multiple repetition maximum testing and anthropometry. *J Strength Cond Res.* 2006;20(3):584–92.

50. Amarante do Nascimento M, Januário R, Gerage A, Mayhew J, Cheche Pina F, Cyrino E. Familiarization and reliability of one repetition maximum strength testing in older women. *J Strength Cond Res.* 2013;27(6):1636–42.

51. Seo D, Kim E, Fahs C, et al. Reliability of the one-repetition maximum test based on muscle group and gender. *J Sports Sci Med.* 2012;11(2):221–5.

52. Lyons T, McLester J, Arnett S, Thoma M. Specificity of training modalities on upper-body one repetition maximum performance: free weights vs. hammer strength equipment. *J Strength Cond Res.* 2010;24(11):2984–8.

53. Faigenbaum A, McFarland J. Resistance training for kids: right from the start. *ACSMs Health Fit J.* 2016;20(5):16–22.

54. Bompa T, Haff G. *Periodization: Theory and Methodology of Training.* Champaign (IL): Human Kinetics; 2009. 411 p.

55. Baechle T, Earle R. Learning how to manipulate training variables to maximize results. *Weight Training: Steps to Success.* 4th ed. Champaign (IL): Human Kinetics; 2012. p. 177–8.

56. Ralston G, Kilgore L, Wyatt F, Baker J. The effect of weekly set volume on strength gain: a meta-analysis. *Sports Med.* 2017;47(12):2585–601.

57. Grgic J, Schoenfeld B, Davies T, Lazinica B, Krieger J, Pedisic Z. Effect of resistance training frequency on gains in muscular strength: a systematic review and meta-analysis. *Sports Med.* 2018;48(5):1207–20.

58. Sousa A, Neiva H, Izquierdo M, Cadore E, Alves A, Marinho D. Concurrent training and detraining: brief review on the effect of exercise intensities. *Int J Sports Med.* 2019;40(12):747–55.

59. Kraemer WJ, Ratamess NA. Fundamentals of resistance training: progression and exercise prescription. *Med Sci Sports Exerc.* 2004;36(4):674–88.

60. La Scala Teixeira C, Evangelista A, Pereira P, Da Silva-Grigoletto M, Bocalini D, Behm D. Complexity: a novel load progression strategy in strength training. *Front Physiol.* 2019;10:839.

61. Morgan F, Battersby A, Weightman A, et al. Adherence to exercise referral schemes by participants — what do providers and commissioners need to know? A systematic review of barriers and facilitators. *BMC Public Health.* 2016;16:227.

62. Sylvester B, Standage M, McEwan D, et al. Variety support and exercise adherence behavior: experimental and mediating effects. *J Behav Med.* 2016;39(2):214–24.

63. Jafarnezhadgero A, Madadi-Shad M, McCrum C, Karamanidis K. Effects of corrective training on drop landing ground reaction force characteristics and lower limb kinematics in older adults with genu valgus: a randomized controlled trial. *J Aging Phys Act.* 2019;27(1):9–17.

64. Faro J, Wright J, Hayman L, Hastie M, Gona P, Whiteley J. Functional resistance training and affective response in female college-age students. *Med Sci Sports Exerc.* 2019;51(6):1186–94.

65. Williams T, Tolusso D, Fedewa M, Esco M. Comparison of periodized and non-periodized resistance training on maximal strength: a meta-analysis. *Sports Med.* 2017;47(10):2083–100.

66. Ratamess N, Rosenberg J, Klei S, et al. Comparison of the acute metabolic responses to traditional resistance, bodyweight, and battling rope exercise. *J Strength Cond Res.* 2015;29(1):47–57.

67. Pesce C. Shifting the focus from quantitative to qualitative exercise characteristics in exercise and cognition research. *J Sport Exerc Psychol.* 2012;34(6):766–86.

68. Suchomel T, Nimphius S, Bellon C, Stone M. The importance of muscular strength: training considerations. *Sports Med.* 2018;48(4):765–85.

69. Kuroda Y, Sato Y, Ishizaka Y, Yamakado M, Yamaguchi N. Exercise motivation, self-efficacy, and enjoyment as indicators of adult exercise behavior among the transtheoretical model stages. *Glob Health Promot.* 2012;19(1):14–22.

70. McPhate L, Simek E, Haines T, Hill K, Finch C, Day L. "Are your clients having fun?" The implications of respondents' preferences for the delivery of group exercise programs for falls prevention. *J Aging Phys Act.* 2016;24(1):129–38.

71. Elsangedy H, Machado D, Krinski K, et al. Let the pleasure guide your resistance training intensity. *Med Sci Sports Exerc.* 2018;50(7):1472–9.

72. Rhodes R, Lubans D, Karunamuni N, Kennedy S, Plotnikoff R. Factors associated with participation in resistance training: a systematic review. *Br J Sports Med.* 2017;51(20):1466–72.

73. Csikszentmihalyi M, Abuhamdeh S, Nakamura J. Flow. In: Elliot A, Dweck C, editors. *Handbook of Competence and Motivation.* New York (NY): Guilford Press; 2005. p. 598–698.

74. Reilly T, Morris T, Whyte G. The specificity of training prescription and physiological assessment: a review. *J Sports Sci.* 2009;27(6):575–89.

75. Ramírez-Campillo R, Martínez C, de La Fuente C, et al. High-speed resistance training in older women: the role of supervision. *J Aging Phys Act.* 2017;25(1):1–9.

76. Mazzetti SA, Kraemer WJ, Volek JS, et al. The influence of direct supervision of resistance training on strength performance. *Med Sci Sports Exerc.* 2000;32(6):1175–84.

77. Gentil P, Bottaro M. Influence of supervision ratio on muscle adaptations to resistance training in nontrained subjects. *J Strength Cond Res.* 2010;24(3):639–43.

78. Mann S, Jimenez A, Steele J, Domone S, Wade M, Beedie C. Programming and supervision of resistance training leads to positive effects on strength and body composition: results from two randomised trials of community fitness programmes. *BMC Public Health.* 2018;18(1):420.

79. Ratamess NA, Faigenbaum AD, Hoffman JR, Kang J. Self-selected resistance training intensity in healthy women: the influence of a personal trainer. *J Strength Cond Res.* 2008;22(1):103–11.

80. Elsangedy H, Krause M, Krinski K, Alves R, Hsin Nery Chao C, da Silva S. Is the self-selected resistance exercise intensity by older women consistent with the American College of Sports Medicine guidelines to improve muscular fitness? *J Strength Cond Res.* 2013;27(7):1877–84.

81. Dias M, Simão R, Saavedra F, Buzzachera C, Fleck S. Self-selected training load and RPE during resistance and aerobic training among recreational exercisers. *Percept Mot Skills.* 2018;125(4):769–87.

82. Cotter J, Garver M, Dinyer T, Fairman C, Focht B. Ratings of perceived exertion during acute resistance exercise performed at imposed and self-selected loads in recreationally trained women. *J Strength Cond Res.* 2017;31(8):2313–8.

83. Conlon J, Newton R, Tufano J, et al. Periodization strategies in older adults: impact on physical function and health. *Med Sci Sports Exerc.* 2016;48(12):2426–36.

84. Cormie P, McGuigan M, Newton R. Developing maximal neuromuscular power: part 2 — training considerations for improving maximal power production. *Sports Med.* 2011;41(2):125–46.

85. Pontes S, de Carvalho A, Almeida K, et al. Effects of isokinetic muscle strengthening on muscle strength, mobility, and gait in post-stroke patients: a systematic review and meta-analysis. *Clin Rehabil.* 2019;33(3):381–94.

86. Hickey J, Timmins R, Maniar N, Williams M, Opar D. Criteria for progressing rehabilitation and determining return-to-play clearance following hamstring strain injury: a systematic review. *Sports Med.* 2017;47(7):1375–87.

87. Englund D, Sharp R, Selsby J, Ganesan S, Franke W. Resistance training performed at distinct angular velocities elicits velocity-specific alterations in muscle strength and mobility status in older adults. *Exp Gerontol.* 2017;91:51–6.

88. Zinke F, Warnke T, Gäbler M, Granacher U. Effects of isokinetic training on trunk muscle fitness and body composition in world-class canoe sprinters. *Front Physiol.* 2019;10:21.

89. Chu D, Myer G. *Plyometrics.* Champaign (IL): Human Kinetics; 2013. 248 p.

90. Sáez de Villarreal E, Requena B, Cronin J. The effects of plyometric training on sprint performance: a meta-analysis. *J Strength Cond Res.* 2012;26(2):575–84.

91. Oxfeldt M, Overgaard K, Hvid L, Dalgas U. Effects of plyometric training on jumping, sprint performance, and lower body muscle strength in healthy adults: a systematic review and meta-analyses. *Scand J Med Sci Sports.* 2019;29(10):1453–65.

92. Vetrovsky T, Steffl M, Stastny P, Tufano J. The efficacy and safety of lower-limb plyometric training in older adults: a systematic review. *Sports Med.* 2019;49(1):113–31.

93. Holm L, Reitelseder S, Pedersen T, et al. Changes in muscle size and MHC composition in response to resistance exercise with heavy and light loading intensity. *J Appl Physiol (1985).* 2008;105(5):1454–61.

94. Vingren J, Kraemer W, Ratamess N, Anderson J, Volek J, Maresh C. Testosterone physiology in resistance exercise and training: the up-stream regulatory elements. *Sports Med.* 2010;40(12):1037–53.

95. Hooper D, Kraemer W, Focht B, et al. Endocrinological roles for testosterone in resistance exercise responses and adaptations. *Sports Med.* 2017;47(9):1709–20.

96. Kerr Z, Collins C, Comstock R. Epidemiology of weight training-related injuries presenting to United States emergency departments, 1990 to 2007. *Am J Sports Med.* 2010;38(4):765–71.

97. Quatman C, Myer G, Khoury J, Wall E, Hewett T. Sex differences in "weightlifting" injuries presenting to United States Emergency Rooms. *J Strength Cond Res.* 2009;23(7):2061–7.

98. Pirruccio K, Kelly J. Weightlifting shoulder injuries presenting to U.S. emergency departments: 2000–2030. *Int J Sports Med.* 2019;40(8):528–34.

99. Suchomel T, Comfort P, Stone M. Weightlifting pulling derivatives: rationale for implementation and application. *Sports Med.* 2015;45(6):823–39.

100. Haff G, Triplett T. *Essentials of Strength Training and Conditioning.* 4th ed. Champaign (IL): Human Kinetics; 2016. 752 p.

101. Huynh A, Leong K, Jones N, et al. Outcomes of exertional rhabdomyolysis following high-intensity resistance training. *Inter Med J.* 2016;46(5):602–8.

102. Cunanan A, DeWeese B, Wagle J, et al. The general adaptation syndrome: a foundation for the concept of periodization. *Sports Med.* 2018;48(4):787–97.

103. Coulombe B, Games K, Neil E, Eberman L. Core stability exercise versus general exercise for chronic low back pain. *J Athl Train.* 2017;52(1):71–2.

104. Sasaki S, Tsuda E, Yamamoto Y, et al. Core-muscle training and neuromuscular control of lower limb and trunk. *J Athl Train*. 2019;54(9):959–69.

105. De Blaiser C, Roosen P, Willems T, Danneels L, Bossche L, De Ridder R. Is core stability a risk factor for lower extremity injuries in an athletic population? A systematic review. *Phys Ther Sport*. 2018;30:48–56.

106. Granacher U, Gollhofer A, Hortobágyi T, Kressig R, Muehlbauer T. The importance of trunk muscle strength for balance, functional performance, and fall prevention in seniors: a systematic review. *Sports Med*. 2013;43(7):627–41.

107. Granacher U, Lacroix A, Muehlbauer T, Roettger K, Gollhofer A. Effects of core instability strength training on trunk muscle strength, spinal mobility, dynamic balance and functional mobility in older adults. *Gerontology*. 2013;59(2):105–13.

108. Borde R, Hortobágyi T, Granacher U. Dose-response relationships of resistance training in healthy old adults: a systematic review and meta-analysis. *Sports Med*. 2015;45(12):1693–720.

109. Schoenfeld B, Wilson J, Lowery R, Krieger J. Muscular adaptations in low-versus high-load resistance training: a meta-analysis. *Eur J Sport Sci*. 2016;16(1):1–10.

110. Schoenfeld B, Grgic J, Ogborn D, Krieger J. Strength and hypertrophy adaptations between low- vs. high-load resistance training: a systematic review and meta-analysis. *J Strength Cond Res*. 2017;31(12):3508–23.

111. Feito Y, Heinrich K, Butcher S, Poston W. High-Intensity functional training (HIFT): definition and research implications for improved fitness. *Sports (Basel)*. 2018;6(3):E76.

112. Meeusen R, Duclos M, Foster C, et al. Prevention, diagnosis, and treatment of the overtraining syndrome: joint consensus statement of the European College of Sport Science and the American College of Sports Medicine. *Med Sci Sports Exerc*. 2013;45(1):186–205.

113. Carroll K, Bazyler C, Bernards J, et al. Skeletal muscle fiber adaptations following resistance training using repetition maximums or relative intensity. *Sports (Basel)*. 2019;7(7):E169.

114. Carroll K, Bernards J, Bazyler C, et al. Divergent performance outcomes following resistance training using repetition maximums or relative intensity. *Int J Sports Physiol Perform*. 2018;14(1):46–54.

115. Shimano T, Kraemer W, Spiering B, et al. Relationship between the number of repetitions and selected percentages of one repetition maximum in free weight exercises in trained and untrained men. *J Strength Cond Res*. 2006;20(4):819–23.

116. Schoenfeld B, Ogborn D, Krieger J. Effects of resistance training frequency on measures of muscle hypertrophy: a systematic review and meta-analysis. *Sports Med*. 2016;46(11):1689–97.

117. Grgic J, Schoenfeld B, Skrepnik M, Davies T, Mikulic P. Effects of rest interval duration in resistance training on measures of muscular strength: a systematic review. *Sports Med*. 2018;48(1):137–51.

118. Grgic J, Lazinica B, Mikulic P, Krieger J, Schoenfeld B. The effects of short versus long inter-set rest intervals in resistance training on measures of muscle hypertrophy: a systematic review. *Eur J Sport Sci*. 2017;17(8):983–93.

119. Grgic J, Schoenfeld B, Latella C. Resistance training frequency and skeletal muscle hypertrophy: a review of available evidence. *J Sci Med Sport*. 2019;22(3):361–70.

120. Schoenfeld B, Grgic J, Krieger J. How many times per week should a muscle be trained to maximize muscle hypertrophy? A systematic review and meta-analysis of studies examining the effects of resistance training frequency. *J Sports Sci*. 2019;37(11):1286–95.

121. Ralston G, Kilgore L, Wyatt F, Buchan D, Baker J. Weekly training frequency effects on strength gain: a meta-analysis. *Sports Med Open*. 2018;4(1):36.

122. Strohacker K, Fazzino D, Breslin W, Xu X. The use of periodization in exercise prescriptions for inactive adults: a systematic review. *Prev Med Rep*. 2015;2:385–96.

123. De Souza E, Tricoli V, Rauch J, et al. Different patterns in muscular strength and hypertrophy adaptations in untrained individuals undergoing nonperiodized and periodized strength regimens. *J Strength Cond Res*. 2018;32(5):1238–44.

5

Flexibility Assessments and Exercise Programming for Apparently Healthy Participants

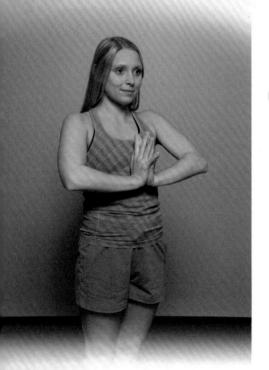

OBJECTIVES

- To understand the context of flexibility as it relates to health and wellness.
- To describe the basic anatomy and physiology of the musculoskeletal system related to flexibility.
- To differentiate methods of range of motion exercises and classify their strengths and weaknesses.
- To select appropriate assessment protocols for flexibility and analyze the results of those assessments.
- To formulate appropriate programs for development of whole-body flexibility.

INTRODUCTION

The development and maintenance of flexibility has long been a recommended component of health-related fitness (1). The President's Council on Sports, Fitness & Nutrition was in part prompted by the report of Kraus and Hirschland (2), indicating American children performed poorly compared with European children in a fitness assessment, especially on flexibility. The American College of Sports Medicine (ACSM) released its first position stand on cardiorespiratory and muscular fitness in 1981; however, recommendations for flexibility exercises were not included until 1998.

Similar to other components of fitness, it is important to maintain an adequate range of motion (ROM) necessary for activities of daily living and improved functional mobility — particularly in older individuals (3). In addition, stretching a specific muscle group may have positive "global" ROM effects on other body parts (4,5). However, the increase in ROM through flexibility training does not necessarily decrease the incidence of injuries associated with physical activity (4). Further, two recent review articles have concluded that when using static stretching (SS) with a duration of >60 seconds or when using proprioceptive neuromuscular facilitation (PNF) prior to physical activity, there appears to be a decrement in subsequent muscle performance. Such an effect on muscle performance was not evident when dynamic stretching (DS) was applied (4,6). Current evidence suggests that a <30-second DS session does not impede muscle performance, and >30 seconds may improve muscle performance (4).

Flexibility requirements are specific to the demands of individual activities, with some activities requiring more than average ROM at particular joints (*e.g.*, gymnastics and ballet) (7). Recent evidence indicates that increases in flexibility do not necessarily correlate with an increase in mobility. Regular physical activity has been shown to be the best way to improve mobility — particularly in older individuals (8).

Basic Principles of Flexibility

Flexibility is defined as the ROM of a joint or group of joints, as determined by the surrounding skeletal muscles and not influenced by any external forces (9). The flexibility of any given movable joint includes both static and dynamic components. Static flexibility is the full ROM of a given joint due to external forces. It can be achieved by the use of gravitational force, a partner, or specific exercise equipment (10). In contrast, dynamic flexibility is the full ROM of a given joint achieved by the voluntary use of skeletal muscles in combination with external forces (11). Although it is recognized that dynamic flexibility is greater than static flexibility for a given joint, the two may be independent of each other (12). Each movable joint has its own anatomical structure that helps define the ROM in which that joint can move. Due to this joint specificity, the ROM of one particular joint may not predict the ROM of other joints, although individuals participating in a full-body ROM program or performing activities that move several joints through their full ROM will generally have greater full-body flexibility (13).

> Visit ⊙ Lippincott® Connect to watch video 5.1, which demonstrates dynamic arm circles.

Factors Affecting Flexibility

ROM of a given joint is determined by several factors, including muscle properties, physical activity and exercise, anatomical structure, age, and gender.

Muscle properties: The inherent properties of muscle tissue play a major role in the ROM of a given joint. Skeletal muscles, when stretched, exhibit both viscous and elastic properties (viscoelastic properties), which allow them to lengthen under applied long constant tension (creep), and stress relaxation. The response of these properties enables progressive deformation over time, thus increasing ROM (14). Furthermore, research has suggested that the viscoelastic properties of skeletal muscle may be altered and lead to an increase in ROM by either an external thermal modality (*i.e.*, heat pad) or a physically active warm-up (15).

Physical activity and exercise: Both single and multiple bouts of physical activity can lead to greater flexibility of the affected joints, primarily by moving joints through a fuller ROM during exercise than would normally occur (12,16,17). In addition, resistance training programs that incorporate full-ROM exercises may also increase flexibility of the affected joints (18,19), assuming both agonist and antagonist muscles around the joint are being trained (20). For instance, pull-ups or chin-ups move the shoulder through a ROM not normally encountered in day-to-day activities, thereby increasing shoulder ROM. Furthermore, athletes who regularly perform ROM exercise during aerobic, resistance, or flexibility exercise improve performance, at least in part, through an enhanced level of flexibility (21–23). Nonetheless, discrepancies exist in the level of flexibility necessary for a variety of activities (24), such as athletes in the same sport but at different competitive levels (collegiate vs. professional) (25) and athletes in the same sport but at different positions (26). Additionally, there is also a difference in the level of flexibility between dominant and nondominant limbs in athletes who participate in sports that involve bilateral asymmetrical motions such as tennis and baseball (27,28).

Anatomical structures: The ROM of a given joint is influenced by its structure and the anatomical structures surrounding it. Freely moveable joints (synovial) are classified into one of six groups, each with a specific permissible plane or planes of movement (Fig. 5.1) (13,29). Furthermore, joint flexibility is not affected equally by connective tissues around joints. Johns and Wright (30) demonstrated that relative contributions of various soft tissues to joint stiffness are as follows: joint capsule (47%), muscles (41%), tendons (10%), and the skin (2%). In addition, soft tissue

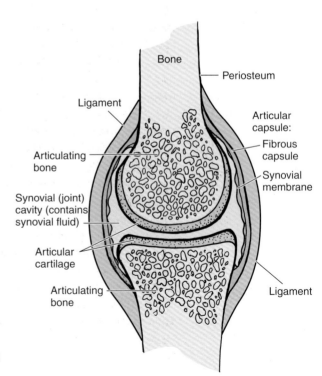

FIGURE 5.1. Classification of synovial joints. (From Bushman B, Battista R, Swan P, Ransdell L, Thompson WR, editors. *ACSM's Resources for the Personal Trainer*. 4th ed. Philadelphia [PA]: Lippincott Williams & Wilkins; 2014. 592 p.)

bulk including muscle and subcutaneous fat tissues may affect joint flexibility because of potential movement restriction (29,31).

Age and gender: Several studies have examined the relationship between the degree of flexibility within a given joint relative to age and gender. These studies have demonstrated that with aging, there is a reduction in collagen solubility, which may lead to increases in tendon rigidity and therefore reduction in joint ROM (21). This reduction may be further exacerbated by age-related conditions such as past injuries, degenerative joint disease, and decreased levels of physical activity (21–23). Normative data collected on thousands of men and women at The Cooper Institute show that women consistently have greater ROM across almost all measured joints compared with men (32). Some of the reasons for increased female flexibility include smaller muscles and wider hips (33) and differences in hormonal levels (34). A study by Park et al. (34) demonstrated that changes in estradiol and progesterone levels during ovulation led to a greater degree of knee joint laxity. Furthermore, it was also demonstrated that women have a more compliant Achilles tendon, resulting in greater ankle flexibility and lower muscle stiffness (35).

> Visit ◯ Lippincott® Connect to watch video 5.2, which demonstrates the soldier walk.

Modes of Flexibility Training

There are four types of flexibility training modes. Three of these modes — static, ballistic, and PNF — are considered "traditional" flexibility training modes (27). Dynamic flexibility training is becoming more common especially as part of the warm-up routine (28,29) to better prepare the body for activity (36). Of all the different modes, static flexibility training is most commonly used and can be further subdivided into three categories: (a) slow and constant stretch with a partner (passive), (b) slow and constant stretch without any assistance, or "self-stretching," and (c) slow and constant stretch against a stationary object (isometric) (25).

Static Flexibility

SS is the most commonly used flexibility protocol of all due to the fact that it can be easily administered without assistance (25), and regardless of the type of SS, each involves a slow and constant motion that is held in the terminal ROM of the muscle, or point of mild discomfort, for 10–30 seconds (31). To achieve an optimal degree of ROM, it is recommended that each exercise is repeated no more than four times. Taylor et al. (37) found that little alteration of the musculotendinous unit occurred with more than four repetitions and that the first few stretches were responsible for the muscle elongation. The advantage of using this method involves both relaxation and concurrent elongation of the stretched muscle without stimulation of the stretch reflex (14). Several studies have demonstrated that SS can lead to both short- and long-term gains in flexibility (38–40) through a decrease in muscle/tendon stiffness and viscoelastic stress relaxation (41,42). Although many researchers and practitioners view SS as effective and beneficial (Fig. 5.2) (7,38,39), others have raised concerns as to the effectiveness prior to sport performance (3,4,43). Because SS is slow and controlled, it does not provide an increase in muscle temperature and blood flow redistribution that is needed before exercise particularly prior to competitive sports performance (44–46). In addition, the view that SS may improve performance is ambiguous, with several studies reporting an increase (46–49), several reporting a decrease (40,43,50,51), and others reporting no changes (37,52) in performance.

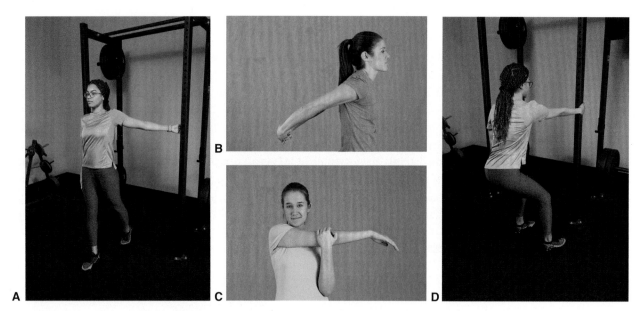

FIGURE 5.2. Examples of static stretches: pectoral wall stretch **(A)**, posterior shoulder hyperextension **(B)**, anterior cross-arm stretch **(C)**, and lat stretch **(D)**. (**B** and **C** from Ratamess N. *ACSM's Foundations of Strength Training and Conditioning*. Philadelphia [PA]: Lippincott Williams & Wilkins; 2012. 560 p.)

Ballistic Flexibility

Ballistic stretching involves rapid and bouncing-like movements in which the resultant momentum of the body or body segments is used to extend the affected joint through the full ROM (13). This type of stretching technique, as opposed to SS and PNF, is no longer advocated as common practice for most individuals (53) to improve a joint's ROM. However, ballistic stretching is still used by some athletes and coaches to increase blood flow to the muscle prior to competition or practice. Current research in this area indicates that properly performed ballistic stretching is equally as effective as SS in increasing joint ROM and may be considered for adults who engage in activities that involve ballistic movements such as basketball (31,54,55). However, given the nature of the movements, this type of stretching produces a rapid and high degree of tension inside the muscle, which may potentially lead to muscle and tendon injuries by stimulating a myotatic reflex (also referred to as the stretch reflex) in the muscle (14,15,27). The stimulation of a myotatic reflex increases muscle tension and does not allow enough time to reduce tension or increase length which is common with this mode of stretching (13,56). However, the hypothesis that ballistic stretching leads to muscle or connective tissue injury has never been supported by the scientific literature (57,58). Although not recommended for the general population, recent research has indicated that ballistic stretching can improve vertical jump height, which can be important for performance in sporting events such as basketball, soccer, and volleyball (56,59). Yet, for the general population, it is recommended to use techniques that are viewed as safer and may potentially be more effective such as SS, DS, and PNF (28).

Proprioceptive Neuromuscular Facilitation

Originated in the 1940s and 1950s by Herman Kabat and Margaret Knott, PNF was developed to treat patients with paralysis to improve the strength and flexibility of a weaker, more distal muscle by increasing irradiation of strength from the stronger more proximal muscle that was related in function (60). It was later adopted for use by athletes as a technique to increase ROM (Fig. 5.3) (11).

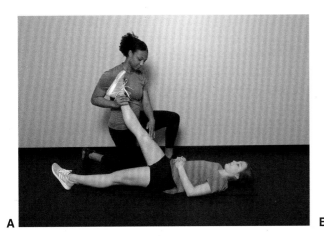
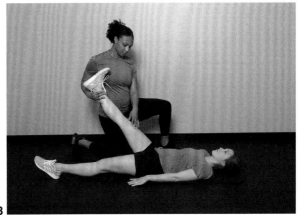
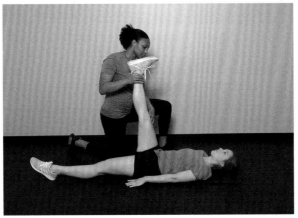

FIGURE 5.3. Linear PNF stretching.

Traditionally, movement consists of specific spiral and diagonal patterns to mimic functional motion in the joint and use Sherrington's (61) principles of successive induction, reciprocal inner-vation and inhibition, and irradiation. This diagonal movement of the limb has been shown to produce changes in the cortical hemispheres of the brain leading to a more permanent functional motion (62,63). There are two pairs of diagonal patterns when working with the upper and lower extremity to improve functional motion. These are diagonal 1 (D1) and diagonal 2 (D2) with either a flexion or an extension component associated with the motion and are used in both the upper and lower extremities (Fig. 5.4) (60,64).

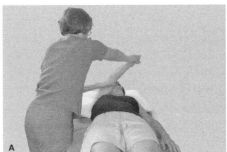
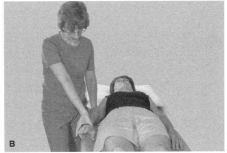

FIGURE 5.4. D1 flexion **(A)** and D1 extension **(B)** PNF stretching. (From O'Sullivan SB, Schmitz TJ. *Improving Functional Outcomes in Physical Rehabilitation*. 2nd ed. Philadelphia [PA]: F.A. Davis; 2016. 384 p.)

In addition to diagonal movements, the use of sensory cues such as proprioceptive, visual, auditory, and tactile sensation are used to augment motor responses (60,61,64). The techniques most commonly used to improve flexibility include hold–relax (HR), agonist contraction (AC), and hold–relax with agonist contraction (HR-AC). These combine passive stretch with isometric and concentric muscle actions designed to use the autogenic and reciprocal inhibition responses of the Golgi tendon organs (GTOs) (13,28). It is hypothesized that through the responses of the GTO, the muscle and tendon are able to elongate and achieve greater ROM, thus increasing neuromuscular efficiency (28,65).

> Visit ⊙ Lippincott® Connect to watch video 5.3, which demonstrates PNF stretching.

Each technique comprises three phases: (a) a passive prestretch, (b) passive stretch, and (c) contraction. The HR technique is most commonly used and begins with passively moving the limb to a point of resistance, holding that position for a couple of seconds, followed by a submaximal isometric contraction of the target muscle (*i.e.*, muscle to be stretched). The contraction is held for ~5 seconds and is followed by a voluntary relaxation of the target muscle (66). One repetition has been shown to be sufficient to increase ROM with subsequent repetitions producing minor gains (60,64,66). In the AC technique, the "agonist" is considered the muscle opposite of the target muscle. In this case, the individual concentrically contracts the muscle *opposite* the target muscle and holds it at the end range for several seconds. Movement is performed independently and controlled. After brief relaxation, the individual repeats the procedure. There have been reports of improved ROM with this technique. As an example, to improve the ROM in the hamstrings, the individual would concentrically shorten the quadriceps to move the lower limb toward the body and hold at the end range. This technique has had best results with individuals who are unable to produce a pain-free maximal isometric contraction necessary for HR. Additionally, this technique can be performed without the assistance of another person (64,65). HR-AC combines the HR and AC techniques where the limb is passively moved to an endpoint of resistance, holding that position for a couple of seconds followed by a submaximal isometric contraction. Upon relaxation, the individual immediately concentrically contracts the opposite muscle to a greater ROM and holds in this new range for a few seconds. When PNF is compared with other stretching techniques with respect to effectiveness of improving ROM, the data are inconsistent. Some studies have demonstrated that PNF is superior to both static and ballistic stretching techniques (9,67,68), whereas others have found no difference (20,69–71). Despite the wide support that PNF stretching has among researchers and practitioners, there are some limitations with these techniques such as the need for a trained partner and the potential risk for musculoskeletal injury (72,73).

Dynamic Flexibility

As opposed to the previously mentioned stretching techniques, dynamic flexibility uses slow and controlled, sport-specific movements designed to increase core temperature, leading to increased neuromuscular conduction and compliance and enzymatic activity, which may accelerate energy production and enhance activity-related flexibility and balance (7,29,31,74). In view of the fact that these exercises are sport specific, there is no comprehensive list of dynamic exercises. The design of such exercises is only limited by the knowledge and resourcefulness of the coach/trainer (74). In the past few years, several studies have examined the effectiveness of dynamic flexibility in relation to the degree of flexibility and athletic performance and the effects of preexercise SS and DS on anaerobic performance in different populations. One study demonstrated that both static

EXERCISE IS MEDICINE CONNECTION

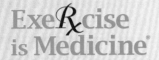

Moonaz S, Bingham C III, Wissow L, Bartlett S. Yoga in sedentary adults with arthritis: effects of a randomized controlled pragmatic trial. *J Rheumatol.* 2015:42(7);1194–202.

Yoga has been used for more than 5,000 years around the world as a means of improving health and preparation for meditation, with well-documented studies showing increased flexibility and ROM, a key aspect of health-related fitness. Yoga's use has increased dramatically as a popular exercise modality in the United States in the recent past. It is estimated that the number of Americans that practice yoga increased by 29% between the years 2008 and 2012.

In addition to the benefits to flexibility, yoga has often been used to ease pain and dysfunction associated with arthritis, a debilitating condition that results in inflammation, stiffness, and pain at and around the joints and affects over 50 million Americans. Recent evidence suggests that yoga training may improve physical activity adherence and physical and psychological health through a series of postures referred to as asanas.

Moonaz et al. randomly assigned 75 physically inactive adults with rheumatoid arthritis (RA) or knee osteoarthritis (OA) to an 8-week yoga program group or a control group. Per week, the yoga program group completed two 60-minute classes and one home practice. Outcome measures included physical and mental components representing health-related quality of life (HRQL) domains and disease activity. In the yoga group, the researchers followed the participants for an additional 9 months to examine the long-term effects of the program. The results of this study demonstrated that an 8-week yoga program led to improved physical and mental components, improved walking capacity, and reduced depressive symptoms. It was also demonstrated that most of these benefits were maintained 9 months after cessation of the program.

In summary, appropriately designed yoga programs can be an effective treatment for improving physical and psychological health and physical abilities in patients with RA and OA.

Visit ⊙ Lippincott® Connect to watch videos 5.4 and 5.5, which demonstrate the kneeling cat and modified cobra positions, respectively.

and dynamic stretches improve the ROM of the hamstring muscle; yet, SS was more effective (7). Furthermore, whereas some studies have demonstrated that a warm-up that included DS was superior for improving sport performance to one that included SS (75–77), others have failed to show those differences (58,78,79). Also related to DS, eccentric training was recently introduced as a new technique that is designed to reduce the occurrence of injuries and improve flexibility and performance. Using this technique, the participant is instructed to resist flexion in a given joint by eccentrically contracting the antagonist muscles during the entire ROM (57). Two studies examining this technique have demonstrated some merit when compared with SS. The available evidence suggests that short sessions of dynamic stretches (<30 s) do not adversely affect exercise bout performance, and prolonged sessions (>30 s) may facilitate performance (4,80). Therefore, DS is recommended both prior to more vigorous exercise and also as a potential adjunct to improving sport performance.

● Muscle and Tendon Proprioceptors

There are two types of joint receptors that provide muscular dynamic and limb movement information to the central nervous system (81). These joint receptors, muscle spindles (Fig. 5.5), and GTOs (Fig. 5.6) must be considered when discussing stretching and flexibility. Muscle spindles are a collection of 3–10 intrafusal, specialized muscle fibers that are innervated by γ motor neurons and provide information about the rate of change in muscle length. The intrafusal muscle fibers run parallel to the extrafusal muscle fibers (regular muscle fibers), which are innervated by α motor neurons and are responsible for tension development (see Fig. 5.5) (13,82). When muscle spindles are stimulated, there is a dual response in which rapid tension development is initiated in the stretched muscle and inhibited in the antagonist muscle. The response in the stretched muscle is known as a stretch or myotatic reflex, and the response in the antagonist muscle is known as reciprocal inhibition (13,20,83). These responses serve an important role in both SS and PNF. Because the myotatic reflex is less likely to occur in slow and controlled movements, static stretch is viewed as a safer and more effective technique than ballistic stretch (13). During PNF stretching when there is an increase in tension in the antagonist muscle with a concurrent elongation of the agonist muscle, a further lengthening of the stretched muscle is thought to be mediated by reciprocal inhibition (28,60).

GTOs are located in the musculotendinous junction and respond to changes in muscle tension (see Fig. 5.6). These organs are encapsulated in a series with 10–15 muscle fibers and can identify and provide a response to changes in the amount of tension (static) and the rate of tension (dynamic) development. When the GTOs are stimulated, there is a dual response in which tension development is inhibited in the contracting muscle (autogenic inhibition) and initiated in the antagonist muscles to protect the muscle tissue from damage (13,82). Similar to the muscle spindles' response, the GTO plays an important role in PNF. The active tension development in the muscle prior to a stretch elicits autogenic inhibition, which promotes further lengthening of the affected muscle (20,82,83).

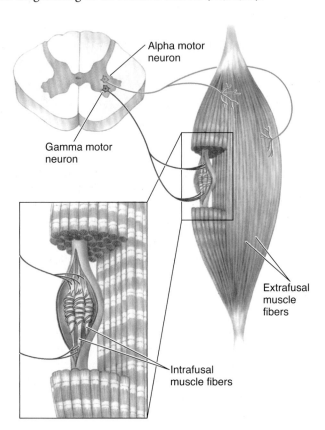

Alpha motor neuron

Gamma motor neuron

Extrafusal muscle fibers

Intrafusal muscle fibers

FIGURE 5.5. Structure and location of the muscle spindles. (From Bear MF, Connors BW, Parasido MA. *Neuroscience: Exploring the Brain.* 2nd ed. Philadelphia [PA]: Lippincott Williams & Wilkins; 2001. 855 p.)

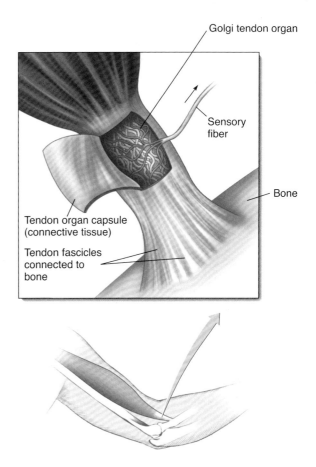

FIGURE 5.6. Structure and location of the GTO. (From Premkumar K. *The Massage Connection: Anatomy & Physiology.* 2nd ed. Baltimore [MD]: Lippincott Williams & Wilkins; 2004. 341 p.)

Flexibility Assessment Protocols

Flexibility and ROM can be assessed dynamically or statically. However, dynamic flexibility testing is mostly used in research settings as functional movement. Static flexibility can be assessed either directly or indirectly. Directly, flexibility can be measured using goniometers, Leighton flexometers, or inclinometers. The most common method used to measure flexibility indirectly is the sit-and-reach test. Although previous editions of this text described various versions of the sit-and-reach test, it was removed from this edition due to several reasons. First, the sit-and-reach test is an indirect measure with several different published versions, which at times may cause confusion (31). Second, several studies have suggested that although the sit-and-reach test is established to measure low back and hamstring flexibility, the relationship to low back pain and hamstring flexibility is questionable (84,85). Presently, more commonly used tools are goniometers and functional movement screenings.

Goniometers and Inclinometers

Quantitative assessment of ROM is necessary to identify deficiencies resulting from injury or the need for a flexibility training program relative to the individual's needs. Given that ROM is joint specific, knowing the ROM ranges for the specific joint will help to address any problematic areas that need attention. The most useful method for determining individual joint flexibility is using a goniometer (Fig. 5.7). Once established, an appropriate flexibility prescription with the goal of increasing or maintaining ROM can be implemented.

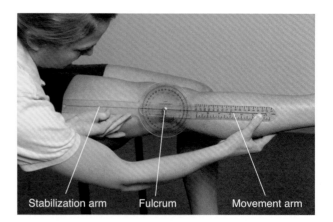

FIGURE 5.7. A goniometer includes the body axis or fulcrum, a stabilization arm, and a movement arm.

A goniometer is similar to a protractor and is used to measure a joint's ROM expressed in degrees. Proper procedures followed by an ACSM Certified Exercise Physiologist® (ACSM-EP®) provide both valid and reliable results (31). Proper positioning of the instrument includes first identifying the specific joint line and placing the axis (pin) of the goniometer at the joint's axis of rotation. Second, line up the arms with the given anatomical reference points on the body. The goniometer consists of two arms: a stabilization arm that is fixed and aligned with specific anatomical reference points on the proximal body segment and a movement arm that aligns with specific anatomical reference points that follow the distal body segment as it is moved through its ROM (84,85).

An inclinometer is a type of gravity-dependent goniometer. The inclinometer measures the angle between the movement arm and the line of gravity while the tester holds the device on the distal end of the of the body segment. As seen in Figure 5.8 and as recommended by the American Medical Association, a double inclinometer should be used (64,86,87).

Procedures for goniometry assessment of commonly measured joints are listed in Table 5.1. General guidelines for proper goniometry and inclinometer assessments include the following (see ACSM [31] Box 3.12):

1. Client should participate in a general warm-up followed by SS prior to ROM testing.
2. If using a goniometer, the axis of the goniometer should be placed at the center of the joint being evaluated. The fixed arm of the goniometer should be aligned with the appropriate bony landmark of the stationary body part, and the movable arm of the goniometer should be aligned with the specified bony landmark of the body segment that is going to be moving. For anatomical landmarks, refer to Gibson et al. (87). If using an inclinometer, it should be held on the distal end of the moveable body segment.
3. Record the ROM in degrees.
4. Administer multiple trials; three are recommended.
5. Use the best score to compare to reference values.

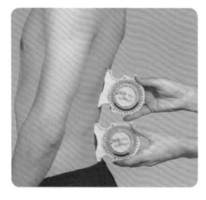
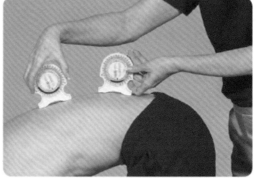

FIGURE 5.8. An inclinometer and a double inclinometer. (From Gibson AL, Wagner DR, Heyward VH. *Advanced Fitness Assessment and Exercise Prescription.* 8th ed. Champaign [IL]: Human Kinetics; 2019. 560 p.)

TABLE 5.1 Procedures for Goniometry Assessment of Joints Commonly of Concern to Health and Fitness Professionals

Movement	Plane of Motion	Axis of Motion	Average Range	Goniometer Position	Stabilization	Starting/Ending Body Position	
Spine							
					Upper Body		
Lumbar flexion (Fig. 5.9)	Sagittal	Bilateral	4-in increase	Tape measure position 1. Top point: spinous process C7 2. Bottom point: level to posterior superior iliac spine (PSIS)	Client is seated on floor or table with pelvis stabilized to prevent anterior/posterior tilting with legs extended.	Client is in good posture with a stabilized cervical, thoracic, and lumbar spine in 0° of flexion, extension, rotation, or lateral flexion. Head is in neutral position. Client performs lumbar flexion until first sign of resistance.	FIGURE 5.9. Lumbar flexion and extension. (From Bushman B, Battista R, Swan P, Ransdell L, Thompson WR, editors. *ACSM's Resources for the Personal Trainer.* 4th ed. Philadelphia [PA]: Lippincott Williams & Wilkins; 2014. 592 p.)
Lumbar extension (see Fig. 5.9)	Sagittal	Bilateral	2-in difference as spine extends	Tape measure position 1. Top point: spinous process C7 2. Bottom point: level to PSIS	Client is seated on floor or table with pelvis stabilized to prevent anterior/posterior tilting with legs extended.	Client is in good posture with a stabilized cervical, thoracic, and lumbar spine in 0° of flexion, extension, rotation, or lateral flexion. Head is in neutral position. Client performs lumbar extension until first sign of resistance.	

Continued

Table 5.1 Procedures for Goniometry Assessment of Joints Commonly of Concern to Health and Fitness Professionals (continued)

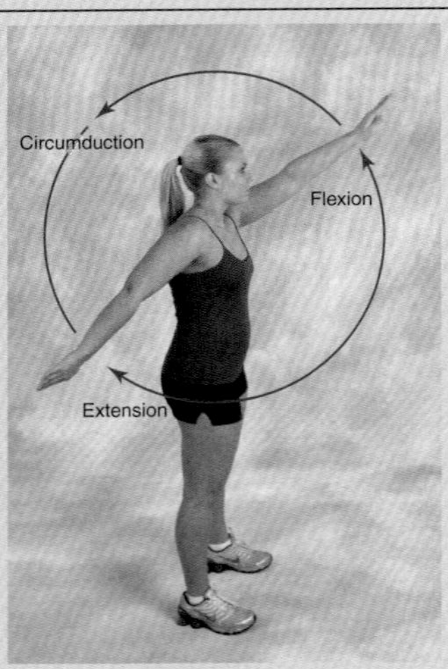

FIGURE 5.10. Glenohumeral flexion and extension. (From Bushman B, Battista R, Swan P, Ransdell L, Thompson WR, editors. *ACSM's Resources for the Personal Trainer.* 4th ed. Philadelphia [PA]: Lippincott Williams & Wilkins; 2014. 592 p.)

Movement	Plane of Motion	Axis of Motion	Average Range	Goniometer Position	Stabilization	Starting/Ending Body Position
Upper Body						
Shoulder						
Glenohumeral flexion (Fig. 5.10)	Sagittal	Bilateral	0°–180°	1. Axis point: lateral aspect of greater tubercle 2. Stabilization arm: perpendicular to the floor 3. Movement arm: Align with midline of humerus and reference the lateral epicondyle.	Client is in good posture with a stabilized scapula (retracted), thoracic, and lumbar spine. Stabilize scapula to prevent tilting, rotation, or elevation.	Client is seated with glenohumeral in 0° of flexion, extension, abduction, or adduction. Head is in neutral position. Palm of hand should be facing the body. Elbow should be extended completely. Client performs glenohumeral flexion until the first sign of resistance.
Glenohumeral extension (see Fig. 5.10)	Sagittal	Bilateral	0°–60°	1. Axis point: lateral aspect of greater tubercle 2. Stabilization arm: perpendicular to the floor 3. Movement arm: Align with midline of humerus and reference the lateral epicondyle.	Client is in good posture with a stabilized scapula (retracted), thoracic, and lumbar spine. Stabilize scapula to prevent tilting, rotation, or elevation. Place towel under humerus to stabilize and align with acromion process.	Client is prone on table with glenohumeral in 0° of flexion, extension, abduction, or adduction. Head is in neutral position. Palm of hand should face the body. Elbow should be extended completely. Client performs glenohumeral extension until the first sign of resistance.

FIGURE 5.11. Glenohumeral internal rotation and external rotation. (From Bushman B, Battista R, Swan P, Ransdell L, Thompson WR, editors. *ACSM's Resources for the Personal Trainer.* 4th ed. Philadelphia [PA]: Lippincott Williams & Wilkins; 2014. 592 p.)

Glenohumeral internal rotation (Fig. 5.11)	Transverse	Longitudinal 0°–70°	1. Axis point: olecranon process of the elbow 2. Stabilization arm: perpendicular to the floor 3. Movement arm: Align with lateral midline of ulna and reference the ulnar styloid.	Client is in good posture with a stabilized scapula (retracted), thoracic, and lumbar spine. Stabilize scapula to prevent tilting, rotation, or elevation. Place towel under humerus to stabilize and align with acromion process.	Client is supine on table with humerus abducted at 90° and elbow is flexed at 90°. Elbow is at 0° of supination and pronation. Client performs glenohumeral internal rotation until the first sign of resistance. 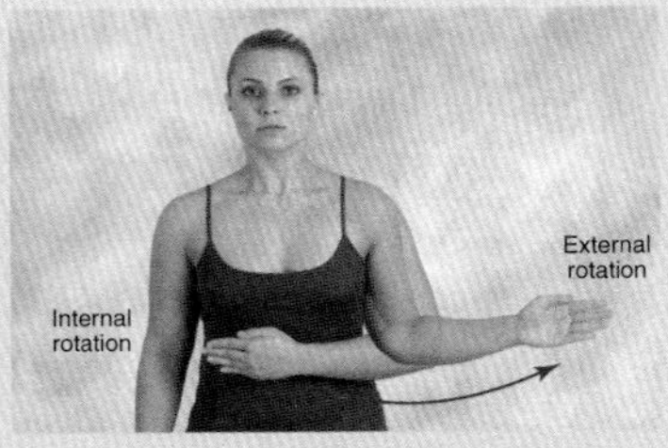
Glenohumeral external rotation (see Fig. 5.11)	Transverse	Longitudinal 0°–90°	1. Axis point: olecranon process of the elbow 2. Stabilization arm: perpendicular to the floor 3. Movement arm: Align with lateral midline of ulna and reference the ulnar styloid.	Client is in good posture with a stabilized scapula (retracted), thoracic, and lumbar spine. Stabilize scapula to prevent tilting, rotation, or elevation. Place towel under humerus to stabilize and align with acromion process.	Client is supine on table with humerus abducted at 90° and elbow is flexed at 90°. Elbow is at 0° of supination and pronation. Client performs glenohumeral external rotation until the first sign of resistance.

Continued

Table 5.1 Procedures for Goniometry Assessment of Joints Commonly of Concern to Health and Fitness Professionals (continued)

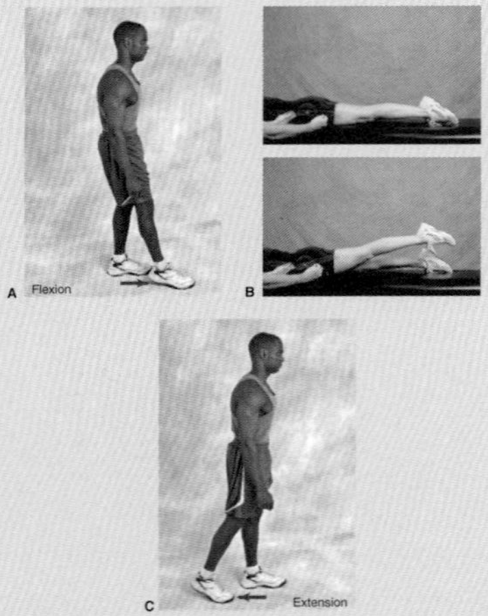

FIGURE 5.12. Hip flexion with the testing leg fully extended (A) and with the testing knee and hip both flexed 90° (B); hip extension with the testing leg fully extended (C). (A and C from Bushman B, Battista R, Swan P, Ransdell L, Thompson WR, editors. *ACSM's Resources for the Personal Trainer.* 4th ed. Philadelphia [PA]: Lippincott Williams & Wilkins; 2014. 592 p. B from Kaminsky L. *ACSM's Health-Related Physical Fitness Assessment Manual.* 4th ed. Philadelphia [PA]: Lippincott Williams & Wilkins; 2014. 192 p.)

Movement	Plane of Motion	Axis of Motion	Average Range	Goniometer Position	Stabilization	Starting/Ending Body Position
Hip						
Hip flexion (testing leg fully extended) (Fig. 5.12A)	Sagittal	Bilateral	0°–90°	1. Axis point: greater trochanter of the lateral thigh 2. Stabilization arm: lateral midline of the pelvis 3. Movement arm: lateral midline of the femur, using the lateral epicondyle as a reference	Client is in good posture with a stabilized scapula, thoracic, lumbar spine, and pelvic area. Pelvis should not rise off table. Opposite leg not being assessed should have knee flexed and foot flat on table for added stability and protection for the back.	Client is supine on table with hip in 0° of flexion, extension, abduction, adduction, and rotation. Testing leg has knee fully extended. Client performs hip flexion until the first sign of resistance or until the pelvis rotates or knee breaks extension.
Hip flexion (testing knee flexed 90° and hip flexed 90°) (Fig. 5.12B)	Sagittal	Bilateral	0°–120°	1. Axis point: greater trochanter of the lateral thigh 2. Stabilization arm: lateral midline of the pelvis 3. Movement arm: lateral midline of the femur, using the lateral epicondyle as a reference	Client is in good posture with a stabilized scapula, thoracic, lumbar spine, and pelvic area. Pelvis should not rise off table. Opposite leg not being assessed should have knee flexed and foot flat on table for added stability and protection for the back.	Client is supine on table with knee flexed at 90° and hip flexed at 90°, and hip is in 0° of abduction, adduction, and rotation. Knee is flexed to reduce contraction of hamstrings. Client performs hip flexion until the first sign of resistance or until the pelvis rotates.

Movement	Plane		Range	Client posture	Measurement points	Procedure
Hip extension (testing leg fully extended) (Fig. 5.12C)	Sagittal	Bilateral	0°–30°	Client is in good posture with a stabilized scapula, thoracic, lumbar spine. Pelvis and pelvic area. Pelvis should not rise off table. Opposite leg not being assessed should have leg fully extended on table for added stability.	1. Axis point: greater trochanter of the lateral thigh 2. Stabilization arm: lateral midline of the pelvis 3. Movement arm: lateral midline of the femur, using the lateral epicondyle as a reference	Client is prone on table with a hip in 0° of flexion, extension, abduction, adduction, and rotation. Testing leg has knee fully extended. Client performs hip extension until the first sign of resistance or until the pelvis rotates.
Hip abduction (Fig. 5.13)	Frontal	Anterior/posterior	0°–45°	Client is in good posture with a stabilized scapula, thoracic, lumbar spine, and pelvic area. Stabilize for lateral trunk flexion on both sides.	1. Axis point: locate anterior superior iliac spine (ASIS) 2. Stabilization arm: imaginary line connecting axis point ASIS to other ASIS 3. Movement arm: anterior midline of the femur, using the midline of the patella as a reference	Client is supine on table with hip in 0° of flexion, extension, abduction, adduction, and rotation. Testing leg has knee fully extended. Client performs hip abduction until the first sign of resistance or lateral trunk flexion occurs on either side.

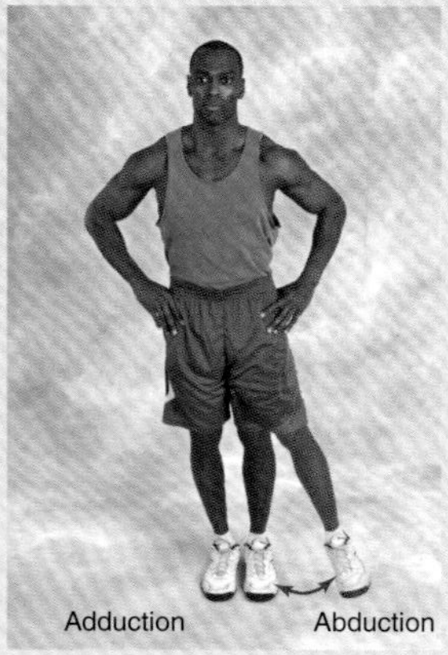

FIGURE 5.13. Hip adduction and abduction. (From Bushman B, Battista R, Swan P, Ransdell L, Thompson WR, editors. *ACSM's Resources for the Personal Trainer.* 4th ed. Philadelphia [PA]: Lippincott Williams & Wilkins; 2014. 592 p.)

Continued

Table 5.1 Procedures for Goniometry Assessment of Joints Commonly of Concern to Health and Fitness Professionals (continued)

Movement	Plane of Motion	Axis of Motion	Average Range	Goniometer Position	Stabilization	Starting/Ending Body Position
Lower Body						
Hip						
Hip adduction (see Fig. 5.13)	Frontal	Anterior/posterior	0°–30°	1. Axis point: located at the ASIS 2. Stabilization arm: imaginary horizontal line connecting axis point ASIS to other ASIS 3. Movement arm: anterior midline of the femur, using the midline of the patella as a reference	Client is in good posture with a stabilized scapula, thoracic, lumbar spine, and pelvic area. Opposite leg not being tested should be abducted fully to allow for testing hip to be assessed.	Client is supine on table with hip in 0° of flexion, extension, and rotation. Testing leg has knee fully extended. Client performs hip adduction until the first sign of resistance or lateral trunk flexion or pelvic rotation occurs.

Flexibility Program Design

The framework for developing and maintaining whole-body ROM is structured around the same underlying principles that all health-related fitness components use: progressive overload, specificity of training, individual differences, and reversibility. The components of a health-related fitness program consisting of frequency, intensity, time, and type (FITT) are the foundation for which flexibility programs are developed (46,51).

Assessment of ROM at specific joints helps determine the need for a flexibility program. Healthy individuals with inadequate ROM for particular activities should engage in a program that caters to their specific needs.

Once adequate ROM is achieved, a maintenance program should be prescribed. For individuals with hypermobility in joint ROM, there does not seem to be a benefit of participation in a flexibility training program (24,88–91).

The principle of progressive overload in the context of flexibility demonstrates that for ROM to improve, it must be stressed beyond its normal range. This may be accomplished by completing the flexibility exercises recommended below or by participating in activities that elicit greater ROM in targeted joints.

The principle of overload for flexibility training may be applied by the following:

- Increasing frequency (sessions per day or week)
- Increasing intensity (point of stretch)
- Increasing time for each session

Individual differences as it relates to neuromuscular function and structure should be taken into consideration in the design of a flexibility program. However, to date, there are no specific guidelines for optimal progression (31,54). The principle of reversibility should also be considered with respect to flexibility training as with other modes of exercise. Feland et al. (92) demonstrated that flexibility gains are lost within 4–8 weeks of ceasing flexibility exercises.

After assessment of flexibility, a training program may be necessary to increase or maintain ROM relative to individual goals. See Table 5.2 for an evidence-based flexibility exercise program

Table 5.2	Flexibility Exercise Evidence-Based Recommendations
FITT	**Evidence-Based Recommendation**
Frequency	■ $\geq$2–3 d · wk^{-1} with daily being most effective
Intensity	■ Stretch to the point of feeling tightness or slight discomfort.
Time	■ Holding a static stretch for 10–30 s is recommended for most adults.
	■ In older individuals, holding a stretch for 30–60 s may confer greater benefit.
	■ For PNF stretching, a 3- to 6-s light-to-moderate contraction (*e.g.*, 20%–75% of maximum voluntary contraction) followed by a 10- to 30-s assisted stretch is desirable.
Type	■ A series of flexibility exercises for each of the major muscle-tendon units is recommended.
	■ Static flexibility (*i.e.*, active or passive), dynamic flexibility, ballistic flexibility, and PNF are each effective.

Adapted with permission from American College of Sports Medicine. *ACSM's Guidelines for Exercise Testing and Prescription.* 11th ed. Philadelphia (PA): Wolters Kluwer; 2021. 548 p. (Table 5.6).

recommendation. To improve ROM, two to three training sessions per week for at least 3–4 weeks may be required (92–94), although daily stretching exercises may be more effective (54). During each of the training sessions, each exercise should include two to four repetitions in which the stretch is held between 10 and 30 seconds, with 30–60 seconds in older individuals, with a goal of accumulating 60 seconds of stretch across two to four repetitions (31,54,95). Increasing the duration of each repetition beyond 30–60 seconds does not seem to lead to improved ROM benefits except perhaps in an elderly population (54,92,96). Generally, joints of the neck, shoulders, upper and lower back, pelvis, hips, and legs will need to be trained as it relates to daily activity and performance (37).

Flexibility training should be conducted when a muscle is warm and therefore should be completed after an aerobic warm-up of at least 5 minutes and some general ROM exercises. Similarly, testing may occur subsequent to cardiovascular or strength sessions. Because some researchers have demonstrated that acute preexercise flexibility training may have negative effects on ensuing performance, postexercise flexibility training may be more beneficial (88–91). The intensity of flexibility training is dependent on the individual; recommendations suggest that a given stretch be held to the point of tightness or slight discomfort (97). The duration of the training session may vary based on the mode of the flexibility exercise. An SS session should be at a minimum of 10 minutes, and if PNF stretching is being employed, a 20%–75% maximum voluntary contraction should be held for 3- to 6-second contraction followed by either a 10- to 30-second assisted stretch or opposing muscle contraction to another position show similar results in the short term (31,64,66).

The mode of the flexibility program should depend on the individual and available equipment. Generally, increased ROM has been demonstrated in all modes of flexibility training (98,99). Table 5.3 lists some static stretches for the major muscle groups.

Numerous examinations have reported no link between ROM training and prevention of low back pain, injury, or postexercise muscle soreness (100–104). However, individuals with ROM imbalances may be at an increased risk for injury during activity (105) and therefore benefit from stretching exercises when combined with other forms of exercise (106). This benefit, however, may be limited to those with ROM imbalances and not be effective as a simple means of injury prevention. Furthermore, there has been recent research suggesting a link between antibiotics and musculotendinous injuries. Individuals who are using fluoroquinolone antibiotics are at an increased risk for tendon rupture and joint and muscle damage and therefore should approach flexibility exercises with extreme caution (107).

> Visit ⊙ Lippincott® Connect to watch videos 5.7 and 5.8, which demonstrate pendulum leg swings and dynamic hip rotation, respectively.

Overall Range of Motion Recommendations

To determine an appropriate program design, one must discern between flexibility training with the sole purpose of increasing ROM (often using SS) and/or flexibility exercises with the primary purpose of preparing for fitness training or sport-specific training. The former may be necessary for someone who has limited ROM due to genetics or disuse due to injury or lack of activity. The latter is generally part of a dynamic warm-up prior to more intense or skill-dependent exercise and therefore allows for better preparation for optimal performance (103,108). However, ROM warm-up activities that do not include a dynamic component (and therefore do not tend to increase body temperature, blood flow, etc.) have not shown a benefit to performance or reduction in injury rate during subsequent activity (89–91,100–103).

Table 5.3 Static Stretches for the Major Muscle Groups

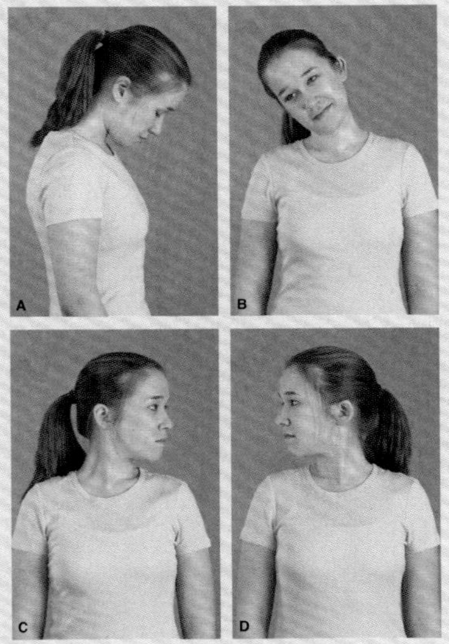

FIGURE 5.14. Neck flexion **(A)**, extension **(B)**, lateral flexion **(C)**, and rotation **(D)**. (From Ratamess N. *ACSM's Foundations of Strength Training and Conditioning.* Philadelphia [PA]: Lippincott Williams & Wilkins; 2012. 560 p.)

Continued

Stretch	Muscle Involved	Starting Position	Description
Neck			
			Upper Body
Flexion for stretching extensors (Fig. 5.14A)	■ Obliquus capitis superior Rectus capitis superior major Rectus capitis superior minor Obliquus capitis inferior Semispinalis capitis Splenius cervicis Longissimus capitis Levator scapulae	Standing or sitting	Starting with the superior segments, first retract your chin and then slowly flex your cervical spine so that your chin moves toward your chest. Maintain your chest and shoulders in a static position.
Lateral bending (Fig. 5.14C)	■ Upper trapezius Anterior, middle, and posterior scalene Sternocleidomastoid Splenius capitis	Standing or sitting	Take your right hand and reach over the top of your head, placing it palm down on your head so that your middle two fingers touch your left ear. Carefully, pull your head directly toward the right side, being careful not to let your head move forward or back. Repeat to the left.
Rotation (Fig. 5.14D)	■ Sternocleidomastoid Longissimus capitis Splenius capitis Obliquus capitis inferior	Standing or sitting	Use your left hand to reach behind your back and pull your right forearm gently inferiorly and toward the left, depressing your right shoulder. Carefully turn your head toward the left. Repeat toward the right.

Table 5.3 Static Stretches for the Major Muscle Groups (continued)

Upper Body

Stretch	Muscle Involved	Starting Position	Description
Shoulder			
Extension for stretching flexors	■ Pectoralis major Anterior deltoid Long head of biceps brachii Coracobrachialis	Standing	Lock your hands together behind back with elbows only slightly flexed. Lift interlocked hands up behind your back, extending your shoulders. No need to bend your back forward.
Flexion for stretching extensors	■ Latissimus dorsi Teres major Posterior deltoid Long head of the triceps brachii Rhomboid major and minor through their action on the scapula	Standing in front of a chair	Place both hands on the back of a chair or object of similar height. Then, carefully bend at the waist until arms are straightened overhead with a roughly 90° angle at the waist. Be careful to keep your lower back straight, allowing the forward bend to come from flexion at the hips.
Adduction for abductors (Fig. 5.15)	■ Middle deltoid Supraspinatus Upper trapezius through its action in superiorly rotating the scapula (a necessary and integral motion in abducting the shoulder)	Standing	Reach your right hand behind your back. Grasp your right forearm with your left hand. Adduct your right arm by carefully pulling it toward the left until a gentle stretch is felt at the right shoulder. Then slowly lean your head toward the left, increasing the stretch at both your right shoulder and your upper trapezius. Repeat toward the right.
Abduction for adductors (see Fig. 5.15)	■ Pectoralis major Latissimus dorsi Teres major Rhomboids major and minor via their action on the scapula	Standing	Extend your right arm overhead, palm facing to the left. Reach your entire arm directly toward the left and continue with left side bending of your torso. Repeat to the right leading with your left hand.

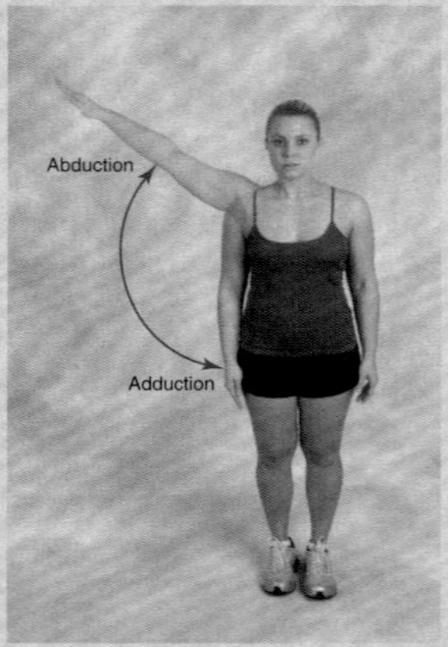

FIGURE 5.15. Shoulder abduction and adduction. (From Bushman B, Battista R, Swan P, Ransdell L, Thompson WR, editors. *ACSM's Resources for the Personal Trainer*. 4th ed. Philadelphia [PA]: Lippincott Williams & Wilkins; 2014. 592 p.)

FIGURE 5.16. Shoulder horizontal adduction and horizontal abduction. (From Bushman B, Battista R, Swan P, Ransdell L, Thompson WR, editors. *ACSM's Resources for the Personal Trainer.* 4th ed. Philadelphia [PA]: Lippincott Williams & Wilkins; 2014. 592 p.)

Continued

Stretch	Muscles	Position	Instructions
Horizontal abduction for horizontal adductors (Fig. 5.16)	Anterior deltoid, Sternal portion of pectoralis major, Coracobrachialis	Standing	Abduct arms to shoulder level with palms facing upward. Horizontally abduct both shoulders, keeping them at shoulder level. You may use a doorway to help assist with this movement. Ideally, both sides can be stretched simultaneously (as the tension from one side stabilizes the origin on the other side); however, this is not necessary, and effective stretches can be performed unilaterally. 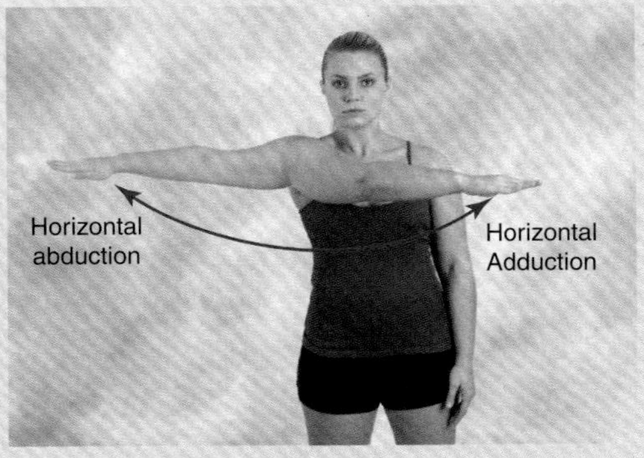
Horizontal adduction for horizontal abductors (see Fig. 5.16)	Posterior deltoid, Teres minor, Infraspinatus, Upper and middle trapezius, Rhomboid major and minor via their attachment to the scapula	Standing	To stretch your left shoulder horizontal abductors, grasp the posterior aspect of your left elbow with your right hand. Horizontally adduct your left shoulder by pulling your left elbow horizontally across toward your right shoulder just beneath the chin. Repeat with the right.
External rotation for internal rotators	Subscapularis, Latissimus dorsi, Pectoralis major, Teres major, Anterior deltoid	Standing in a doorway, right arm at your side, elbow flexed to 90°, and palm facing forward against the doorframe	To stretch your right shoulder internal rotators, keep your right elbow at your side and right hand against the door frame and then carefully turn your body toward the left until you feel a gentle stretch. Repeat for your left shoulder.

Table 5.3	Static Stretches for the Major Muscle Groups (continued)		
Stretch	**Muscle Involved**	**Starting Position**	**Description**
Upper Body			
Shoulder			
Internal rotation for external rotators	Infraspinatus Teres minor Posterior deltoid	Standing	Internally rotate your left shoulder by placing your left hand behind your back with the palm facing posteriorly. Place the palm of your right hand over the anterior aspect of your left shoulder. Back into a doorway with the posterior surface of the left elbow against the door jam. While maintaining firm support of the anterior shoulder with the left palm and hand (do not let the shoulder push forward), carefully move your entire body backward, forcing the elbow forward, until an easy stretch is felt in your left shoulder. Repeat on the opposite side to stretch your right shoulder.
Elbow			
Extension for flexors (Fig. 5.17)	Long and short heads of the biceps brachii Brachialis Brachioradialis	Standing	Clasp your hands together behind your lower back, extend your elbows completely, and then externally rotate your arms so that your palms are facing your buttocks. Now, extend both shoulders by lifting the hands up and away from your buttocks.

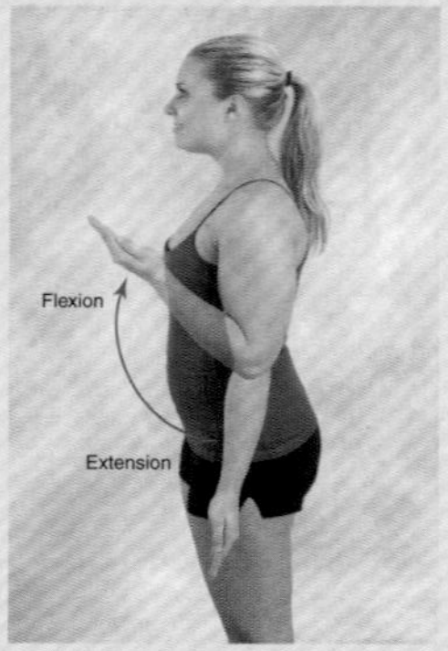

FIGURE 5.17. Elbow flexion and extension. (From Bushman B, Battista R, Swan P, Ransdell L, Thompson WR, editors. *ACSM's Resources for the Personal Trainer.* 4th ed. Philadelphia [PA]: Lippincott Williams & Wilkins; 2014. 592 p.)

Flexion for extensors (see Fig. 5.17)	▪ Long, medial, and middle heads of the triceps brachii Anconeus	Standing	Extend your right arm overhead and flex your elbow maximally. Place the palm of your left hand against your right forearm just distal to the elbow, with your fingers curving over your right elbow. Squeeze your elbow joint to keep it maximally flexed and then slowly pull it posteriorly and medially. Repeat with the left arm.
Pronation for supinators (Fig. 5.18)	▪ Supinator Biceps brachii	Standing with arms relaxed at sides	To stretch the supinators of your right arm, flex your right elbow slightly and pronate your right forearm so that the palm is facing down. Using your left hand, grasp your right forearm just proximal to your wrist. Pronate your right forearm while externally rotating your right humerus. Repeat with the left forearm. 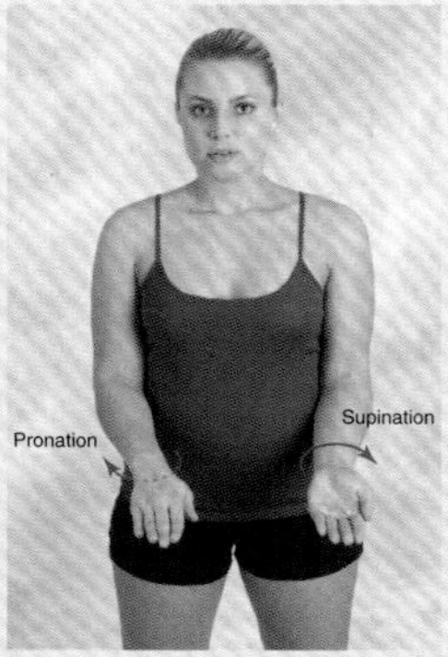
Supination for pronators (see Fig. 5.18)	▪ Pronator teres Pronator quadratus	Standing	To stretch the pronators of your right forearm, extend your right elbow and supinate your right hand. With your left hand, grasp your right forearm just proximal to the wrist. Using your left hand, rotate your right wrist externally, further supinating your right forearm. Be sure to keep your upper arm from externally rotating as well — this may require an active contraction of the shoulder internal rotators. Repeat with the left forearm.

FIGURE 5.18. Elbow supination and pronation. (From Bushman B, Battista R, Swan P, Ransdell L, Thompson WR, editors. *ACSM's Resources for the Personal Trainer.* 4th ed. Philadelphia [PA]: Lippincott Williams & Wilkins; 2014. 592 p.)

Continued

Table 5.3 Static Stretches for the Major Muscle Groups (continued)

Upper Body

Stretch	Muscle Involved	Starting Position	Description
Wrist and Hand			
Flexion for extensors (Fig. 5.19)	Extensor carpi radialis Extensor digitorum Extensor indicis Extensor digiti minimi Extensor carpi radialis Extensor pollicis longus Extensor pollicis brevis	Sitting or standing	To stretch the extensors of your left arm and hand, extend your left arm out in front of you with your elbow extended, forearm pronated. Flex your left wrist and then attempt to flex fingers 2–5 into a fist. Repeat on the right arm.
Extension for flexors (see Fig. 5.19)	Flexor carpi radialis Flexor digitorum profundus Flexor digitorum superficialis Palmaris longus Flexor pollicis longus Flexor carpi ulnaris	Sitting or standing	To stretch the flexors of your left wrist and hand, extend your left arm out in front of you with your elbow extended and palm supinated. Use your right hand to extend the fingers and the wrist of your left hand by carefully pulling the fingers back toward you. Repeat with the right.

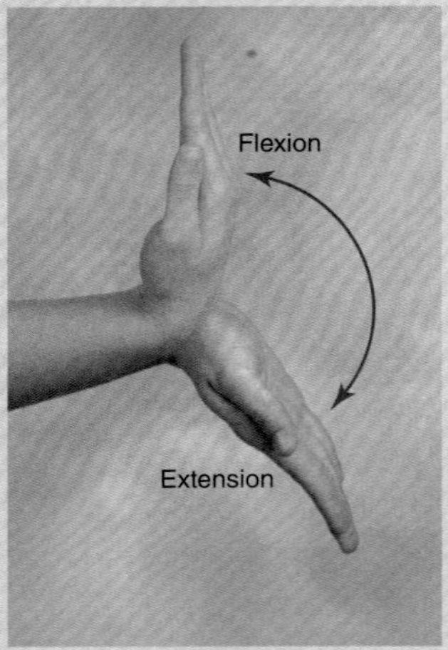

FIGURE 5.19. Wrist extension and flexion. (From Bushman B, Battista R, Swan P, Ransdell L, Thompson WR, editors. *ACSM's Resources for the Personal Trainer.* 4th ed. Philadelphia [PA]: Lippincott Williams & Wilkins; 2014. 592 p.)

Fingers

Extension and abduction for flexors and adductors (Fig. 5.20)	▪ Umbricales Interossei (plantar adductors, dorsal abductors) Flexor pollicis brevis Abductor pollicis brevis Abductor pollicis longus Flexor digiti minimi Opponens pollicis Opponens digiti minimi	Sitting or standing with upper arms at sides, elbows flexed, and palms together	Place your hands together in front of you, matching your palms and fingers as if you are about to pray. With elbows flexed and wrists and fingers extended, elevate both elbows by flexing both shoulders while lowering both hands extending the wrists. Keep palms together and finger matched. Now, maximally abduct all fingers.

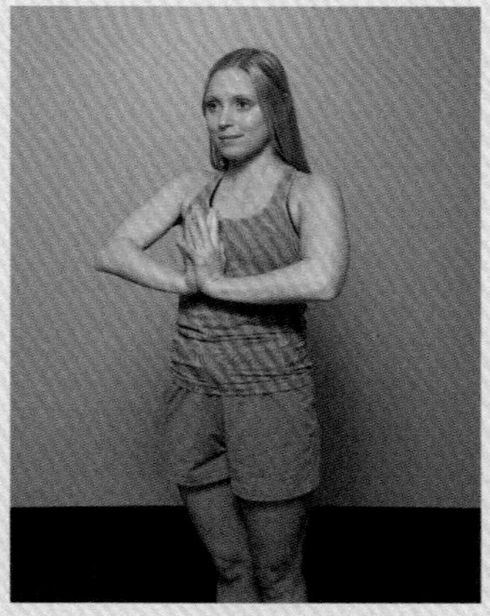

FIGURE 5.20. Finger flexion and adduction.

Trunk

Flexion for extensors (Fig. 5.21A)	▪ Multifidus Spinalis thoracis Longissimus thoracis Iliocostalis thoracis Quadratus lumborum Erector spinae	Lying on the floor, supine	Bring both of your knees up to your chest flexing both hips. Using your arms and hands, pull both of your knees closer to your chest. Continue pulling until your buttocks are off the floor, flexing your mid and lower spine. You may carefully flex your cervical and upper thoracic spine by pulling your head up toward your knees.

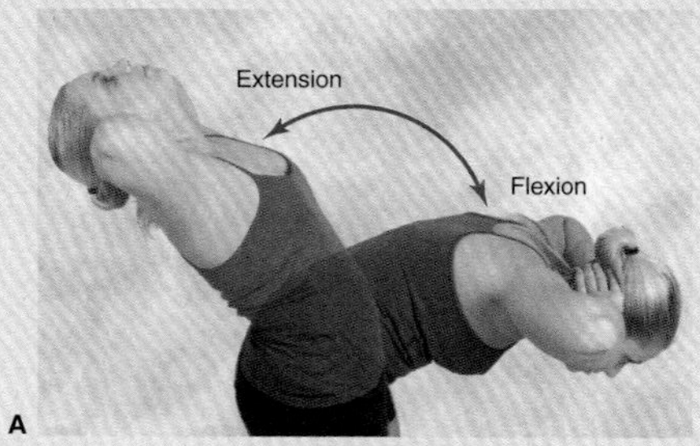

FIGURE 5.21. **A.** Trunk extension and flexion. (continued)

Continued

Table 5.3 Static Stretches for the Major Muscle Groups (continued)

Upper Body

Stretch	Muscle Involved	Starting Position	Description
Trunk			
Extension for flexors (see Fig. 5.21A)	▪ Rectus abdominis External oblique Internal oblique	Lying on the floor, prone, with elbows flexed and palms on the floor just beneath the shoulders	Slowly attempt to press your chest and shoulders up and forward while taking care not to extend your head and neck. Your hip bones (ASIS) should remain in contact with the floor.
Lateral flexors bending (Fig. 5.21B)	▪ Internal oblique External oblique Iliocostalis lumborum Multifidus Quadratus lumborum	Lying on the floor on your left side	To stretch the lateral flexors on your left side, laterally flex your torso toward the right by pressing up with your left arm and hand. Be sure to bend directly sideways, staying in the frontal plane. Repeat on the right side.
Rotation (Fig. 5.21C)	▪ Internal and external oblique Rotators Semispinalis Multifidus	Sitting on the floor with both legs extended	Straighten your spine and then step your left foot over and place it on the right side of your right knee. Now, rotate your upper body and head toward the left, placing your right elbow against the lateral side of your left knee. Continue turning to the left by applying pressure against your left knee with your right elbow. Repeat on the opposite side.

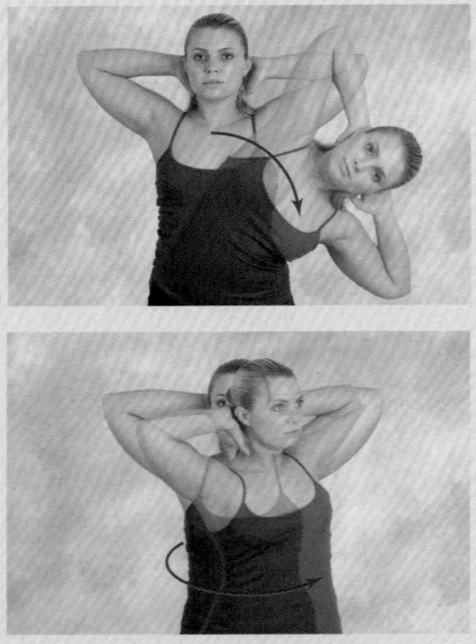

FIGURE 5.21. *(continued)* **B.** Trunk lateral flexion. **C.** Trunk rotation. (From Bushman B, Battista R, Swan P, Ransdell L, Thompson WR, editors. *ACSM's Resources for the Personal Trainer.* 4th ed. Philadelphia [PA]: Lippincott Williams & Wilkins; 2014. 592 p.)

Continued

Lower Body

Hip

Flexors (Fig. 5.22)	■ Psoas major and minor Iliacus Rectus femoris Sartorius Tensor fasciae latae	Standing	To stretch the hip flexors on your right side, first step forward about 2 ft with your left foot. While keeping your torso and hips facing forward, move your upper body and hips anteriorly over your left foot by flexing your left knee and allowing a relaxed flexion in your right knee and ankle. You may allow your right heel to come off the floor. Contract your abdominals to keep your lower back from extending. Repeat on your left side.
Extensors (see Fig. 5.22)	■ Gluteus maximus Hamstrings Semimembranosus Semitendinosus Long head of biceps femoris	Lying supine	To stretch the hip extensors on your left side, grasp your left knee with your right hand. Using your right arm and hand, pull your left knee up and across your torso toward your right shoulder, flexing and adducting your left hip. While keeping your knee in this position, actively extend your left knee to add stretch to the hamstrings, which also extend the hip. Repeat on the opposite side.
Adductors	■ Adductor magnus Adductor longus Adductor brevis Pectineus gracilis	Lying on the floor with knees extended and legs abducted	Using the abductors of your hips, abduct your legs to their end range. You may assist this stretch by placing the medial borders of your feet against a wall. As you achieve a stretching sensation, you can scoot your feet slightly farther apart on the wall.
Abductors	■ Gluteus medius Gluteus minimus Tensor fasciae latae	Standing	To stretch your left hip abductors, place your left hand onto a wall or chair to the left, step forward and toward the left with your right foot so that your right foot rests just ahead and to the left of your left foot. Bend to the right pushing your left hip toward the wall or chair. Continue bending toward the right with your upper body to achieve a stretch in the left hip.

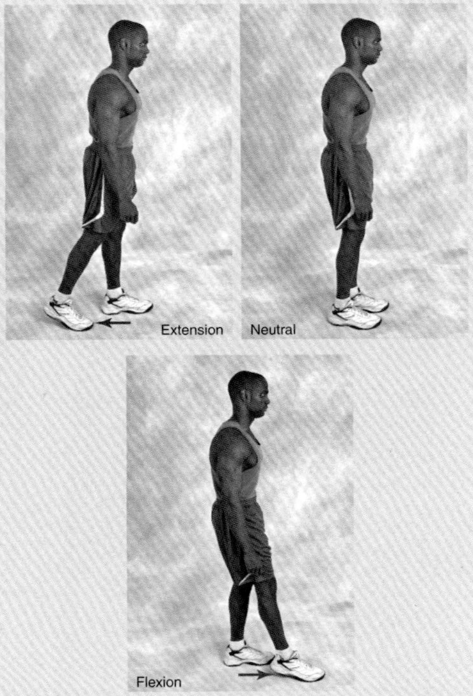

FIGURE 5.22. Hip flexion and extension. (From Bushman B, Battista R, Swan P, Ransdell L, Thompson WR, editors. *ACSM's Resources for the Personal Trainer.* 4th ed. Philadelphia [PA]: Lippincott Williams & Wilkins; 2014. 592 p.)

Table 5.3	Static Stretches for the Major Muscle Groups (continued)

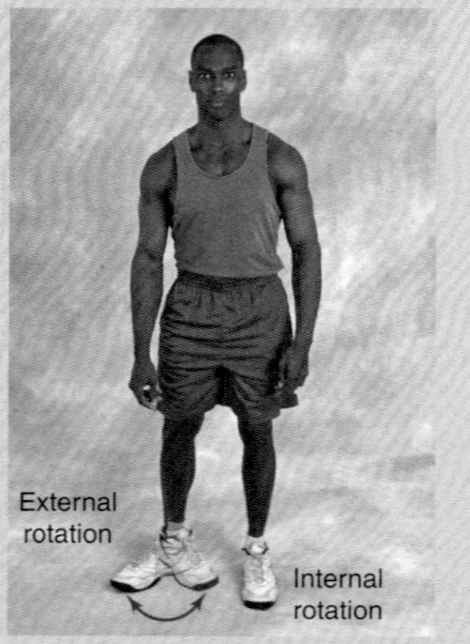

FIGURE 5.23. Hip internal rotation and external rotation. (From Bushman B, Battista R, Swan P, Ransdell L, Thompson WR, editors. *ACSM's Resources for the Personal Trainer.* 4th ed. Philadelphia [PA]: Lippincott Williams & Wilkins; 2014. 592 p.)

Stretch	Muscle Involved	Starting Position	Description
Hip			
Internal rotators (Fig. 5.23)	Anterior fibers of the gluteus medius Hip adductors and medial hamstrings (semimembranosus and semitendinosus)	Lying supine, with the left knee flexed to 90°	To stretch the internal rotators of your left hip, place the ankle of your left leg on top of and across the right thigh, making sure that the lateral lower left leg is lying on top of the right femur. Now, place your left hand on your left knee and carefully press it toward the floor, taking care not to let your hips twist. Repeat on the right.
External rotators (see Fig. 5.23)	Piriformis Gluteus maximus Posterior fibers of gluteus medius Inferior and superior gemelli Obturator internus and externus Quadratus femoris	Lying on the floor, supine	To stretch the external rotators of your left hip, flex your left hip to just above 90°. Next, adduct your left hip by pulling your left knee over toward the right by pulling with your right hand. You may allow your left hip/buttock to come slightly off the floor. Repeat for the right hip.

FIGURE 5.24. Knee flexion and extension. (From Bushman B, Battista R, Swan P, Ransdell L, Thompson WR, editors. *ACSM's Resources for the Personal Trainer.* 4th ed. Philadelphia [PA]: Lippincott Williams & Wilkins; 2014. 592 p.)

Knee

Flexors (Fig. 5.24)	■ Semimembranosus Semitendinosus Long and short heads of biceps femoris Popliteus Gastrocnemius	Standing	To stretch the knee flexors of your left leg, stand facing a chair so that you can comfortably straighten your leg and place your heel on top of the chair. Choose a chair or similar object that will allow you to keep your spine straight once you have lifted your leg onto it. (Note: Many people will have to choose a lower surface.) Carefully lean forward while keeping your spine straight. 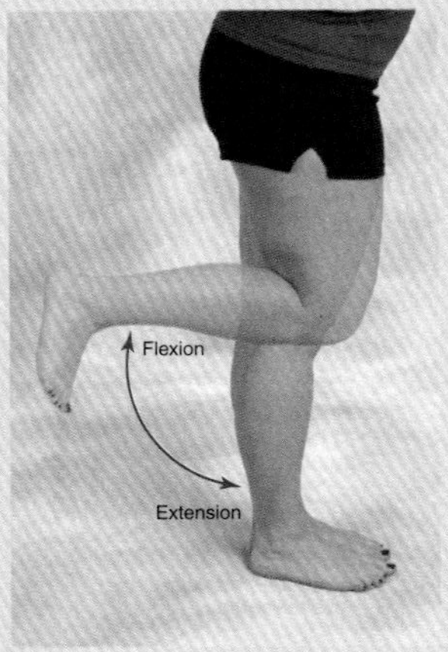
Extensors (see Fig. 5.24)	■ Rectus femoris Vastus intermedius Vastus lateralis Vastus medialis	Standing	To stretch the extensors of the right knee, holding onto a chair, wall, or partner with the left hand for stabilization, flex your right knee and grab your right shin just proximal to the ankle with your right hand. Tighten your abdominals and concentrate on not allowing your back to arch (extend). Now, pull your right ankle posteriorly and then superiorly toward your buttock. Repeat for the left knee.

Continued

Table 5.3 Static Stretches for the Major Muscle Groups (continued)

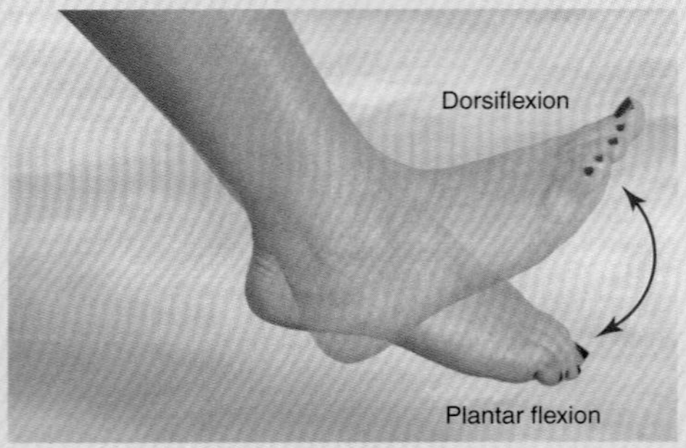

FIGURE 5.25. Ankle dorsiflexion and plantarflexion. (From Bushman B, Battista R, Swan P, Ransdell L, Thompson WR, editors. *ACSM's Resources for the Personal Trainer.* 4th ed. Philadelphia [PA]: Lippincott Williams & Wilkins; 2014. 592 p.)

Stretch	Muscle Involved	Starting Position	Description
Lower Body			
Ankle and Foot			
Extensors (dorsiflexors) (Fig. 5.25)	Anterior tibialis Extensor digitorum longus Extensor digitorum brevis Extensor hallucis longus Extensor hallucis brevis Peroneus tertius	Seated	To stretch the extensors of the right ankle, foot, and toes, while seated in a chair, flex the right knee and plantarflex the foot and toes. Place the dorsum of your right foot and toes on the floor about 6 in under or beside the chair. Apply gentle pressure on the distal end of the foot to achieve a stretch. Repeat on the left.
Flexors (plantar flexors) (see Fig. 5.25)	Gastrocnemius Soleus Peroneus brevis Posterior tibialis Flexor digitorum longus Flexor digitorum brevis Flexor hallucis longus Flexor hallucis brevis	Standing	To stretch the flexors of the ankle, foot, and toes of your right leg, step forward about 18 in with your left foot. Flex both knees while keeping your right heel on the ground. Maintain a neutral-to-high right arch (this may require a slight external rotation of your right tibia). Repeat to stretch the left ankle, foot, and toes.

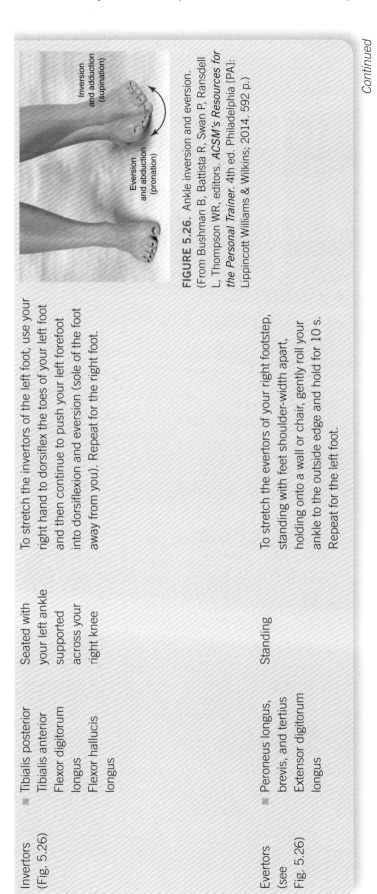

FIGURE 5.26. Ankle inversion and eversion. (From Bushman B, Battista R, Swan P, Ransdell L, Thompson WR, editors. *ACSM's Resources for the Personal Trainer*. 4th ed. Philadelphia [PA]: Lippincott Williams & Wilkins; 2014. 592 p.)

Invertors (Fig. 5.26)	▪ Tibialis posterior Tibialis anterior Flexor digitorum longus Flexor hallucis longus	Seated with your left ankle supported across your right knee	To stretch the invertors of the left foot, use your right hand to dorsiflex the toes of your left foot and then continue to push your left forefoot into dorsiflexion and eversion (sole of the foot away from you). Repeat for the right foot.
Evertors (see Fig. 5.26)	▪ Peroneus longus, brevis, and tertius Extensor digitorum longus	Standing	To stretch the evertors of your right footstep, standing with feet shoulder-width apart, holding onto a wall or chair, gently roll your ankle to the outside edge and hold for 10 s. Repeat for the left foot.

Continued

Table 5.3	Static Stretches for the Major Muscle Groups (continued)

Stretch	Muscle Involved	Starting Position	Description
Lower Body			
Toes			
Extensors (Fig. 5.27A)	▪ Extensor digitorum longus Extensor digitorum brevis Extensor hallucis longus Extensor hallucis brevis Extensor digiti minimi	Seated with left ankle crossed over your right knee	To stretch the extensors of your left foot and toes, place your right hand over the dorsal surface of the toes of your left foot. Carefully flex all five toes toward dorsal surface of your foot. Repeat for the right foot.
Flexors (Fig. 5.27B)	▪ Flexor digitorum longus Flexor digitorum brevis Flexor hallucis longus Flexor hallucis brevis Flexor digiti minimi brevis	Seated with your left ankle crossed over the right knee	To stretch the toe flexors of your left foot, grasp the toes of your left foot with the fingers and palm of your right hand. Extend all five toes and dorsiflex your ankle by pushing the toes toward the shin and allowing the ankle to dorsiflex. Repeat for your right foot.

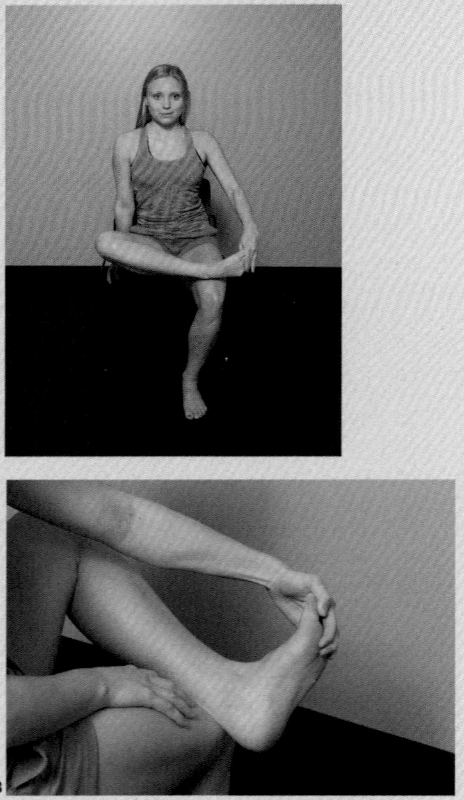

FIGURE 5.27. Toe extension (**A**) and flexion (**B**).

Acute beneficial effects from static flexibility exercise as it relates to performance are not well supported. Preactivity static flexibility training has been shown to decrease strength, sprint performance, endurance performance, and efficiency because it relates to energy expenditure and power output (88–91,105). With the demonstrated detrimental effects of SS on dynamic performance, it is therefore recommended that preactivity ROM be dynamic and/or flexibility programming occur postactivity or during the training session. Dynamic exercise during the warm-up period with the purpose of increasing body temperature and blood flow will naturally increase ROM during the activity. To date, there is not sufficient evidence to advocate against routine flexibility exercises, especially those following, or separate from, other exercise sessions (96), as chronic increases in ROM have yielded conflicting results related to injury prevention and performance. Moreover, some research has demonstrated a reduction of overuse injuries among individuals with improved flexibility (109), whereas others demonstrate that typical muscle stretching programs do not produce a reduction in exercise-related injuries (102). Ultimately, the most prudent recommendation to the health professional is to assess the needs of the individual based on the goals and desired outcomes to achieve the desired activity level. Initial assessment of joint-specific ROM in the individual would be the first step in the development of a flexibility program. If the client is in need of increased ROM, it would be prudent to implement a flexibility training program as previously described. A client with adequate or hyper ROM may be placed on a maintenance program or focus on other areas of health-related fitness until time for reassessment.

> Visit ◉ Lippincott® Connect to watch videos 5.9 through 5.11, which demonstrate goniometry assessment, arm hugs, and dynamic warm up.

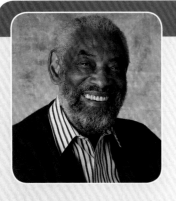

The Case of Allen

Submitted by **Stephanie Marie Otto, PhD, ACSM EP-C, Assistant Professor, Gustavus Adolphus College, St. Peter, MN**

Allen is a retired Navy officer who experienced tightening in his chest and dizziness during a recent walk.

Narrative

Allen retired from the Navy 10 years ago and is currently not working. He spends his days gardening and playing with his four grandchildren. Every morning, he walks along the beach for 20 minutes, and he regularly engages in strength-training activities from his Navy days, but he never has done much flexibility exercise. Allen has played bingo twice a week at the local bingo hall for the past year, but his wife complains because he comes home smelling of smoke. Over the last few years, Allen feels that his hip joint is not as limber as he used to be during his active duty times. He comes to you for advice and guidance. After some preliminary testing and information gathering, you discover that Allen's blood pressure is 160/88 mm Hg, and he also revealed to you that his father passed away from a heart attack at the age of 53 years. His total cholesterol is 190 mg · dL^{-1}, non–high-density lipoprotein cholesterol (non–HDL-C) is 149 mg · dL^{-1}, and HDL-C is 43 mg · dL^{-1}. Allen is 58 years old, and his body mass index is 23. Allen came in a year ago for an assessment, and his results were as follows.

Aerobic fitness ($\dot{V}O_{2max}$): 40.3 mL · kg^{-1} · min^{-1} (no chest pain reported during this exercise test)
Upper body strength (bench press weight ratio): 0.98
Leg strength (leg press weight ratio): 1.97
Hip extension ROM testing: 12°
Hip flexion ROM testing: 122°
Push-ups: 32
Skinfold: 19.1%

Allen is worried about his reduced hip flexibility and comes to you for advice about his current activity participation and lifestyle.

Goals

Goal 1: Flexibility assessment and improve flexibility if needed
Goal 2: Risk factor assessment
Goal 3: Maintain current weight

QUESTIONS

- How would you proceed after this initial conversation with Allen?
- Assuming Allen is cleared for exercise, how would you plan for his next session with you, and what flexibility exercise would you recommend, if any?
- What other lifestyle factors would you want to discuss with Allen that are contributing to his risk of developing cardiovascular disease?
- Assuming Allen is cleared for exercise, and considering his goals, what would you recommend as an activity plan?

References

1. American College of Sports Medicine. *ACSM's Guidelines for Exercise Testing and Prescription.* 8th ed. Philadelphia (PA): Lippincott Williams & Wilkins; 2010. 400 p.
2. Neiman D. *Exercise Testing and Prescription: A Health-Related Approach.* 7th ed. New York (NY): McGraw Hill; 2011. 672 p.
3. Garber CE, Blissmer B, Deschenes MR, et al. American College of Sports Medicine position stand. Quantity and quality of exercise for developing and maintaining cardiorespiratory, musculoskeletal, and neuromotor fitness in apparently healthy adults: guidance for prescribing exercise. *Med Sci Sports Exerc.* 2011;43(7):1334–59.

SUMMARY

Development and maintenance of flexibility is one of the five components of health-related fitness, and maintaining an adequate ROM is important for activities of daily living. Nevertheless, controversy exists regarding the overall benefits of flexibility training for injury prevention or sport performance. Because flexibility training involves multiple modes, the ACSM-EP can choose which is best for each client and implement these as part of a dynamic warm-up or during the cool-down phase of exercise. Many different methods and tools are used to assess ROM and flexibility. Among the most common are the use of goniometers for the measurement of ROM and functional movement assessments. Overall, flexibility exercise prescription depends on the mode of the exercise and should be set on the basis of established ACSM guidelines.

STUDY QUESTIONS

1. Characterize the various modes of flexibility training, including the advantages and disadvantages of each.
2. Differentiate between the two types of sensory organs that provide muscular dynamic and limb movement information to the central nervous system with respect to location and function.
3. Design a sample static flexibility exercise prescription based on the FITT principle.
4. Assess the controversy that surrounds the need for flexibility training with respect to health and athletic performance.

REFERENCES

1. Friedrich LJ. Gymnastick exercises. In: Friedrich LJ, editor. *A Treatise on Gymnasticks.* Northampton (MA): Simeon and Butler; 1828. p. 1–7.
2. Kraus H, Hirschland R. Minimum muscular fitness tests in school children. *Res Q.* 1954;25(2):178–88.
3. Batista LH, Vilar AC, de Almeida Ferreira JJ, Rebelatto JR, Salvini TF. Active stretching improves flexibility, joint torque, and functional mobility in older women. *Am J Phys Med Rehabil.* 2009;88(10):815–22.
4. Behm DG, Blazevich AJ, Kay AD, McHugh M. Acute effects of muscle stretching on physical performance, range of motion, and injury incidence in healthy active individuals: a systematic review. *Appl Physiol Nutr Metab.* 2016;41(1):1–11.

5. Chaouachi A, Padulo J, Kasmi S, Othmen AB, Chatra M, Behm DG. Unilateral static and dynamic hamstrings stretching increases contralateral hip flexion range of motion. *Clin Physiol Funct Imaging.* 2017;37(1):23–9.
6. Lima CD, Ruas CV, Behm DG, Brown LE. Acute effects of stretching on flexibility and performance: a narrative review. *J Sci Sport Exerc.* 2019;1(1):29–37.
7. Bandy WD, Irion JM, Briggler M. The effect of static stretch and dynamic range of motion training on the flexibility of the hamstring muscles. *J Orthop Sports Phys Ther.* 1998;27(4):295–300.
8. 2018 Physical Activity Guidelines Advisory Committee. *2018 Physical Activity Guidelines Advisory Committee*

Scientific Report. Washington (DC): U.S. Department of Health and Human Services; 2018. 779 p.

9. Holt LE, Travis TM, Okita T. Comparative study of three stretching techniques. *Percept Mot Skills.* 1970;31(2):611–6.

10. Jeffreys I. Warm-up and stretching. In: Baechle TR, Earle R, editors. *Essentials of Strength Training and Conditioning.* 3rd ed. Champaign (IL): Human Kinetics; 2008. p. 296–305.

11. Shellock FG, Prentice WE. Warming-up and stretching for improved physical performance and prevention of sports-related injuries. *Sports Med.* 1985;2(4):267–78.

12. Hubley CL, Kozey JW, Stanish WD. The effects of static stretching exercises and stationary cycling on range of motion at the hip joint. *J Orthop Sports Phys Ther.* 1984;6(2):104–9.

13. Hall SJ. *Basic Biomechanics.* 6th ed. Boston (MA): WCB/McGraw Hill; 2011. 577 p.

14. Noakes T. *Lore of Running.* 4th ed. Champaign (IL): Human Kinetics; 2003. 931 p.

15. Noonan TJ, Best TM, Seaber AV, Garrett WE Jr. Thermal effects on skeletal muscle tensile behavior. *Am J Sports Med.* 1993;21(4):517–22.

16. Getchell B. *Physical Fitness: A Way of Life.* 2nd ed. New York (NY): Wiley; 1979. 352 p.

17. Raab DM, Agre JC, McAdam M, Smith EL. Light resistance and stretching exercise in elderly women: effect upon flexibility. *Arch Phys Med Rehabil.* 1988;69(4):268–72.

18. Leighton JR. A study of the effect of progressive weight training on flexibility. *J Assoc Phys Ment Rehabil.* 1964;18:101–4.

19. Tanigawa MC. Comparison of the hold-relax procedure and passive mobilization on increasing muscle length. *Phys Ther.* 1972;52(7):725–35.

20. Church JB, Wiggins MS, Moode FM, Crist R. Effect of warm-up and flexibility treatments on vertical jump performance. *J Strength Cond Res.* 2001;15(3):332–6.

21. O'Brien M. Functional anatomy and physiology of tendons. *Clin Sports Med.* 1992;11(3):505–20.

22. Bell DR, Blackburn JT, Hackney AC, Marshall SW, Beutler AI, Padua DA. Jump-landing biomechanics and knee-laxity change across the menstrual cycle in women with anterior cruciate ligament reconstruction. *J Athl Train.* 2014;49(2):154–62.

23. Houck JC, De Hesse C, Jacob R. The effect of ageing upon collagen metabolism. *Symp Soc Exp Biol.* 1967;21:403–25.

24. Gleim GW, McHugh MP. Flexibility and its effects on sports injury and performance. *Sports Med.* 1997;24(5):289–99.

25. Sprague HA. Relationship of certain physical measurements to swimming speed. *Res Q.* 1976;47(4):810–4.

26. Oberg B, Ekstrand J, Möller M, Gillquist J. Muscle strength and flexibility in different positions of soccer players. *Int J Sports Med.* 1984;5(4):213–6.

27. Shrier I. Does stretching improve performance? A systematic and critical review of the literature. *Clin J Sport Med.* 2004;14(5):267–73.

28. Haff GG. Roundtable discussion: flexibility training. *Strength Cond J.* 2006;28(2):64–85.

29. Mann DP, Jones MT. Guidelines to the implementation of a dynamic stretching program. *Strength Cond J.* 1999;21(6):53.

30. Johns RJ, Wright V. Relative importance of various tissues in joint stiffness. *J Appl Physiol.* 1962;17(5):824–8.

31. American College of Sports Medicine. *ACSM's Guidelines for Exercise Testing and Prescription.* 11th ed. Philadelphia (PA): Wolters Kluwer; 2022. 548 p.

32. The Cooper Institute. *Physical Fitness Assessments and Norms.* Dallas (TX): The Cooper Institute; 2005. 44 p.

33. Liguori G, Carroll-Cobb S. *FitWell: Questions and Answers.* New York (NY): McGraw Hill; 2011. 499 p.

34. Park SK, Stefanyshyn DJ, Loitz-Ramage B, Hart DA, Ronsky JL. Changing hormone levels during the menstrual cycle affect knee laxity and stiffness in healthy female subjects. *Am J Sports Med.* 2009;37(3):588–98.

35. Kato E, Oda T, Chino K, et al. Musculotendinous factors influencing difference in ankle joint flexibility between men and women. *Int J Sport Health Sci.* 2005;3:218–25.

36. Chatzopoulos D, Galazoulas C, Patikas D, Kotzamanidis C. Acute effects of static and dynamic stretching on balance, agility, reaction time and movement time. *J Sports Sci Med.* 2014;13(2):403–9.

37. Taylor DC, Dalton JD Jr, Seaber AV, Garrett WE Jr. Viscoelastic properties of muscle-tendon units. The biomechanical effects of stretching. *Am J Sports Med.* 1990;18(3):300–9.

38. Bandy WD, Irion JM. The effect of time on static stretch on the flexibility of the hamstring muscles. *Phys Ther.* 1994;74(9):845–2.

39. Depino GM, Webright WG, Arnold BL. Duration of maintained hamstring flexibility after cessation of an acute static stretching protocol. *J Athl Train.* 2000;35(1):56–9.

40. Marek SM, Cramer JT, Fincher AL, et al. Acute effects of static and proprioceptive neuromuscular facilitation stretching on muscle strength and power output. *J Athl Train.* 2005;40(2):94–103.

41. Magnusson SP, Simonsen EB, Aagaard P, Sørensen H, Kjaer M. A mechanism for altered flexibility in human skeletal muscle. *J Physiol.* 1996;497(Pt 1):291–8.

42. Magnusson SP, Simonsen EB, Dyhre-Poulsen P, Aagaard P, Mohr T, Kjaer M. Viscoelastic stress relaxation during static stretch in human skeletal muscle in the absence of EMG activity. *Scand J Med Sci Sports.* 1996;6(6):323–8.

43. Manoel ME, Harris-Love MO, Danoff JV, Miller TA. Acute effects of static, dynamic, and proprioceptive neuromuscular facilitation stretching on muscle power in women. *J Strength Cond Res.* 2008;22(5):1528–34.

44. McGlynn GH, Laughlin NT, Rowe V. Effect of electromyographic feedback and static stretching on artificially induced muscle soreness. *Am J Phys Med.* 1979;58(3):139–48.

45. Smith LL, Brunetz MH, Chenier TC, et al. The effects of static and ballistic stretching on delayed onset muscle soreness and creatine kinase. *Res Q Exerc Sport.* 1993;64(1):103–7.

46. Simic L, Sarabon N, Markovic G. Does pre-exercise static stretching inhibit maximal muscular performance? A meta-analytical review. *Scand J Med Sci Sports.* 2013;23(2):131–48.

47. Hunter JP, Marshall RN. Effects of power and flexibility training on vertical jump technique. *Med Sci Sports Exerc.* 2002;34(3):478–86.

48. Kerrigan DC, Xenopoulos-Oddsson A, Sullivan MJ, Lelas JJ, Riley PO. Effect of a hip flexor-stretching program

on gait in the elderly. *Arch Phys Med Rehabil.* 2003; 84(1):1–6.

49. Worrell TW, Smith TL, Winegardner J. Effect of hamstring stretching on hamstring muscle performance. *J Orthop Sports Phys Ther.* 1994;20(3):154–9.

50. Behm DG, Bambury A, Cahill F, Power K. Effect of acute static stretching on force, balance, reaction time, and movement time. *Med Sci Sports Exerc.* 2004;36(8):1397–402.

51. Cramer JT, Housh TJ, Weir JP, Johnson GO, Coburn JW, Beck TW. The acute effects of static stretching on peak torque, mean power output, electromyography, and mechanomyography. *Eur J Appl Physiol.* 2005;93(5–6):530–9.

52. Young W, Clothier P, Otago L, Bruce L, Liddell D. Acute effects of static stretching on hip flexor and quadriceps flexibility, range of motion and foot speed in kicking a football. *J Sci Med Sport.* 2004;7(1):23–31.

53. Lamontagne A, Malouin F, Richards CL. Viscoelastic behavior of plantar flexor muscle-tendon unit at rest. *J Orthop Sports Phys Ther.* 1997;26(5):244–52.

54. Garber CE, Blissmer B, Deschenes MR, et al. American College of Sports Medicine position stand. Quantity and quality of exercise for developing and maintaining cardiorespiratory, musculoskeletal, and neuromotor fitness in apparently healthy adults: guidance for prescribing exercise. *Med Sci Sports Exerc.* 2011;43(7):1334–59.

55. Woolstenhulme MT, Griffiths CM, Woolstenhulme EM, Parcell AC. Ballistic stretching increases flexibility and acute vertical jump height when combined with basketball activity. *J Strength Cond Res.* 2006;20(4):799–803.

56. Opplert J, Babault N. Acute effects of dynamic stretching on muscle flexibility and performance: an analysis of the current literature. *Sports Med.* 2018;48(2):299–325.

57. Nelson RT. A comparison of the immediate effects of eccentric training vs static stretch on hamstring flexibility in high school and college athletes. *N Am J Sports Phys Ther.* 2006;1(2):56–61.

58. Unick J, Kieffer HS, Cheesman W, Feeney A. The acute effects of static and ballistic stretching on vertical jump performance in trained women. *J Strength Cond Res.* 2005;19(1):206–12.

59. Kirmizigil B, Ozcaldiran B, Colakoglu M. Effects of three different stretching techniques on vertical jumping performance. *J Strength Cond Res.* 2014;28(5):1263–71.

60. Voss DE, Ionta MK, Myers BJ. *Proprioceptive Neuromuscular Facilitation: Patterns and Techniques.* 3rd ed. Philadelphia (PA): Harper & Row; 1985. 370 p.

61. Sherrington CS. On plastic tonus and proprioceptive reflexes. *Exp Physiol.* 1909;2(2):109–56.

62. Lial L, Moreira R, Correia L, et al. Proprioceptive neuromuscular facilitation increases alpha absolute power in the dorsolateral prefrontal cortex and superior parietal cortex. *Somatosens Mot Res.* 2017;34(3):204–12.

63. Moreira R, Lial L, Teles Monteiro MG, et al. Diagonal movement of the upper limb produces greater adaptive plasticity than sagittal plane flexion in the shoulder. *Neurosci Lett.* 2017;643:8–15.

64. Kisner C, Colby LA, Borstad J. *Therapeutic Exercise: Foundations and Techniques.* 7th ed. Philadelphia (PA): F.A. Davis; 2018. 1088 p.

65. Hindle KB, Whitcomb TJ, Briggs WO, Hong J. Proprioceptive neuromuscular facilitation (PNF): its mechanisms and effects on range of motion and muscular function. *J Hum Kinet.* 2012;31:105–13.

66. Sharman MJ, Cresswell AG, Riek S. Proprioceptive neuromuscular facilitation stretching: mechanisms and clinical implications. *Sports Med.* 2006;36(11):929–39.

67. Sady SP, Wortman M, Blanke D. Flexibility training: ballistic, static or proprioceptive neuromuscular facilitation? *Arch Phys Med Rehabil.* 1982;63(6):261–3.

68. Wallin D, Ekblom B, Grahn R, Nordenborg T. Improvement of muscle flexibility. A comparison between two techniques. *Am J Sports Med.* 1985;13(4):263–8.

69. Chen C-H, Nosaka K, Chen H-L, Lin M-J, Tseng K-W, Chen TC. Effects of flexibility training on eccentric exercise-induced muscle damage. *Med Sci Sports Exerc.* 2011;43(3):491–500.

70. Godges JJ, Macrae H, Longdon C, Tinberg C, Macrae PG. The effects of two stretching procedures on hip range of motion and gait economy. *J Orthop Sports Phys Ther.* 1989;10(9):350–7.

71. Lucas RC, Koslow R. Comparative study of static, dynamic, and proprioceptive neuromuscular facilitation stretching techniques on flexibility. *Percept Mot Skills.* 1984;58(2):615–8.

72. Cornelius WL. Flexibility exercise: effective practices. *NSCA J.* 1989;11(6):61–2.

73. Hedrick A. Flexibility: flexibility and the conditioning program. *NSCA J.* 1993;15(4):62–7.

74. Hedrick A. Dynamic flexibility training. *Strength Cond J.* 2000;22(5):33–8.

75. McMillian DJ, Moore JH, Hatler BS, Taylor DC. Dynamic vs. static-stretching warm up: the effect on power and agility performance. *J Strength Cond Res.* 2006;20(3):492–9.

76. Needham RA, Morse CI, Degens H. The acute effect of different warm-up protocols on anaerobic performance in elite youth soccer players. *J Strength Cond Res.* 2009;23(9):2614–20.

77. Thompsen AG, Kackley T, Palumbo MA, Faigenbaum AD. Acute effects of different warm-up protocols with and without a weighted vest on jumping performance in athletic women. *J Strength Cond Res.* 2007;21(1):52–6.

78. Clark L, O'Leary CB, Hong J, Lockard M. The acute effects of stretching on presynaptic inhibition and peak power. *J Sports Med Phys Fitness.* 2014;54(5):605–10.

79. Handrakis JP, Southard VN, Abreu JM, et al. Static stretching does not impair performance in active middle-aged adults. *J Strength Cond Res.* 2010;24(3):825–30.

80. Behm DG, Chaouachi A. A review of the acute effects of static and dynamic stretching on performance. *Eur J Appl Physiol.* 2011;111(11):2633–51.

81. McArdle WD, Katch FI, Katch VL. *Exercise Physiology: Energy, Nutrition, & Human Performance.* 6th ed. Philadelphia (PA): Lippincott Williams & Wilkins; 2007. 1068 p.

82. Guyton AC, Hall JE. *Textbook of Medical Physiology.* 11th ed. Philadelphia (PA): Elsevier Saunders; 2006. 1116 p.

83. Moore MA, Hutton RS. Electromyographic investigation of muscle stretching techniques. *Med Sci Sports Exerc.* 1980;12(5):322–9.

84. Clarkson HM. *Musculoskeletal Assessment: Joint Motion and Muscle Testing.* 3rd ed. Baltimore (MD): Lippincott Williams & Wilkins; 2012. 656 p.

85. Palmer ML, Epler M. *Fundamental of Musculoskeletal Assessment Techniques.* 2nd ed. Baltimore (MD): Lippincott Williams & Wilkins; 1998. 432 p.

86. American Medical Association. *Guides to the Evaluation of Permanent Impairment.* 4th ed. Chicago (IL): American Medical Association; 1993. 350 p.

87. Gibson AL, Wagner DR, Heyward VH. *Advanced Fitness Assessment and Exercise Prescription.* 8th ed. Champaign (IL): Human Kinetics; 2019. 560 p.

88. Kistler BM, Walsh MS, Horn TS, Cox RH. The acute effects of static stretching on the sprint performance of collegiate men in the 60-and 100-m dash after a dynamic warm-up. *J Strength Cond Res.* 2010;24(9):2280–4.

89. Knudson D, Noffal G. Time course of stretch-induced isometric strength deficits. *Eur J Appl Physiol.* 2005;94(3):348–51.

90. Knudson DV, Noffal GJ, Bahamonde RE, Bauer JA, Blackwell JR. Stretching has no effect on tennis serve performance. *J Strength Cond Res.* 2004;18(3):654–6.

91. Wilson JM, Hornbuckle LM, Kim J-S, et al. Effects of static stretching on energy cost and running endurance performance. *J Strength Cond Res.* 2010;24(9):2274–9.

92. Feland JB, Myrer JW, Schulthies SS, Fellingham GW, Measom GW. The effect of duration of stretching of the hamstring muscle group for increasing range of motion in people aged 65 years or older. *Phys Ther.* 2001;81(5):1110–7.

93. de Weijer VC, Gorniak GC, Shamus E. The effect of static stretch and warm-up exercise on hamstring length over the course of 24 hours. *J Orthop Sports Phys Ther.* 2003;33(12):727–33.

94. Decoster LC, Cleland J, Altieri C, Russell P. The effects of hamstring stretching on range of motion: a systematic literature review. *J Orthop Sports Phys Ther.* 2005;35(6):377–87.

95. Roberts JM, Wilson K. Effect of stretching duration on active and passive range of motion in the lower extremity. *Br J Sports Med.* 1999;33(4):259–63.

96. Bandy WD, Irion JM, Briggler M. The effect of time and frequency of static stretching on flexibility of the hamstring muscles. *Phys Ther.* 1997;77(10):1090–6.

97. Freitas SR, Vilarinho D, Rocha Vaz J, Bruno PM, Costa PB, Mil-homens P. Responses to static stretching are dependent on stretch intensity and duration. *Clin Physiol Funct Imaging.* 2015;35(6):478–84.

98. Mahieu NN, McNair P, De Muynck M, et al. Effect of static and ballistic stretching on the muscle-tendon tissue properties. *Med Sci Sports Exerc.* 2007;39(3):494–501.

99. Yuktasir B, Kaya F. Investigation into the long-term effects of static and PNF stretching exercises on range of motion and jump performance. *J Bodyw Mov Ther.* 2009;13(1):11–21.

100. Herbert RD, Gabriel M. Effects of stretching before and after exercising on muscle soreness and risk of injury: systematic review. *BMJ.* 2002;325(7362):468.

101. Park DY, Chou L. Stretching for prevention of Achilles tendon injuries: a review of the literature. *Foot Ankle Int.* 2006;27(12):1086–95.

102. Pope RP, Herbert RD, Kirwan JD, Graham BJ. A randomized trial of preexercise stretching for prevention of lower-limb injury. *Med Sci Sports Exerc.* 2000;32(2):271–7.

103. Thacker SB, Gilchrist J, Stroup DF, Kimsey CD Jr. The impact of stretching on sports injury risk: a systematic review of the literature. *Med Sci Sports Exerc.* 2004;36(3):371–8.

104. Pieber K, Herceg M, Quittan M, Csapo R, Müller R, Wiesinger GF. Long-term effects of an outpatient rehabilitation program in patients with chronic recurrent low back pain. *Eur Spine J.* 2014;23(4):779–85.

105. Knapik JJ, Bauman CL, Jones BH, Harris JM, Vaughan L. Preseason strength and flexibility imbalances associated with athletic injuries in female collegiate athletes. *Am J Sports Med.* 1991;19(1):76–81.

106. Wendt M, Cieślik K, Lewandowski J, Waszak M. Effectiveness of combined general rehabilitation gymnastics and muscle energy techniques in older women with chronic low back pain. *Biomed Res Int.* 2019;2019:2060987.

107. Huston KA. Achilles tendinitis and tendon rupture due to fluoroquinolone antibiotics. *N Engl J Med.* 1994;331(11):748.

108. Harvey L, Herbert R, Crosbie J. Does stretching induce lasting increases in joint ROM? A systematic review. *Physiother Res Int.* 2002;7(1):1–13.

109. Hartig DE, Henderson JM. Increasing hamstring flexibility decreases lower extremity overuse injuries in military basic trainees. *Am J Sports Med.* 1999;27(2):173–6.

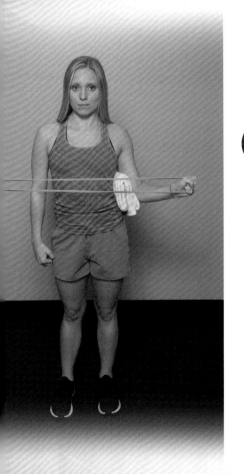

6

Functional Movement Assessments and Exercise Programming for Apparently Healthy Participants

- To understand the integration of the motor system and the sensory system in developing motor patterns.
- To examine the importance of stability, mobility, and proprioception within the context of progressive exercise programing.
- To understand the relevance of optimizing posture for improved neuromuscular function.
- To identify the muscles commonly affected by neuromuscular imbalances.
- To describe appropriate assessments and exercise prescription and self-myofascial release strategies to improve movement potential.

INTRODUCTION

One of the most salient features of successful strength and conditioning programs is progressively overloading the body to the extent that adaptation occurs. This progression is optimized when three fundamental features are present: sensory acuity, optimal stabilization strategies, and mobility. There are, however, a number of pervasive issues, including obesity and overweight, sedentary lifestyles, poor posture, improper training, and aging that are known to compromise these preconditions of progression. With knowledge of biomechanics, motor control, and optimal alignment, the American College of Sports Medicine (ACSM) Exercise Physiologist (ACSM-EP®) is in a position to make the necessary program adjustments and offer lifestyle recommendations to accommodate for these ever-present issues. Ultimately, these accommodations can lay the foundation for optimal gains in functional capacity, strength, and performance.

 ## Sensorimotor Control

Motor Learning

During early phases of motor learning, performance is largely under conscious control, meaning a great deal of focus and concentration is needed in order to successfully perform the movement. On repeated practice, control of individual movements becomes integrated into motor patterns. These motor patterns are stored in the central nervous system (CNS), not unlike saving a document on a computer. Once motor patterns are integrated and stored, they become automatic and are fine-tuned by unconscious sensory feedback. The saving of motor patterns makes the neuromuscular system more efficient when the body is exposed to similar demands in the future. For this reason, after sufficient practice, we do not really have to think about riding a bike, hitting a golf ball, or performing a clean and jerk. The problem lies in the saving of faulty motor patterns because, once stored, motor patterns can be challenging to correct.

Proprioception

The sensory system and the motor control system, collectively known as the sensorimotor system, work together to control movement, balance, posture, and joint stability (1–3). Essentially, in order for optimal movement to occur, the body requires the brain to process afferent sensory information from multiple sources. Dr. Charles Sherrington (4) was the first to characterize this input as proprioception. Currently, proprioception is understood to be the sense of knowing where one's body is in space and is composed of static (joint position sense) and dynamic (kinesthetic movement sense) (5). Proprioception enables us, with closed eyes, to estimate the size of our feet, describe the width of our pelvis, and scratch our noses. Table 6.1 describes common movements that are derived from proprioceptive acuity. This sensory input is gathered from specialized nerve endings, termed *mechanoreceptors*, that are located within the skin, muscles, fascia, and joints (6). Information collected from visual and vestibular centers further supports

Key Point

Motor control is developed through enhancing proprioceptive acuity and grooving proper movement patterns through practice.

Table 6.1	Salient Features of Proprioceptive Acuity
Characteristic	**Example**
Postural control	Maintaining balance during perturbations (a force, such as a gentle tap or vibration, that is applied with the intention of altering balance)
Precise calibration of limb position in space	Threading a needle
Maintenance of steady muscle force production/movement amplitudes	Unbroken, smooth motion during the eccentric and concentric phases of a dumbbell chest press
Discrimination of object weight	Tailoring the effort required to lift a 5-lb weight and a 25-lb weight
Production of coordinated gait patterns	Biomechanically efficient walking; running
Controlling the timing of muscular contraction for dynamic stabilization and multisegmental movement	Executing a tennis serve or a clean and jerk
Feedback and feed-forward motor control	Reaction time and anticipatory responses in a soccer game

proprioception, and when taken together, the result is precise body awareness and well-adapted motor actions (Fig. 6.1).

Proprioception is an important mediator of joint stability and mobility and ultimately the calibration of movement (7). It follows that this sensory acuity is central to safely perform many of the resistance training exercises that are included in conventional exercise programs. If there are disturbances in proprioception, reactive (feedback) and preparatory/anticipatory (feed-forward) motor control and stability will be altered, increasing the risk of injury (8). It is also important to note that problems with stability and/or mobility issues will perpetuate proprioceptive deficits. Figure 6.2 describes the afferent and efferent pathways involved in the sensorimotor system.

Stability and Mobility

There is a good reason why we prefer driving a car with aligned tires, lug nuts tightened, and fan belts secured. For example, if the fan belt is secured (stability), it can move at a very high speed (mobility) for many miles without wear and tear. If these requisite features are not present, we can

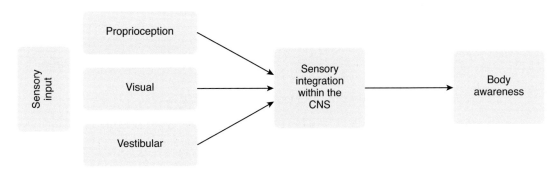

FIGURE 6.1. Sensory input from vestibular, visual, and proprioception is integrated within the CNS resulting in relatively keen body awareness.

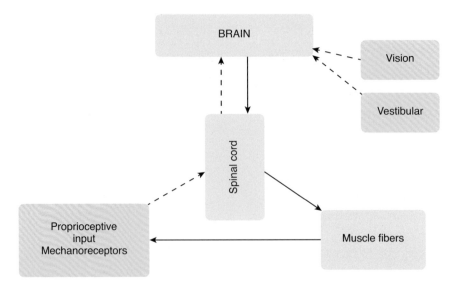

FIGURE 6.2. The sensorimotor system integrates all sensory (afferent) and muscular (efferent) activity. Afferent activity is indicated by the dotted lines, whereas the solid lines indicate efferent activity. (Adapted from Riemann BL, Lephart SM. The sensorimotor system, part I: the physiologic basis of functional joint stability. *J Athl Train.* 2002;37[1]:71–9.)

expect to shell out money for repairs far sooner than the manufacturer originally predicted. We might also expect far-reaching changes to the overall structure and function of the car. The factors that contribute to the mechanical efficiency and the long life of our cars are akin to the features needed for optimal function in the body, stability, and mobility.

Stability has been defined as the state of remaining unchanged, even in the presence of forces that would normally change the state or condition (9). Others have defined stability as the state of a joint remaining or promptly returning to proper alignment through an equalization of forces (10). Joint stabilization then occurs through coordinated muscle coactivation, creating a suitable amount of stiffness to maintain joint alignment (11).

Stabilization strategies are managed at the subcortical level, where the generation of stability is somewhat automatic and requires quality proprioceptive input. For example, a tennis player does not consciously consider the use of the rotator cuff muscles (glenohumeral stabilizers) while serving; rather, the player is more focused on the voluntary actions of the ball toss and the service motion. Ideally, the muscles of the rotator cuff perform the job of joint centration (keeping the humeral head in an optimal position within the glenoid fossa) in an anticipatory manner, described as glenohumeral stabilization (12). To this end, the sensorimotor system is responsible for providing awareness, coordination, and feedback to maintain optimal positioning of the shoulder joint, thereby enhancing the quality of movement and reducing the chance of injury (13,14). Conversely, if the stabilizing rotator cuff muscles are not recruited with proper timing and speed and proper muscle patterns, the humeral head is subject to the pulling forces of the deltoid muscles, which can cause the humeral head to shift upward within the socket. The upward translation is problematic

Key Point

Optimal stabilization strategies require the following:

1. A stable base from which forces are transferred

2. Adequate muscular capacity (strength and endurance)

3. CNS motor programming (integration of sensory input) that produces synchronous activation of the muscles

Table 6.2	Muscle Classification
Mobilizers	**Stabilizers**
Upper trapezius	Deep cervical flexors
Levator scapulae	Lower trapezius
Pectoralis major and minor	Serratus anterior
Deltoids	Rotator cuff (infraspinatus, supraspinatus, teres minor, subscapularis)
Erector spinae	Middle and lower trapezius
Iliopsoas	Transversus abdominis
Quadriceps	Multifidus
Rectus abdominis	Gluteus medius and maximus

in that several musculotendinous structures (*e.g.*, biceps tendon and rotator cuff tendons) that are located in this area can become impinged between the acromion process and the head of the humerus. Other illustrations of the automation of healthy stabilization strategies are the anticipatory bracing that occurs when a dog unexpectedly pulls on the leash, the bracing of the neck and trunk when cyclist rides over a pothole, or the postural adjustments that are made during abrupt change directions on the tennis court.

Some researchers have categorized muscles as two distinct yet interdependent systems: stabilizers or mobilizers (15,16). Categorization is largely based on their relative contributions to movement and maintaining posture and position in the body (Table 6.2).

Classifying muscles in this way is beneficial for the exercise physiologist because stabilizing muscles have unique characteristics (Table 6.3) that require specialized training approaches, which is described later in this chapter. Generally speaking, mobilizing muscles are superficially located and responsible for controlling locomotion, alignment, and balancing forces imposed on the spine. Stabilizing muscles are more centrally located and largely function to create stiffness across joints. These muscles are shorter in length and respond to changes in posture and extrinsic loads. Conversely, mobilizers, or global muscles, comprise long lever arms, allowing greater force production, torque, and gross multiplanar movements.

Table 6.3	Mobilizer and Stabilizer Characteristics
Mobilizers	**Stabilizers**
Fast twitch	Slow twitch
Fatigues easily	Resistant to fatigue
Superficial	Deep
Relatively small proprioceptive role	Major contributor to proprioception
High force production	Low force production
Prone to hold excess tension/shorten	Prone to inhibition/weakness
Concentric	Isometric/eccentric
Gross movement	Joint stabilization

What Is the Core?

Perhaps, the most common discussion of stabilization relates to core function. This is because the hips and the trunk serve as our center of mass and attempts to centralize the strength and coordination of the core are believed to yield optimal force production through the limbs. The principle of core stability can be illustrated in a simple comparison: shooting a canon off of a canoe versus a stable surface. To date, there is no universally accepted definition of the core, where some researchers describe the core as a muscular cylinder with the abdominals comprising the front, the multifidus and gluteals the back, the diaphragm as the roof, and the pelvic floor as the base of the cylinder (11,15,17,18). Tse et al. (19) defined the core as all muscles of the trunk and pelvis that contribute to maintaining a stable spine. Other researchers suggest that the core is an integrated system composed of passive structures (*e.g.*, ligaments and bone), the active spinal muscles and thoracolumbar fascia, and the neural control unit (20,21). Precise definition notwithstanding, there is universal agreement that the core is central to all kinetic chains and that upper and lower extremity movement is optimized in conditions where there is sufficient endurance and neuromuscular control of the core (15,17,18). Moreover, proper core function improves the spine's ability to withstand the various loads and directional forces that it encounters during daily activities, sport, and exercise.

Mediators of the Proprioception, Mobility, and Stability

Overweight and Obesity and Physical Inactivity

Overweight and obesity is a worldwide epidemic and is associated with elevated risk for a number of chronic diseases such as diabetes, hypertension, and the metabolic syndrome. Among adult men and women, obesity and overweight has been shown to be associated with alterations in motor function and postural control, possibly due to reductions in muscular strength and endurance, postural distortion, discomfort with movement, and the perception of stiffness (22,23). Unfortunately, associations of poor motor control and elevated body mass index (BMI) have also been reported in children and adolescents (24–26). Moreover, obesity and overweight in growth and developmental stages is believed to contribute to aberrant motor patterning, which extends to adulthood (23).

Propensity for Inhibition of Stabilizing Muscles

Dr. Vladimir Janda, a key figure in twentieth century rehabilitation and one of the first to characterize the sensorimotor system, suggested that certain muscles had an inherent propensity for weakening or inhibition, whereas other muscles were prone to hypertonicity (2). Ultimately, the tendencies of certain muscles to weaken or tighten may lead to postural distortion and alterations in motor control (2). This altered regulation of the sensorimotor system may occur due to participation in sports involving repetitive actions, overtraining, poor ergonomics, sedentary lifestyle, trauma, or disease.

Previous Injury and Pain

Disturbances in the motor control system often follow injury and leave residual effects (27,28). In other words, although the client is pain free, mobility and stability problems and sensory deficits remain. This sets the stage for a perpetuating cycle of motor control impairment and mobility and stability limitations. Specifically, these alterations lead to inappropriate magnitudes of muscle forces and stiffness across joints, allowing for a joint to buckle or undergo shear translation (as described in the rotator cuff example earlier) (11). The loss of stability may be due to damage incurred to the passive structures of the joint (*e.g.*, tendons, ligaments) where they can no longer support joint integrity. Additionally, sensory receptors within the joints may be compromised, which will result in the delayed action of stabilizing muscles (28). The delay in action changes the order of muscle activation that is necessary for joint centration (16,29).

Everyday Posture and Limited Variety of Movement

Sahrmann (30) proposes that movement impairment stems from a biomechanical cause. In which case, repeated movements in one direction or sustained postures result in the remodeling of sarcomeres, whereby muscle lengths adaptively shorten or lengthen. The adaptive shortening represents a loss of sarcomeres, whereas muscle lengthening represents the addition of sarcomeres in series, taken together results in overall muscle imbalance (30). In effect, we stray from a neutral position and begin to adopt the posture that we are in most of the time (31). The muscle length adaptations then influence length tension and force-coupling relationships, motor control, and ultimately how we are able, or in many cases unable, to move (31). This set of circumstances is often seen in individuals who are sedentary, where the muscles of the anterior torso and the internal rotators of the shoulder tend to shorten. Athletes are also susceptible to development of faulty stabilization strategies and mobility particularly those who perform repeated unvaried or unidirectional movement patterns (*e.g.*, cyclists, runners, golfers, overhead athletes).

From a performance standpoint, a tight and shortened agonist (prime mover) has a lowered activation threshold and is described as hypertonic. This simply means that it will not take much stimulus to activate the muscle. In which case, hypertonic muscles suppress (decrease neural activity via reciprocal inhibition) the activity of lengthened antagonists and cause further weakening of that muscle (32). For example, hypertonic iliopsoas muscles often result from repeated hip flexion as seen in long-distance cycling or running or from prolonged seated postures. The hypertonicity of the hip flexors then contributes to the progressive weakening of the gluteus maximus via reciprocal inhibition. The gluteus maximus is an important hip extensor; thus, when forceful hip extension is necessary, the hamstrings (a synergist of the gluteus maximus) will compensate for the weakened gluteus maximus. This compensatory pattern is problematic for two main reasons. First, the pattern overworks the synergists (in the example, the hamstrings), which increases the risk for injury. Second, this compensatory pattern becomes etched within the sensorimotor system and will alter quality proprioception, mobility, and stability. These alterations then tend to perpetuate further postural distortion. For example, when the hamstrings become hypertonic (also due to sedentary posture), they exert a downward force on the proximal attachment site at the ischial tuberosity of the pelvis. This force rotates the pelvis posteriorly, which reduces the neutral curvature of the lumbar spine (flattens the low back) (31).

Joint Structure

Mobility and stability are partly derived from the articular geometry, or the shape and depth of joints. It is important to realize that some clients will present with structural anomalies that will prohibit full range of motion (ROM) on certain exercises. For example, an individual's hip joint may have a capsular structure that prevents performing a deep squat with the feet pointed in a neutral alignment. In such cases, the ACSM professional should encourage movement that is most comfortable for the client and not attempt to stretch through this nonmodifiable limitation.

Age

The adverse effects of aging on proprioception, stability, and mobility are well established (7,33). This is particularly relevant for the exercise physiologist because the percentage of individuals older than the age of 60 years continues to increase and the risk of falls, due to diminished kinesthesia and postural control, increases with age. These factors highlight the functional significance of balance and stability training in older populations. The reasons behind proprioceptive decline in the elderly include a reduction in the number of joint mechanoreceptors, changes to the structure and sensitivity of mechanoreceptors, and inadequate processing of proprioceptive input within the CNS (34–37).

Key Points

Alterations in movement quality can stem from multiple factors including obesity and overweight, sedentary behavior, poor postures, unvaried movement, joint structure, propensity for certain muscles to become inhibited, and age. It follows that fitness practitioners must consider each of these omnipresent factors when designing exercise programs.

What Is Neutral Position and Why Is It So Important?

Panjabi (21) describes neutral position as "the posture of the spine in which the overall internal stresses in the spinal column and muscular effort to hold the posture are minimal." A nice illustration of mechanical importance of neutral can be seen in a tent that has supporting wires equally tight around the structure. Conversely, if one set of support wires is tighter in comparison to the

Implications for Exercise Physiologist

Context for the Principles of Overload, Specificity, and Other Training Variables
The principle of overload is a fundamental construct of resistance training design (38). The overload principle suggests that in order to enhance muscular fitness, the body must exercise at an intensity that exceeds what it is normally accustomed to. It is important to recognize that overload represents a specific threshold that must be met in order for adaptation to occur. The way in which we introduce overload, however, must consider a superseding principle, which is quality movement should not be compromised, as flawed motor patterns can be easily ingrained and are difficult to correct once they take hold. To put it another way, overload should not outpace the client's sensory awareness, capacity to stabilize, and ability to move through a full ROM without compensation.

The principle of specificity suggests that specific adaptations occur upon application of specific demands. Accordingly, to improve proprioceptive acuity, sensory-specific training is necessary. More to the point, strength training is not the most effective way to improve sensory deficits.

In summary, fundamental principles of exercise prescription must be taken within context of quality movement. This means the adjustment of resistance training variables, including exercise selection, velocity of movement, and the number of repetitions and sets, should all be based on the client's sensorimotor capacity.

other side, the tent will likely collapse. In humans, maintaining neutral is important because it organizes the body into its most biomechanically efficient posture (20,21). More specifically, neutral position (a) optimizes ideal muscle length tension and force-coupling relationships, (b) minimizes compressive and shear forces imposed on the joint, and (c) optimizes the timing and speed of contraction of stabilizing muscles.

 ## Assessment and Prescription

Establishing a Movement Baseline

A widely held belief is that simple body weight movement is an appropriate place to begin a strength and conditioning program. This logic is based on the assumption that the client already has sufficient proprioceptive acuity, mobility, and appropriate command of the stabilizing muscles to maintain optimal alignment. Given the pervasive contributors of muscle imbalance described earlier, this assumption is a chancy supposition, whereby further exploration into the client's true movement baseline is likely needed (31).

Considering the majority of fitness assessments will take place in fitness centers, gyms, and studios, without the use of sophisticated laboratory equipment, the most pragmatic strategies for the exercise physiologist are left to observation of static and dynamic postures and symmetry of movement. It is important to note that if pain is present during any of the following assessments or exercises, the ACSM practitioner should recommend a medical exam by a qualified medical professional.

Assessment of Static Neutral Posture

Although static posture does not necessarily capture how an individual moves, it does provide the exercise physiologist some insight regarding specific muscle imbalances. This information can then be used in the selection of stabilization exercises and stretching and self-myofascial release (SMR) strategies. Static postural assessments also help clients develop an awareness of neutral posture, which holds great relevance when clients are performing dynamic movements that require maintenance of neutral while under load (*e.g.*, squat, lunge, deadlift, farmer's carries).

Plumb Line Assessment
Use of a plumb line or a static posture app is useful in identifying deviations from a neutral position. Clients should be barefoot, wear form-fitting clothing that enables the assessor to identify bony landmarks, and be encouraged to assume their everyday, relaxed posture during the assessment. Table 6.4 describes a basic plumb line postural assessment.

Wall Test
In addition to the plumb line assessment, a wall assessment of normal lumbar curvature and forward head posture is helpful. Instruct the client to stand with his or her back against a wall and feet approximately 6 in from the wall. Ideally, the back of the head should be positioned against the wall and the assessor's hand should be able to fit snugly in between the wall of the client's lumbar spine and the wall. Taken together, these static postural assessments expose areas of tightness and/or weakness. There are occasions where simply drawing the client's attention to the postural distortion and offering verbal cues will prove helpful (Table 6.5). Additionally, Table 6.5 offers specific stretching targets that correspond to the listed postural deviations.

Progressive Approach to Developing Postural Awareness
Unfortunately, due to various sensory, mobility, and stability limitations, the ability to distinguish neutral spine may be challenged. To begin, the ACSM practitioner should cue the client,

Table 6.4	Basic Plumb Line Static Postural Assessment	
View	**Setup for Assessment**	**Alignment Checkpoints**[a]
Sagittal	Client should stand sideways to the plumb line, with the line positioned slightly anterior to the client's ankle (lateral malleolus).	External auditory meatus (ear canal) Acromioclavicular joint Greater trochanter of the femur Tibial tuberosity
Anterior	Client should stand facing the plumb line, with feet equidistant from the line. Align the plumb line with the pubis.	Navel Sternum Chin Nose Eyes are equidistant from the line. Additionally, the shoulder girdle should be level.

[a]The plumb line should pass through these anatomical landmarks.

Adapted from Kendall FP, McCreary EK, Provance PG, Rodgers MM, Romani WA. *Muscles: Testing and Function with Posture and Pain*. 5th ed. Baltimore (MD): Lippincott Williams & Wilkins; 2005. 560 p.

both manually and verbally, to arch the low back and then flatten the low back (see Table 6.6 for progressive postural staging of this process). This should be repeated several times, on which the client should be asked to find the middle of the two extremes. Once neutral alignment is found, the client should be instructed to hold this posture for several seconds and then lose neutral by arching or flattening the low back, only to regain neutral position again. The client should begin performing each stage with eyes open and then eyes closed. When more dynamic movements, such as hip hinging and squatting, are introduced, a dowel placed along the spine provides valuable tactile feedback for the client. The client should be encouraged to maintain three points of contact with the dowel: the back of the head, the upper thoracic spine, and the pelvis.

Table 6.5	Postural Corrective Suggestions	
Postural Deviation	**Suggestive Verbal Cues**	**Stretching Target**
Forward head posture	"Tuck the chin."	Pectoralis major and minor; latissimus dorsi; abdominals
Increased thoracic curvature	"While tucking your chin, stand or sit as tall as possible."	Pectoralis major and minor; latissimus dorsi; abdominals
Internal rotation of the shoulders	"Create as much width between your shoulders."	Pectoralis major and minor; latissimus dorsi
Posterior pelvic tilt	"Align your rib cage over your pelvis."	Hamstrings; abdominals
Hyperextension of lumbar spine	"Gently contract your glute muscles." "Lock your ribcage on top of your pelvis."	Erector spinae; quadratus lumborum; quadriceps; iliopsoas

Table 6.6	**Progressive Stages for Neutral Posture**

Stage 1 Lying on the ground

Stage 2 Seated

Stage 3 Standing

Stage 4 Standing and adding in hip hinging

Stage 5 Farmer carries with bilateral loading

Stage 6 Farmer carries with unilateral loading

Integrative Assessments and Corrections

As muscles rarely work in isolation, assessments that consider the body as an integrated system, involving various segments of the body responding to movements in a synchronous coordinated fashion, are quite valuable (19). Although the following patterns may seem rudimentary, keep in mind that poor posture, fatigue, repeated asymmetrical movements, stress, and poor exercise practices have the potential to corrupt even the most primal motor patterns (2,11,31,39,40). Reclaiming these basic patterns then feeds the reflexive and intentional stabilization strategies needed for more functional movements such as the deadlift, squat, lunges, etc. (41,42).

Wall Plank-and-Roll

The wall plank-and-roll (WPR) is not only an assessment of lumbar stability but can also serve as an exercise to enhance lumbar torsional (antirotational) control (43). The client should be instructed to face a wall, with feet positioned approximately 2 ft from the wall. The client's elbows should be positioned on the wall, with forearms lying one on top of the other. The client should then be instructed to "brace" or stiffen the trunk (11) and pivot on the balls of his or her feet while pulling one elbow off the wall ending in a side plank position. The client should be encouraged to rotate the entire body as a single unit. No lumbar or pelvic motion should be observed while pivoting from side to side. Once the client demonstrates sufficient stability for the wall roll, progressions include side planks on the floor, initially performed on the knees and ultimately performed in a full-body side plank position. Of practical relevance, in order to optimize the effectiveness of isometric endurance exercises such as the side plank (also called the side bridge), Dr. Stuart McGill (11) recommends performing repeated sets of short-duration holds (8–10 s) rather than having the client perform one set of a prolonged (>30 s).

Teaching How to Brace

With respect to teaching clients how to brace, a few concepts are important to emphasize. First, the client should be instructed to precontract, or brace, the abdominal wall prior to performing isometric exercises such as a plank or isotonic movements such as squatting movements. Stuart McGill (11) suggests the use of the simple cue of "pretend you are about to be hit in the stomach." It is worth mentioning that the "hit" is not necessarily a full force strike to the stomach rather only intended to create the image of creating sufficient stability to maintain neutral alignment but not too much stiffness where motion is prevented (11). In other words, *the intensity of the brace should be tailored to the **relative intensity** of the exercise*, where the resultant coactivation of the trunk muscles is ample to protect the spine during lifting tasks but does not encumber proper mobility. For example, a client performing a body weight squat may require a low level of bracing intensity; however, when performing a one repetition maximum (1-RM) squat, the client should be encouraged to brace with closer to a maximal effort to maintain spinal integrity.

Diaphragmatic Breathing Assessment and Corrective Methods

Evaluation of diaphragmatic control is important for several reasons. First, the diaphragm muscles are not only the prime muscles of respiration but are also a vital muscle of core stabilization. To this end, if proper diaphragmatic control is not present, the generation of intra-abdominal pressure required to stabilize the spine during lifting tasks can be compromised (42,44). Second, breathing pattern problems have been shown to result in muscular imbalance, motor control alterations, and chronic low back pain (11,42,45). Third, as with proper conditioning of any muscle in the body, improving the endurance of the respiratory muscles enables these muscles to perform at higher capacities, ultimately leading to improved work capacity and prolonged time to fatigue (46). Fourth, those who tend to breathe at quicker rates, described as hyperventilation, exceed the gas exchange needs of metabolism. To this end, overbreathing has the potential to drastically lower carbon dioxide (CO_2) levels, which can raise pH levels (46). Not only is this a performance-limiting issue, if hyperventilation is severe enough, light-headedness and possibly unconsciousness can result. Finally, alterations in breathing mechanics have been correlated with low scores on the Functional Movement Screen (41), an evaluation of movement quality that explores seven different movement patterns.

Healthy breathing patterns, or diaphragmatic breathing, involve the expansion of the rib cage and abdomen and involves proper recruitment and endurance of the diaphragm muscles (47). Conversely, altered breathing involves breathing from the upper chest, as shown by rib cage elevation, and often involves shallow and quick breathing rates (45). The Hi-Lo Assessment is a simple assessment of proper diaphragmatic control during breathing and is detailed in Table 6.7.

Ideally, the hand on the upper abdomen should rise before the hand on the chest. Additionally, the hand on the chest should move slightly forward and not upward toward the chin (45). Conveniently, this simple assessment also serves as a means to correct the breathing pattern problem. The basic approach, detailed in Table 6.8, involves the client practicing a diaphragmatic breathing pattern while progressing through more challenging postures and movements. Clients demonstrating improper breathing habits should be encouraged to regularly practice breathing (using the same hand positions) that is focused on expansion of the rib cage and upper abdomen prior to any chest movement and to increase the length of each breath, in particular the client should be encouraged to fully exhale. Routine follow-up breathing pattern assessment should be

Table 6.7	Hi-Lo Assessment

Client places one hand on his or her sternum and one hand on his or her upper abdomen.

The client is then instructed to perform 10 breathing cycles.

The client reports which hand moved first at the beginning of the inhalation phase during the majority of the assessment. In addition, the practitioner should observe the hand movements of the client.

Adapted from Chaitow L. Breathing pattern disorders, motor control, and low back pain. *Int J Osteopath Med.* 2004;7(1):33–40.

Table 6.8	Diaphragmatic Breathing Pattern Progression	
Stage	**Description**	**Postural Progression**
Static	Maintenance of postural stability while breathing diaphragmatically	Supine on stable surface Seated Standing
Dynamic	Simultaneous limb movement while maintaining postural stability and diaphragmatic breathing patterns	Supine on floor with arm or leg movement Supine on foam roller with arm or leg movement Seated with arm or leg movement Standing with arm or leg movement
Advanced	Increase ventilation by performing any type of aerobic exercise	Immediately stop the aerobic exercise and perform an isometric exercise (*e.g.*, side plank, bird dog, curl-up). This will assist in improve the coordination of the diaphragm during tasks of core stabilization. Note: For these low-loading challenges, abdominal bracing should occur in concert with diaphragmatic breathing.

Adapted from Nelson N. Diaphragmatic breathing: the foundation of core stability. *Strength Cond J.* 2012;34(5):34–40; McGill SM. *Low Back Disorders: Evidence-Based Prevention and Rehabilitation.* 2nd ed. Champaign (IL): Human Kinetics; 2007. 328 p.

performed to monitor for changes and to emphasize the relevance of diaphragmatic breathing patterns in optimizing core stability and overall health.

Rolling Patterns: Assessment and Correction

Although infants can roll with relative efficiency by 6–8 months of age, the pattern may become altered later in life due to mobility deficits or insufficient core stabilization patterning (48). More specifically, demonstration of efficient rolling patterns reveals proper recruitment sequencing of the core stabilizing muscles (*i.e.*, initiated with the deeper trunk stabilizers, including the transversus abdominis, multifidus, diaphragm, and pelvic floor, and followed by recruitment of the more superficial or global muscles including the internal and external obliques, rectus abdominis, quadratus lumborum, and erector spinae). However, given the lack of variety of daily movement among many individuals (including athletes performing motions in one direction), symmetrical rotational efficiency may be altered. The objective of the assessment is to observe the rolling strategy of the client in eight different patterns, leading from all four quadrants of the body. Ideally, the client should be able to roll with equal ease in all directions. When first performing the rolling assessments, use limited cues (Table 6.9) because the goal is to observe his or her movement plan and "cheating" methods.

There are times where clients will have difficulty completing rolling patterns. In which case, Table 6.10 and the following figures provide some of the common associated mobility and stability limitations and corresponding corrections. The rolling pattern itself can also be modified by placing a foam roller under one side of the trunk (just lateral to the spine); this will assist the client in rolling away from the bolstered side.

The client should be encouraged to practice each of the patterns (particularly the patterns where coordination and symmetry of movement was poor) while keeping the cues offered in Table 6.11 in mind.

Table 6.9	Assessment of Rolling Patterns	
Rolling Direction[a]	**Beginning Position**	**Cues**
Supine to prone leading with the right or left arm	Supine; legs straight and slightly abducted; arms overhead and slightly abducted; when looking down at the client, he or she should resemble an "X."	"With no help from the legs, roll onto your belly."
Supine to prone leading with the right or left leg	Supine; legs straight and slightly abducted; arms overhead and slightly abducted	"With no help from your arms, roll onto your belly."
Prone to supine leading with the right or left arm	Prone; legs straight and slightly abducted; arms overhead and slightly abducted	"With no help from your legs, roll onto your back."
Supine to prone leading with the right or left leg	Prone; legs straight and slightly abducted; arms overhead and slightly abducted	"With no help from your arms, roll onto your back."

[a]Each pattern should be performed right to left and left to right, totaling eight patterns.

Table 6.10	Correctives for Those Who Are Initially Unable to Perform Rolling Patterns
Exercise Progression for Rolling Patterns	
Strength or Mobility Limitation	**Corrective Stretch or Exercise**
Thoracic spine mobility	Modified cobra stretch (Fig. 6.3); doorway pectoralis major stretch
Gluteus maximus weakness	Bird dog (Fig. 6.4) or quadruped exercises; glute bridges (Fig. 6.5)
Gluteus medius weakness	Lateral band walks (Fig. 6.6); clam shell exercises (Fig. 6.7)
Core endurance	WPR; side plank performed on knees (Fig. 6.8)

Table 6.11	Verbal Cues for Rolling Patterns
Rolling Direction[a]	**Verbal Cues**
Supine to prone leading with the right arm	"Begin by looking to the left, lead with the eyes and head; lift the right arm; look into the left shoulder and roll over like a rag doll."
Supine to prone leading with the right leg	"Flex the hip and then cross the right leg over the left and roll."
Prone to supine leading with the right arm	"Lift the right arm, look up and over the opposite shoulder and roll."
Prone to supine leading with the right leg	"Bend the right knee, lift the foot toward the ceiling, cross the right leg over the left and roll."

[a]These sample cues are for rolling from right to left. Simply reverse the cuing when rolling from left to right.

Adapted from Hoogenboom BJ, Voight ML, Cook G, Gill L. Using rolling to develop neuromuscular control and coordination of the core and extremities of athletes. *N Am J Sports Phys Ther.* 2009;4(2):70–82.

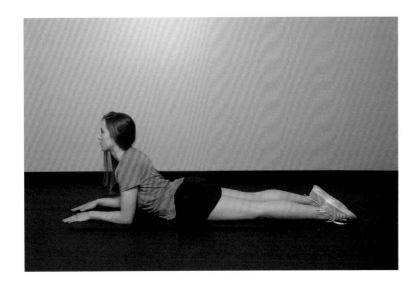

FIGURE 6.3. Modified cobra stretch.

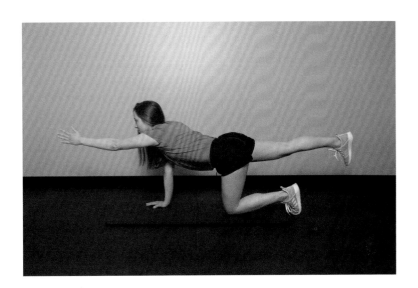

FIGURE 6.4. Bird dog.

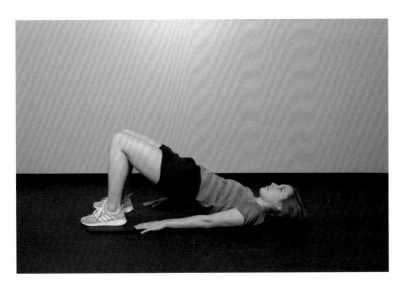

FIGURE 6.5. Glute bridge.

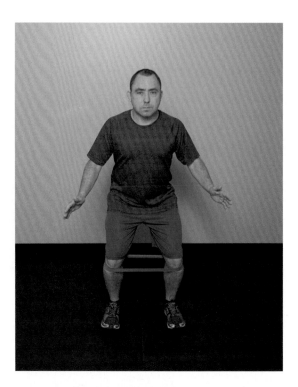

FIGURE 6.6. Lateral band walks.

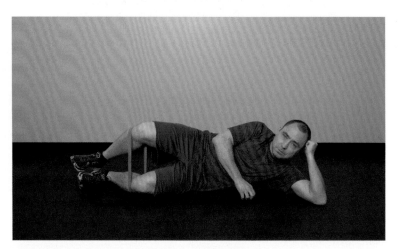

FIGURE 6.7. Clam shell.

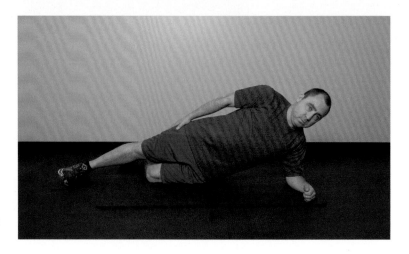

FIGURE 6.8. Side plank
performed on the knees.

Table 6.12	Alignment Fault Checklist

Loss of cervical neutral — head positioned in front of the body or tilting up or down

Loss of thoracic extension — rounding of the thoracic spine

Internal rotation of the shoulders

Posterior pelvic tilt — loss of neutral lordosis in the lumbar spine or flattening of lumbar spine

Anterior pelvic tilt — excessive arching of low back

Knee valgus — knees collapsing inward

Addressing Alignment Issues

It is essential for the ACSM-EP to be able to critically appraise the quality of movement during an exercise session. In the fitness center setting, this evaluation will often rely on observing any alignment faults that may present during the performance of an exercise (Table 6.12). Many times, verbal and manual cuing can correct the problem; however, there are occasions where alignment faults are the result of low endurance, timing issues of the stabilizing muscles, and/or tightness in the mobilizing muscles that were outlined earlier in this chapter (Table 6.13).

The training goal is to improve the endurance and functional stabilization capacity of these muscles. In which case, a good place to start is incorporating isometric exercises applied at various joint-specific angles for the weakened or inhibited muscles (49), with short duration hold and relax cycles (5–8 s). For example, if weakness is noted in the rhomboid muscles (demonstrated by excessive thoracic kyphosis), an effective approach might involve the following:

- Instruct the client to maintain a tall neutral posture while retracting and depressing the scapula, holding this position for 5–8 seconds and then relaxing.
- Progression 1: Have the client perform multiple sets of this exercise, still using 5- to 8-second holds.

Table 6.13	Common Alignment Faults Along with Corresponding Inhibited or Weak Stabilizing Muscles	
Alignment Fault	**Associated Weak or Inhibited Muscles**	**Suggested Corrective Exercises**
Loss of cervical neutral	Deep cervical flexors (longus colli, capitis)	Chin tucks (Fig. 6.9); isometric cervical exercise (*e.g.*, using hands on forehead resisting neck flexion effort)
Loss of thoracic extension	Middle and lower trapezius	Scapular retraction with no weight (Fig. 6.10); progressing to seated rows
Internal rotation of the shoulders	External rotators of the shoulder (infraspinatus)	Band or dumbbell shoulder external rotation (Fig. 6.11)
Posterior pelvic tilt	Gluteus medius and maximus; multifidus	Glute bridges; quadruped or bird dog
Anterior pelvic tilt	Gluteus medius and maximus; transversus abdominis	Curl-up; side plank/bridge
Knee valgus	Gluteus medius and maximus	Lateral band walks; clam shells; glute bridges; bird dog

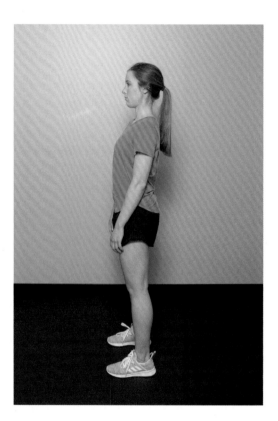

FIGURE 6.9. Chin tucks.

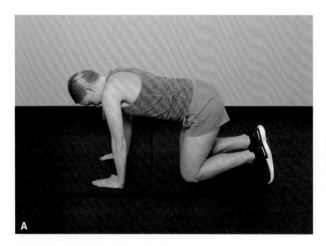

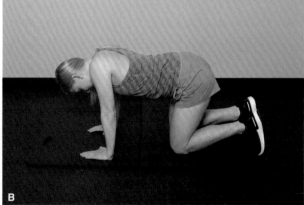

FIGURE 6.10. Scapular retraction.

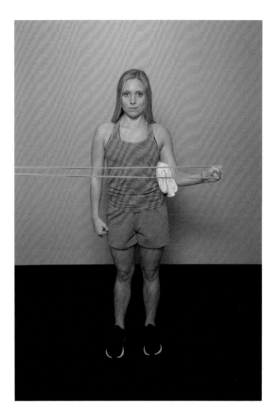

FIGURE 6.11. Band external rotation.

- Progression 2: Have the client perform the same isometric hold against light resistance tubing.
- Progression 3: As the client develops endurance and greater recruitment efficiency of the rhomboids, introduce more dynamic movements, such as a seated row or single-arm dumbbell row. In this case, repetitions schemes should be focused on enhancing muscular endurance (12–15 repetitions).

Instability Training

Instability training is a method of training that challenges a client's ability to maintain balance while challenging the client's center of gravity. This is often accomplished by narrowing the client's base of support (*e.g.*, by moving the legs closer together, maintaining single leg postures, or performing exercises on unstable surfaces). By challenging posture in this way, instability training is thought to improve feed-forward and feedback mechanisms, ultimately improving stability and proprioception. It is worth noting that the goal of instability training is to improve stability and sensory acuity, not necessarily to improve strength in the extremities, and thus should involve low load tasks. When planning instability training, it is essential to tailor the difficulty of the exercise to the client's relative functional capacity. In effect, the client should be able to demonstrate some level of postural control, but at the same time, the exercise should require a great deal of concentration. Once the client has mastered one level, the client should progress to the next level of difficulty. Table 6.14 illustrates a systematic approach to instability training. Once the client can adequately perform the exercise on the floor, the next stage would involve having the client perform the same sequence of exercises, only on an unstable surface, such as a cushioned surface or an Airex pad. The next stage might incorporate the use of an elevated surface, as the client performs functional challenges such as medicine ball tosses or sport-specific tasks (Figs. 6.14 and 6.15).

Table 6.14	Instability Training Progression Example	
Exercise	**Position**	**Demonstration of Mastery**
A1. Wide staggered stance on the floor Eyes open (Fig. 6.12)	Client stands on the floor with one foot in front of the other, wide stance to increase the base of support.	Maintains optimal alignment without significant swaying for 30 s
A2. Wide staggered stance on the floor Eyes closed	Client stands on the floor with one foot in front of the other, wide stance to increase the base of support.	Maintains optimal alignment without significant swaying for 30 s
A3. Wide staggered stance on the floor with weight shift Eyes closed	Client stands on the floor with one foot in front of the other, wide stance to increase the base of support. Instruct client to shift majority of weight onto front foot and then to back foot.	Maintains optimal alignment without significant swaying for 30 s
B1. Narrow staggered stance Eyes open	Client stands on the floor with one foot directly in front of the other as if standing on a balance beam.	Maintains optimal alignment without significant swaying for 30 s
B2. Narrow staggered stance Eyes closed	Client stands on the floor with one foot directly in front of the other as if standing on a balance beam.	Maintains optimal alignment without significant swaying for 30 s
B3. Narrow staggered stance Eyes closed with weight shift	Client stands on the floor with one foot directly in front of the other as if standing on a balance beam. Instruct client to shift majority of weight onto front foot then to back foot.	Maintains optimal alignment without significant swaying for 30 s
C1. Single-leg stance Eyes open	Client stands on one foot on the floor.	Maintains optimal alignment without significant swaying for 30 s
C2. Single-leg stance Eyes closed (Fig. 6.13)	Client stands on one foot on the floor.	Maintains optimal alignment without significant swaying for 30 s
C3. Single-leg stance with reach	Client stands on one foot on floor and reaches with opposite hand to a specific target.	Able to perform several reaches without losing balance

Self-Myofascial Release and Stretching

Another important component of a well-rounded exercise prescription is managing hypertonic muscles and soft tissue restriction that compromise mobility. Although stretching approaches such as proprioceptive neuromuscular facilitation (PNF) and static stretching are known to improve ROM, several reviews have reported significant deleterious effects on neuromuscular performance when done prior to activity (50,51). Conversely, several recent investigations have shown that SMR elicits improvements in ROM without concomitant performance decrements when done prior to activity (52–54).

SMR is based on a form of manual therapy believed to alleviate the discomfort associated with tender spots within the myofascia, known as trigger points (55,56), and relax hypertonic areas

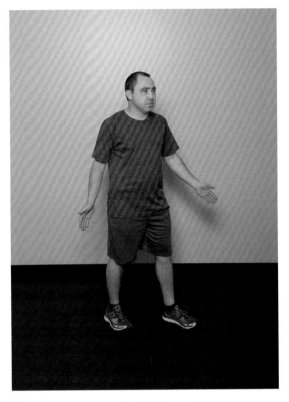

FIGURE 6.12. Wide staggered stance, eyes open.

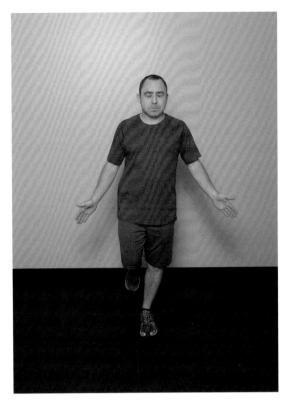

FIGURE 6.13. Single-leg stance, eyes closed.

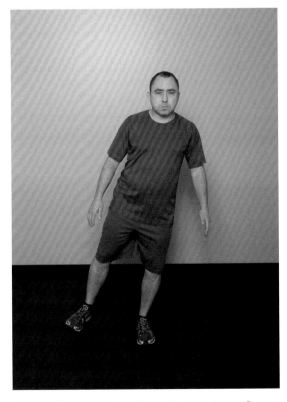

FIGURE 6.14. Progression option: one leg on floor.

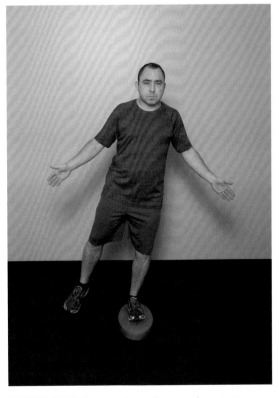

FIGURE 6.15. Progression option: one leg on an elevated surface.

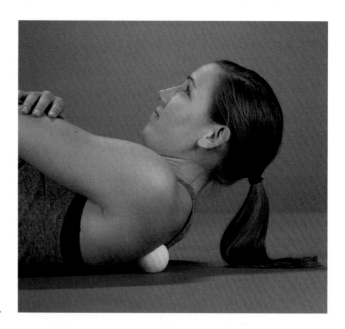

FIGURE 6.16. Lacrosse ball on upper back.

within soft tissue (57). SMR involves the compression of soft tissue using tools such as foam rollers, roller massagers, or tennis balls and is performed by the individual rather than by a therapist (Figs. 6.16 and 6.17). Currently, the mechanisms behind SMR are unclear, although prevailing theories suggest that the compressive forces imposed on the myofascia stimulate various mechanoreceptors that reduce muscle-firing rates (58–60). Additionally, mechanical pressure induced by SMR may improve the viscous and fluid qualities of fascia, described as thixotropism (59). Other theories have proposed that the myofascia becomes restricted due to local inflammation (61). Although it is unclear how SMR might reduce inflammation, there is evidence indicating that SMR transiently increases local blood flow (62,63). To this end, the increased blood flow may aid in the reduction of inflammation. Table 6.15 includes a few suggested SMR and stretching targets for common alignment issues.

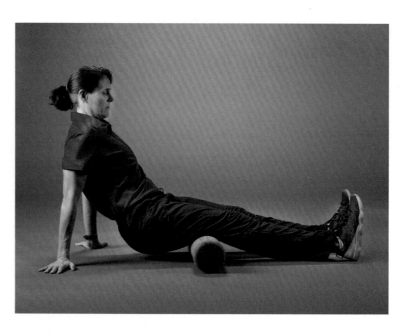

FIGURE 6.17. Foam rolling hamstrings.

Table 6.15	Alignment Issues and Soft Tissue Targets
Alignment Fault	**Self-Myofascial Release and Stretching Targets**
Excessive kyphosis of the thoracic spine	Pectoralis major and minor; latissimus dorsi; abdominals
Internal rotation of the shoulders	Pectoralis major and minor; latissimus dorsi
Posterior pelvic tilt	Hamstrings (see Fig. 6.17); abdominals
Hyperextension of the lumbar spine	Quadratus lumborum; quadriceps; iliopsoas

Lifestyle Recommendations

Stability, mobility, and sensory issues develop over long periods of time and are often mediated by lifestyle habits. Although exercise sessions are a critical piece of the repatterning process, the ACSM-EP should also offer recommendations that address lifestyle issues known to perpetuate muscle imbalance. Suggestions might include improving the ergonomics of the work environment, setting a recurring alarm to serve as a reminder to stand and walk around the office, practice of diaphragmatic breathing, and foam rolling while watching television.

SUMMARY

Although progressive overload is essential for improvements in strength and endurance outcomes, it should not come at the expense of proper movement patterning. To this end, it is critical for the ACSM practitioner to recognize that stability, mobility, and proprioception are requisite features of motor patterning and collectively serve as the foundation for strength and functional development. Unfortunately, pervasive issues such as sedentary behavior, obesity and overweight, and limited variety in movement impair these foundational components of fitness. If insufficient stabilizing strategies, lack of mobility, and low proprioceptive acuity are observed, practitioners must incorporate a systematic, progressive approach to improve baseline function prior to advancing the client into more conventional exercise prescription.

REFERENCES

1. Franklin DW, Wolpert DM. Computational mechanisms of sensorimotor control. *Neuron*. 2011;72(3):425–42.

2. Jull GA, Janda V. Muscles and motor control in low back pain: assessment and management. In: Twomey LT, Taylor JR, editors. *Physical Therapy of the Low Back*. New York (NY): Churchill Livingstone; 1987. p. 253–78.

3. Lephart S, Fu F. *Proprioception and Neuromuscular Control in Joint Stability*. Champaign (IL): Human Kinetics; 2000. 439 p.

4. Sherrington C. *The Integrative Action of the Nervous System*. New Haven (CT): Yale University Press; 1906. 128 p.

5. Gandevia SC, Refshauge KM, Collins DF. Proprioception: peripheral inputs and perceptual interactions. *Adv Exp Med Biol*. 2002;508:61–8.

6. Rothwell J. *Control of Human Voluntary Movement*. London (United Kingdom): Chapman and Hall; 1994. 325 p.

7. Goble DJ, Coxon JP, Wenderoth N, Van Impe A, Swinnen SP. Proprioceptive sensibility in the elderly: degeneration, functional consequences and plastic-adaptive processes. *Neurosci Biobehav Rev*. 2009;33(3):271–8.

8. Röijezon U, Clark NC, Treleaven J. Proprioception in musculoskeletal rehabilitation. Part 1: basic science and principles of assessment and clinical interventions. *Man Ther*. 2015;20(3):368–77.

9. Kersey R. Taber's Cyclopedic Medical Dictionary, 20th ed. *Athl Ther Today*. 2006;11(3):47.

10. Riemann BL, Lephart SM. The sensorimotor system, part I: the physiologic basis of functional joint stability. *J Athl Train.* 2002;37(1):71–9.

11. McGill SM. *Low Back Disorders: Evidence-Based Prevention and Rehabilitation.* 2nd ed. Champaign (IL): Human Kinetics; 2007. 328 p.

12. Myers J, Wassinger C, Lephart S. Sensorimotor contribution to shoulder stability: effect of injury and rehabilitation. *Man Ther.* 2006;11(3):197–201.

13. Ionta S, Heydrich L, Lenggenhager B, et al. Multisensory mechanisms in temporo-parietal cortex support self-location and first-person perspective. *Neuron.* 2011;70(2):363–74.

14. Tripp B, Yochem E, Uhl T. Functional fatigue and upper extremity sensorimotor system acuity in baseball athletes. *J Athl Train.* 2007;42(1):90–8.

15. Bergmark A. Stability of the lumbar spine: a study in mechanical engineering. *Acta Orthop Scand Suppl.* 1989;230:1–54.

16. Richardson C, Hodges PW, Hides J. *Therapeutic Exercise for Lumbopelvic Stabilization: A Motor Control Approach for the Treatment and Prevention of Low Back Pain.* 2nd ed. Edinburgh (United Kingdom): Churchill Livingstone; 2004. 271 p.

17. Bliss L, Teeple P. Core stability: the centerpiece of any training program. *Curr Sports Med Rep.* 2005;4(3):179–83.

18. Borghuis J, Hof A, Lemmink K. The importance of sensory-motor control in providing core stability. *Sports Med.* 2008;38(11):893–916.

19. Tse MA, McManus AM, Masters RSW. Development and validation of a core endurance intervention program: implications for performance in college-age rowers. *J Strength Cond Res.* 2005;19(3):547–55.

20. Panjabi MM. The stabilizing system of the spine. Part I. Function, dysfunction, adaptation, and enhancement. *J Spinal Disord.* 1992;5(4):383–9.

21. Panjabi MM. The stabilizing system of the spine. Part II. Neutral zone and instability hypothesis. *J Spinal Disord.* 1992;5(4):390–7.

22. Kováčiková Z, Svoboda Z, Neumannová K, Bizovská L, Cuberek R, Janura M. Assessment of postural stability in overweight and obese middle-aged women. *Acta Gymnica.* 2014;44(3):149–53.

23. Shultz S, Byrne N, Hills A. Musculoskeletal function and obesity: implications for physical activity. *Curr Obes Rep.* 2014;3(3):355–60.

24. Cattuzzo MT, Henrique R, Ré A, et al. Motor competence and health related physical fitness in youth: a systematic review. *J Sci Med Sport.* 2016;19(2):123–9.

25. Đokić Z, Međedović. Relationship between overweight, obesity and the motor abilities of 9-12 year old school children. *Phys Cult.* 2013;67(2):91–102.

26. Duncan MJ, Stanley M, Wright SL. The association between functional movement and overweight and obesity in British primary school children. *BMC Sports Sci Med Rehabil.* 2013;5:11.

27. Richardson C, Jull G, Hodges P, Hides J. *Therapeutic Exercise for Spinal Segmental Stabilisation in Low Back Pain: Scientific Basis and Clinical Approach.* Edinburgh (United Kingdom): Churchill Livingstone; 1999. 191 p.

28. Switlick T, Kernozek TW, Meardon S. Differences in joint-position sense and vibratory threshold in runners with and without a history of overuse injury. *J Sport Rehabil.* 2015;24(1):6–12.

29. Hodges PW, Richardson CA. Altered trunk muscle recruitment in people with low back pain with upper limb movement at different speeds. *Arch Phys Med Rehabil.* 1999;80(9):1005–12.

30. Sahrmann S. *Diagnosis and Treatment of Movement Impairment Syndromes.* St. Louis (MO): Mosby; 2002. 384 p.

31. MacIntosh BR, Gardiner P, McComas AJ. *Skeletal Muscle: Form and Function.* 2nd ed. Champaign (IL): Human Kinetics; 2006. 432 p.

32. Whittle MW. *Gait Analysis: An Introduction.* 4th ed. Edinburgh (Scotland): Butterworth Heineman Elsevier; 2007. 255 p.

33. Wingert JR, Welder C, Foo P. Age-related hip proprioception declines: effects on postural sway and dynamic balance. *Arch Phys Med Rehabil.* 2014;95(2):253–61.

34. Adamo D, Martin B, Brown S. Age-related differences in upper limb proprioceptive acuity. *Percept Mot Skills.* 2007;104(3 Pt 2):1297–309.

35. Aydoğ S, Korkusuz P, Doral M, Tetik O, Demirel H. Decrease in the numbers of mechanoreceptors in rabbit ACL: the effects of aging. *Knee Surg Sports Traumatol Arthrosc.* 2006;14(4):325–9.

36. Goble DJ, Brown SH. Task-dependent asymmetries in the utilization of proprioceptive feedback for goal-directed movement. *Exp Brain Res.* 2007;180(4):693–704.

37. Iwasaki T, Goto N, Goto J, Ezure H, Moriyama H. The aging of human Meissner's corpuscles as evidenced by parallel sectioning. *Okajimas Folia Anat Jpn.* 2003;79(6):185–9.

38. Kraemer WJ, Ratamess NA. Fundamentals of resistance training: progression and exercise prescription. *Med Sci Sports Exerc.* 2004;36(4):674–88.

39. Kibler WB, Press J, Sciascia A. The role of core stability in athletic function. *Sports Med.* 2006;36(3):189–98.

40. Lin YH, Li CW, Tsai LY, Liing R. The effects of muscle fatigue and proprioceptive deficits on the passive joint senses of ankle inversion and eversion. *Isokinet Exerc Sci.* 2008;16(2):101–5.

41. Bradley H, Esformes J. Breathing pattern disorders and functional movement. *Int J Sports Phys Ther.* 2014;9(1):28–39.

42. Nelson N. Diaphragmatic breathing: the foundation of core stability. *Strength Cond J.* 2012;34(5):34–40.

43. Yoon C, Lee J, Kim K, Kim H, Chung SG. Quantification of lumbar stability during wall plank-and-roll activity. *PM R.* 2015;7(8):803–13.

44. Key J. 'The core': understanding it, and retraining its dysfunction. *J Bodywork Mov Ther.* 2013;17(4):541–59.

45. Chaitow L. Breathing pattern disorders, motor control, and low back pain. *Int J Osteopath Med.* 2004;7(1):33–40.

46. McArdle WD, Katch FI, Katch VL. *Exercise Physiology: Nutrition, Energy, and Human Performance.* 8th ed. Baltimore (MD): Wolters Kluwer; 2015. 1088 p.

47. Pryor JA, Prasad SA. *Physiotherapy for Respiratory and Cardiac Problems: Adults and Paediatrics.* 3rd ed.

Edinburgh (United Kingdom): Churchill Livingstone; 2002. 552 p.

48. Hoogenboom BJ, Voight ML, Cook G, Gill L. Using rolling to develop neuromuscular control and coordination of the core and extremities of athletes. *N Am J Sports Phys Ther.* 2009;4(2):70–82.

49. Baechle TR, Earle RW. *Essentials of Strength Training and Conditioning.* 2nd ed. Champaign (IL): Human Kinetics; 2000. 672 p.

50. Behm DG, Chaouachi A. A review of the acute effects of static and dynamic stretching on performance. *Eur J Appl Physiol.* 2011;111(11):2633–51.

51. Kay AD, Blazevich AJ. Effect of acute static stretch on maximal muscle performance: a systematic review. *Med Sci Sports Exerc.* 2012;44(1):154–64.

52. Healey KC, Hatfield DL, Blanpied P, Dofrman LR, Riebe D. The effects of myofascial release with foam rolling on performance. *J Strength Cond Res.* 2014;28(1):61–8.

53. Peacock CA, Krein DD, Silver TA, Sanders GJ, von Carlowitz KA. An acute bout of self-myofascial release in the form of foam rolling improves performance testing. *Int J Exerc Sci.* 2014;7(3):202–11.

54. Sullivan KM, Silvey D, Button DC, Behm DG. Roller-massager application to the hamstrings increases sit-and-reach range of motion within five to ten seconds without performance impairments. *Int J Sports Phys Ther.* 2013;8(3):228–36.

55. Bron C, Dommerholt JD. Etiology of myofascial trigger points. *Curr Pain Headache Rep.* 2012;16(5):439–44.

56. Travell JG, Simons DG, Cummings BD. *Myofascial Pain and Dysfunction: The Trigger Point Manual.* Baltimore (MD): Williams & Wilkins; 1983. 628 p.

57. McKenney K, Elder AS, Elder C, Hutchins A. Myofascial release as a treatment for orthopaedic conditions: a systematic review. *J Athl Train.* 2013;48(4):522–7.

58. Roylance DS, George JD, Hammer AM, et al. Evaluating acute changes in joint range-of-motion using self-myofascial release, postural alignment exercises, and static stretches. *Int J Exerc Sci.* 2013;6(4):310–9.

59. Schleip R. Fascial plasticity — a new neurobiological explanation: part 1. *J Bodyw Mov Ther.* 2003;7(1):11–9.

60. Tozzi P. Selected fascial aspects of osteopathic practice. *J Bodyw Mov Ther.* 2012;16(4):503–19.

61. Bednar DA, Orr FW, Simon GT. Observations on the pathomorphology of the thoracolumbar fascia in chronic mechanical back pain: a microscopic study. *Spine (Phila Pa 1976).* 1995;20(10):1161–4.

62. Okamoto T, Masuhara M, Ikuta K. Acute effects of self-myofascial release using a foam roller on arterial function. *J Strength Cond Res.* 2014;28(1):69–73.

63. Queré N, Noël E, Lieutaud A, d'Alessio P. Fasciatherapy combined with pulsology touch induces changes in blood turbulence potentially beneficial for vascular endothelium. *J Bodyw Mov Ther.* 2009;13(13):239–45.

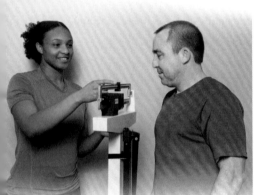

CHAPTER **7**

Body Composition and Weight Management

OBJECTIVES

- To understand and apply the various methods of anthropometric measurements and body composition assessment.
- To understand current best practices for the treatment of obesity and prevention of weight gain.
- To understand the key nutrition messages as described by the 2015–2020 U.S. Department of Agriculture (USDA) Dietary Guidelines (1).
- To understand and apply the American College of Sports Medicine's (ACSM) metabolic calculations.

INTRODUCTION

The prevalence of overweight and obesity has been increasing in the United States and in developed countries around the world. Recent estimates indicate that approximately 72% of the U.S. population are classified as either overweight or obese (body mass index [BMI] $\geq$25.0 kg · m^{-2}), with approximately 40% classified as obese (BMI $\geq$30.0 kg · m^{-2}), including 7% with severe obesity (BMI $\geq$40 kg · m^{-2}) (2). The prevalence of obesity varies by sex, race, and Hispanic origin, with higher rates found in Hispanic and Mexican American men and women and in non-Hispanic black women compared with non-Hispanic white men and women (2). Obesity rates among children aged 2–5 years, children aged 6–11 years, and adolescents are 14%, 18%, and 21%, respectively (3). Obesity is a worldwide problem with global obesity rates nearly tripling between 1975 and 2016. In 2016, the World Health Organization estimated that more than 1.9 billion adults are overweight; of those, 650 million or 13% of the adult population are obese (4).

Overweight and obesity are characterized by high amounts of body fat in relation to overall lean body mass and are linked to premature mortality and numerous chronic diseases, including hypertension, cardiovascular disease (CVD), dyslipidemia, respiratory problems, Type 2 diabetes, some cancers, sleep apnea, arthritis, and other musculoskeletal disorders (5,6). Central (abdominal) obesity is associated with the metabolic syndrome, a clustering of metabolic factors that increase the risk of CVD, Type 2 diabetes, and stroke (7).

It is estimated that obesity-related conditions account for more than 7% of total health care costs in the United States (8). Adults with obesity spend 42% more on direct health care costs than adults with a healthy weight (9). The two most frequently mentioned obesity-related disorders included in health cost calculations are CVD and diabetes (10). Individuals with moderate obesity (BMI between 30.0 and 35.0 kg · m^{-2}) are more than twice as likely as individuals with a healthy weight to be prescribed prescription pharmaceuticals to manage medical conditions (11), whereas per capita health care costs for adults with severe obesity are 81% higher than for adults with a healthy weight (12). Several medical conditions exist that promote inadequate energy expenditure.

Body composition is an important component of health-related physical fitness. It is important that the American College of Sports Medicine Certified Exercise Physiologist® (ACSM-EP®) Understands how to properly measure body composition, make sound weight loss goals, prescribe appropriate exercise programs, and provide appropriate nutritional recommendations for weight loss and weight management. Due to the high prevalence of obesity, the percentage of body fat is often emphasized. However, it is equally important to consider the changes in body composition that accompany aging. Sarcopenia is the age-related loss of muscle mass that is accompanied by a decrease in strength. The body composition assessments completed in most health fitness settings do not provide a precise measurement of muscle mass, but muscle mass is a major component of the fat-free mass that is estimated and should be discussed with the client.

This chapter discusses the different methods for measuring body composition, reviews ACSM exercise guidelines for individuals who are overweight and obese, and provides sound physical activity (PA) and nutritional information regarding weight management.

Anthropometric Measurements

Anthropometrics are a set of noninvasive, quantitative techniques for determining body size by measuring, recording, and analyzing specific dimensions of the body, such as height, weight, and body circumference.

Height and Weight

Height is measured using a calibrated wall-mounted stadiometer (a vertical ruler mounted on a wall with a wide horizontal headboard). The clients should remove their shoes and hair ornaments, stand straight with their heels together, and look straight ahead. Before taking the measurement, ask that the clients take a deep breath and hold it. Height is recorded in either inches or centimeters. Weight is measured using either a calibrated balance beam or an electronic scale. The clients should wear only light clothing, remove their shoes, empty their pockets, void the bladder if necessary, and stand in the center of the platform with weight distributed evenly on both feet. Weight is recorded in either pounds or kilograms.

Body Mass Index

BMI is a measure of weight in relation to a person's height. It is calculated by dividing body weight in kilograms by height in meters squared (refer to the "How to Calculate Body Mass Index" box) or can be determined with a BMI table (Table 7.1) or by using an online BMI calculator (*e.g.*, https://www.nhlbi.nih.gov/health/educational/lose_wt/BMI/bmicalc.htm) (13).

BMI is used to classify individuals as underweight (<18.5 kg $\cdot$ m^{-2}), normal weight ($18.5–24.9$ kg $\cdot$ m^{-2}), overweight ($25.0–29.9$ kg $\cdot$ m^{-2}), or obese (≥30 kg $\cdot$ m^{-2}) (14) and to identify individuals at risk for obesity-related diseases (Table 7.2). For most individuals, obesity-related health problems increase with a BMI ≥25.0 kg $\cdot$ m^{-2}. A BMI ≥30.0 kg $\cdot$ m^{-2} is associated with

Table 7.1				Body Mass Index Chart										
BMI (kg · m^{-2})	19	20	21	22	23	24	25	26	27	28	29	30	35	40
Height (in)							Weight (lb)							
58	91	96	100	105	110	115	119	124	129	134	138	143	167	191
59	94	99	104	109	114	119	124	128	133	138	143	148	173	198
60	97	102	107	112	118	123	128	133	138	143	148	153	179	204
61	100	106	111	116	122	127	132	137	143	148	153	158	185	211
62	104	109	115	120	126	131	136	142	147	153	158	164	191	218
63	107	113	118	124	130	135	141	146	152	158	163	169	197	225
64	110	116	122	128	134	140	145	151	157	163	169	174	204	232
65	114	120	126	132	138	144	150	156	162	168	174	180	210	240
66	118	124	130	136	142	148	155	161	167	173	179	186	216	247
67	121	127	134	140	146	153	159	166	172	178	185	191	223	255
68	125	131	138	144	151	158	164	171	177	184	190	197	230	262
69	128	135	142	149	155	162	169	176	182	189	196	203	236	270
70	132	139	146	153	160	167	174	181	188	195	202	207	243	278
71	136	143	150	157	165	172	179	186	193	200	208	215	250	286
72	140	147	154	162	169	177	184	191	199	206	213	221	258	294
73	144	151	159	166	174	182	189	197	204	212	219	227	265	302
74	148	155	163	171	179	186	194	202	210	218	225	233	272	311
75	152	160	168	176	184	192	200	208	216	224	232	240	279	319
76	156	164	172	180	189	197	205	213	221	230	238	246	287	328

Adapted from U.S. Department of Health and Human Services, National Health, Lung, and Blood Institute, People Science Health. Body Mass Index Table 1 [Internet]. [cited 2017 Feb 23]. Available from: http://www.nhlbi.nih.gov/guidelines/obesity/bmi_tbl.htm

Table 7.2	Classification of Disease Risk Based on BMI and Waist Circumference (5)		
		Disease Risk[a] Relative to Normal	
		Waist Circumference	
		Men ≤102 cm	**Men >102 cm**
Weight	**BMI**	**Women ≤88 cm**	**Women >88 cm**
Underweight	<18.5	—	—
Normal	18.5–24.9	—	—
Overweight	25.0–29.9	Increased	High
Obesity			
Class I	30.0–34.9	High	Very high
Class II	35.0–39.9	Very high	Very high
Class III	≥40	Extremely high	Extremely high

[a]Disease risk for Type 2 diabetes, hypertension, and cardiovascular disease. Dashes (—) indicate that no additional risk at these levels of BMI was assigned. Increased waist circumference can also be a marker for increased risk even in persons of normal weight.

hypertension, dyslipidemia, coronary heart disease, and mortality (15). A BMI of $<18.5 \ \text{kg} \cdot \text{m}^{-2}$ also increases mortality risk (16). BMI can be used to classify children and adolescents as either overweight or obese using the standard BMI formula along with a BMI for age growth chart provided by the Centers for Disease Control and Prevention (17). In children and adolescents, overweight is defined as the ≥85th to <95th percentile of BMI for age and sex, whereas obesity is defined as ≥95th percentile for age and sex (17).

BMI is a useful screening tool that indicates the level of body fatness. However, BMI does not differentiate between fat and fat-free mass, so it is not a true measure of adiposity, and a wide variation in body fat percentage can occur in individuals with the same BMI (18). Limitations of using BMI to

HOW TO   Calculate Body Mass Index

The following example can be used to learn how to calculate BMI. An individual weighing 150 lb (or 68.18 kg [divide weight in pounds by 2.2]), standing 66 in tall (or 1.68 m tall [multiply height in inches by 0.0254]) has a BMI of

$$BMI = \text{weight (kg)} / \text{height (m}^2)$$
$$= 68.18 \ \text{kg} / (1.68 \ \text{m})^2$$
$$= 68.18 / 2.82$$
$$= 24.2 \ \text{kg} \cdot \text{m}^{-2}$$

An alternative formula eliminates the need to convert pounds and inches to kilograms and meters, respectively. Using the same example,

$$BMI = (\text{weight [lb]} / \text{height [in}^2]) \times 704.5$$
$$= (150 \ \text{lb} / 66 \ \text{in}^2) \times 704.5$$
$$= (0.0344352) \times 704.5$$
$$= 24.2 \ \text{kg} \cdot \text{m}^{-2}$$

classify individuals as normal, overweight, or obese must be recognized. Individuals with high levels of muscle mass can be misclassified as overweight or, in extreme cases, obese (*e.g.*, elite body builder). BMI can underestimate body fat in persons who have lost muscle mass (*e.g.*, older adults), have low bone mineral density (19), or are of a non-white lineage (20,21). High BMI in very short individuals (under 5 ft) may not reflect fatness. When possible, the ACSM-EP should combine the use of BMI with measures of body composition for a more complete profile of an individual. It is possible to predict percentage body fat from BMI, but this is not recommended because of the high margin of error associated with this technique ($\pm$5% fat) (22). Although BMI by itself is unable to differentiate body fat from lean mass, the BMI-based categories of overweight (25.0–29.9 $kg \cdot m^{-2}$) and obesity ($\geq$30 $kg \cdot m^{-2}$) are linked to premature mortality and numerous chronic, obesity-related diseases (23).

Circumference Measures

Circumference measures are a beneficial adjunct to other anthropometric measures. They are easily understood by clients and can be used with severely obese individuals, particularly when skinfold thicknesses are too large for standard skinfold calipers. Circumference measures can be used to determine localized adipose tissue deposition and body fat distribution, an important predictor of the health risks of obesity (23). Specifically, central obesity (also referred to as abdominal or android obesity) is associated with a higher risk of hypertension, metabolic syndrome, Type 2 diabetes mellitus, dyslipidemia, CVD, and premature death compared to gynoid obesity, which is characterized by a greater proportion of fat distributed on hips and thighs (24). The standard circumference sites are described in Table 7.3 and shown in Figure 7.1. Although the waist and hip

Table 7.3	Standardized Description of Circumference Sites (25)
Site	**Location Description**
Abdomen	With the subject standing upright and relaxed, a horizontal measure is taken at the height of the iliac crest, usually at the level of the umbilicus.
Arm	With the subject standing erect and arms hanging freely at the sides with hands facing the thigh, a horizontal measure is taken midway between the acromion and the olecranon processes.
Buttocks/hips	With the subject standing erect and feet together, a horizontal measure is taken at the maximal circumference of buttocks. This measure is used for the hip measure in a waist/hip measure.
Calf	With the subject standing (feet apart ~20 cm), a horizontal measure is taken at the level of the maximum circumference between the knee and the ankle, perpendicular to the long axis.
Forearm	With the subject standing, arms hanging downward but slightly away from the trunk and palms facing anteriorly, a measure is taken perpendicular to the long axis at the maximal circumference.
Hips/thigh	With the subject standing, legs slightly apart (~10 cm), a horizontal measure is taken at the maximal circumference of the hip/proximal thigh, just below the gluteal fold.
Midthigh	With the subject standing and one foot on a bench, so the knee is flexed at 90°, a measure is taken midway between the inguinal crease and the proximal border of the patella, perpendicular to the long axis.
Waist	With the subject standing, arms at the sides, feet together, and abdomen relaxed, a horizontal measure is taken at the narrowest part of the torso (above the umbilicus and below the xiphoid process). Note: The National Obesity Task Force (NOTF) suggests obtaining a horizontal measure directly above the iliac crest as a method to enhance standardization. Unfortunately, current formulas are not predicated on the NOTF suggested site.

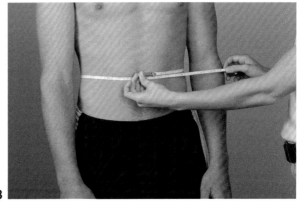

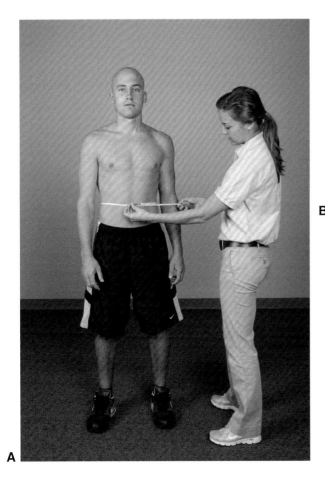

FIGURE 7.1. Measuring waist circumference. The waist is measured at the smallest circumference above the umbilicus (usually 1–2 in).

are the most commonly measured sites, other circumference sites can be also used to track changes that occur in a client.

Body fat distribution can be determined using the waist-to-hip ratio (WHR). This assessment helps the ACSM-EP identify individuals with higher amounts of abdominal fat. To determine the WHR, divide the circumference of the waist by the circumference of the hips (buttocks/hips; see Table 7.3). If a female client has a waist circumference of 31.0 in and a hip circumference of 42.0 in, her WHR is 35.0 / 42.0 = 0.83. Health risks increase as WHR increases, and standards for risk vary with age and sex (Table 7.4).

Waist circumference alone can be used as an indicator of health risk because it reflects the level of abdominal obesity (8). Health risks are high when the waist circumference is ≥35.0 in (88.0 cm) for women and ≥40.0 in (102.0 cm) for men. Furthermore, waist circumference can be combined with BMI to more precisely classify disease risk (see Table 7.2). It is important to note that these risk criteria are based on data derived from white men and women. African American men and women may have different BMI and waist circumference cut points (27–29). One study found that BMI and WHR correlated with mortality in whites but not in African Americans; however, the risk of mortality associated with waist circumference was almost identical between races (28).

Waist-to-height ratio (WHtR) is an additional screening tool for central obesity. The risk of cardiometabolic disease is increased when the WHtR is ≥0.5. WHtR is calculated by dividing waist circumference by height, both of which can be easily measured by the ACSM-EP. As a general rule, the waist measurement should be less than half of the height measurement (30–32).

Circumference measurements should be taken using a flexible yet inelastic tape measure with a spring-loaded handle (*e.g.*, Gulick tape measure) that standardizes the tension of the tape on

Table 7.4	Waist-to-Hip Ratio Norms for Men and Women (26)		
Age	**Low Risk**	**Moderate Risk**	**High Risk**
Men (yr)			
20–29	<0.83	0.83–0.88	>0.88
30–39	<0.84	0.84–0.91	>0.91
40–49	<0.88	0.88–0.95	>0.95
50–59	<0.90	0.90–0.96	>0.96
60–69	<0.91	0.91–0.98	>0.98
Women (yr)			
20–29	<0.71	0.71–0.77	>0.77
30–39	<0.72	0.72–0.78	>0.78
40–49	<0.73	0.73–0.79	>0.79
50–59	<0.74	0.74–0.81	>0.81
60–69	<0.76	0.76–0.83	>0.83

the skin. Each site should be measured twice in a rotational order, and an average of the two measures is used to represent the circumference value. The ACSM-EP should retest if duplicate measures are not within 5 mm (or 0.5 cm).

> Visit ⊙ the Point to watch video 7.1, which explains how to measure waist circumference for men and women.

Measuring Body Composition

Anthropometric measurements provide important information about the relationship between obesity and health but do not provide precise estimates of body composition. Body composition is the relative proportion of fat and fat-free tissues in the body. Determining body composition, or percentage body fat, helps the ACSM-EP (a) identify individuals with high and low levels of body fat that are associated with increased health risks, (b) design appropriate exercise programs, (c) formulate dietary recommendations, (d) assess the progress of a client in response to a weight management program, and (e) develop weight loss goals. Body composition can be measured using various techniques that vary in terms of accuracy, cost, and complexity. The more common body composition measurements that are used in health/fitness settings include skinfolds and bioelectrical impedance. The most commonly used laboratory measures include hydrostatic weighing (HW), plethysmography, and dual-energy x-ray absorptiometry (DXA).

Tables 7.5 and 7.6 provide percentile values for percentage body fat in men and women, respectively. Experts have not agreed on an exact percentage body fat value associated with optimal health risk; however, a range of 10%–22% for men and 20%–32% for women is considered satisfactory for health (33). Although research generally supports these ranges, age and race may also impact what is considered a health percentage body fat (34,35).

Table 7.5	Body Composition (% Body Fat) for Men						

	Age (yr)						
% Body Fat	20–29	30–39	40–49	50–59	60–69	70–79	
99	4.2	7.3	9.5	11.1	12.0	13.6	VL[a]
95	6.4	10.3	13.0	14.9	16.1	15.5	
90	7.9	12.5	15.0	17.0	18.1	17.5	E
85	9.1	13.8	16.4	18.3	19.2	19.0	
80	10.5	14.9	17.5	19.4	20.2	20.2	
75	11.5	15.9	18.5	20.2	21.0	21.1	G
70	12.6	16.8	19.3	21.0	21.7	21.6	
65	13.8	17.7	20.1	21.7	22.4	22.3	
60	14.8	18.4	20.8	22.3	23.0	22.9	
55	15.8	19.2	21.4	23.0	23.6	23.6	F
50	16.7	20.0	22.1	23.6	24.2	24.1	
45	17.5	20.7	22.8	24.2	24.9	24.5	
40	18.6	21.6	23.5	24.9	25.6	25.2	
35	19.8	22.4	24.2	25.6	26.4	25.7	P
30	20.7	23.2	24.9	26.3	27.0	26.3	
25	22.1	24.1	25.7	27.1	27.9	27.1	
20	23.3	25.1	26.6	28.1	28.8	28.0	
15	25.1	26.4	27.7	29.2	29.8	29.3	VP
10	26.6	27.8	29.1	30.6	31.2	30.6	
5	29.3	30.2	31.2	32.7	33.5	32.9	
1	33.7	34.4	35.2	36.4	37.2	37.3	
n =	1,938	10,457	16,032	9,976	3,097	571	

VL, very lean; E, excellent; G, good; F, fair; P, poor; VP, very poor.

Total n = 42,071. Norms are based on Cooper Clinic patients.

[a]Very lean — No less than 3% body fat is recommended for males.

Reprinted with permission from The Cooper Institute, Dallas, Texas. Updated 2013. For more information: www.cooper institute.org

Skinfold Measurements

Skinfold measurements are used to determine the amount of subcutaneous adipose tissue, that is, the fat located directly below the skin. Skinfold measures can be used to estimate the percentage of body fat and correlate well with body composition determined by underwater weighing and DXA. The skinfold technique is based on the assumptions that (a) approximately one-third of total body fat is located subcutaneously (36) and (b) the amount of subcutaneous fat is proportional to total body fat (25). However, these assumptions vary with sex, age, and ethnicity, which introduce some error into the prediction of percentage body fat from skinfold measurements. Other factors that may contribute to measurement error include poor technique and/or an inexperienced evaluator, a severely obese or extremely lean client, and an improperly calibrated caliper. In severely obese

Table 7.6	Fitness Categories for Body Composition (% Body Fat) for Women by Age						
	Age (yr)						
% Body Fat	**20–29**	**30–39**	**40–49**	**50–59**	**60–69**	**70–79**	
99	11.4	11.0	11.7	13.5	13.8	13.7	VL[a]
95	14.1	13.8	15.2	16.9	17.7	16.4	
90	15.2	15.5	16.8	19.1	20.1	18.8	E
85	16.1	16.5	18.2	20.8	22.0	21.2	
80	16.8	17.5	19.5	22.3	23.2	22.6	
75	17.7	18.3	20.5	23.5	24.5	23.7	G
70	18.6	19.2	21.6	24.7	25.5	24.5	
65	19.2	20.1	22.6	25.7	26.6	25.4	
60	20.0	21.0	23.6	26.6	27.5	26.3	
55	20.7	22.0	24.6	27.4	28.3	27.1	F
50	21.8	22.9	25.5	28.3	29.2	27.8	
45	22.6	23.7	26.4	29.2	30.1	28.6	
40	23.5	24.8	27.4	30.0	30.8	30.0	
35	24.4	25.8	28.3	30.7	31.5	30.9	P
30	25.7	26.9	29.5	31.7	32.5	31.6	
25	26.9	28.1	30.7	32.8	33.3	32.6	
20	28.6	29.6	31.9	33.8	34.4	33.6	
15	30.9	31.4	33.4	34.9	35.4	35.0	VP
10	33.8	33.6	35.0	36.0	36.6	36.1	
5	36.6	36.2	37.0	37.4	38.1	37.5	
1	38.4	39.0	39.0	39.8	40.3	40.0	
n =	1,342	4,376	6,392	4,496	1,576	325	

VL, very lean; E, excellent; G, good; F, fair; P, poor; VP, very poor.

Total *n* = 18,507. Norms are based on Cooper Clinic patients.

[a]Very lean — No less than 10%–13% body fat is recommended for women.

Reprinted with permission from The Cooper Institute, Dallas, Texas. Updated 2013. For more information: www.cooper institute.org

individuals, the skinfold thickness may exceed the maximum aperture of the caliper. To avoid embarrassing the client, the ACSM-EP can use circumference measures only or use a different technique for measuring body composition, if available. The accuracy of predicting the percentage body fat from skinfolds is ±3.5%, assuming that proper technique is used when taking measures and that an appropriate regression equation is used to estimate percentage body fat (37). Overall, the skinfold method provides reasonable accuracy for predicting the percentage of body fat in a field setting (38).

Various regression equations have been developed to predict body density or body fat percentage from skinfold measurements. Table 7.7 lists generalized equations that allow calculation of body density for a wide range of individuals. Other population-specific equations that are sex, age, ethnicity, fatness, and sport specific are available and may provide a more accurate estimate

Table 7.7	Generalized Skinfold Equations to Determine Body Density (39,40)	
	Men	**Women**
Seven-site formula (chest, midaxillary, triceps, subscapular, abdomen, suprailiac, and thigh)	BD = 1.112 − 0.00043499 (sum of seven skinfolds) + 0.00000055 (sum of seven skinfolds)^2 − 0.00028826 (age) *[See 0.008 g/cc or ~3.5% fat]*	BD = 1.097 − 0.00046971 (sum of seven skinfolds) + 0.00000056 (sum of seven skinfolds)^2 − 0.00012828 (age) *[See 0.008 g/cc or ~3.5% fat]*
Three-Site Formula		
Chest, abdomen, and thigh	BD = 1.10938 − 0.0008267 (sum of three skinfolds) + 0.0000016 (sum of three skinfolds)^2 − 0.0002574 (age) *[See 0.008 g/cc or ~3.4% fat]*	NA
Chest, triceps, and subscapular	BD = 1.1125025 − 0.0013125 (sum of three skinfolds) + 0.0000055 (sum of three skinfolds)^2 − 0.000244 (age) *[See 0.008 g/cc or ~3.6% fat]*	NA
Triceps, suprailiac, and thigh	NA	BD = 1.099421 − 0.0009929 (sum of three skinfolds) + 0.0000023 (sum of three skinfolds)^2 − 0.0001392 (age) *[See 0.009 g/cc or ~3.9% fat]*
Triceps, suprailiac, and abdominal	NA	BD = 1.089733 − 0.0009245 (sum of three skinfolds) + 0.0000025 (sum of three skinfolds)^2 − 0.0000979 (age) *[See 0.009 g/cc or ~3.9% fat]*

BD, body density; NA, not applicable.

of body composition (37). Most regression equations use two or three skinfolds to predict body density, which can then be converted to percentage body fat. The following are two of the most commonly used prediction equations to estimate percentage body fat from body density (41,42):

Brozek equation: % body fat = (495 / body density) − 450
Siri equation: % body fat = (457 / body density) − 414.2

Bioelectrical Impedance

Bioelectrical impedance analysis (BIA) is a rapid, noninvasive body composition assessment tool. When using a single-frequency BIA analyzer, a harmless electrical current is passed through the body, and the impedance to that current is measured. Multifrequency BIA analyzers are similar but use a range of electrical currents. Electrical impedance is related to the percentage of water contained in various body tissues. Lean tissue, which is composed of mostly water and electrolytes, is a good electrical conductor, whereas fat tissue, which contains much less water, acts as an impedance to the electrical current. BIA estimates total body water and relies on regression equations to estimate body fat percentage and fat-free mass.

The accuracy of predicting the percentage of body fat from BIA ranges between ±2.7% and ±6.3% (44). Selecting an appropriate regression equation and controlling potential sources of

HOW TO   Measure Skinfolds

Skinfolds are measured at standardized sites, described in Table 7.8 and shown in Figure 7.2. The skinfold sites must be precisely located using anatomical landmarks, and the following procedures must be followed for the accurate determination of body composition (25):

- Take all measurements on the right side of the client's body with the client standing upright. The client's skin should be dry and lotion free. Do not take skinfold measurements immediately after exercise.

- Identify and mark all sites before measuring skinfold thickness.

- Firmly grasp the skinfold (two layers of skin and subcutaneous fat) between the thumb and the index finger of the left hand, 1 cm above the site to be measured. To grasp the skinfold, place the thumb and index finger about 3 in apart on a line that is perpendicular to the long axis of the skinfold. Pull the skinfold up and away from the body.

- Keep the fold elevated while the measurement is being taken. Keep pinching the fold with the left hand throughout the entire measurement.

- Hold the caliper in the right hand with the dial facing up. Place the jaws of the calipers perpendicular to the fold 1 cm below the fingers and halfway between the crest and the base of the fold and release all pressure on the lever while keeping the caliper perpendicular to the skinfold.

- Record the skinfold measurement to the nearest 0.5 mm, 1–2 seconds after releasing the lever.

- Take skinfold measures in rotational order to allow time for the skinfold to regain its normal thickness.

- Take a minimum of two measurements at each site. If duplicate measurements are not within 1 or 2 mm (or 10%), retest this site.

- Average the correct measurements for each skinfold site. Using the client's measurements and validated skinfold equations, percentage body fat can be estimated.

measurement error help keep estimates in the lower end of this range. The type (*e.g.*, hand-to-hand, foot-to-foot, or hand-to-foot), range of electrical currents, and manufacturer of the BIA instrument may also affect the accuracy of the results. Regardless of the BIA analyzer used, factors that alter hydration status are a major source of error (45); therefore, it is essential for the client to follow pretesting guidelines. These guidelines will assist in attaining an accurate prediction of percentage body fat using BIA (46):

- No eating or drinking within 4 hours of the test
- No exercise within 12 hours of the test
- Completely void the bladder within 30 minutes of the test.
- No alcohol consumption within 48 hours of the test
- No diuretic medication within 7 days of the test (Clients should not discontinue use of prescribed diuretic medication unless approved by their personal physician.)
- Avoid taking measurements prior to menstruation to avoid the possible effects of water retention in women.
- Use the same BIA analyzer when measuring change in a client's body composition over time.
- Complete measurements in a thermoneutral environment.

Table 7.8	Standardized Descriptions of Skinfold Sites (25)
Site	**Location Description**
Abdominal	Vertical fold; 2 cm to the right side of the umbilicus
Triceps	Vertical fold; on the posterior midline of the upper arm, halfway between the acromion and the olecranon processes, with the arm held freely to the side of the body
Biceps	Vertical fold; on the anterior aspect of the arm over the belly of the biceps muscle, 1 cm above the level used to mark the triceps site
Chest/pectoral	Diagonal fold; one-half the distance between the anterior axillary line and the nipple (men), or one-third of the distance between the anterior axillary line and the nipple (women)
Medial calf	Vertical fold; at the maximum circumference of the calf on the midline of its medial border
Midaxillary	Vertical fold; on the midaxillary line at the level of the xiphoid process of the sternum; an alternate method is a horizontal fold taken at the level of the xiphoid/sternal border in the midaxillary line.
Subscapular	Diagonal fold (at a 45° angle); 1–2 cm below the inferior angle of the scapula
Suprailiac	Diagonal fold; in line with the natural angle of the iliac crest taken in the anterior axillary line immediately superior to the iliac crest
Thigh	Vertical fold; on the anterior midline of the thigh, midway between the proximal border of the patella and the inguinal crease (hip)

Laboratory Methods for Measuring Body Composition

There are a number of sophisticated methods that can be used to determine percentage body fat. These methods tend to be more precise than the methods described earlier but require highly trained technicians and expensive specialized equipment that is not available in most health/fitness settings. However, the ACSM-EP should have knowledge of these advanced techniques because they are often used as the reference standard for field measures of body composition.

HW (underwater weighing) is a widely used technique for determining body composition. This technique calculates body density from body volume, based on Archimedes's principle, which states that the weight under water is directly proportional to the volume of water displaced by the body volume. The protocol requires that a person be weighed on land and under water. The densities of muscle and bone are higher than the density of water, whereas fat is less dense than water. A person with high levels of muscle and bone will be heavier (more dense) in water compared with a person with higher levels of fat. HW has a standard error of the estimate of ±2.0%–2.8% body fat for young adults (47).

Air displacement plethysmography (ADP) is an alternative to HW for determining body composition. ADP measures body volume by determining the volume of air the body displaces in a closed chamber (plethysmograph). ADP has many advantages over HW, in that it is quick and noninvasive; does not require submersion in water; and accommodates children, adults, and older

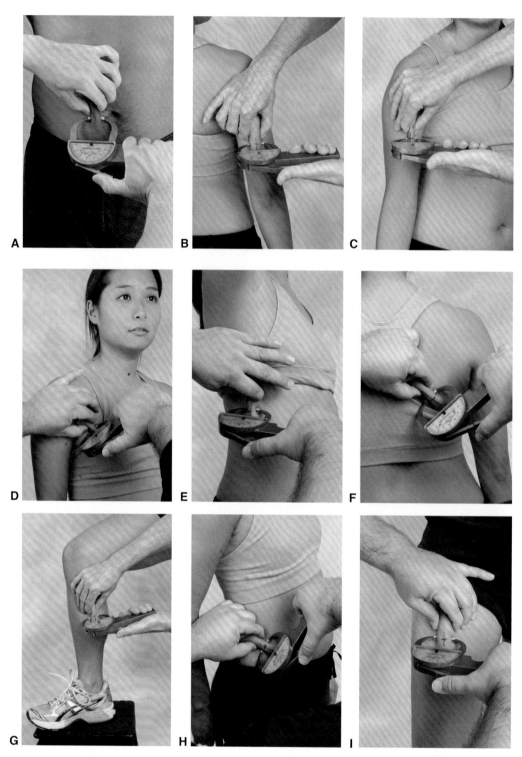

FIGURE 7.2. Common skinfold sites. **A.** Abdominal: vertical fold, 2 cm to the right side of the umbilicus. **B.** Triceps: vertical fold on the posterior midline of the upper arm, halfway between the acromion and the olecranon processes, with the arm held freely to the side of the body. **C.** Biceps: vertical fold on the anterior aspect of the arm over the belly of the biceps muscle, 1 cm above the level used to mark the triceps site. **D.** Chest: diagonal fold, one-half the distance between the anterior axillary line and the nipple (men) or one-third of the distance between the axillary line and the nipple (women). **E.** Midaxillary: vertical fold on the midaxillary line at the level of the xiphoid process of the sternum. **F.** Subscapular: diagonal fold (at a 45° angle), 1–2 cm below the inferior angle of the scapula. **G.** Medial calf: vertical fold at the maximum circumference of the calf on the midline of its medial border. **H.** Suprailium: diagonal fold in line with the natural angle of the iliac crest taken in the anterior axillary line immediately superior to the iliac crest. **I.** Thigh: vertical fold, on the anterior midline of the thigh, midway between the proximal border of the patella and the inguinal crease (hip) (43).

adults as well as individuals who are obese or disabled. There is one commercial system currently available (BOD POD, Life Measurement Instruments; Concord, CA). The accuracy of ADP is similar to that of HW (25).

DXA uses very low-current x-rays at two energy levels to measure bone mineral content, body fat, and lean soft tissue mass. This method requires an individual to lie supine on a table while being scanned from head to toe. DXA is safe and easy to use, but the instrumentation can be very expensive. This method can be used across the lifespan (children, adults, and older adults); however, DXA should not be used in women who are either pregnant or lactating. As a result, females who are of childbearing age need to be screened to ensure that they are not pregnant. With appropriate standards and methodology, the reproducibility of DXA is ±1.7% for percentage body fat (48).

Weight Management

The causes of obesity are complex and multifactorial and are a mixture of genetic, behavioral, physiological, geographical, economic, and social factors. Although many factors contribute to an individual's body weight, a healthy diet and regular PA are critical for attaining and/or maintaining a healthy weight. For example, the *F as in Fat* report (49) noted that the states with the highest levels of physical inactivity and the lowest levels of fruit and vegetable consumption had the highest rankings of obesity.

Energy Balance

The management of body weight is dependent on energy balance: energy intake (the amount of calories consumed) and energy expenditure (the amount of calories expended). To reduce body weight, energy expenditure must exceed energy intake, referred to as a negative energy balance. Conversely, an individual gains weight when in a positive energy balance, that is, when energy intake exceeds energy expenditure. Body weight is maintained when an individual is in energy balance — expending the same number of calories as they are consuming.

Although the concept of energy balance is simple in theory, weight regulation in free living individuals is very challenging because genetic and environmental conditions must also be considered (50). It is hypothesized that humans developed physiological mechanisms that promote the storage of fat during periods of feast, so they could survive periods of famine (51). Although these mechanisms were useful in the past, the genetic predisposition to store fat is a liability in the current environment where food production and access is stable and daily PA requirements have decreased (52). For example, low levels of peptide YY and cholecystokinin stimulate appetite and higher levels of insulin, neuropeptide Y, and leptin increase fat storage (53–55). Regardless of this "thrifty gene" hypothesis, recent changes to the environment where inexpensive high-fat food is readily available and in which there is little need for PA has made it difficult to manage body weight. In addition to environmental factors making weight loss challenging, there are physiological changes that occur as a result of weight loss. For instance, ghrelin and neuropeptide Y levels increase with weight loss, which stimulates appetite and promotes fat storage (56). Furthermore, weight loss also reduces resting energy expenditure (REE) and reduces the amount of energy expended for a given activity (53).

Total daily energy expenditure (TDEE) is the total number of calories expended each day and reflects the amount of energy required to carry out all metabolic processes within the body. Examples of these metabolic processes include growth of new cells, maintaining the functions of

HOW TO   Estimate Target Body Weight

An individual's current percentage body fat, current body weight, and desired percentage of body weight can be used to develop weight loss goals using the following equations:

1. Estimate percentage body fat (using one of the methods discussed earlier in this chapter).

2. Fat mass = Total body mass × (Percentage body fat / 100)

3. Fat-free mass = Total body mass − Fat mass

4. Desired weight = Fat-free mass / [1 − (Desired percentage body fat / 100)]

Example

1. Percentage body fat = 31%; Total body mass = 213 lb; Desired percentage body fat = 25%

2. Fat mass = Total body mass × (Percentage body fat / 100)
$$= 213 \times 0.31$$
$$= 66.03 \text{ lb}$$

3. Fat-free mass = Total body mass − Fat mass
$$= 213 - 66.03$$
$$= 146.97 \text{ lb}$$

4. Desired weight = Fat-free mass / [1 − (Desired percentage body fat / 100)]
$$= 146.97 / [1 - 0.25]$$
$$= 146.97 / 0.75$$
$$= 195.96 \ (\sim 196 \text{ lb})$$

body tissues, and providing fuel for movement of the body, including exercise. There are three components and reported contributions to TDEE (57):

- REE (*or* resting metabolic rate [RMR]): 55%–75% of TDEE
- Thermic effect of food (TEF): 7%–15% of TDEE
- Thermic effect of PA (TEPA): 15%–30% of TDEE

REE is the energy required to maintain normal regulatory balance and body functions at rest. In the simplest terms, REE is an estimate of how many calories a person uses if he or she were to do nothing but rest for 24 hours. There are several factors that influence REE. To some degree, everyone's "metabolism" is determined by their genes; however, there are several other factors within the individual that contribute to energy expenditure. The heart, lungs, kidneys, brain, and liver represent approximately 80% of daily energy expenditure (58). Skeletal muscle is more metabolically active than fat, with a metabolic rate of about 10–15 kcal $\cdot$ kg^{-1} $\cdot$ d^{-1} (58). A person's age, gender, and ethnicity also influence REE, primarily because of the impact on lean body mass.

The TEF is the energy required for the digestion, absorption, transport, metabolism, and storage of consumed food. The final component of energy expenditure, TEPA, is the most variable and depends on an individual's PA level (PAL), including structured exercise and nonexercise activity thermogenesis (NEAT), which reflects the energy expended for everything we do that is not sleeping, eating, or exercise.

To determine an individual's total energy needs, REE must first be measured or estimated using prediction equations. Next, an activity factor is used to calculate TDEE for that individual.

Table 7.9	Common Resting Energy Expenditure (kcal · d⁻¹) Predictive Equations for Adults	
	Men	**Women**
Harris-Benedict (for adults)	66.47 + 13.75 (weight in kg) + 5 (height in cm) − 6.8 (age in yr)	665 + 9.6 (weight in kg) + 1.8 (height in cm) − 4.7 (age in yr)
Mifflin-St. Jeor (for obese adults)	10 (weight in kg) + 6.3 (height in cm) − 5 × age + 5	10 (weight in kg) + 6.3 (height in cm) − 5 × age − 161

REE can be measured using indirect calorimetry, which measures an individual's oxygen consumption or predicted using equations. Prediction equations take into account an individual's age, gender, height, and weight or fat-free mass; equations that incorporate fat-free mass provide the most accurate prediction of REE (59). Although prediction equations can be useful, caution should be advised as REE can be overestimated in these equations, which could make losing and maintain weight loss challenging (60). Table 7.9 provides the Harris-Benedict and Mifflin-St. Jeor (61) predictive equations, which are commonly used in adults. Another method uses the Institute of Medicine (IOM) total energy expenditure (TEE) equations (62). Regardless of the equation used, a person's PAL is factored in to determine total calories needed for TDEE (Table 7.10).

The following is an example for determining TEE prediction for a 35-year-old man, who is 6 ft, weighs 180 lb, and is lightly active. Using the Mifflin-St. Jeor equation, the calculated REE would be

$$1{,}781 \text{ kcal (REE)} \times 1.375 \text{ (lightly active)} = 2{,}448 \text{ kcal} \cdot \text{day}^{-1}$$

The individual needs about 2,500 kcal · d⁻¹ to maintain his or her weight at a low activity level (see Table 7.10). To achieve 1 lb of weight loss per week, this person's caloric requirements would be approximately 2,000 kcal · d⁻¹, or a 500-cal daily deficit. It should be noted that it is not recommended for an individual to consume less than 1,200 kcal · d⁻¹ unless medically indicated because this low calorie intake is not likely to meet basic nutrient needs.

The following are the equations to be used with the IOM method to quantify a client's TEE. Unlike the PAL used for other questions, the PALs for the IOM are based on gender (64).

Table 7.10	Common Activity Factors Used with Resting Energy Expenditure to Calculate Total Daily Calorie Needs for Weight Maintenance in Adults (63)	
Level of Physical Activity		**Common Activity Factor**
Sedentary (little to no activity)		1.2
Light activity		1.375
Moderate activity		1.55
Very active		1.725
Exceedingly active		1.9

Table 7.11	Estimated Calorie Needs per Day by Age, Gender, and Physical Activity Level (1,65)		
		Physical Activity Level		
Gender	**Age (yr)**	**Sedentary**	**Moderately Active**	**Active**
Female	2–3	1,000	1,000–1,200	1,000–1,400
	4–8	1,200–1,400	1,400–1,600	1,400–1,800
	9–13	1,400–1,600	1,600–2,000	1,800–2,200
	14–18	1,800	2,000	2,400
	19–30	1,800–2,000	2,000–2,200	2,400
	31–50	1,800	2,000	2,200
	51+	1,600	1,800	2,000–2,200
Male	2–3	1,000	1,000–1,400	1,000–1,400
	4–8	1,200–1,400	1,400–1,600	1,600–2,000
	9–13	1,600–2,000	1,800–2,200	2,000–2,600
	14–18	2,000–2,400	2,400–2,800	2,800–3,200
	19–30	2,400–2,600	2,600–2,800	3,000
	31–50	2,200–2,400	2,400–2,600	2,800–3,000
	51+	2,000–2,200	2,200–2,400	2,400–2,800

PAL for men:
Sedentary: PA = 1.0, when $1.0 \leq PAL < 1.4$
Low active: PA = 1.12, when $1.4 \leq PAL < 1.6$
Active: PA = 1.27, when $1.6 \leq PAL < 1.9$
Very active: PA = 1.54, when $1.9 \leq PAL < 2.5$

PAL for women:
Sedentary: PA = 1.0, when $1.0 \leq PAL < 1.4$
Low active: PA = 1.14, when $1.4 \leq PAL < 1.6$
Active: PA = 1.27, when $1.6 \leq PAL < 1.9$
Very active: PA = 1.45, when $1.9 \leq PAL < 2.5$

Thus, PA is entered into the TEE equation in the following text to give total daily energy requirements for an individual:

For men:
TEE = $864 - 9.72 \times$ age (yr) + PA $\times$ [($14.2 \times$ weight (kg) + $503 \times$ height (m)]

For women:
TEE = $387 - 7.31 \times$ age (yr) + PA $\times$ [($10.9 \times$ weight (kg) + $660.7 \times$ height (m)]

It is important to consider that using either method of determining an individual's energy needs gives total calories needed for weight maintenance. When calculating for weight loss, the recommended rate in adults is 1–2 lb · wk^{-1}, which is equal to a daily caloric deficit of 500–1,000 cal. Table 7.11 shows the estimated range of daily energy needs for various population groups.

Preventing Weight Gain

On average, American adults gain 1–2 lb annually (66), suggesting a chronic positive energy balance. In 2019, ACSM published a systematic review focusing on PA and its role in the prevention of weight gain in adults based, in part, on the *2018 Physical Activity Guidelines for Americans* and the accompanying scientific report (67–69). The evidence suggests that PA helps prevent weight gain and the development of obesity, particularly if performed at a moderate to vigorous intensity for more than 150 min $\cdot$ wk^{-1}. There is less evidence to support that lighter intensity activities will prevent weight gain. Although decreasing sedentary time may positively impact some cardiometabolic risk factors, interventions that focus solely on this behavior will likely not prevent either weight gain or obesity. A more effective approach for preventing weight gain is to replace sedentary activities with moderate- to vigorous-intensity PA (69).

Treatment of Obesity

The most effective weight loss interventions include diet, exercise, and behavior change strategies and often result in a 5%–10% reduction in body weight. A sustained weight loss of only 3%–5% can improve CVD risk factors, making a positive impact on overall health (6). PA has a modest impact on initial weight loss compared to reductions in energy intake, but programs that combine diet and exercise result in a 20% greater weight loss compared to diet alone, unless the reduction in energy intake is severe (70,71). For most overweight and obese individuals, moderate reductions in energy intake and adequate levels of PA maximize weight loss in individuals who are overweight or obese (25). Maintaining weight loss is challenging, with people regaining, on average, 33%–50% of their initial weight loss within 1 year of the end of an intervention. PA is an important part of weight loss maintenance and improved health, but it may take more than the public health recommendations of 150 min $\cdot$ wk^{-1} (25,71). To promote long-term weight loss maintenance, ACSM recommends that individuals progress to at least 250 min $\cdot$ wk^{-1} ($\geq$2,000 kcal $\cdot$ wk^{-1}) of moderate- to vigorous-intensity exercise (25).

FITT Recommendations

The goals of exercise during weight loss are to maximize the amount of caloric expenditure and to integrate exercise into an individual's lifestyle to prepare them for successful weight loss maintenance (25). When possible, exercise should be done at a moderate to vigorous intensity for a prolonged period of time (see "FITT Recommendations for Individuals Who Are Overweight and Obesity"). The types of exercise activities that work well for the individuals who are overweight and obese include walking, swimming, water aerobics, jogging/walking in water, biking, and elliptical and rowing machines. All these activities can be done at an appropriate intensity and for a long duration without negatively impacting the knee and hip joints. Resistance training is also important to include after an aerobic activity has been incorporated into a person's routine, as it will not only improve muscular strength and endurance but will also provide other health benefits, such as improvements in blood glucose levels and insulin sensitivity.

Depending on the amount of excess body weight and the aerobic fitness of the client, FITT recommendations can be adjusted to meet the needs of the client. If an ACSM-EP is working with a client who has not exercised in a long time, has never exercised, or is severely obese, initially doing short bouts of exercise completed multiple times a day may be necessary. The client may exercise for longer durations as his or her fitness level increases. This is also a good strategy to use if the client has a very busy schedule and cannot fit in one longer bout.

The FITT principle for weight loss following ACSM guidelines is as follows (25):

FITT Recommendations for Individuals Who Are Overweight and Obese

	Aerobic	Resistance	Flexibility
Frequency	$\geq$5 d · wk^{-1}	2–3 d · wk^{-1}	$\geq$2–3 d · wk^{-1}
Intensity	Initial intensity should be moderate (40%–59% $\dot{V}O_2R$ or HRR); progress to vigorous ($\geq$60% %$\dot{V}O_2R$ or HRR) for greater health benefits.	60%–70% of 1-RM. Gradually increase to enhance strength and muscle mass.	Stretch to the point of feeling tightness or slight discomfort.
Time	30 min · d^{-1} (150 min · wk^{-1}); increase to 60 min · d^{-1} or more (250–300 min · wk^{-1}).	2–4 sets of 8–12 repetitions for each of the major muscle groups	Hold static stretch for 10–30 s; 2–4 repetitions of each exercise
Type	Prolonged, rhythmic activities using large muscle groups (*e.g.*, walking, cycling, swimming).	Resistance machines and/or free weights	Static, dynamic, and/or PNF

$\dot{V}O_2R$, oxygen uptake reserve; HRR, heart rate reserve; 1-RM, one repetition maximum; %$\dot{V}O_2R$, percentage of oxygen uptake reserve; PNF, proprioceptive neuromuscular facilitation.

Training Considerations

Demonstrating exercises to clients is a critical element to program implementation. Exercise demonstration allows the client to see what has been verbally explained and also allows key aspects of the exercise to be highlighted. Depending on the severity of obesity, it may also be necessary to identify suitable equipment. Keep in mind that some equipment has a maximum weight limit or the person may not fit or be comfortable while exercising on the equipment. Furthermore, certain basic activities may be difficult, such as going down and getting up from the floor or bending over. Thus, specific exercises in a person's exercise program may need to be modified or removed. All these aspects should be considered when designing an exercise program for an overweight and obese client.

Although there are numerous approaches to planning exercise for weight loss, the basic principles of exercise prescription are outlined in Chapter 3. In addition, Chapter 8 provides detailed information about exercise prescription in people with cardiovascular, metabolic, and pulmonary disease, which are often present in individuals who are overweight or obese. Most important, if someone is overweight, obese, and currently sedentary, the ACSM-EP needs to use caution and empathy in the early stages of an exercise program. The sedentary overweight or obese person is likely to find exercise initially uncomfortable and accompanied by soreness the following day or two (delayed-onset muscle soreness or DOMS). These feelings may also bring about lower levels of self-efficacy and a lower desire to achieve the intended weight loss goals. Therefore, prescribing exercise becomes just as much art as science when working with this population.

When working with clients who are overweight or obese, it may be of considerable value to incorporate opportunities to work with registered dietitians or other health care professionals. Further, the ACSM-EP can become familiar with the *2018 Physical Activity Guidelines for*

Americans (68), *ACSM's Guidelines for Exercise Testing and Prescription* (25), and the *2015-2020 Dietary Guidelines for Americans* to help individualize specific exercise programs and weight loss plans (1).

Weight Loss Goals

Developing realistic short- and long-term weight loss goals is important when working with those who are trying to lose weight. Research suggests that lifestyle interventions often result in a weight loss of 5%–10% of initial weight, which does not return most people to a nonobese state. This may be disappointing for the client, but this weight loss, if sustained, improves overall health.

When an ACSM-EP works with a client who is overweight or obese, the goal is to ensure that the person loses fat while either maintaining or increasing lean muscle mass. Weight loss should occur at a rate of 1–2 lb $\cdot$ wk^{-1} (15). Although this is a feasible goal at the beginning of a weight loss program, it is difficult for many clients to continue to lose weight at this rate. Consequently, multiple short-term (*i.e.*, three to four) goals may need to be created until the person reaches the desired percentage body fat and weight, especially if the client is trying to achieve more than a 10% weight reduction.

Measuring body weight is a good method to use for weekly tracking because depending on which percentage body fat method is used, there could be a 3%–6% error in the estimated value. Therefore, if percentage body fat was measured each week, it would be difficult to determine either whether a change has actually occurred or whether it is a reflection of measurement error. This problem does not exist with absolute weight, although it is best to measure weight at a consistent time of day. Also, a person can weigh himself or herself each week without having to see a specialist to be measured (72).

Metabolic Equations

The ACSM metabolic equations can be used to estimate the number of calories that will be expended during a workout or to estimate the length of time an individual has to exercise to expend a certain number of calories. A calorie, also known as a kilocalorie (kcal), is an expression of energy intake and expenditure. It takes approximately 3,500 cal to make and store 1 lb of body weight. The following is an example of using metabolic equations to determine caloric expenditure. Either of these yield a reasonable estimate of calories expended and can be useful in setting exercise and dietary goals with a client.

These metabolic calculations yield a range of caloric expenditures that can be expected while performing the exercise. Keep in mind also that this value of kcal $\cdot$ min^{-1} includes the calories that would have been expended at rest, so this is the "gross" caloric expenditure for the 30 minutes. Refer to Chapters 3 and 8 to determine "net" caloric expenditure or the calories strictly from the exercise.

Weight Management Myths

When working with someone who is trying to lose weight, he or she may ask about some common myths.

Myth 1: Fat Turns into Muscle

Fat and muscle are two separate tissues in the body. It is impossible to change fat into muscle or muscle into fat. During weight loss, fat mass in the body typically decreases while the amount of muscle mass may increase if exercise is of sufficient intensity (overload principle).

HOW TO   Calculate Metabolic Equations (Weight Management)

Here is an example calculating caloric expenditure using metabolic equations.
Female — height: 63 in, weight: 68 kg, BMI: 26.6 kg · m^{-2}
Client walks on a treadmill at 3.5 mph and a 5% grade for 30 min.
What is the client's total caloric expenditure?

$$\text{mph} \times (26.8 \text{ m} \cdot \text{min}^{-1}) = \text{m} \cdot \text{min}^{-1}$$

$$(3.5 \text{ mph}) \times (26.8 \text{ m} \cdot \text{min}^{-1}) = 93.8 \text{ m} \cdot \text{min}^{-1}$$

$$5\% \text{ grade} = 0.05$$

$$\dot{V}O_2 \text{ (mL} \cdot \text{kg}^{-1} \cdot \text{min}^{-1}) = (0.1 \times \text{m} \cdot \text{min}^{-1}) + (1.8 \times \text{m} \cdot \text{min}^{-1} \times \text{grade}) + 3.5$$

$$\dot{V}O_2 \text{ (mL} \cdot \text{kg}^{-1} \cdot \text{min}^{-1}) = (0.1 \times 93.8) + (1.8 \times 93.8 \times 0.05) + 3.5$$

$$\dot{V}O_2 \text{ (mL} \cdot \text{kg}^{-1} \cdot \text{min}^{-1}) = 9.38 + 8.44 + 3.5$$

$$\dot{V}O_2 = 21.32 \text{ mL} \cdot \text{kg}^{-1} \cdot \text{min}^{-1}$$

$$[(\text{mL} \cdot \text{kg}^{-1} \cdot \text{min}^{-1}) \times \text{kg}] / 1{,}000 = \dot{V}O_2 \text{ (L} \cdot \text{min}^{-1})$$

$$(21.32 \times 68) / 1{,}000 = 1.45 \text{ L} \cdot \text{min}^{-1}$$

$$\text{L} \cdot \text{min}^{-1} \times 5 = \text{kcal} \cdot \text{min}^{-1}$$

Note: Approximately 5 kcal are consumed for every liter of oxygen.

$$1.45 \times 5 = 7.25 \text{ kcal} \cdot \text{min}^{-1}$$

$$7.25 \text{ kcal} \cdot \text{min}^{-1} \times 30 \text{ min} = 217.5 \text{ kcal}$$

Total caloric expenditure on treadmill = 217.5 kcal for 30 min
This information can then be used to determine how many minutes, over how many days, the client will need to exercise to achieve her weight loss goals.

Myth 2: Spot Reducing Works

It is not possible to reduce fat in a chosen region of the body. Fat reduction occurs in a somewhat random fashion and is not likely to be the same for any two persons. Often, clients want to target "problem areas" such as the abdomen, arms, or upper thighs. They have the false belief that training a specific muscle will result in fat loss in that same area and often think localized fatigue signifies fat utilization. Although the exercises may help to strengthen the targeted muscle, it will not reduce fat in that area of the body.

Myth 3: Gaining Weight at the Start of an Exercise Program Is from Increased Muscle

Muscle hypertrophy occurs only after 6–8 wk of higher intensity resistance training, and therefore, it is highly unlikely to see any muscle gain in the first 2 months of an exercise program. Even beyond that point, most people will not exercise at an intensity high enough to produce significant increases in muscle mass. More likely, those who are new to exercise may overcompensate their calorie intake, thinking their newfound exercise "allows" them to eat more, thereby increasing their overall body weight.

Table 7.12	Recommended Macronutrient Proportions by Age (73)		
	Carbohydrate (%)	Protein (%)	Fat (%)
Young children (1–3 yr)	45–65	5–20	30–40
Older children and adolescents (4–18 yr)	45–65	10–30	25–35
Adults (≥19 yr)	45–65	10–35	20–35

Treatment of Obesity through Nutrition

Every 5 years, a new edition of the *Dietary Guidelines for Americans* is available to the public. It is intended to help Americans aged 2 years to older adults improve overall health through evidence-based recommendations for healthy food choices (Table 7.12). The *2015-2020 Dietary Guidelines for Americans* builds on the *2010 Dietary Guidelines* and provides five Guidelines with associated Key Recommendations. A key expansion of the *Dietary Guidelines* is that the focus is now related to healthy eating patterns rather than individual food groups or nutrients. As stated in the *2015-2020 Dietary Guidelines Executive Summary*, "These Guidelines also embody the idea that a healthy eating pattern is not a rigid prescription, but rather, an adaptable framework in which individuals can enjoy foods that meet their personal, cultural, and traditional preferences and fit within their budget" (1).

The guidelines for the *2015-2020 Dietary Guidelines for Americans* are as follows (1):

1. **Follow a healthy eating pattern across the lifespan.** All food and beverage choices matter. Choose a healthy eating pattern at an appropriate calorie level to help achieve and maintain a healthy body weight, support nutrient adequacy, and reduce the risk of chronic disease.
2. **Focus on variety, nutrient density, and amount.** To meet nutrient needs within calorie limits, choose a variety of nutrient-dense foods across and within all the food groups in recommended amounts.
3. **Limit calories from added sugars and saturated fats and reduce sodium intake.** Adopt an eating pattern low in added sugars, saturated fats, and sodium. Cut back on foods and beverages higher in these components that fit within a healthy eating pattern.
4. **Shift to healthier food and beverage choices.** Choose nutrient-dense foods and beverages across and within all food groups in place of less healthy choices.
5. **Support healthy eating patterns for all.** Everyone has a role in helping to create and support healthy eating patterns in multiple settings nationwide, from home to school to work to communities.

The Key Recommendations provide individuals with more guidance on how to follow the mentioned Guidelines:

Adopt a healthy eating pattern that accounts for all foods and beverages within an appropriate calorie level.

A healthy eating pattern includes

- A variety of vegetables from all of the subgroups — dark green, red and orange, legumes (beans and peas), starchy and other
- Fruits, especially whole fruits

- Grains, at least half of which are whole grains
- Fat-free or low-fat dairy, including milk, yogurt, cheese, and/or fortified soy beverages
- A variety of proteins, including seafood, lean meats and poultry, eggs, legumes (beans and peas), and nuts, seeds, and soy products
- Limiting the amount of oils that are from saturated fats and *trans* fats
- Limiting foods that have added sugars and sodium

Specifically,

- Consume less than 10% of calories per day from added sugars.
- Consume less than 10% of calories per day from saturated fats.
- Consume less than 2,300 mg · d^{-1} of sodium.
- If alcohol is consumed, it should be consumed in moderation — up to one drink per day for women and up to two drinks per day for men — and only by adults of legal drinking age.

The MyPlate concept is still a very useful way to visualize a healthy eating pattern and is in accordance with the updated *Dietary Guidelines* (Fig. 7.3). The ChooseMyPlate Web site can be an evidence-based resource for all health, nutrition, and exercise professionals: http://www.choose-myplate.gov/dietary-guidelines (74).

Another key message of the *2015-2020 Dietary Guidelines for Americans* is that there are relationships among individual food choices and the context and settings within which these choices are made to include the family environment, social and work settings, living situations, and communities. Thus, this edition of the *Dietary Guidelines* encourages efforts among health professionals, communities, businesses and industries, organizations, governments, and other areas of society to help support individuals in making healthy food choices and in meeting PA recommendations that are recommended in the *Dietary Guidelines*. It is the responsibility of the ACSM-EP to keep abreast of changes that occur with the *Dietary Guidelines*. The ACSM-EP should also be aware of their professional scope of practice, particularly when clients ask for a diet plan or nutritional advice. In many states, only a registered dietitian can create diet plan for a person (see https://www.nutritioned.org/state-requirements.html). The ACSM-EP can use the nutritional information earlier to help educate/direct clients on ways to improve their nutrition choices without prescribing a specific diet plan.

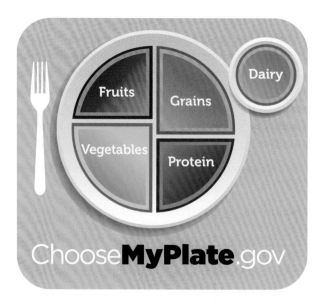

FIGURE 7.3. MyPlate: the new healthy eating guide (74).

Table 7.13	Inappropriate Weight Loss Methods and Consequences (75–79)
Method	**Negative Consequences**
Saunas	Dehydration, only lose water weight, low amount of weight loss, temporary weight loss
Vibrating belts	No weight loss
Body wraps	Small weight loss, temporary weight loss, skin irritation
Overexercising	Overuse injury, unhealthy amount of weight loss
Electric muscle stimulators	No change in body composition, bruising, and skin irritation
Sweat suits	Dehydration, only lose water weight, low amount of weight loss, temporary weight loss
Dietary supplements	Not regulated by FDA, so dosage may not be known; may have nutrient drug interactions, drug–drug interactions, and other side effects such as nausea, dizziness, and racing heart
Very low calorie diets	May not meet nutrient needs of the individual promoting deficiencies in specific nutrients (*e.g.*, calcium deficiency leads to brittle, broken bones, hip fractures); could lead to dehydration, constipation, or fatigue
Fad diets	Often "cut out" a food group, which leads to specific nutrient, vitamin, and mineral deficiencies; not sustainable for long periods; could lead to "yo-yo" dieting (*i.e.*, intervals of weight loss followed by weight gain); low-carbohydrate diets do not meet body's requirement for a minimum of 130 g of carbohydrates a day; could lead to fatigue and lack of energy; could lead to dehydration and/or constipation; not recommended

FDA, U.S. Food and Drug Administration.

Treatment of Obesity through Other Methods

Different strategies exist for modifying a person's body composition and promoting weight loss. Although many of these strategies are effective, some are considered unsafe and should not be used by individuals trying to lose weight. Inappropriate weight loss methods include saunas, electric stimulators, sweat suits, vibrating belts, body wraps, overexercising, very low calorie diets, fad diets, and using dietary supplements (Table 7.13).

Appropriate weight loss methods include exercise, dietary changes, behavioral strategies, and bariatric surgery. Bariatric surgery rates have increased 31% from 158,000 to 228,000 between 2011 and 2017 (80). Although this surgery is very effective at producing weight loss (81), recent research indicates that incorporating exercise training after bariatric surgery enhances the amount of overall weight loss and fat mass loss in addition to improving physical function (82). Although more research exists on the impact exercise has after bariatric surgery, the limited research related to exercise before surgery suggests that engaging in exercise prior to surgery improves fitness, self-efficacy, and quality of life and results in higher activity levels after surgery (83,84). Research is underway to determine the appropriate amount of exercise for people who have undergone bariatric surgery; currently, it is recommended that those who completed bariatric surgery follow the FITT prescription discussed earlier in this chapter (25). For many people, bariatric surgery is medically indicated because of severe obesity and/or comorbidities threatening their health. The ACSM-EP should recognize that weight loss is not easy, and for some people, the health risk of being either overweight or obese is such that medical care should be sought. However, for those either not interested or indicated for surgery, adding a behavioral component to their exercise and diet plan may aid them in achieving their weight loss goals and/or increase activity levels (85).

Behavioral Strategies

Interventions that combine diet, PA, and behavior therapy are the most effective programs for weight loss and weight maintenance (5). Behavioral weight loss programs not only target dietary intake and PA but also provide clients with strategies to help them make the necessary lifestyle changes. Key strategies used in behavioral weight loss programs include the following:

- Self-monitoring — keeping food or PA logs or monitoring body weight on a regular basis
- Goal setting — setting realistic goals for the number of minutes of exercise one will accomplish during the next week or month
- Stimulus control — modifying one's environment to enhance successful behavior change such as removing "risky" foods from the refrigerator or hanging an exercise adherence calendar in a prominent spot
- Problem solving — identifying situations that pose a problem for overeating (such as holidays) and developing a solution to eat healthy and avoid excess caloric intake

There are many additional behavioral strategies that clients can use to enhance a weight management program. See Chapter 12 for more information on behavioral strategies that can assist with weight loss goals.

Weight Loss Supplements

The ACSM-EP has a responsibility to encourage healthy weight loss, when indicated, by eating a balanced diet including adequate fruit and vegetables, limiting sugary beverages and energy-dense foods, and including regular exercise and activity. Taking this approach is considered safe and reasonable and should provide sufficient nutrition to meet daily needs. However, despite this, many different weight loss products and supplements are available to the public, often with little or no evidence to support their value. One of the most reputable resources for information on vitamins, minerals, supplements, and herbal products is the Office of Dietary Supplements (86). Although medications and drugs prescribed by a doctor are regulated by the U.S. Food and Drug Administration (FDA), supplements and herbal products are not regulated by the government in terms of efficacy, safety, dosing, and purity of the product. The FDA Web site does list updates and warnings related to supplements (both dietary and herbal) and is an important resource for an ACSM-EP and his or her clients (87). The rating on effectiveness is based on available research (88). Some advertised physiological mechanisms for dietary supplements include increased energy expenditure, modified carbohydrate metabolism, decreased fat production, and blocked absorption of dietary fat. However, numerous safety concerns have been raised with some supplements (*e.g.*, ephedra, bitter orange, and chitosan), occasionally resulting in their removal from the consumer market.

People of all ages experiment with weight loss products, including caffeine and energy drinks. Although a safe upper limit has been established for adults and caffeine ($250–300$ mg $\cdot$ d^{-1}), there is no recommendation for adolescents. Therefore, as a general rule, caffeine and energy drinks should be consumed with caution, particularly in the younger/adolescent population. Many energy drinks are also high in sugar and calories, so regardless of age, the consumption of these drinks may be a source of excess calories and not "cost-effective" in terms of the benefits outweighing the risks. Side effects of energy drinks and caffeine depend on the individual's sensitivity but may include sleeplessness, nervousness, irritability, and anxiety. There are a wide variety of resources the ACSM-EP can use for additional information on supplements and herbal products. Some of these resources include the National Center for Complementary and Alternative Medicine, Center for Food Safety and Applied Nutrition (FDA), ConsumerLab.com, and Dietary Supplement Verified U.S. Pharmacopeia (USP).

Dieting

Although many people may also experiment with "dieting" for weight loss, in general, most popular diets are to be approached with caution. Ideally, individuals interested in the current popular diet fads should first seek the advice of a registered dietitian or other health care professional trained in nutrition to determine the safety and effectiveness of the diet. Diets to be cautious of include those promoting low carbohydrates, excessive protein intake, or any meal pattern that eliminates or emphasizes any one particular food group. For instance, the IOM recommends at least 130 g of carbohydrate each day for all age groups (73). Thus, diets prescribing low carbohydrate intake may fall short of this requirement and likely lead to cravings. Individuals need a variety of foods from each food group to meet their needs for growth, development, and maintenance throughout the lifespan. Any client who wishes to "go on a diet" should first consider his or her optimal health/dietary needs. A more prudent approach may be to consider permanent dietary changes (such as eating more fruits and vegetables) as opposed to "going on a diet."

Medications

Medications that are taken for common health issues such as high blood pressure, diabetes, depression, seizure disorders, and allergies can result in either weight gain or weight loss (88,89). Therefore, it is important that the ACSM-EP be aware of the medications a client is taking as they may inhibit the client's ability to manage his or her weight.

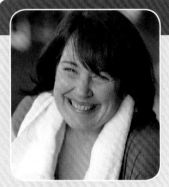

The Case of Lisa

Narrative

Lisa, a 56-year-old female nonsmoker, was inactive and thin most of her life but started gaining weight when she turned 40 years old. The weight gain accelerated after menopause, and Lisa now finds herself "50 lb overweight" (height 5 ft 4 in, weight 190 lb). Her resting heart rate is 64 bpm, her resting blood pressure is 142/88 mm Hg, and she has 38% body fat. A recent blood test revealed that Lisa's low-density lipoprotein (LDL) cholesterol is 168 mg $\cdot$ dL^{-1}, high-density lipoprotein (HDL) cholesterol is 38 mg $\cdot$ dL^{-1}, and glycolated hemoglobin (HbA1C) is 6.3%. Lisa is concerned because her mother had a heart attack when she was 60 years old, just 4 years older than Lisa is now. Based on her doctor's advice, Lisa is seeking guidance from an ACSM-EP.

The ACSM-EP suggested that Lisa engage in immediate lifestyle changes, including regular PA and dietary changes. Lisa's blood pressure is categorized as stage 2 hypertension, and her fasting glucose levels fall into the prediabetic category. She also has multiple risk factors for heart disease including age, family history, physical inactivity, obesity, hypertension, and dyslipidemia. Lifestyle changes accompanied by weight loss can impact Lisa's overall health profile. Because Lisa has no history of PA, the ACSM-EP recommended a walking program, starting with 20 minutes, 5 times per week at a moderate intensity (40%–59% of HRR). The goal is to gradually progress to 6–7 d $\cdot$ wk^{-1} for 30–60 min $\cdot$ d^{-1} at a moderate to vigorous intensity to maximize caloric expenditure. A resistance training program, starting at two sets of 8–10 exercises at 50%–60% of the one repetition maximum (1-RM) two to three times per week was also recommended, with a goal to gradually progress to 70%–80% of the 1-RM. Lisa should also engage in flexibility exercises 2–3 d $\cdot$ wk^{-1}.

The ACSM-EP had Lisa complete a 3-day dietary log that included a weekend day. Prescribing a diet for Lisa is beyond the scope of practice for the ACSM-EP. However, upon review of the dietary log, the ACSM-EP was able to make important suggestions to Lisa's about her eating habits, such as (a) suggesting a decrease in the intake of sweets, (b) educating Lisa about the caloric content of the muffins that she purchases for breakfast each morning, and (c) helping Lisa understand places where she can substitute lower calorie foods for higher calorie foods. The dietary log also allowed the ACSM-EP to understand Lisa's eating behaviors. For example, she noted that Lisa often eats in the car and in front of the TV and eats fast food three to four times per week. Based on all of the information that the ACSM-EP gathered about Lisa's diet and exercise habits, they were able to implement some behavioral strategies that will contribute to Lisa's success in changing her diet and exercise habits and losing weight. These strategies included putting up an adherence calendar that was marked with a red star each day Lisa exercised, learning more about the health benefits of exercise, and committing to eating only when sitting at the dining room table.

QUESTIONS

- Calculate the baseline TEE, lean body mass (lb), and fat mass (lb) for Lisa.
- Lisa has an initial weight loss goal of 6% of her body weight. How many pounds does she need to lose?
- What other type of aerobic exercise is appropriate for Lisa?
- Calculate a heart rate for Lisa for exercise that would fit the ACSM recommendations for moderate intensity.
- What other behavioral strategies might be useful for Lisa to engage in?

SUMMARY

Overweight and obesity have reached epidemic levels in the United States and around the world. Because the ACSM-EP will regularly encounter individuals who wish to lose weight, they must develop the knowledge and skills needed to help people manage their weight. The ACSM-EP must be skilled in anthropometric measurements and body composition analysis in order to develop safe and effective weight loss goals and monitor changes over time. Further, the ACSM-EP should be familiar with ACSM's FITT recommendations for overweight and obesity so that they design the most effective exercise program. It is also important to remember the art of exercise prescription when working with this population including modifying the FITT principle when needed, helping the client set realistic goals, individualizing and tailoring the program, modifying exercises that are difficult to perform, and being sensitive to the unique challenges exercise has for this population. Although prescribing a diet is beyond the scope of practice for the ACSM-EP, providing sound nutritional advice and helping a client adopt new eating habits is also critical for success. The awareness of adverse weight loss strategies clients might want to employ and the ability to educate clients on healthy alternatives to lose and maintain weight loss are also important skills for the ACSM-EP. Weight management is a challenging endeavor, but clients can be successful when they incorporate exercise, healthy dietary changes, and behavioral strategies into their lifestyle.

STUDY QUESTIONS

1. Discuss the pros and cons of the different percentage body fat measurement methods in individuals with a BMI $>35.0 \text{ kg} \cdot \text{m}^{-2}$.
2. State the critical components to a weight loss strategy.
3. Identify the key aspects of the *2015-2020 Dietary Recommendations*.
4. Robert walked on a treadmill at a speed 2.5 mph and a grade of 10% for 40 minutes. How many kilocalories did he expend?

REFERENCES

1. U.S. Department of Agriculture. 2015-2020 Dietary guidelines for Americans: executive summary [Internet]. Washington (DC): U.S. Department of Agriculture; [cited 2019 Jul 17]. Available from: http://health.gov/dietaryguidelines/2015/guidelines/executive-summary.
2. Fryar CD, Carroll MD, Ogden CL. *Prevalence of Overweight, Obesity, and Extreme Obesity Among Adults Aged 20 and Over: United States, 1960–1962 Through 2015–2016.* Hyattsville (MD): National Center for Health Statistics; 2018. 6 p.
3. National Center for Health Statistics. Health, United States, 2017: *With Special Feature on Mortality.* Hyattsville (MD): National Center for Health Statistics; 2018. 87 p.
4. World Health Organization. Obesity and overweight [Internet]. Geneva (Switzerland); [cited 2019 Jul 12]. Available at: https://www.who.int/news-room/fact-sheets/detail/obesity-and-overweight.
5. U.S. Department of Health and Human Services. *Clinical Guidelines on the Identification, Evaluation, and Treatment of Overweight and Obesity in Adults: The Evidence Report* (NIH Publication No. 98-4083). Bethesda (MD): National Heart, Lung, and Blood Institute; 1998. 262 p.
6. Jensen MD, Ryan DH, Apovian CM, et al. 2013 AHA/ACC/TOS guideline for the management of overweight and obesity in adults: a report of the American College of Cardiology/American Heart Association Task Force on Practice Guidelines and The Obesity Society. *J Am Coll Cardiol.* 2014;63:2985–3023.
7. Churilla JR, Zoeller R. Physical activity: physical activity and the metabolic syndrome: a review of the evidence. *Am J Lifestyle Med.* 2008;2:118–25.
8. Canoy D. Distribution of body fat and risk of coronary heart disease in men and women. *Curr Opin Cardiol.* 2008;23(6):591–8.

9. Finkelstein EA, Trogdon JG, Cohen JW, Dietz W. Annual medical spending attributable to obesity: payer- and service-specific estimates. *Health Aff.* 2009;28(5):w822–31.

10. Tremmel M, Gerdtham U, Nilsson PM, Saha S. Economic burden of obesity: a systematic literature review. *Int J Environ Res Public Health.* 2017:14(4):435.

11. Teuner CM, Menn P, Heier M, Holle R, John J, Wolfenstetter SB. Impact of BMI and BMI change on future drug expenditures in adults: results from the MONICA/KORA cohort study. *BMC Health Serv Res.* 2013:13;424.

12. Arterburn DE, Maciejewski ML, Tsevat J. Impact of morbid obesity on medical expenditures in adults. *Int J Obes.* 2005;29(3):334–9.

13. National Heart, Lung, and Blood Institute. Calculate your body mass index [Internet]. Bethesda (MD): National Heart, Lung, and Blood Institute; [cited 2019 Jul 12]. Available at: https://www.nhlbi.nih.gov/health/educational/lose_wt/BMI/bmicalc.htm.

14. Flegal KM, Carroll MD, Odgen CL, Curtin LR. Prevalence and trends in obesity among US adults. *JAMA.* 2010;303(3):235–41.

15. U.S. Department of Health and Human Services. *The Practical Guide: Identification, Evaluation, and Treatment of Overweight and Obesity in Adults* (NIH Publication No. 00-4084). Bethesda (MD): National Heart, Lung, and Blood Institute; 2000. 94 p.

16. Flegal KM, Graubard BI, Williamson DF, Gail MH. Excess deaths associated with underweight, overweight, and obesity. *JAMA.* 2005;293(15):1861–7.

17. Centers for Disease Control and Prevention. Defining childhood obesity [Internet]. Centers for Disease Control and Prevention; [cited 2020 Sep 16]. Available from: https://www.cdc.gov/obesity/childhood/defining.html.

18. Lahey R, Khan SS. Trends in obesity and risk of cardiovascular disease. *Curr Epidemiol Rep.* 2018;5(3):243–51.

19. Nahar VK, Nelson KM, Ford MA, et al. Predictors of bone mineral density among Asian Indians in northern Mississippi: a pilot study. *J Res Health Sci.* 2016;16(4):228–32.

20. Jih J, Mukherjea A, Vittinghoff E, et al. Using appropriate body mass index cut points for overweight and obesity among Asian Americans. *Prev Med.* 2014;65:1–6.

21. Misra A. Ethnic-specific criteria for classification of body mass index: a perspective for Asian Indians and American Diabetes Association position statement. *Diabetes Technol Ther.* 2015;17(9):667–1.

22. Duren DL, Sherwood RJ, Czerwinski SA, et al. Body composition methods: comparisons and interpretation. *J Diabetes Sci Technol.* 2008;2(6):1139–46.

23. Ross R, Neeland IJ, Yamashita S, et al. Waist circumference as a vital sign in clinical practice: a consensus statement from the IAS and ICCR Working Group on Visceral Obesity. *Nature Rev Endocrinol.* 2020;16:177–89.

24. Pi-Sunyer FX. The epidemiology of central fat distribution in relation to disease. *Nutr Rev.* 2004;62(7 Pt 2):S120–6.

25. American College of Sports Medicine. *ACSM's Guidelines for Exercise Testing and Prescription.* 11th ed. Philadelphia (PA): Wolters Kluwer; 2022. 548 p.

26. Bray GA, Gray DS. Obesity. Part 1 — pathogenesis. *West J Med.* 1988;149:429–41.

27. Camhi SM, Bray GA, Bouchard C, et al. The relationship of waist circumference and BMI to visceral, subcutaneous, and total body fat: sex and race differences. *Obesity.* 2011;19(2):402–8.

28. Katzmarzyk PT, Mire E, Bray GA, Greenway FL, Heymsfield SB, Bouchard C. Anthropometric markers of obesity and mortality in white and African American adults: the Pennington Longitudinal Study. *Obesity.* 2013;21(5):1070–5.

29. Staiano AE, Bouchard C, Katzmarzyk PT. BMI-specific waist circumference thresholds to discriminate elevated cardiometabolic risk in White and African American adults. *Obes Facts.* 2013;6:317–24.

30. Ashwell M, Gibson S. Waist-to-height ratio as an indicator of early health risk: simpler and more predictive than using a matrix based on BMI and waist circumference. *BMJ Open.* 2016;6(3)6:e010159.

31. Shen S, Lu Y, Qi H, et al. Waist-to-height ratio is an effective indicator for comprehensive cardiovascular health. *Sci Rep.* 2017;7:43046.

32. Rezende AC, Souza LG, Jardim TV, et al. Is waist-to-height ratio the best predictive indicator of hypertension incidence? A cohort study. *BMC Public Health.* 2018;18(1):281.

33. Lohman TG. Body composition methodology in sports medicine. *Phys Sports Med.* 1982;10(12):46–7.

34. Gallagher D, Heymsfield SB, Heo M, Jebb SA, Murgatroyd PR, Sakamoto Y. Healthy percentage body fat ranges: an approach for developing guidelines based on body mass index. *Am J Clin Nutr.* 2000;72(3):694–701.

35. Kelly TL, Wilson KE, Heymsfield SB. Dual energy x-ray absorptiometry body composition reference values from NHANES. *PLoS One.* 2009:4(9):e7038.

36. Lohman TG. Skinfolds and body density and their relations to body fatness: a review. *Hum Biol.* 1981;53(2):181–225.

37. Heyward VH, Wagner DR. *Applied Body Composition Assessment.* 2nd ed. Champaign (IL): Human Kinetics; 2004. 280 p.

38. Nickerson BS, Fedewa MV, Cicone Z, Esco MR. The relative accuracy of skinfolds compared to four-compartment estimates of body composition. *Clin Nutr.* 2020;39:1112–6.

39. Jackson AW, Pollock M. Practical assessment of body composition. *Phys Sportsmed.* 1985;13(5):76–90.

40. Pollack ML, Schmidt DH, Jackson AS. Measurement of cardiorespiratory fitness and body composition in the clinical setting. *Compr Ther.* 1980;6(9):12–27.

41. Brozek J, Grande F, Anderson JT, Keys A. Densitometric analysis of body composition: revision of some quantitative assumptions. *Ann N Y Acad Sci.* 1963;110:113–40.

42. Siri WE. Body composition from fluid spaces and density: analysis of methods. 1961. *Nutrition.* 1993;9(5):480–92.

43. American College of Sports Medicine. *ACSM's Resources for the Personal Trainer.* 4th ed. Baltimore (MD): Lippincott Williams Wilkins; 2014. 592 p.

44. Graves JE, Kanaley JA, Garzareooa L, Pollock ML. Anthropometry and body composition assessment. In: Maud PJ, Foster C, editors. *Physiological Assessment of Human Fitness.* 2nd ed. Champaign (IL): Human Kinetics; 2006. p. 185–226.

45. Lemos, T, Gallagher D. Current body composition measurement techniques. *Curr Opin Endocrinol Diabetes Obes.* 2017;24(5):310–4.

46. Gibson AL, Wagner DR, Heyward VH. *Advanced Fitness Assessment and Exercise Prescription.* 8th ed. Champaign (IL): Human Kinetics; 2019. 552 p.

47. Lohman TG. *Advances in Body Composition Assessment.* Champaign (IL): Human Kinetics; 1992. 150 p.

48. Bray GA. *A Guide to Obesity and the Metabolic Syndrome.* Boca Raton (FL): CRC Press; 2011. 412 p.

49. Levi J, Vinter S, St. Larent R, Segal LM. *F as in Fat: How Obesity Threatens America's Future.* Washington (DC): Trust for American's Health, Robert Wood Johnson Foundation; 2010. 124 p.

50. Lahney R, Khan SS. Trends in obesity risk of cardiovascular disease. *Curr Epidemiol Rep.* 2018;5(3):243–51.

51. Chakravathy MV, Booth FW. Eating, exercise, and "thrifty" genotypes: connecting the dots toward an evolutionary understanding of modern chronic diseases. *J Apply Physiol (1985).* 2004;96(1):3–10.

52. Piaggi P, Vinales KL, Santini F, Krakoff J. Energy expenditure in the etiology of human obesity: spendthrift and thrifty metabolic phenotypes and energy-sensing mechanisms. *J Endocrinol Invest.* 2018;41(1):83–9.

53. Cooper JA. Factors affecting circulating levels of peptide YY in humans: a comprehensive review. *Nutr Res Rev.* 2014;27(1):186–97.

54. Knuth ND, Johannsen DL, Tamboli RA, et al. Metabolic adaptation following massive weight loss is related to the degree of imbalance and change in circulating leptin. *Obesity.* 2014;22(12):2563–9.

55. Farr OM, Gavrieli A, Mantzoros CS. Leptin applications in 2015: what have we learned about leptin and obesity? *Curr Opin Endocrinol Diabetes Obes.* 2015;22(5):353–9.

56. Greenway FL. Physiological adaptations to weight loss and factors favouring weight regain. *Int J Obes (Lond).* 2015;39(8):1188–96.

57. Soares MJ, Müller MJ. Resting energy expenditure and body composition: critical aspects for clinical nutrition. *Eur J Clin Nutr.* 2018;72:1208–14.

58. Elia M. Organ and tissue contribution to metabolic weight. In: Kinney JM, Tucker HN, editors. *Energy Metabolism: Tissue Determinants and Cellular Corollaries.* New York (NY): Raven Press; 1999. p. 61–79.

59. Frankenfield D, Roth-Yousey L, Compher C. Comparison of predictive equations for resting metabolic rate in healthy non-obese and obese adults: a systematic review. *J Am Diet Assoc.* 2005;105(5):775–89.

60. McLay-Cooke RT, Gray AR, Jones LM, Taylor RW, Skidmore PM, Brown RC. Prediction equations overestimate the energy requirements more for obesity-susceptible individuals. *Nutrients.* 2017;9(9):1012.

61. Frankenfield D. Bias and accuracy of resting metabolic rate equations in non-obese and obese adult. *Clin Nutr.* 2013;32(6):976–82.

62. Institute of Medicine. *Dietary Reference Intakes (DRIs): Acceptable Macronutrient Distribution Ranges* [Internet]. Washington (DC): National Academies Press; 2011 [cited 2016 Jan 15]. Available from: http://fnic.nal.usda.gov/ sites/fnic.nal.usda.gov/files/uploads/recommended_intakes_individuals.pdf.

63. Lutz C, Mazur E, Litch N. *Nutrition and Diet Therapy.* 6th ed. Philadelphia (PA): F.A. Davis; 2015. 672 p.

64. Gerrior S, Juan W, Basiotis P. An easy approach to calculating estimated energy requirements. *Prev Chronic Dis.* 2006;3(4):A129.

65. U.S. Department of Agriculture. Appendix 2. Estimated calorie needs per day, by age, sex, & physical activity level [Internet]. Washington (DC): U.S. Department of Agriculture; [cited 2019 Aug 21]. Available from: http://health.gov/dietaryguidelines/2015/guidelines/appendix-2/.

66. Dutton GR, Kim Y, Jacobs DR, et al. 25-Year weight gain in a racially balanced sample of U.S. adults: the CARDIA study. *Obesity.* 2016;24(9):1962–8.

67. 2018 Physical Activity Guidelines Advisory Committee. *2018 Physical Activity Guidelines Advisory Committee Scientific Report.* Washington (DC): U.S. Department of Health and Human Services; 2018. 779 p.

68. U.S. Department of Health and Human Services. *2018 Physical Activity Guidelines for Americans.* 2nd ed. Washington (DC): U.S. Department of Health and Human Services; 2018. 118 p.

69. Jakicic JM, Powell KE, Campbell WW, et al. Physical activity and the prevention of weight gain in adults: a systematic review. *Med Sci Sport Exerc.* 2019;51(6);1262–9.

70. Curioni CC, Lourenco PM. Long-term weight loss after diet and exercise: a systematic review. *Int J Obes.* 2005;29:1168–74.

71. Donnelly JE, Blair SN, Jakicic JM, Manore MM, Rankin JW, Smith BK. Appropriate physical activity intervention strategies for weight loss and prevention of weight regain for adults. *Med Sci Sports Exerc.* 2009;41(2):459–71.

72. Klem ML, Wing RR, McGuire MT, Seagle HM, Hill JO. A descriptive study of individuals successful at long-term maintenance of substantial weight loss. *Am J Clin Nutr.* 1997;66(2):239–46.

73. Institute of Medicine. *Dietary Reference Intakes (DRI) for Energy, Carbohydrate, Fiber, Fat, Fatty Acids, Cholesterol, Protein, and Amino Acids* [Internet]. Washington (DC): National Academies Press; 2005 [cited 2019 Aug 12]. Available from: https://www.nal.usda.gov/fnic/dri-nutrient-reports.

74. ChooseMyPlate Web site [Internet]. Washington (DC): U.S. Department of Agriculture; [cited 2019 Aug 21]. Available from: http://www.choosemyplate.gov.

75. Porcari JP, McLean KP, Foster C, Kernozek T, Crenshaw B, Swensen C. Effects of electrical muscle stimulation on body composition, muscle strength, and physical appearance. *J Strength Cond Res.* 2002;16(2):165–72.

76. Hayter TL, Coombes JS, Knez WL, Brancato TL. Effects of electrical muscle stimulation on oxygen consumption. *J Strength Cond Res.* 2005;19(1):98–101.

77. Turocy PS, DePalma BF, Horswill AC, et al. National Athletic Trainers' Association position statement: safe weight loss and maintenance practices in sport and exercise. *J Athl Train.* 2011;46(3):322–36.

78. Khawandanah J, Tewfik I. Fad diets: lifestyle promises and health challenges. *J Food Res.* 2016;5(6):80–94.

79. Barrea L, Altieri B, Polese B, et al. Nutritionist and obesity: brief overview on efficacy safety and drug interactions of the main weight-loss dietary supplements. *Int J Ob Suppl.* 2019;9;32–49.

80. American Society for Metabolic and Bariatric Surgery. Estimate of bariatric surgery numbers, 2011-2018. Newberry (FL): American Society for Metabolic and Bariatric Surgery; [cited 2019 Dec 30]. Available from: https://asmbs .org/resources/estimate-of-bariatric-surgery-numbers.

81. Schauer PR, Burgera B, Ikramuddin S, et al. Effect of laparoscopic Roux-en Y gastric bypass on type 2 diabetes mellitus. *Ann Surg.* 2003;238(4):467–84.

82. Bellicha A, Ciangura C, Poitou C, Portero P, Oppert JM, Effectiveness of exercise training after bariatric surgery — a systematic literature review and meta-analysis. *Obes Rev.* 2018;19(11):1544–56.

83. Baillot A, Audet M, Baillargeon JP, et al. Impact of physical activity and fitness in class II and III obese individuals: a systemic review. *Obes Rev.* 2014;15(9):721–39.

84. Bond DS, Graham TJ, Vithiananthan S, et al. Changes in enjoyment, self-efficacy and motivation during a randomized trial to promote habitual physical activity adoption in bariatric surgery patients. *Surg Obes Relat Dis.* 2016;15(5):1072–9.

85. Powell SM, Fasczewski KS, Gill DL, Davis PG. Got with the FLOW: implementation of a psychological skills intervention in an exercise program for post-bariatric surgery patients. *J Health Psychol.* 2020;25(13–14):2260–71.

86. Office of Dietary Supplements, National Institutes of Health. Vitamin B12 [Internet]. Bethesda (MD): U.S. Department of Health and Human Services; [cited 2019 Aug 21]. Available from: http://ods.od.nih.gov/factsheets /vitaminb12/.

87. U.S. Food and Drug Association Web site [Internet]. Silver Spring (MD): U.S. Food and Drug Association; [cited 2019 Aug 21]. Available from: http://www.fda.gov/.

88. Mayo Clinic. Dietary supplements for weight loss. Melt away fat. Lose weight naturally. Tempting claims, but do the products deliver? [Internet]. Scottsdale (AZ): Mayo Clinic; [cited 2011 Jul 21]. Available from: https://www .mayoclinic.org/healthy-lifestyle/weight-loss/in_depth /weight-loss/art-20046409.

89. MedicineNet. Prescription drugs causing weight gain? [Internet]. San Clemente (CA): MedicineNet; [cited 2018 Aug 21]. Available from: http://www.medicinenet.com /script/main/art.asp?articlekey=56339&page=2.

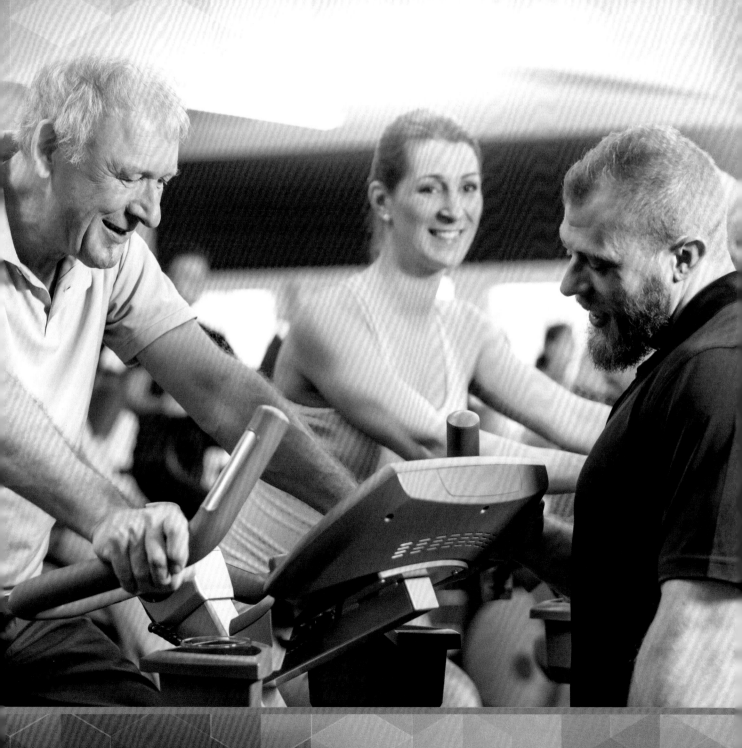

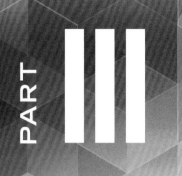

PART

III

Exercise Programming for Special Populations

Exercise for Individuals with Controlled Cardiovascular, Metabolic, Pulmonary, and Chronic Kidney Disease

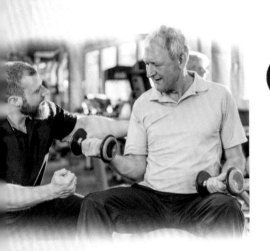

OBJECTIVES

- To describe the pathophysiology of common chronic diseases.
- To describe the role medication plays in altering the exercise response in various chronic diseases.
- To explain the nuances of exercise prescription in various chronic diseases compared with apparently healthy individuals.

INTRODUCTION

The ACSM Certified Exercise Physiologist® (ACSM-EP®) is responsible for developing exercise prescriptions for healthy clients and individuals with medically controlled diseases who are cleared by their physician for independent exercise. The role of physical activity and exercise training in primary and secondary disease prevention/treatment is well established (1–4). The amount of physical activity and exercise recommended for health and fitness benefits varies between the different chronic diseases and is provided within structured and well-developed guidelines. Individuals with chronic diseases often present unique and challenging exercise limitations, but physical activity and exercise should not be avoided. Instead, exercise should become part of their medical management plan. Individuals with a chronic disease can experience health fitness benefits such as reduced disease symptoms, reduced medication reliance, and restoration of mental well-being (2). Because disease states usually cause exercise limitations and restrictions, the ACSM-EP must know these limitations to ensure a safe and effective exercise prescription. ACSM-EPs must also recognize when to refer someone back to his or her physician or to more specialized exercise training with clinical supervision. This chapter reviews disease pathology, exercise considerations and contraindications, and the process for developing a proper frequency, intensity, time, and type (FITT) plan to allow optimal health outcomes for the client with a cardiovascular, metabolic, pulmonary, and chronic kidney disease (CKD) after physician clearance has been established.

 Pathophysiology

Cardiovascular Disease

Cardiovascular diseases (CVDs) account for more American deaths than any other disease, with nearly 860,000 total deaths annually (5). Due to the financial cost, prevalence, and the associated morbidity and mortality, the ACSM-EP should understand CVD pathology and exercise measures for working with this population. A strong understanding of the disease pathology and specific exercise nuances will allow the ACSM-EP to effectively design an exercise prescription to lessen the effects of CVD and improve the client's health fitness status and quality of life.

Coronary Heart Disease

Coronary artery disease (CAD) is one of the most prevalent forms of CVD and accounts for the most cardiovascular deaths (5). CAD often results in ischemia present in myocardial tissue due to arterial stenosis (narrowing of the coronary arteries). Several factors contribute to this process, including a buildup of atherosclerotic plaques, vascular remodeling causing luminal stenosis, dyslipidemia, hypertension (HTN), and numerous inflammatory factors. Central to CAD is the formation of atherosclerotic plaque in the elastic and smooth lining inside of arteries (Fig. 8.1). Plaque formations in the coronary arteries obstruct blood flow to cardiac muscle tissue initiating reduced cardiac function and/or tissue death (necrosis) due to lack of oxygen (6,7). Atherosclerosis is the process of fat deposit on the interior wall of an artery causing the wall to thicken while reducing luminal diameter, creating a buildup of fat and fibrous plaques. The arterial narrowing is progressive and dangerous. The atherosclerotic process begins with a focal injury to the lining of the artery, eventually causing damage to the endothelium. The endothelium becomes more permeable to lipids, allowing low-density lipoprotein cholesterol (LDL-C) to easily move through the damaged endothelium and into the arterial intima layer. Once inside the intima, macrophages oxidize LDL-C and form arterial foam cells. As these foam cells evolve and develop, fatty streaks start to form around the initial injury site and the plaque formation process begins (8). Fatty streak

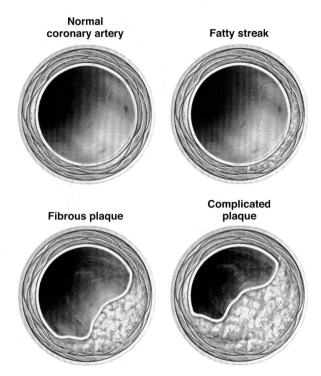

FIGURE 8.1. Depiction of the typical progression for plaque buildup in a coronary artery. The disease process begins with a normal coronary artery and the progression to fatty streak to an artery with complicated plaque. (Asset provided by Anatomical Chart Co.)

formation starts a repeating cycle of repair and remodeling to the artery wall in which luminal diameter is progressively reduced until either a partial or complete occlusion of the lumen occurs (9). Partial impairment of coronary artery blood flow and oxygen delivery to cardiac tissue is referred to as myocardial ischemia. The complete obstruction of blood flow to the cardiac myocardial tissue is referred to as a myocardial infarction (MI) or commonly referred to as a heart attack resulting in tissue death or necrosis (6).

Myocardial ischemia is an imbalance between myocardial oxygen demand and supply. Myocardial ischemia is differentiated into two categories: stable and unstable ischemia. Stable ischemia is a lack of oxygen to myocardial tissue during times of increased oxygen demand in the heart as seen with exercise. The impaired ability to deliver blood to cardiac tissue during exercise causes an oxygen deficit or imbalance in the tissue, causing chest pain, referred to as angina, and reduced exercise capacity (10). The symptoms of stable ischemia lessen as the oxygen supply of the heart improves and stabilizes, or when exercise eases or ceases, allowing the coronary arteries to effectively provide the cardiac tissue with adequate blood flow and oxygen. Unstable ischemia is more severe and is often observed with symptoms at rest and during times of little exertional stress. Individuals with unstable ischemia need to seek medical treatment immediately, as unstable ischemia may be a warning sign that a heart attack is imminent (10). In no case should individuals with unstable ischemia perform exercise or an exercise test.

Hypertension

HTN is common among patients with CAD. HTN is considered the "silent killer" because the signs and symptoms often go unnoticed. The severity of HTN, however, cannot be overlooked. If left untreated, HTN is a major risk factor for developing multiple complications such as atherosclerosis, stroke, heart attack, chronic heart failure, kidney failure, and blindness (11).

The American College of Cardiology/American Heart Association Task Force defines HTN as an elevation in either systolic blood pressure (SBP) (>130 mm Hg) or diastolic blood pressure (DBP)

(>80 mm Hg) (12). Diagnosis is confirmed when elevated blood pressure (BP) measurements are recorded on at least two separate days or when the patient is known to be taking antihypertensive medication (12). The etiology of HTN is categorized as either primary or secondary. Primary HTN accounts for 90%–95% of all cases, has no established pathology, and is thus considered idiopathic (arising spontaneously or from an obscure or unknown cause) (9). Secondary HTN, which accounts for very few cases, is associated with identifiable causes such as renal disease, stress, drug-induced side effects, sleep apnea, neurological disorders, and others (9).

BP is regulated by two factors: cardiac output (a product of heart rate [HR] and stroke volume [SV]) and total peripheral vascular resistance. Increased peripheral resistance is the most common characteristic of primary and secondary HTN and is caused by chronic vasoconstriction (narrowing of the peripheral arterioles) or by vascular plaque buildup. When HTN is present, arterioles lose elasticity due to the increased presence of fibrous collagen tissue. Collagen buildup causes improper arteriole constriction and relaxation, which is important in normal blood flow regulation. In time, this condition leads to increased vascular resistance, increased BP, and eventually accelerated atherosclerosis development (9).

Current guidelines for the management of HTN provide specific instructions on the implementation of pharmacological therapies in addition to emphasizing lifestyle modifications including habitual physical activity as the initial therapy to lower BP and to prevent or attenuate progression to HTN in individuals with pre-HTN (13,14).

Peripheral Artery Disease

The pathological development of peripheral artery disease (PAD) mimics CAD with the primary difference being the location of the affected blood vessels. Specifically, PAD is characterized by occlusion or narrowing of peripheral arteries of the upper and lower limbs as a result of the buildup of atherosclerotic plaques (15). Although blood vessels of the upper limbs may be affected, most cases of PAD are observed in the arterial network of the lower limbs (16). As a result of this vascular remodeling and subsequent dysfunction, the occlusion causes a reduction of blood flow to the distal limbs. This reduced blood flow leads to a mismatch between oxygen supply and demand, leading to the development of ischemia, and manifests as pain and easy fatigability (17).

The most common symptom of PAD is intermittent claudication, characterized by a repeatable aching, cramping sensation, or fatigue in the muscles of the calf in one or both legs. These sensations are often triggered by weight-bearing exercises and normally dissipate with terminating activity (16). The severity of PAD is based on the extent of claudication and is quantified using the ankle/brachial systolic pressure index (ABI), which is the ratio of SBP measurements taken in a supine position at rest at the level of the ankle. Brachial artery pressure is calculated with the equation: ABI = ankle SBP / brachial SBP (18,19). Values of >0.90 are considered normal, whereas ≤0.90 is the threshold for PAD confirmation. Although limitations in the use of ABI as a diagnostic criterion for PAD exist (15,20), ABI is generally accepted as an effective predictive measurement (21). PAD severity is rated on a 4-point scale: grade 0 = asymptomatic, grade 1 = intermittent claudication, grade 2 = ischemic rest pain, and grade 4 = minor/major tissue loss in the limbs.

Metabolic Diseases

Metabolic diseases have varying genetic or environmental causes that alter normal metabolic function. The most common of these causes are diabetes mellitus (DM), dyslipidemia, and obesity, each of which responds well to exercise therapy. If not treated properly, each condition can lead to more severe health issues including CAD.

Diabetes

Type 1 and Type 2 diabetes are defined by a decrease in the production, release and/or effectiveness, and action of insulin. Either form of diabetes results in increased blood glucose levels, a condition referred to as hyperglycemia (22,23). If untreated, diabetes can cause vasculature damage and starves the cell of needed glucose.

Type 1 diabetes is less common, found in only 5%–10% of all patients with diabetes, and is characterized by an absolute deficiency in blood insulin release because of the destruction of pancreatic insulin-secreting beta cells (24). Generally, the destruction of the beta cells is idiopathic. Patients with Type 1 diabetes are referred to exercise professionals with more specialized training to prescribe and monitor exercise.

Patients with Type 2 diabetes have hyperglycemia, which is typically a result of decreased insulin sensitivity. Excessive abdominal fat is a leading risk factor for Type 2 diabetes. The disease responds well to exercise therapy and pharmacological treatments that either increase insulin sensitivity or decrease blood glucose levels.

Dyslipidemia

Dyslipidemia, defined as abnormal blood cholesterol and triglyceride levels, is caused by a combination of genetic and/or environmental factors. Because lipids are hydrophobic, lipids must combine with proteins to travel through the cardiovascular system. Cholesterol and triglyceride are packaged inside transports known as lipoproteins and are classified by their density: chylomicrons, very low-density lipoproteins (VLDLs), low-density lipoproteins (LDLs), and high-density lipoproteins (HDLs) (25). Total cholesterol is the total amount of cholesterol found circulating in the blood, and if total cholesterol levels rise above 200 mg $\cdot$ dL^{-1}, cholesterol is considered a risk factor for CAD. HDL is responsible for aiding in the removal of lipids from the circulation through reverse cholesterol transport. Hence, HDL cholesterol (HDL-C) is referred to as the "good" cholesterol. Healthy circulating HDL-C levels are greater than 40 mg $\cdot$ dL^{-1}. If HDL-C levels are less than 40 mg $\cdot$ dL^{-1}, very little reverse cholesterol transport occurs, leading to further vascular lipid accumulation and accelerated atherosclerosis rates. Excessive amounts of LDL-C, or "bad" cholesterol (>130 mg $\cdot$ dL^{-1}), is associated with increased risk of atherosclerosis and CAD. Subfractions exist within these four lipoprotein classifications: intermediate-density lipoprotein (IDL; an intermediate step in VLDL catabolism), lipoprotein(a) (Lp[a]) (an LDL subfraction highly related to CAD), small and large LDL subfractions, and two HDL subfractions (HDL$_2$ and the more dense HDL$_3$). Both small and large LDL particles are associated with increased risk for CAD. However, small LDL particles are more atherogenic than large particles because of their greater oxidation potential. The other metabolic abnormalities, primarily high levels of triglyceride-rich lipoproteins such as VLDL and low serum HDL-C concentrations, are also associated with increased CAD risk.

Obesity

Obesity is defined as an excessive accumulation of body fat and is associated with a body mass index (BMI) of $\geq$30 kg $\cdot$ m^{-2} (26). Although the causes for obesity are complex and multifaceted, the primary contributors are the combination of high caloric consumption and low daily physical activity (27). Regardless of the etiology, obesity is associated with multiple comorbidities, including insulin resistance, reduced growth hormone secretion, increased cholesterol synthesis and excretion, and an increased incidence of all-cause mortality (28).

Metabolic Syndrome

Metabolic syndrome involves a clustering of metabolic risk factors including hyperglycemia (or current blood glucose medication use), elevated BP (or current HTN medication use), dyslipidemia (or current lipid-lowering medication use), and central adiposity based on waist circumference (29,30). Causes for the metabolic syndrome are multifactorial where genetics and health behavior are critical components. Mortality rates caused by CVD are substantially higher in those individuals with metabolic syndrome (31).

Pulmonary Diseases

Most pulmonary diseases are grouped into two categories: chronic obstructive pulmonary diseases (COPDs) and chronic restrictive pulmonary diseases (CRPDs). However, patients with pulmonary disease can present a multitude of unique challenges for exercise therapy and therefore are typically referred to more specialized pulmonary care clinics.

Chronic Obstructive Pulmonary Disease

COPD is an umbrella term for a collection of pulmonary diseases, including chronic bronchitis, emphysema, and asthma (Fig. 8.2) (6). COPD is characterized by progressive airflow limitations associated with an abnormal inflammatory lung response, limiting the lung's ability to move air during inhalation and exhalation (6). Chronic bronchitis is characterized by a cough lasting for at least 3 months (32), causing chronic pulmonary inflammation, which damages the bronchial lining and impedes lung function and airflow obstruction (33). Emphysema is the permanent enlargement of airspaces along with necrosis of alveolar walls, causing an accumulation of air in the lung tissue (9).

Since 2000, asthma rates have steadily increased in the United States with a 3% increase in cases per year and resulting in a prevalence of approximately 26 million people (34). Asthma consists of both inflammation and increased smooth muscle constriction in the lungs in response to various stimuli (35). Triggers for asthma include environmental, biochemical, autonomic, immunological, infectious, endocrine, exercise, and psychological factors (9). During an asthmatic episode, inflammatory mediators are released, bronchial smooth muscle spasms develop, edema builds up, and the production of mucus causes vascular congestion.

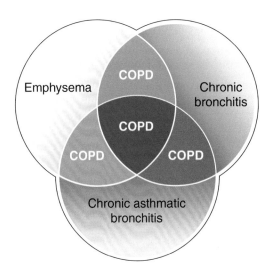

FIGURE 8.2. The relationships among emphysema, chronic bronchitis, chronic asthmatic bronchitis, and COPD. Most clients with COPD have a combination of these diseases. (From McConnell TH. *The Nature of Disease: Pathology for the Health Professions.* Philadelphia [PA]: Lippincott Williams & Wilkins; 2007. 739 p.)

Chronic Restrictive Pulmonary Disease

CRPDs are a large group of pulmonary disorders that are characterized by a reduction in lung volume (36). CRPDs are further categorized into two groups: extrinsic and intrinsic. As the name implies, extrinsic diseases have a restriction in lung volume that originates outside of the lungs, whereas intrinsic CRPDs have an issue specifically the lungs. Generally, extrinsic CRPD arises from weakness or atrophy in the muscles that control respiration (*e.g.*, myasthenia gravis, muscular dystrophy, or severe obesity). Intrinsic CRPDs are typically associated with stiffening of lung tissue (*e.g.*, pulmonary fibrosis, sarcoidosis, and interstitial lung disease). Clients with COPD or CRPD have limited gas exchange within the lungs, frequent shortness of breath, and difficulty breathing. The ACSM-EP's scope of practice does not include most aspects of pulmonary disease, given the unique physiological challenges of each disease. Therefore, individuals with most pulmonary disorders are referred to more specialized care. However, an important caveat to this assertion are asthmatic patients. In general, asthmatic patients are not considered high risk, respond well to exercise, and benefit from a consistent exercise programming (37).

Chronic Kidney Disease

CKD arises from complications with numerous diseases resulting in a change in the structure and functional ability of the kidneys (38,39). Typically, the glomeruli, tubules, interstitium, and blood vessels of the kidneys are damaged, leading to tissue scaring and ultimately a change in kidneys functionality. The best indicator of overall kidney function is glomerular filtration rate (GFR) and is defined as the total amount of fluid filtered through the nephrons per unit of time (40). International guidelines define CKD as a GFR of $<$60 mL $\cdot$ min^{-1} $\cdot$ 1.73 m^{-2}, or with blood markers of kidney damage such as elevated albumin levels, or both, for at least 3 months in duration (41). A GFR below 15 mL $\cdot$ min^{-1} $\cdot$ 1.73 m^{-2} is categorized end-stage kidney disease. At this point, kidney function in no longer able to sustain life, and other therapy options such as dialysis or kidney transplant area considered (38). CKD classification is often separated into three distinct stages: predialysis, receiving dialysis, and posttransplant. In clients with CKD, comorbidities such as CVD, diabetes, and HTN are common (39). The risk of comorbidities and overall health of renal patients has led ACSM to designating renal patients as high risk.

Role of Exercise Training

Exercise is known to have positive effects on both primary and secondary disease prevention/treatment (4,42). In 2010, nearly 50% of Americans had a chronic disease with over 30% having two or more chronic diseases (43). By 2020, the prevalence increased to nearly 60% of Americans having at least one chronic disease and 40% having two or more chronic diseases (44). Even considering the increased prevalence of disease, many people are unaware of the potential disease-altering benefits that exercise provides (45). Therefore, the ACSM-EP is in a unique position to use this knowledge for collective improvement of health through an appropriately exercise prescription.

Cardiovascular Diseases

Exercise training is beneficial for individuals with a history of or at high risk for an MI (2). Exercise has been shown to decrease coronary inflammatory markers (*e.g.*, C-reactive protein [CRP] and lipoprotein-associated phospholipase A2 [PLAC or Lp-PLA2]) (46), reduce stress, damage to the coronary arteries, increase new blood vessel growth (angiogenesis), and vascular regeneration, all factors promoting a faster MI recovery (47). Regular exercise also decreases blood platelet adhesiveness, fibrinogen levels, and blood viscosity, all of which reduce the risk of clotting and the likelihood for a second MI. In addition, regular exercise improves self-efficacy and psychosocial well-being (2). Patients who engage in exercise after an MI can restore their health to near or above pre-MI fitness status and are able to return their lives to a pre-MI state (2). For clients suffering from ischemia and at high MI risk, the effect of exercise can help reduce the risk of an initial MI while also raising the overall quality of life (6). Exercise may also prevent, slow, and even reverse atherosclerotic plaque development, allowing for an increase in the ischemic threshold during daily activities or exercise.

For individuals with PAD, regular exercise training may have a profound impact on alleviating claudication by increasing the ischemic threshold, allowing affected persons to work longer and at higher work intensities before exhibiting symptoms. Patients experience improvements in pain-free walking time (48), pain-free walking distance (49), and maximal walking distance (50). In addition, regular exercise in patients with PAD can improve ABI scores (51) and decrease mortality risk (52).

Endurance exercise does lower resting SBP and DBP values by 5–7 mm Hg in persons with HTN. For individuals at risk for developing HTN, endurance exercise is thought to slow BP

EXERCISE IS MEDICINE CONNECTION

Exe**R**cise is Medicine®

Milani RV, Lavie CJ, Mehra MR. Reduction in C-reactive protein through cardiac rehabilitation and exercise training. *J Am Coll Cardiol.* 2004;43(6):1056–61.

Milani and colleagues (2004) studied the effects of a 3-month formal phase II cardiac rehabilitation and exercise training program on CRP levels. The study consisted of two groups with the populations of both groups having diagnosed CAD. The exercise group underwent a 3-month phase II cardiac rehabilitation program, and the control group did not. Patients in the exercise group received formalized exercise instruction, met three times a week for a duration of an hour each session, and were encouraged to exercise on their own (one to three times a week) in between sessions. Patients also received individual and group counseling from a registered dietitian who stressed dietary management as recommended by the Adult Treatment Panel III guidelines and placed special emphasis on the Mediterranean diet. Results showed people who engaged in the cardiac rehabilitation program had significant decreases in the levels of CRP and blood triglycerides and a significant increase in HDL-C. Because many of the patients in the exercise group were also taking medications, the data were analyzed to determine whether the medications or the exercise (or a combination) caused reduced CRP levels. Also found was that patients taking a statin medication had significant decrease in CRP levels over the course of the rehabilitation program. Also, exercising patients who were not taking a statin medication showed the same decreases in CRP levels as the statin users. The authors reported the favorable effects of exercise training on CRP levels independent of statin therapy. This study demonstrates that therapeutic lifestyle modifications, promoted by a 3-month cardiac rehabilitation and dietary management can produce significant improvements in CRP levels and other cardiac risk factors, such as blood lipids, and can increase exercise capacity, which in turn can promote health and overall well-being.

rise and delay HTN development (53). Although not fully understood, possible mechanisms for exercise-induced BP reductions include an alteration in renal functioning, a decrease in plasma norepinephrine levels, and an increase in circulating vasodilator substances (14,54).

Metabolic Diseases

Patients with Type 2 diabetes gain health fitness benefits rather quickly once an exercise program is initiated. Perhaps the most beneficial aspect is the improved insulin sensitivity reported with exercise training (55,56), which may cause a lower medication requirement and greater control of blood glucose levels. In addition, if body fat is reduced as an indirect effect of exercise, further increases in insulin sensitivity are found (55,56).

Dyslipidemic clients engaging in physical activity and exercise reduce postprandial lipidemia or the amount of cholesterol in their blood after a meal (57). Exercise also provides a positive benefit on other blood lipid values by lowering blood concentrations of LDL-C and increasing concentrations of HDL-C (58–61).

The role of exercise in treating obesity is most effective when used in combination with caloric restriction (62,63). As expected, increased exercise training in an obese client promotes regional fat loss, especially abdominal fat deposits (28), which can also improve psychological well-being (28). However, even when reductions in body fat or weight do not occur, exercise participation will still produce other positive health fitness benefits (64). As an additional benefit, noticeable reductions in body weight and fat can increase self-image and self-esteem.

Risk factors associated with the metabolic syndrome are improved by engaging in physical activity and modifying dietary behaviors (65). Exercise is effective for lowering BP, blood glucose, and body mass while improving blood lipid levels. Treating individuals with the metabolic syndrome is consistent with guidelines for healthy adults. Generally, both aerobic and resistance exercises are recommended as part of the exercise prescription. However, cardiovascular risk factors must be considered by the ACSM-EP as each risk factor is for individually when designing the exercise prescription.

Ultimately, regular exercise yields improvement in many obesity comorbidities, including lowered BP, improved glucose tolerance, reduced triglyceride levels, and decreased CAD risk factors (66). The ACSM-EP is expected to understand the basic mechanisms involved in these positive changes to better prescribe individual exercise to each client.

Pulmonary Diseases

The scientific literature is mixed regarding the role exercise plays in reducing the pathologies of pulmonary diseases (67). Although exercise does not cure pulmonary diseases, a noticeable increase in quality of life is observed in the pulmonary client. In fact, the overall benefit of exercise allows the pulmonary client to exercise longer at higher exercise intensities (68).

Chronic Kidney Disease

Historically, exercise as a therapy for CKD has been largely overlooked, and as a result, rehabilitation programs and the impact of exercise in the scientific literature fall far behind that of cardiovascular and pulmonary diseases (69). Presently, the scientific knowledge concerning the impact of exercise on CKD has increased with many studies supporting a positive impact on health, specifically in reducing risk factors associated with CVD. Exercise in patients with CKD lowers SBP and DBP (70), reduces the number of antihypertensive drugs required to control HTN (71), and lowers resting HR (72). Patients with CKD often experience muscle wasting or cachexia (73), and resistance exercise can increase muscular strength in the predialysis (74), dialysis (74), and transplant populations (75). Literature on the impact of exercise on kidney function is mixed (76), but resistance exercise when combined with a low-protein diet may result in a slower decline in GFR (77).

The Art and Science of Exercise Prescription and Programming in Controlled Disease Populations

A "one-size-fits-all" approach is not an effective method to creating exercise prescriptions or programs. Rather, the successful ACSM-EP should create specific and individualized programs to meet the client's needs and health goals, especially when referring to patients suffering from chronic diseases.

The body of scientific information regarding exercise prescription for individuals with chronic disease has increased significantly in the past 25 years (1,78). Nevertheless, the application of these principles should not be completed in an exceedingly rigid and precise fashion. Rather, the procedures presented in this chapter are only principles and should be used with flexibility and careful attention to the contraindications, limitations, health history, and goals of the individual. Because exercise responses and adaptations vary considerably across individuals, and particularly in those individuals with chronic disease, the ACSM-EP must be prepared to modify exercise prescriptions accordingly. The ACSM-EP uses the basic scientific process, knows the individual's specific needs, and develops and implements an appropriate exercise prescription with an overarching goal of promoting a more physically active lifestyle.

Chronic diseases present unique and challenging limitations for the ACSM-EP in developing an appropriate exercise program. ACSM-EPs must be aware of such limitations and use scientific principles in conjunction with their own experiences to adapt and implement a properly designed exercise prescription that is effective in optimizing health fitness benefits and ensures safety. Thus, the ACSM-EP must recognize the process of making an exercise prescription is an art as well as a science.

Special FITT Considerations for Persons with Chronic Diseases

Clients with cardiovascular, metabolic, pulmonary, or CKD need to include physical activity and exercise as part of their lifestyle. The ACSM recommends the use of the FITT principle. However, an important note is that total exercise volume and progression of exercise programming are extremely important in an individual with chronic disease. Many individuals may only be able to maintain minimal volumes of exercise and must progress to improve their condition (1). However, when considering chronic disease populations presented in this chapter, the focus of the "FITT" components is discussed more thoroughly with each disease. The ACSM-EP must be diligent in using the FITT principle carefully to develop an individualized exercise program, ensuring patient safety while maximizing functional capacity, and developing optimal health fitness benefits. Tables 8.1 and 8.2 present general aerobic and resistance exercise guidelines for patients diagnosed with chronic diseases, respectively.

High-Intensity Interval Training

High-intensity interval training (HIIT) is an exercise training protocol consisting of alternating high- and low-intensity exercise intervals with an underlying premise that participants complete greater exercise volumes at a higher intensity than during sustained, continuous exercise (79–82). HIIT programming is flexible and allows for the adjustment of duration and intensity of both the high- and low-intensity exercise intervals, generally altered to meet individual fitness levels and goals. The high-intensity periods are typically 80%–90% of heart rate reserve (HRR), with the low-intensity intervals roughly 60%–70% of HRR. HIIT is an effective exercise training method

Table 8.1	General Aerobic Training Guidelines to Be Applied in the Effective Development of Exercise Prescriptions for the Treatment of a Population with Chronic Disease
Frequency (d · wk^{-1})	CVD: 3–7 (3 d if all are vigorous)
	PAD: 3–5
	DM: 3–7
	Pulmonary: 3–5
	CKD: 3–5
Intensity	CVD: moderate 40%–59% HRR or RPE <11–14 (6–20 scale); vigorous 60%–89% HRR; or deconditioned 30%–39% HRR
	PAD: 40%–59% $\dot{V}O_2$ reserve or to the exercise intensity in which the patient experiences moderate pain (*e.g.*, 3–4 out of 5 points on the claudication pain scale)
	DM: 50%–80% HRR or RPE = 12–16 (6–20 scale)
	Pulmonary: prescribed on an individual basis, based on GXT with scale for dyspnea
	CKD: 40%–59% $\dot{V}O_2$ reserve or RPE = 12–13 (6–20 scale)
Time	CVD: achieve 1,500–2,000 kcal of energy expenditure each week or 20–60 min per session
	PAD: 30–50 min per session (excluding rest periods)
	DM: 20–60 min per session
	At least 150 min · wk^{-1} at moderate intensity (*e.g.*, 600 METs · min · wk^{-1}) or 90 min · wk^{-1} at vigorous intensity (*e.g.*, 540 METs · min · wk^{-1})
	Pulmonary: 20–60 min a session
	CKD: 20–60 of continuous activity, can use 3- to 5-min bouts to accumulate 20–60 min · d^{-1} if needed
Type	CVD: large dynamic muscle group exercises
	PAD: weight bearing: walking or treadmill
	DM: walk, bicycle, jogging, water aerobics activities
	Pulmonary: Walking and cycling are most strongly recommended.
	CKD: rhythmic activities using large muscle groups

GXT, graded exercise test; METs, metabolic equivalents.

Data from Cooper CB. Exercise in chronic pulmonary disease: aerobic exercise prescription. *Med Sci Sports Exerc*. 2001;33(7 suppl): S671–9; Liguori G. *ACSM's Guidelines for Exercise Testing and Prescription*. 11th ed. Philadelphia (PA): Wolters Kluwer; 2021; Rooke TW, Hirsch AT, Misra S, et al. 2011 ACCF/AHA Focused Update of the Guideline for the Management of Patients With Peripheral Artery Disease (updating the 2005 guideline): a report of the American College of Cardiology Foundation/American Heart Association Task Force on Practice. *J Am Coll Cardiol*. 2011;58(19):2020–45; Schairer JR. Exercise prescription in patients with cardiovascular disease. In: Swain DP, editor. *ACSM's Resource Manual for Guidelines for Exercise Testing and Prescription*. 7th ed. Philadelphia (PA): Lippincott Williams & Wilkins; 2014. p. 624; Verity L. Exercise prescription in patients with diabetes. In: Ehrman J, editor. *ACSM's Resource Manual for Guidelines for Exercise Testing and Prescription*. 6th ed. Philadelphia (PA): Lippincott Williams & Wilkins; 2010. p. 600–17.

producing beneficial changes in various physiological, performance, and health-related factors, which are similar or superior to those improvements reported for steady-state moderate-intensity continuous exercise training (79–81). The use of HIIT also provides functional benefits for clients with chronic diseases and is a valuable tool of every comprehensive medical management plan (80,83). HIIT improves health-related factors such as exercise capacity and quality of life for CVD (84,85), pulmonary disease (86,87), and diabetes (88,89). The use of HIIT protocols or any exercise

Table 8.2	General Resistance Training Guidelines to Be Applied in the Effective Development of Exercise Prescriptions for the Treatment of a Chronic Diseased Population
Frequency (d · wk^{-1})	CVD: 2–3
	PAD: 2–4, performed on nonconsecutive days
	DM: 2–3, performed on nonconsecutive days
	Pulmonary: 2–3 (4–5 d · wk^{-1} for respiratory muscles)
	CKD: 2–3
Intensity	CVD: 60%–80% 1-RM low to moderate
	PAD: 60%–80% 1-RM low to moderate
	RPE: ~14–16 (6–20 scale)
	DM: 50%–85% 1-RM low to moderate
	RPE: ~14–16 (6–20 scale)
	Pulmonary: 50%–80% 1-RM low to moderate
	RPE: ~12–15 (6–20 scale) (possibly lower depending on severity of COPD)
	CKD: 65%–75% 1-RM. Performance of 1-RM is not recommended unless medical clearance is obtained. ≥3-RM test can be used to estimate 1-RM value.
Time	CVD: 8–12 exercises
	1–4 sets per exercise
	PAD: 8–12 exercise
	1–3 set per exercise, 10–15 repetitions
	DM: 8–12 exercises
	2–3 sets per exercise
	Pulmonary: 8–12 exercises
	2–3 sets per exercise
Type	CVD: elastic bands, light (1–5 lb) hand weights, light free weights with wall pulleys, and machines
	PAD: all major muscle groups; emphasis on lower limbs if time is limited
	DM: all major muscle groups
	Upper body: 4–5 exercises
	Lower body: 4–5 exercises
	Pulmonary: free weights, elastic bands, body weight exercises, and machine exercises
	CKD: 8–10 exercises
	Minimum 1 set with goal of multiple sets; 10–15 repetitions

Data from Cooper CB. Exercise in chronic pulmonary disease: aerobic exercise prescription. *Med Sci Sports Exerc.* 2001;33(7 suppl): S671–9; Liguori G. *ACSM's Guidelines for Exercise Testing and Prescription.* 11th ed. Philadelphia (PA): Wolters Kluwer; 2021; Rooke TW, Hirsch AT, Mirsa S, et al. ACC/AHA Focused Update of the Guideline for the Management of Patients with Peripheral Artery Disease (updating the 2005 guideline): a report of the American College of Cardiology Foundation/American Heart Association Task Force on Practice. *J Am Coll Cardiol.* 2011;58(19):2020–45; Schairer JR. Exercise prescription in patients with cardiovascular disease. In: Swain DP, editor. *ACSM's Resource Manual for Guidelines for Exercise Testing and Prescription.* 7th ed. Philadelphia (PA): Lippincott Williams & Wilkins; 2014. p. 624; Verity L. Exercise prescription in patients with diabetes. In: Ehrman J, editor. *ACSM's Resource Manual for Guidelines for Exercise Testing and Prescription.* 6th ed. Philadelphia (PA): Lippincott Williams & Wilkins; 2010. p. 600–17; Johansen KL, Painter P. Exercise in individuals with CKD. *Am J Kidney Dis.* 2012;59(1):126–34.

programming does require medical concern for client safety. However, existing scientific evidence supports that HIIT presents little risk for stable clients with a chronic health disease when exercise protocols are followed (82,84–86,88).

Cardiovascular Disease

CVD pathology is associated with reduced functional capacity and exercise tolerance, and in general, patients with CVD have higher sedentary rates than most other individuals (42). In addition, other factors such as medications (*e.g.*, β-blockers, β-adrenergic blocking agents, central α_2-agonists, nitrates, nitroglycerin, calcium channel blockers [CCBs], cardiac glycosides, and angiotensin-converting enzyme [ACE] inhibitors), intermittent claudication, and angina due to myocardial ischemia all impact the application of the FITT principle when developing an exercise prescription for clients with CVD.

Some clients with CVD may choose to enroll in a cardiac rehabilitation program to initiate an exercise program. Cardiac rehabilitation programming reduces disease symptoms and risk of a second cardiovascular event (90). However, regardless of the exercise setting, the ACSM-EP can safely prescribe exercise in a stable client with CVD. Exercise frequency is usually prescribed as 5 or more days each week. In a very low fit person, multiple daily exercise periods lasting as little as 10 minutes and totaling at least 30 minutes could provide numerous health benefits. Clients with CVD usually have limited functional capacities; therefore, shorter exercise periods of 10–15 minutes performed two or three times each day may be useful and improve exercise tolerance. In addition, intermittent work (alternating higher and lower intensity exercise) is useful (42). When making lifestyle modifications to include physical activity and exercise, clients with CVD may experience concerns regarding program adherence and motivation. The ACSM-EP has a significant role in helping facilitate motivation and support the program adherence. Refer to Chapters 11 and 12 for client behavioral adaptations and changes.

Typically, exercise intensity is measured as a percentage of oxygen volume consumed per unit of time ($\dot{V}O_2$ reserve) or HRR; however, using these variables may be difficult in many CVD cases because of the effect of HR-modifying medications and/or HR-altering medical conditions. In these cases, rating of perceived exertion (RPE) as an alternative measurement of exercise intensity is useful. Exercise intensity is always prescribed below the myocardial ischemic threshold; however, any client experiencing ischemia should exercise in the presence of someone with more specific training.

Exercise duration varies with the disease severity. The overall exercise goal for clients with CVD is to progress to 60 minutes of aerobic conditioning per day. However, starting with shorter exercise duration is often necessary (10- to 15-min periods). When a shorter duration is initially applied, a progression of 1–5 minutes per session depending on individual exercise tolerance is recommended (42).

Resistance training also offers health fitness benefits beyond that of aerobic conditioning alone. The use of the FITT principle for resistance training is beneficial for the client with CVD when compared to the general population. However, ensure that contraindications before beginning the program are considered. Note that most cardiac patients will likely start at a low level. Therefore, potential exercise equipment for completing these exercises includes elastic bands, light (1–5 lb) hand weights, light free weights with wall pulleys, and exercise machines. Refer to Chapter 4 for more information on resistance training programming.

Metabolic Disease

When compared with other metabolic diseases, clients with Type 2 diabetes receive the most benefit by incorporating physical activity and exercise as part of their management plan (55). In addition, Type 2 diabetes is currently the most common metabolic disorder in the world (91). Therefore, this section focuses on exercise prescriptions for those with Type 2 diabetes. The ACSM-EP can safely work with clients if their Type 2 diabetes is well controlled. However, the ACSM recommends that any individual with diabetes whose condition is uncontrolled or has been sedentary should be referred to a physician prior to starting an exercise program independent of desired intensity. In addition, if a client with Type 2 diabetes continues to experience frequent uncontrolled changes in blood glucose levels, he or she should be referred to a health care professional and encouraged to exercise under the supervision of more skilled personnel. When developing an exercise prescription for the client with Type 2 diabetes, an important consideration is often the need to reduce overall body fat. However, if the client is taking a glycemic lowering agent, blood glucose can potentially drop beyond a safe level when combining medication with exercise (1,55,56). The ACSM-EP must therefore balance the appropriate exercise prescription with the effect of the medication to avoid any diabetes-related complications (1).

Because weight loss is so important in most individuals with Type 2 diabetes, special consideration is given to physical activity and exercise volume and frequency to maximize weight loss (92). Being physically active and exercising $3–7 \text{ d} \cdot \text{wk}^{-1}$ is recommended for individuals with Type 2 diabetes (1). Exercise intensity usually ranges between 50% and 80% HRR and $\dot{V}O_2$ reserve and corresponds to an RPE of 12–16 (1). Exercise duration will depend on the fitness level and exercise tolerance of the client. Most individuals with Type 2 diabetes can begin with a daily accumulation of 20 minutes with the ultimate goal of progressing to 60 minutes of daily aerobic conditioning. The time for a client to reach 60 minutes of daily accumulated exercise variables and may take weeks or months. Similar to clients with CVD, multiple daily physically activity or exercise periods of 10 minutes or more may be used as well as the use of intermittent work or HIIT (lower exercise intensity mixed with higher exercise intensity). The overall goal is to obtain the health fitness benefits associated with 150–300 minutes of total physical activity and exercise each week (4). Aerobic exercise emphasizing the rhythmic motion of large muscle groups is recommended, although the type of exercise chosen should reflect the individual's interest and goals.

Resistance training for clients with diabetes is recommended if there is an absence of contraindications such as retinopathy and recent laser treatment (1). Exercise frequency and intensity recommendations for diabetics are no different from those recommendations used for healthy sedentary individuals. Exercise intensity is set at 50%–85% of one repetition maximum (1-RM) with one to three sets of 10–15 repetitions (1,56). Exercise duration is usually set at 8–10 multiple-joint exercises involving most if not all major muscle groups and is often performed in one whole-body session or split into multiple sessions (1). Exercise type or mode is based on the presence of exercise limitations and includes free weights, elastic bands, body weight exercises, and any variety of machines.

In addition, individuals with diabetes must always wear medical identification. Maintaining proper foot care to reduce foot sores and blisters is vital especially in clients with peripheral neuropathy. Foot sores and blisters are more likely to become infected and result in more serious complications due to the lack of feeling in the lower extremities. Exercising clients with diabetes must have an available source of easily ingestible carbohydrates. Exercising with a partner is often recommended for individuals with diabetes. Finally, exercise in the early evening should be completed with caution as exercising at this time could cause hypoglycemic conditions later in the night and could lead to dire consequences (93).

Pulmonary Disease

Clients with advanced stages of COPD or CRPD are especially unique among the chronic diseases presented in this chapter (32,94). In most cases, these clients are unlikely to ever fully vanquish their symptoms, and their functional capacity and exercise tolerance will progressively become more restricted (32). The scope of practice for the ACSM-EP does not warrant working with this population and instead encourages referral to the appropriate health care personnel.

The ACSM-EP is prepared to work with clients with well-controlled asthma and should encourage these individuals to perform aerobic exercise at least $3–5 \text{ d} \cdot \text{wk}^{-1}$. Unfortunately, a consensus does not exist regarding the optimal aerobic intensity for the client with asthma, and therefore, guidelines for older adults are often used (see Chapter 10). Another guiding technique used in developing appropriate exercise intensity is the use of the dyspnea scale rating which focuses on a value in the range of 4–6 on a scale of 0–10. For the client with pulmonary disease, exercise recommendations are to obtain at least 20 minutes each session and, in the long term, move progressively toward 60 minutes of continuous or intermittent physical aerobic conditioning.

Chronic Kidney Disease

Clients with CKD possess several challenges for the ACSM-EP in developing a proper exercise prescription. The CKD population is often diagnosed with other pathologies such as cardiovascular and metabolic diseases; as a result, the ACSM-EP needs to be vigilant in identifying all barriers to exercise in this population. An ideal FITT principle for clients with CKD has not been fully developed but modifying the recommendations for the general population to meet the needs of this unique population is warranted (1).

Clients with CKD tend to be sedentary, so continuous aerobic exercise may be difficult to achieve. The use of intermittent exercise with 3 minutes of exercise followed by 3 minutes of rest is beneficial. As the client adapts, the amount of time spent exercising can increase, and the rest periods can decrease. Most importantly, the client with CKD should be instructed to reduce the daily time spent doing sedentary behaviors (95).

For resistance exercise, the FITT guidelines for clients with CKD are similar to individuals with CVD and metabolic diseases. Special consideration is warranted when prescribing the proper weight for exercises as a 1-RM test is often not performed in this population. The ACSM-EP should consider other submaximal effort tests when assessing strength and prescribing the proper exercise intensity.

Effects of Myocardial Ischemia, Myocardial Infarction, and Hypertension on Cardiorespiratory Responses during Exercise

CVD continues to be the leading cause of death in the United States for men and women alike (96–98). The prevalence of CVD continues to rise even as medical technology finds new ways to improve overall survival rates (26). An MI survivor has likely a significant level of myocardial ischemia as one key predisposing factor and a limited exercise tolerance and functional capacity.

HTN is a common disorder with a prevalence of about 1 in 3 adults reported in the United States (26). Although HTN may go undetected for many years, this disease possesses medical considerations when physical activity and exercise are performed. Therefore, because of the high prevalence of CVD and HTN, the ACSM-EP must be keenly aware of these conditions, their etiology, and their impact on an individual's exercise and functional performance.

Myocardial Ischemia

Myocardial ischemia indicates a shortage of oxygenated blood flow to the heart myocardium. The prevalence of ischemia in the United States is approximately 7%, although the proportion of individuals suffering from ischemia increases with age. Ischemia is an imbalance of oxygen supply and demand. Impaired blood supply is a result of several mechanisms, the most common being atherosclerosis, congestive heart failure (CHF), or both. Oxygen demand is elevated dramatically during physical or emotional exertion. If oxygen supply fails to meet an increased demand, even briefly, then ischemia is present. If ischemia is prolonged, then any viable myocardium becomes at risk for necrosis and infarction. Oftentimes, ischemia is associated with chest discomfort/pain or angina.

In a typical exercise session, myocardial oxygen demand is increased, which is met by an increased frequency and vigor of the heart pumping action. This linear relationship between oxygen demand and HR continues until an individual reaches maximum exercise capacity. However, in the client with ischemia, maximum exercise capacity is limited by insufficient myocardial oxygen supply. If oxygen delivery to target muscle is impaired, such as in the case of CHF or atherosclerosis, exercise capacity is limited, and the client will reach the "ischemic threshold" sooner. Avoiding this ischemic threshold is a critical concern in prescribing exercise. However, as previously stated, any client experiencing ischemia should exercise in the presence of someone with more specific training.

Myocardial Infarction

An MI occurs when prolonged ischemia causes heart tissue death or necrosis (7). The ischemia duration necessary to produce an infarct varies; therefore, the ACSM-EP must design exercise prescriptions that safely avoid the ischemic threshold or the HR at which angina symptoms develop. Also, because necrosis is caused by the loss of heart tissue, any necrosis will negatively impact the movement of an action potential throughout the heart and reduce the contractile state of the heart, lowering ejection fraction, and limiting exercise capacity and tolerance (99).

Initiating exercise in the patient with post-MI should be approached with caution. Known exercise benefits for clients after an MI include reducing the likelihood for a second infarct, decreasing time to return to work, increasing overall functional capacity, and improving self-efficacy (100).

Although post-MI exercise is relatively safe, including vigorous exercise, the ACSM-EP must understand each client's exercise limitations and myocardial oxygen supply. Therefore, the initiation of exercise programming is appropriate only after gaining medical clearance and physician approval for independent exercise. The ACSM-EP likely will work with this type of patient after completing a supervised program of cardiac rehabilitation under the guidance of the medical community and exercise professionals.

Hypertension

Daily physical activity and exercise is part of the treatment for HTN, although such programming should be implemented with caution (101). Normally, a single exercise session causes a linear increase in SBP while a steady constant DBP is maintained (102). In the hypertensive person, it is possible to exhibit an exaggerated BP response during exercise, at relatively low exercise intensities, even if resting BP is controlled (103,104). This dramatic increase in arterial pressure puts undue pressure on the arterial intima, which increases the likelihood of dislodging atherosclerotic plaques and/or thrombi that typically precipitate an MI or a stroke. In addition, repeated periods of high-intensity exercise could further exacerbate endothelial damage.

Given the potential concerns associated with exercise and HTN, the ACSM-EP must be aware of and follow guidelines for initiating and terminating exercise in the client with HTN. By adhering to these standards, the ACSM-EP can guide the client to the safe use of regular physical activity and exercise as an important adjunct to any pharmaceutical therapy in managing BP.

Exercise Concerns, Precautions, and Contraindications

Cardiovascular Disease

The information found in Table 8.3 presents the clinical indications and contraindications for patients in cardiac rehabilitation (inpatient and outpatient). This information and the following summarized points are meant to help the ACSM-EP develop and implement a safe exercise prescription as discussed in this chapter.

- As with any chronic disease, the ACSM-EP must foster a safe environment that facilitates clients' understanding of their disease and exercise limitations.
- Before starting exercise, clients must have the knowledge to define and treat angina, identify CVD symptoms and provoking factors, and understand individual exercise tolerance limits (90).

Table 8.3	Clinical Indications and Contraindications for Inpatient and Outpatient Cardiac Rehabilitation

Indications	Contraindications
■ Medically stable after MI	■ Unstable angina
■ Stable angina	■ Uncontrolled HTN (resting SBP >180 mm Hg and/or resting DBP >110 mm Hg)
■ Coronary artery bypass graft surgery	■ Orthostatic BP drop of >20 mm Hg with symptoms
■ Percutaneous transluminal coronary angioplasty or other transcatheter procedure	■ Significant aortic stenosis (aortic valve orifice area of <1.0 cm² in an average-sized adult)
■ Stable heart failure	■ Acute systemic illness or fever
■ Cardiomyopathy	■ Uncontrolled atrial or ventricular dysrhythmias
■ Heart and/or other organ transplantation	■ Uncontrolled sinus tachycardia (>120 bpm)
■ Other cardiac surgery, including valvular and pacemaker insertion (including implantable cardioverter defibrillator)	■ Uncompensated CHF
	■ Third-degree atrioventricular block without pacemaker
■ Peripheral arterial disease	■ Active pericarditis or myocarditis
■ At risk for CAD with diagnoses of diabetes, dyslipidemia, HTN, obesity, or other diseases and conditions	■ Recent embolism
	■ Thrombophlebitis
	■ Aortic dissection
■ Other patients who may benefit from structured exercise and/or patient education based on physician referral and consensus of the rehabilitation team	■ Resting ST-segment depression or elevation (>2 mm)
	■ Uncontrolled diabetes
	■ Severe orthopedic conditions that would prohibit exercise
	■ Other metabolic conditions, such as acute thyroiditis, hypokalemia, hyperkalemia, or hypovolemia

By knowing this information, clients can better understand their disease, exercise limits, and health implications while fostering safe exercise.

■ A goal for primary exercise programming is to reduce disease risk for the client with CVD and increase the ease in completing activities of daily living. Exercise training will increase functional capacity and exercise tolerance and reduce the likelihood of another cardiovascular event (90).

■ The early stages of the exercise prescription usually begin with the use of lower, more conservative exercise intensities, usually 10–15 heartbeats per minute below the ischemic threshold (105). Although a lower exercise intensity is less than optimal for maximizing cardiorespiratory fitness and optimizing health fitness benefits, increased functional capacity and reduced CVD risk are still achieved (6).

■ As fitness levels and exercise tolerance improve, the ischemic threshold is increased, and exercise intensity can also be increased.

■ The client with controlled HTN can exercise (101). In the presence of uncontrolled HTN (>180/110 mm Hg), exercise is only enforced after initiating drug therapy (106). For resting SBP greater than 180 mm Hg or resting DBP greater than 110 mm Hg, exercise is contraindicated until BP is under control, even if BP medications are being taken (101).

■ During exercise, if SBP becomes greater than 220 mm Hg or DBP greater than 105 mm Hg, exercise is discontinued to allow BP to return toward resting values (107). The next exercise period is completed at lower exercise intensity to ensure BP stays below 220/105 mm Hg (107).

■ Many HTN medications present unique challenges for the ACSM-EP in prescribing proper exercise. For example, β-blockers can attenuate the HR response by as much as 30 bpm and

HOW TO: Initiate Exercise in a Patient with Coronary Artery Disease in Lieu of a Graded Exercise Test

Equipment Needed

1. BP monitoring equipment: stethoscope and BP cuff (sphygmomanometer)
2. Electrocardiogram (ECG) monitoring unit (3- or 12-lead)
3. RPE chart
4. Exercise equipment (*i.e.*, treadmill, recumbent cycle, elliptical)

Important Information and Tips

1. The results of a graded exercise test (GXT) is a valuable tool in the initiation of an exercise prescription (19). However, in certain cases, a GXT may not have been previously administered. Yet, even without the GXT results, a safe and effective exercise prescription can be developed.

2. Reasons for not performing a GXT before starting an exercise prescription include extreme deconditioning, orthopedic limitations, recent successful percutaneous intervention, and uncomplicated or stable MI (29).

3. Because the client's response to exercise is not documented, client safety is of utmost concern, and the exercise prescription should reflect this. Initiation of exercise at a low intensity, slow exercise intensity progression, and constant monitoring of physiological symptoms help ensure client safety.

Example of an Exercise Prescription

FITT framework for a patient with CAD without a GXT (1,29)

1. Frequency: minimum 3 d · wk^{-1} with additional walking on the days off
   a. Intensity: 2–3 metabolic equivalents (METs)
   b. HR: 20–30 bpm above resting value
2. RPE: 11–14
3. Time: Begin with 3- to 5-min intervals. Allow for adequate rest and recovery between intervals. Aim for an overall exercise duration of 30–45 min.
4. Type: low-intensity modes of exercise
   a. Treadmill (0% grade, low speed)
   b. Cycle ergometer
   c. Arm ergometer
   d. Elliptical
5. Progression: 1–2 METs as tolerated by the client
6. Monitoring: ECG, BP, RPE, and signs or symptoms of ischemia

References

1. American College of Sports Medicine. *ACSM's Guidelines for Exercise Testing and Prescription*. 11th ed. Philadelphia (PA): Wolters Kluwer; 2022. 548 p.
2. McConnell TR. Exercise prescription when the guidelines do not work. *J Cardiopulm Rehabil*. 1996;16(1):34–7.
3. McConnell TR, Klinger TA, Gardner JK, Laubach CA, Herman CE, Hauck CA. Cardiac rehabilitation without exercise tests for post-myocardial infarction and post-bypass surgery patients. *J Cardiopulm Rehabil*. 1998;18(6):458–63.

Suggested Readings

ACMS's Clinical Exercise Physiology — provides research-based applications on numerous disease states and covers elements such as screening, pharmacology, and electrography
ACSM's Exercise Management for Persons with Chronic Diseases and Disabilities — provides detailed overview on the approach on the proper development of an exercise prescription for persons in a diseased state
Pollock's Textbook of Cardiovascular Disease and Rehabilitation — provides comprehensive and detailed descriptions of the pathological effects of CAD and effects on the exercise response

may result in the need for using an RPE scale or "beats above resting" as alternative methods for prescribing exercise intensity. Clients taking these medications are advised to have longer cool-down periods, where BP is monitored to ensure the avoidance of unsafe levels (101).

- The use of a claudication pain perception scale is useful when working with the PAD population. A typical 0–4 scale is commonly employed with ratings of 0 = no pain, 1 = onset of pain, 2 = moderate pain, 3 = intense pain, and 4 = maximal pain. Along with the severity of claudication experienced, the time and distance to the onset of symptoms to maximal pain should also be recorded (1).
- In more severe cases of PAD, some clients may need to begin exercising for only a total of 15 min · d^{-1} with gradual increases of 5 min · d^{-1} every 2–4 weeks depending on individual progression (108).
- In persons with PAD, the client may need additional breaks after the onset of severe claudication symptoms. A specific rest-to-work ratio will need to be tailored and continually modified for every client (1).
- Non–weight-bearing exercises, such as cycling, may be used as a warm-up modality but should not be the primary type of activity prescribed to this population (1).
- A cold environment may aggravate symptoms of intermittent claudication. Therefore, a longer warm-up may be needed for persons with PAD (109).

Metabolic Disease

Under normal conditions, blood glucose homeostasis is maintained by a precise coordination of hormones and metabolic events. Diabetes interrupts this delicate balance, and individuals with diabetes do not always respond normally to exercise. Nonetheless, patients with diabetes can exercise but with precaution. Because diabetes does cause complications in multiple body systems, the ACSM-EP must consider the presence and severity of diabetes and associated complications, medication regimens, and the schedule for these medications to ensure client safety.

- Patients with diabetes need constant blood glucose monitoring and the ability to measure before, during, and after exercise (56).
- A readily available source of carbohydrate, such as fruit juice or hard candy, should be available if needed to increase blood glucose levels (110).
- If blood glucose measurements before or during exercise are less than 70 mg · dL^{-1}, a carbohydrate snack (15 g) is administered, and a blood glucose reading of greater than 100 mg · dL^{-1} is obtained before starting or continuing exercise (110).
- When preexercise blood glucose values are greater than 250 mg · dL^{-1} with the presence of blood ketones or are greater than 300 mg · dL^{-1} with or without the presence of ketones, blood glucose should be lowered prior to initiating exercise (55). However, provided the client feels well and is adequately hydrated and ketones are not present, postponing exercise is not compulsory based solely on hyperglycemia (60).
- When an active retinal hemorrhage is present or recent laser corrective surgery for retinopathy is completed, exercise is avoided. Postponing exercise will limit the risk of triggering vitreous hemorrhage and retinal detachment (110).
- Because clients with diabetes experience a slower healing process, good foot care is accomplished by inspecting feet before and after exercise and by wearing proper shoes and cotton socks to avoid foot sores and blisters.
- Exercise with a partner or under the supervision of an ACSM-EP to reduce the risk of problems associated with hypoglycemic events (56).
- Consideration is always given to timing exercise with the taking of insulin or hypoglycemic agents. Exercise is not recommended during peak insulin action because hypoglycemia

may result. Because delayed postexercise hypoglycemia is a known risk, evening exercising is not recommended.

- Always carry medical identification.
- The ACSM-EP must use conservative practices according to each CVD and diabetic risk factor present in individuals with the metabolic syndrome. Refer to the other bullet points regarding each CVD and diabetic risk factors to help guide the exercise prescription.

Dyslipidemia presents few, if any, exercise limitations, and individuals with elevated blood lipid and lipoprotein levels are encouraged to engage in regular physical activity and exercise. To optimize blood lipid concentrations, clients with dyslipidemia are encouraged to exercise for longer durations (59). Presently, clients with dyslipidemia are recommended to set a short-term goal of $150 \, \text{min} \cdot \text{wk}^{-1}$, a long-term goal of greater than $300 \, \text{min} \cdot \text{wk}^{-1}$, and to expend more than 2,000 kcal of expenditure a week (2,111). Both short- and long-term goals are best achieved by exercising $5 \, \text{d} \cdot \text{wk}^{-1}$ or more and, in some cases, by incorporating physical activity and exercise in multiple daily episodes. In general, most lipid-lowering drugs have no impact on exercise responses.

Obesity continues as a growing global health concern (112,113). Both reducing energy intake by dietary restriction and increasing energy expenditure by exercise are targeted interventions for treating obesity (113,114).

- Individuals who are obese are often at risk for other chronic diseases, and these individuals can need additional medical screening and appropriate supervision for exercise testing and programming.
- Individuals who are obese are recommended to engage in moderate physical activity at least 5, if not all, days of the week and progress to accumulating more than 2,000 kcal a week of energy expenditure.
- Because clients who are obese are at an increased risk for orthopedic injury and are usually in a deconditioned state, the exercise prescription should emphasize the use of low-impact or non–weight-bearing exercises such as the water-based, elliptical, and/or recumbent cycling. These types of low-impact exercises are recommended because of the reduced joint stress and the potential for less musculoskeletal injury.
- Because of possible low fitness levels, an exercise prescription that has a lower intensity and duration progression will likely have fewer injuries.
- Clients who are obese may have a propensity for low motivation and drive for making lifestyle change, and thus, additional motivational strategies are often required to help make these changes (114). Incorporating lifestyle strategies such as realistic goal setting and balance sheets is an effective way to provide positive reinforcement and helps develop motivation to start and adhere to lifestyle change.
- Additional considerations for clients who are obese include adequate flexibility, warm-up and cool-down periods, exercising in cool temperatures with low humidity, adequate hydration, and wearing loose-fitting clothing to allow for heat dissipation.

Pulmonary Disease

The primary goal when developing an exercise prescription for clients with COPD is to reduce barriers for activities of daily living and to help increase quality of life (67).

- Present scientific information is mixed whether exercise training has an impact on lessening the COPD state (115), but because exercise training improves muscle functionality, overall exercise tolerance is improved (67).
- Another exercise training goal for the client with COPD is desensitization to dyspnea — a condition characterized by shortness of breath that often limits exercise. The ACSM-EP must

EXERCISE IS MEDICINE CONNECTION

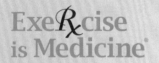

National Institute of Diabetes and Digestive and Kidney Diseases, National Institute of Health. Diabetes prevention program [Internet]. Bethesda (MA): National Institute of Diabetes and Digestive and Kidney Diseases; [cited 2021 Mar 25]. Available from: https://www.niddk.nih.gov/about-niddk/research-areas/diabetes/diabetes-prevention-program-dpp.

The U.S. Diabetes Prevention Program (DPP) was a multicenter trial that compared lifestyle modification with medication in the reduction in incidence of Type 2 diabetes. All participants ($N = 3,234$) at the start of the study were overweight and had either impaired glucose tolerance (IGT) or impaired fasting glucose (IFG). The main outcome measure was the development of Type 2 diabetes. Participants were randomly assigned to one of three groups: control, medication (metformin), or lifestyle modification. The lifestyle group included intensive dietary and physical activity modifications with a weight loss goal (5%–7% of current body weight) and 150 minutes of weekly aerobic activity. The lifestyle modification group reduced Type 2 diabetes incidence by 58%, and this reduction was true across all participating ethnic groups and for both men and women. The metformin group realized a 31% reduction in diabetes incidence and was effective for both men and women, but it was least effective in people aged 45 years and older.

The DPP study provide results indicating weight loss and physical activity lower the risk of Type 2 diabetes by improving the body's ability to use insulin and process glucose.

educate the client with COPD to push past this feeling. Once learned, exercise can continue even when dyspnea is increasing, and thus, greater exercise intensities and durations can be completed resulting in greater health fitness benefits (6,67).

- Early in the exercise program, the client with COPD will need constant monitoring until he or she is able to learn pulmonary triggering symptoms (115).
- To ensure safety, many clients with COPD will need constant oxyhemoglobin saturation monitoring. Blood oxygen saturation should be maintained at greater than 90% (67). However, those patients needing this type of monitoring should exercise with closer medical supervision, which the ACSM-EP is not trained to provide.
- Fast-acting inhalers are always kept available especially while exercising (115).
- A client with CRPD is treated in a similar fashion as a client with COPD because they have similar exercise limitations and considerations (68).
- Additional considerations for patients with COPD include optimal exercise training time being mid to late morning and avoiding extreme temperatures and high humidity as they can trigger symptoms and potentiate a medical incident (67).

Chronic Kidney Disease

Developing a safe and effective exercise prescription for the CKD population is difficult, especially if a client is in the dialysis or posttransplant stage of the disease. Many of the health benefits associated with exercise in this population are linked to reducing the risk or severity of CVD. Presently, no universally accepted exercise recommendations exist for this population, as a result, the ACSM-EP must practice extreme diligence when developing exercise programs for this population.

- Clients who have not participated in regular exercise training in the previous 3 months should be referred for medical clearance prior to starting an exercise program (1).
- In some clients with CKD, prolonged continuous exercise cannot be achieved. Exercise can consist of 1:1 work-to-rest intervals (*i.e.*, 3 min of exercise followed by 3 min of rest — a form of HIIT). Initially, a goal of 15 minutes of exercise be can used; this goal can be increased to 20–60 minutes of continuous exercise (1).
- Dialysis clients are recommended to wait 2 hours before engaging in exercise to allow energy levels to recover after treatment. If energy levels rebound quickly, clients can start exercising at their own discretion (1).
- Measure BP in the arm that does contain the arteriovenous fistula used for dialysis.
- For clients receiving peritoneal dialysis exercise can be performed with the dialysate fluid in their abdomen, but if exercise results in discomfort, the client should drain the fluid before the start of exercise (116).
- In posttransplant clients, exercise may be performed during periods of organ rejection, but exercise intensity should be reduced (117).

Effect of Common Medications on Exercise Capacity and Tolerance

Most individuals with any form of cardiovascular disease, metabolic disease, pulmonary disease, or CKD are likely to take one or more medications (Table 8.4). Whether medications are over-the-counter (OTC) or prescription, many medications impact the exercise response or exercise capacity. The expectation for the ACSM-EP is to have at least a cursory knowledge of the most common medications while keeping an updated drug reference guide handy. This preparation will allow the ACSM-EP to make appropriate and necessary adjustments in the exercise prescription while avoiding ischemic and/or other dangerous thresholds while providing a safe and effective exercise experience.

Over-the-Counter Drugs

OTC drug use is limited in treating individuals with a chronic disease. Aspirin, most commonly used for individuals with CVD, does not pose any concerns when prescribing exercise (87). The same is true with most herbs, natural remedies, and minerals prescribed for CVD, metabolic, or pulmonary diseases. Nonetheless, these preparations are not regulated by the U.S. Food and Drug Administration (FDA) and should be used with extreme caution. The greater risk of OTC medications is drug interaction, and the interactive effect these drugs can have on many chronic diseases. OTC cold and flu medications often contain some form of ephedrine that can increase systemic BP. These medications should be avoided or used cautiously in clients with CVD or HTN. When taken, consider postponing exercise for the day or adjusting exercise intensity and duration accordingly to avoid excessive BP increases.

Patients with diabetes should avoid any OTC drugs containing alcohol or sugar because these medications can affect blood glucose levels. In addition, two common nonsteroidal anti-inflammatory drugs (NSAIDs) — ibuprofen and naproxen — are used cautiously in patients with diabetes because both may increase the risk of hypoglycemia (53). Conflicting evidence exists regarding the effect of NSAIDs on BP; therefore, clients with HTN who are taking NSAIDs are monitored closely (118,119). OTC cough suppressants can impede "productive cough" and are used cautiously in certain patients with pulmonary disease, although the effect on exercise response is negligible.

Table 8.4	Common Medications		
Drug Name	**Mechanism**	**Rest/Exercise Response**	**Special Notes**
OTC cold and flu medication	Vary by class of medication	May effect resting and exercise BP and HR but varies by medication type No significant effect on exercise capacity	Often contain some form of ephedrine that has been shown to increase systemic BP. These medications should be avoided or used cautiously in clients with CVD or HTN. When taken, consider postponing exercise for the day or adjusting exercise intensity and duration accordingly to avoid excessive BP increases.
β-Blockers	Block β receptors May alter myocardial contractility depending on chronic condition	Increases exercise capacity with chronic use Decreased rest and exercise HR and BP	β-Blockers make setting initial exercise intensity difficult, may limit functional capacity, inhibit using HR as an exercise intensity target, and require more rigorous patient self-monitoring. β-Blockers may also block symptoms of hypoglycemia and increase the risk of undetected hypoglycemia during and after exercise.
CCBs and ACE inhibitors	Increase arterial diameter	Decreased rest and exercise BP No significant effect on exercise capacity	ACE inhibitors may produce an irritating dry cough. In these cases, refer client to physician.
Fibrates and statins	Vary by drug class	No significant effect on exercise capacity	Muscle soreness is an indication that a condition referred to as rhabdomyolysis might be evolving. When symptoms of this condition appear, the client should be referred to his or her physician. Clients taking this drug regimen and showing signs of this condition may need increased recovery time or lower exercise intensities.
Digitalis	Increases myocardial contractility	Increases exercise capacity May decrease resting HR Mediates arrhythmias	Can cause ST-segment depression at rest or during exercise
Diuretics	Increase renal water excretion	May increase resting HR May cause premature ventricular contractions (PVCs) May decrease exercise capacity	Individuals taking diuretics should monitor body weight daily. If weight changes considerably on a given day, physician should be advised prior to exercising.

Table 8.4	Common Medications (continued)		
Drug Name	**Mechanism**	**Rest/Exercise Response**	**Special Notes**
Oral medications for treating diabetes	Increase hepatic insulin output. Lower insulin resistance. Decrease absorption of carbohydrates	Minimal effect	The exerciser with diabetes needs to monitor blood glucose closely before, during, and after each exercise session.
NSAIDs	Inhibit COX-1 and/ or COX-2 to reduce inflammation	Conflicting reports, minimal effect	The impact of NSAIDs on the progression of CKD is equivocal. However, chronic exposure of NSAIDs should be avoided in the CKD population.
Proton pump inhibitors (PPI)	Inhibit gastric acid secretion	Minimal effect	PPI use is associated with a higher risk of CKD.

COX, cyclooxygenase.

Data from Ford ES, Giles WH, Dietz WH. Prevalence of the metabolic syndrome among us adults: findings from the third national health and nutrition examination survey. *JAMA*. 2002;287(3):356–9. doi:10.1001/jama.287.3.356; Gooch K, Culleton BF, Manns BJ, et al. NSAID use and progression of chronic kidney disease. *Am J Med*. 2007;120(3):280–e1; Lazarus B, Chen Y, Wilson FP, et al. Proton pump inhibitor use and the risk of chronic kidney disease. *JAMA*. 2016;176(2):238–246.

Prescription Drugs

Many prescription drugs are available to treat CVDs, metabolic diseases, pulmonary diseases, and CKDs, and many of these drugs impact exercise capacity. The most common CVD drugs include β-blockers, CCBs, ACE inhibitors, digitalis, diuretics, and cholesterol-lowering medications. These drug classes are especially common in treating persons with a history of MI, ischemia, and HTN (53,120).

β-Blockers are not only well known for decreasing mortality (121,122) and risk of a second MI (123–125) but also have a profound effect on exercise response. Although β-blockers lower HR and myocardial contractility, these medications may increase exercise capacity (126). This effect makes initial exercise intensity determination difficult, may limit functional capacity, can reduce the use of HR as an exercise intensity target, and requires more rigorous patient self-monitoring. β-Blockers may also block symptoms of hypoglycemia and increase the risk of undetected hypoglycemia during and after exercise.

CCBs (used for treating HTN and angina) and ACE inhibitors (used for treating HTN) both increase arterial diameter, thereby lessening BP and decreasing the work by the heart. CCB's effect is central, whereas ACE inhibitors have a peripheral effect. Although CCBs have some effect on HR and contractility, the extent of this effect is not as great as that found for β-blockers. Therefore, CCBs and ACE inhibitors pose less concern regarding exercise responses, but the ACSM-EP must be aware of unusual changes in BP or HR both before and during exercise. ACE inhibitors do work in the lungs and can produce an irritating dry cough; if this occurs, the ACSM-EP should refer the client to his or her physician.

Niacin and other cholesterol-lowering drugs tend to have very little effect on HR and contractility, and thus, no direct impact on exercise response and exercise capacity or the exercise prescription. Because the liver is the site of action of these drugs, liver function should be checked regularly. Statins alone or in combination with fibric acid are often associated with unusual muscle soreness (127). Muscle soreness potentially indicates the start of a condition referred to as rhabdomyolysis. When symptoms of this condition appear, the client should be referred to his or her physician. Clients taking this drug regimen and showing signs of this condition may need increased recovery time or lower exercise intensities.

Digitalis, commonly used in CHF and for certain persistent arrhythmias, increases contractility, slows HR, and mediates arrhythmias. In the patient with CHF, digitalis typically increases exercise capacity. On the other hand, digitalis can cause ST-segment depression at rest or during exercise, so this medication use should always be noted (59).

Diuretics are used to control HTN and edema by triggering the kidney to excrete water. This increased water excretion may result in an increased resting and submaximal HR. Increased resting HR may be due to decreased blood volume and BP, potentially having a slight negative impact on exercise capacity and thermoregulation. Diuretic use is also associated with increased potassium excretion leading to hypokalemia and potentially cardiac arrhythmias (128). Individuals using diuretics to control edema should check their body weight regularly to monitor fluid loss and prevent dehydration.

In pulmonary disease, β_2-agonists are commonly used as a bronchodilator for both short- and long-term (33) relief and management of asthmatic symptoms. Strong evidence exists for the positive effects of inhaled corticosteroids for managing asthmatic exacerbations and for long-term treatment. However, steroid-based drugs carry long-term complications and are used cautiously.

A variety of oral medications are available to treat diabetes. Mechanisms of action include increasing pancreatic insulin output, lowering insulin resistance, and decreasing absorption of carbohydrates. These drugs may affect exercise capacity as some claim slight improvements in oxygen consumption (106), whereas others report no changes (129). Regardless, the client with diabetes needs to monitor blood glucose closely before, during, and after each exercise session.

Patients with CKD are also commonly diagnosed with other pathologies such as CVD, HTN, and diabetes (39). As a result, the ACSM-EP must be cognizant of the common drugs used in those pathologies and their impact on exercise tolerance and capacity.

Prescribing exercise for clients with CVD, metabolic disease, pulmonary disease, and CKD requires some knowledge of common medications, particularly their effect on exercise response, exercise capacity, and hemodynamics. The ACSM-EP is expected to be familiar with the most commonly prescribed medications and understand how to modify an exercise prescription accordingly. Suggesting medication changes is outside the scope of practice of the ACSM-EP; rather, the ACSM-EP should refer patients back to their attending physician for medication concerns.

Teaching and Demonstrating Safe and Effective Exercise

When developing a physical activity and exercise prescription for a medically cleared client, the ACSM-EP must complete a thorough review of the client's medical record to gain a full understanding of specific health conditions and possible exercise limitations to develop an individualized exercise plan. An orientation session is then scheduled to review the plan, discuss the importance of adherence to gain optimal health benefits and maintain safety, and demonstrate proper execution of all exercises.

Individuals having incurred a recent medical event are encouraged to seek involvement in an organized rehabilitation setting when starting an exercise program (87). The ACSM-EP reviews the medical history, notes, medication history, and any client limitations. The ACSM-EP then has the background information needed to better understand the special needs and health problems surrounding the client's condition(s), to determine exercise contraindications and limitations, and to develop areas of emphasis in the exercise plan to optimize health fitness benefits and maintain safety.

After a complete review of the client's file, the ACSM-EP is ready to meet and discuss all aspects of the plan. Individuals recently diagnosed with a chronic health disease and starting an exercise program are probably concerned with safety and often overwhelmed with making numerous life-style changes. The ACSM-EP is never to assume client's knowledge of any part of the plan, goals, and specific exercise executions. Assumptions concerning client's exercise knowledge may lead to disastrous consequences. For this reason, every aspect of the plan is reviewed, and each exercise is carefully explained and demonstrated with active client participation. Because making lifestyle change is difficult, a thorough explanation of the plan is critical in overcoming potential barriers and increase the client's chance for success. On the other hand, many chronic diseases pose adverse health effects, including unique limitations putting them at higher risk for injury and unwanted medical events. Therefore, if clients do not understand the goals of the program or are confused by incomplete information regarding proper exercise techniques, the likelihood of exercising passed their physical limitations is greatly increased and could result in muscle skeletal injury and excessive fatigue and/or incur an undesirable medical event. Injuries and extreme fatigue can lead to frustration and possible program discontinuation.

Aerobic conditioning is an important component of the exercise program and is relatively easy to describe. Educational sessions provide a vital means for developing patient understanding while enhancing the likelihood in optimizing the FITT principle application. Careful explanation of exercise frequency is essential regarding the number of days per week exercise is performed and providing information on various ways to meet exercise frequency goals. For example, suggesting multiple short exercise episodes per day versus one longer continuous exercise session is often appropriate. Exercise intensity is a measure of exercise difficulty or how hard exercise is being performed. Although several ways to measure intensity exist, HR measurement is most commonly used. A less quantitative means of measuring exercise intensity include the RPE scale or the "talk test" (130). Once the exercise type or mode is selected, the ACSM-EP provides detailed exercise instructions by using demonstrations and includes safety information regarding all exercises and the use of all exercise equipment. For best results, the client performs the exercise while the ACSM-EP observes, and adjustments to the client's program are made. In the early phase of any exercise program, the client is closely monitored for correct exercise movement and appropriate exercise responses. Client records for exercise frequency, intensity, time, and type are developed and kept on file.

Resistance exercise training requires more demonstration than aerobic exercise because different exercises and types of resistance equipment are used for the various muscle groups. Clients with a chronic disease can have numerous resistance exercise contraindications, and the ACSM-EP must have a strong understanding and/or be able to access information regarding various diseases and exercise contraindications to ensure client safety while optimizing health fitness benefits. Like aerobic conditioning, the FITT principle is used for developing a resistance exercise prescription (131). A detailed description of using 1-RM to determine exercise intensity for resistance exercise may be provided. The RPE scale is also an effective indicator of resistance exercise intensity (131). The exercise time or duration is measured by the number of exercise repetitions and sets completed. A set of resistance conditioning exercises is developed for each major muscle group. Each exercise is described and completely demonstrated to show the appropriate range of motion with proper technique, number of repetitions performed, number of sets completed, and proper description of the concentric and eccentric portions of the motion (132). In conjunction with each exercise being demonstrated, the ACSM-EP should explain why each muscle group is exercised, how an exercise movement is beneficial, and what if any potential risks or dangers exist when improper technique is used or the client exercises outside the prescribed recommendations. In addition to the exercises mentioned earlier, all clients should also be engaged in regular flexibility training, which is covered in greater detail in Chapter 5.

The Case of Frank

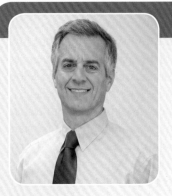

Frank is an unmotivated, sedentary, middle-aged accountant. He has several risk factors for CVD and potential symptoms but has not been clinically diagnosed with a particular disease.

Narrative

From all outward appearances, Frank seems to be an average middle-aged man. He has been an executive accountant for the past 27 years, and since starting this position, Frank has consistently been sedentary. In the past, he has started exercise programs but was very unpredictable and inconsistent with exercising regularly and quit soon after starting. His eating choices are poor and not consistent for good health. He consumes almost no vegetables, but lots of foods with high amounts of saturated fat and low-nutrient densities. In addition, most of his meals are consumed with several beers as his choice of beverage. His most recent endeavor into exercising was spurred on by his daughter, who recommended seeing a qualified professional to help him start and stay faithful to an exercise program. Following his daughter's demand, Frank went to his local college's wellness center to see one of the exercise physiologists on staff. During the initial meeting, a comprehensive assessment was carried out to determine Frank's initial fitness level and his readiness to participate in a program.

Physical Information

Age: 49 years old
Height: 5 ft 10 in
Weight: 203 lb
BMI: 29.19 kg $\cdot$ m^{-2}
Body fat percentage (dual-energy x-ray absorptiometry [DEXA] scan): 29.22%
Resting BP: 138/92 mm Hg
Resting HR: 64 bpm

ACSM Guidelines Risk Factors

Age: 45 years or older male
Family history: His father had a heart attack at the age of 47 years.
Cigarette smoking: does not smoke
Physical activity: sedentary
Obesity: none (but is considered overweight borderline obese by both his body fat and BMI)
Hypertension: SBP and DBP are within hypertensive levels, 138/92 mm Hg.
Dyslipidemia: total cholesterol: 238 mg $\cdot$ dL^{-1}; LDL-C: 161 mg $\cdot$ dL^{-1}; HDL-C: 39 mg $\cdot$ dL^{-1}
Prediabetes: none (resting blood glucose, 88 mg $\cdot$ dL^{-1})

The following results were from exercise testing:

Aerobic fitness ($\dot{V}O_{2max}$) (Balke protocol): approximately 24.8 mL $\cdot$ kg^{-1} $\cdot$ min^{-1}

Bench press weight ratio for 1-RM: 0.77

Leg press weight ratio for 1-RM: 1.55

YMCA bench press test (total lifts): 15

Partial curl-up test (total repetitions): 12

Forward flexion using a sit-and-reach box: 29 cm

Frank's lifestyle is riddled with long periods of sedentary behavior. His low fitness level is affecting his quality of life. He loses his breath and is easily fatigued from menial physical tasks. Unfortunately, Frank isn't too worried about his health, but his daughter is. He only wants to exercise enough to stop his daughter from nagging him.

QUESTIONS

- What is the biggest problem concerning Frank's health right now, and which component of fitness is worst when compared to normative data?
- What sort of disease is Frank setting himself up for, and does he already have symptoms of the disease?
- Is Frank considered high risk, and should he be referred to a physician before starting an exercise program?
- Do you think that Frank's workouts should be supervised?
- Should Frank have his aerobic exercise broken up into intermittent exercise sessions or one longer continuous exercise session?

References

1. American College of Sports Medicine. *ACSM's Exercise Management for Persons with Chronic Diseases and Disabilities*. 4th ed. Champaign (IL): Human Kinetics; 2016. 416 p.
2. American College of Sports Medicine. *ACSM's Guidelines for Exercise Testing and Prescription*. 10th ed. Philadelphia (PA): Wolters Kluwer; 2018. 480 p.
3. American College of Sports Medicine. *ACSM's Resources for Clinical Exercise Physiology*. 2nd ed. Philadelphia (PA): Lippincott Williams & Wilkins; 2010. 368 p.
4. American College of Sports Medicine. *ACSM's Resource Manual for Guidelines for Exercise Testing and Prescription*. 7th ed. Philadelphia (PA): Lippincott Williams & Wilkins; 2014. 896 p.

SUMMARY

Regular physical activity and exercise participation can provide primary and secondary prevention/treatment health fitness benefits. Medications, specialized diets, and surgeries are generally viewed as first options before exercise is considered as an intervention. Nonetheless, daily physical activity and exercise training are effective tools in developing health fitness benefits for persons with chronic diseases. Although exercise is beneficial, the challenges and limitations presented by diseases must be addressed to properly design the most effective and safest physical activity and exercise program. By adapting the ACSM (2) and U.S. physical activity recommendations (4) for prescribing physical activity and exercise programs, the ACSM-EP is better able to meet the exercise needs of the populations in this chapter while also ensuring program safety. The ACSM-EP must know the limitations and challenges these diseases present for the exercising client and how to adapt the physical activity and exercise programs accordingly.

STUDY QUESTIONS

1. Explain the pathophysiology of atherosclerosis, including the role of the major risk factors.
2. Explain why the asthmatic patient has difficulty breathing, particularly during exercise.
3. Explain the major pathological differences between Type 1 and Type 2 diabetes within the context of exercise.
4. Briefly describe the effect of OTC medications on exercise in CAD and pulmonary disease.
5. Explain how the FITT guidelines would differ for the CKD for clients in the predialysis, dialysis, and posttransplant categories.
6. Describe key differences in prescribing exercise for specific clinical populations.

REFERENCES

1. American College of Sports Medicine. *ACSM's Guidelines for Exercise Testing and Prescription*. 11th ed. Philadelphia (PA): Wolters Kluwer; 2022. 548 p.
2. Garber CE, Blissmer B, Deschenes MR, et al. American College of Sports Medicine position stand. Quantity and quality of exercise for developing and maintaining cardiorespiratory, musculoskeletal, and neuromotor fitness in apparently healthy adults: guidance for prescribing exercise. *Med Sci Sports Exerc*. 2011;43(7):1334–59.
3. Riebe D, Franklin BA, Thompson PD, et al. Updating ACSM's recommendations for exercise preparticipation health screening. *Med Sci Sports Exerc*. 2015;47(11):2473–9.
4. Piercy KL, Troiano RP, Ballard RM, et al. The physical activity guidelines for Americans. *JAMA*. 2018;320(19):2020–8.
5. Virani SS, Alonso A, Benjamin EJ, et al. Heart disease and stroke statistics — 2020 update: a report from the American Heart Association. *Circulation*. 2020;141(9):e139–e596.
6. Cooper CB, Doezal BA, Durstine JL, et al. Chronic conditions very strongly associated with tobacco. In: Moore GE, Durstine JL, Painter PL, editors. *ACSM's Management for Persons with Chronic Diseases and Disabilities*. 4th ed. Champaign (IL): Human Kinetics; 2016. p. 95–114.
7. Libby P, Ridker PM. Inflammation and atherothrombosis: from population biology and bench research to clinical practice. *J Am Coll Cardio*. 2006;48(9):A33–46.
8. Mallika V, Goswami B, Rajappa M. Atherosclerosis pathophysiology and the role of novel risk factors: a clinicobiochemical perspective. *Angiology*. 2007;58(5):513–22.
9. Goodman CC, Fuller KS. *Pathology: Implications for the Physical Therapist*. 3rd ed. St. Louis (MO): Saunders Elsevier; 2008. 1760 p.
10. Thompson PD. Exercise and physical activity in the prevention and treatment of atherosclerotic cardiovascular disease. *Arterioscler Thromb Vasc Biol*. 2003;23(8):1319–21.
11. Beevers G, Lip GY, O'Brien E. ABC of hypertension: the pathophysiology of hypertension. *BMJ*. 2001;322(7291):912–6.
12. Arnett DK, Blumenthal RS, Albert MA, et al. 2019 ACC/AHA guideline on the primary prevention of cardiovascular disease: a report of the American College of Cardiology/American Heart Association Task Force on Clinical Practice Guidelines. *Circulation*. 2019;140(11):e596–646.
13. James PA, Oparil S, Carter BL, et al. 2014 Evidence-based guideline for the management of high blood pressure in adults: report from the panel members appointed to the Eighth Joint National Committee (JNC 8). *JAMA*. 2014;311(5):507–20.
14. Greenland P, Peterson E. The new 2017 ACC/AHA guidelines "up the pressure" on diagnosis and treatment of hypertension. *JAMA*. 2017;318(21):2083–4.
15. Serrano Hernando FJ, Martin Conejero A. Peripheral artery disease: pathophysiology, diagnosis and treatment. *Rev Esp Cardiol*. 2007;60(9):969–82.
16. Askew CD, Parmenter B, Leicht AS, Walker PJ, Golledge J. Exercise & Sports Science Australia (ESSA) position statement on exercise prescription for patients with peripheral arterial disease and intermittent claudication. *J Sci Med Sport*. 2014;17(6):623–9.
17. Hiatt WR, Armstrong EJ, Larson CJ, Brass EP. Pathogenesis of the limb manifestations and exercise limitations in peripheral artery disease. *Circ Res*. 2015;116(9):1527–39.
18. Rooke TW, Hirsch AT, Misra S, et al. 2011 ACCF/AHA focused update of the guideline for the management of patients with peripheral artery disease (updating the 2005 guideline): a report of the American College of Cardiology Foundation/American Heart Association Task Force on Practice Guidelines. *J Am Coll Cardiol*. 2011;58(19):2020–45.
19. Aboyans V, Criqui MH, Abraham P, et al. Measurement and interpretation of the ankle-brachial index: a scientific statement from the American Heart Association. *Circulation*. 2012;126(24):2890–909.
20. Stein R, Hrljac I, Halperin JL, Gustavson SM, Teodorescu V, Olin JW. Limitation of the resting ankle-brachial index in symptomatic patients with peripheral arterial disease. *Vasc Med*. 2006;11(1):29–33.
21. Sorensen J, Wilks SA, Jacob AD, Huynh TT. Screening for peripheral artery disease. *Semin Roentgenol*. 2015;50(2):139–47.
22. Baynes HW. Classification, pathophysiology, diagnosis and management of diabetes mellitus. *J Diabetes Metab*. 2015;6(5):541.

23. American Diabetes Association. Classification and diagnosis of diabetes: standards of medical care in diabetes — 2020. *Diabetes Care*. 2020;43(Suppl 1):S14–31.

24. Cnop M, Welsh N, Jonas JC, Jorns A, Lenzen S, Eizirik DL. Mechanisms of pancreatic beta-cell death in type 1 and type 2 diabetes: many differences, few similarities. *Diabetes*. 2005;54(Suppl 2):S97–107.

25. Patsch JR, Sailer S, Kostner G, Sandhofer F, Holasek A, Braunsteiner H. Separation of the main lipoprotein density classes from human plasma by rate-zonal ultracentrifugation. *J Lipid Res*. 1974;15(4):356–66.

26. Benjamin EJ, Muntner P, Alonso A, et al. Heart disease and stroke statistics — 2019 update: a report from the American Heart Association. *Circulation*. 2019;139(10):e56–528.

27. Hill JO, Peters JC. Environmental contributions to the obesity epidemic. *Science*. 1998;280(5368):1371–4.

28. Bouldin MJ, Ross LA, Sumrall CD, Loustalot FV, Low AK, Land KK. The effect of obesity surgery on obesity comorbidity. *Am J Med Sci*. 2006;331(4):183–93.

29. Alberti KG, Eckel RH, Grundy SM, et al. Harmonizing the metabolic syndrome: a joint interim statement of the International Diabetes Federation Task Force on Epidemiology and Prevention; National Heart, Lung, and Blood Institute; American Heart Association; World Heart Federation; International Atherosclerosis Society; and International Association for the Study of Obesity. *Circulation*. 2009;120(16):1640–5.

30. Beilby J. Definition of metabolic syndrome: report of the National Heart, Lung, and Blood Institute/American Heart Association conference on scientific issues related to definition. *Circulation*. 2004;109:433–8.

31. Lakka HM, Laaksonen DE, Lakka TA, et al. The metabolic syndrome and total and cardiovascular disease mortality in middle-aged men. *JAMA*. 2002;288(21):2709–16.

32. Pauwels RA, Buist AS, Calverley PM, Jenkins CR, Hurd SS, Committee GS. Global strategy for the diagnosis, management, and prevention of chronic obstructive pulmonary disease. NHLBI/WHO Global Initiative for Chronic Obstructive Lung Disease (GOLD) workshop summary. *Am J Respir Crit Care Med*. 2001;163(5):1256–76.

33. Barnes PJ. Immunology of asthma and chronic obstructive pulmonary disease. *Nat Rev Immunol*. 2008;8(3):183–92.

34. Moorman JE, Akinbami LJ, Bailey CM, et al. National surveillance of asthma: United States, 2001–2010. *Vital Health Stat 3*. 2012;(35):1–58.

35. Barrios RJ, Kheradmand F, Batts L, Corry DB. Asthma: pathology and pathophysiology. *Arch Pathol Lab Med*. 2006;130(4):447–51.

36. Hsia CC. Cardiopulmonary limitations to exercise in restrictive lung disease. *Med Sci Sports Exerc*. 1999; 31(1 Suppl):S28–32.

37. Rundell K. Asthma. In: Moore GE, Durstine JL, Painter PL, editors. *ACSM's Exercise Management for Person's with Chronic Diseases and Disabilities*. 4th ed. Champaign (IL): Human Kinetics; 2016. p. 183–8.

38. Webster AC, Nagler EV, Morton RL, Masson P. Chronic kidney disease. *Lancet*. 2017;389(10075):1238–52.

39. U.S. Renal Data System. USRDS 2009 annual data report: atlas of chronic kidney disease and end-stage renal disease in the United States [Internet]. Bethesda (MD): National Institutes of Diabetes and Digestive and Kidney Disease. Available from: http://www.usrds.org/atlas09.aspx.

40. Levey AS, Becker C, Inker LA. Glomerular filtration rate and albuminuria for detection and staging of acute and chronic kidney disease in adults: a systematic review. *JAMA*. 2015;313(8):837–46.

41. Kidney Disease: Improving Global Outcomes. KDIGO 2012 clinical practice guideline for the evaluation and management of chronic kidney disease. *Kidney Int Suppl*. 2013;3(1):134–5.

42. Haskell WL, Lee IM, Pate RR, et al. Physical activity and public health: updated recommendation for adults from the American College of Sports Medicine and the American Heart Association. *Med Sci Sports Exerc*. 2007;39(8):1423–34.

43. Gerteis J, Izrael D, Deitz D, et al. Healthcare utilization and costs. In: *Multiple Chronic Conditions Chartbook*. Rockville (MD): Agency for Healthcare Research and Quality; 2014. p. 7–14.

44. Centers for Disease Control and Prevention. Chronic disease in America 2020 [Internet]. Atlanta (GA): Centers for Disease Control and Prevention; [cited]. Available from: https://www.cdc.gov/chronicdisease/resources/infographic/chronic-diseases.htm.

45. Hansen D, Eijnde BO, Roelants M, et al. Clinical benefits of the addition of lower extremity low-intensity resistance muscle training to early aerobic endurance training intervention in patients with coronary artery disease: a randomized controlled trial. *J Rehabil Med*. 2011;43(9):800–7.

46. Kohut ML, McCann DA, Russell DW, et al. Aerobic exercise, but not flexibility/resistance exercise, reduces serum IL-18, CRP, and IL-6 independent of beta-blockers, BMI, and psychosocial factors in older adults. *Brain Behav Immun*. 2006;20(3):201–9.

47. Rehman J, Li J, Parvathaneni L, et al. Exercise acutely increases circulating endothelial progenitor cells and monocyte-/macrophage-derived angiogenic cells. *J Am Coll Cardiol*. 2004;43(12):2314–8.

48. Crowther RG, Leicht AS, Spinks WL, Sangla K, Quigley F, Golledge J. Effects of a 6-month exercise program pilot study on walking economy, peak physiological characteristics, and walking performance in patients with peripheral arterial disease. *Vasc Health Risk Manag*. 2012;8:225–32.

49. Cucato GG, Chehuen Mda R, Costa LA, et al. Exercise prescription using the heart of claudication pain onset in patients with intermittent claudication. *Clinics (Sao Paulo)*. 2013;68(7):974–8.

50. Leicht AS, Crowther RG, Golledge J. Influence of peripheral arterial disease and supervised walking on heart rate variability. *J Vasc Surg*. 2011;54(5):1352–9.

51. Castro-Sanchez AM, Mataran-Penarrocha GA, Feriche-Fernandez-Castanys B, Fernandez-Sola C, Sanchez-Labraca N, Moreno-Lorenzo C. A program of 3 physical therapy modalities improves peripheral arterial disease in diabetes type 2 patients: a randomized controlled trial. *J Cardiovasc Nurs*. 2013;28(1):74–82.

52. Jain A, Liu K, Ferrucci L, et al. Declining walking impairment questionnaire scores are associated with subsequent increased mortality in peripheral artery disease. *J Am Coll Cardiol.* 2013;61(17):1820–9.

53. Rosendorff C. Hypertension and coronary artery disease: a summary of the American Heart Association scientific statement. *J Clin Hypertens (Greenwich).* 2007;9(10): 790–5.

54. Whelton SP, Chin A, Xin X, He J. Effect of aerobic exercise on blood pressure: a meta-analysis of randomized, controlled trials. *Ann Intern Med.* 2002;136(7):493–503.

55. Colberg SR, Albright AL, Blissmer BJ, et al. Exercise and type 2 diabetes: American College of Sports Medicine and the American Diabetes Association: joint position statement. Exercise and type 2 diabetes. *Med Sci Sports Exerc.* 2010;42(12):2282–303.

56. Colberg SR, Sigal RJ, Yardley JE, et al. Physical activity/exercise and diabetes: a position statement of the American Diabetes Association. *Diabetes Care.* 2016;39(11):2065–79.

57. Freese EC, Levine AS, Chapman DP, Hausman DB, Cureton KJ. Effects of acute sprint interval cycling and energy replacement on postprandial lipemia. *J Appl Physiol.* 2011;111(6):1584–9.

58. Durstine JL, Moore GE, Painter PL, Macko R, Gordon BT, Kraus WE. Chronic conditions strongly associated with physical inactivity. In: Moore GE, Durstine JL, Painter PL, editors. *ACSM's Management for Persons with Chronic Diseases and Disabilities.* 4th ed. Champaign (IL): Human Kinetics; 2016. p. 71–94.

59. Fletcher GF, Balady GJ, Amsterdam EA, et al. Exercise standards for testing and training: a statement for healthcare professionals from the American Heart Association. *Circulation.* 2001;104(14):1694–740.

60. Thompson PD, Crouse SF, Goodpaster B, Kelley D, Moyna N, Pescatello L. The acute versus the chronic response to exercise. *Med Sci Sports Exerc.* 2001;33(6 Suppl):S438–45; discussion S52–3.

61. Grundy SM, Stone NJ, Bailey AL, et al. 2018 AHA/ACC/AACVPR/AAPA/ABC/ACPM/ADA/AGS/APhA/ASPC/NLA/PCNA guideline on the management of blood cholesterol: a report of the American College of Cardiology/American Heart Association Task Force on Clinical Practice Guidelines. *J Am Coll Cardiol.* 2019;73(24): e285–350.

62. Gaesser GA, Angadi SS, Sawyer BJ. Exercise and diet, independent of weight loss, improve cardiometabolic risk profile in overweight and obese individuals. *Phys Sportsmed.* 2011;39(2):87–97.

63. Villareal DT, Chode S, Parimi N, et al. Weight loss, exercise, or both and physical function in obese older adults. *N Engl J Med.* 2011;364(13):1218–29.

64. Edmunds J, Ntoumanis N, Duda JL. Adherence and well-being in overweight and obese patients referred to an exercise on prescription scheme: a self-determination theory perspective. *J Sport Exerc Psychol.* 2007;8(5):722–40.

65. Ford ES, Giles WH, Dietz WH. Prevalence of the metabolic syndrome among US adults: findings from the third National Health and Nutrition Examination Survey. *JAMA.* 2002;287(3):356–9.

66. Donnelly JE, Blair SN, Jakicic JM, et al. American College of Sports Medicine position stand. Appropriate physical activity intervention strategies for weight loss and prevention of weight regain for adults. *Med Sci Sports Exerc.* 2009;41(2):459–71.

67. Ries AL, Bauldoff GS, Carlin BW, et al. Pulmonary rehabilitation: joint ACCP/AACVPR evidence-based clinical practice guidelines. *Chest.* 2007;131(5 Suppl):4S–42S.

68. Hsia CC. Chronic restrictive pulmonary disease. In: Moore GE, Durstine JL, Painter PL, editors. *ACSM's Management for Persons with Chronic Diseases and Disabilities.* 4th ed. Champaign (IL): Human Kinetics; 2016. p. 177–82.

69. Smith AC, Burton JO. Exercise in kidney disease and diabetes: time for action. *J Ren Care.* 2012;38(Suppl 1): 52–8.

70. Headley SA, Germain MJ, Milch CM, Buchholz MP, Coughlin MA, Pescatello LS. Immediate blood pressure-lowering effects of aerobic exercise among patients with chronic kidney disease. *Nephrology (Carlton).* 2008;13(7):601–6.

71. Kosmadakis GC, John SG, Clapp EL, et al. Benefits of regular walking exercise in advanced pre-dialysis chronic kidney disease. *Nephrol Dial Transplant.* 2012;27(3): 997–1004.

72. Headley S, Germain M, Milch C, et al. Exercise training improves HR responses and $\dot{V}O_{2peak}$ in predialysis kidney patients. *Med Sci Sports Exerc.* 2012;44(12):2392–9.

73. Workeneh BT, Mitch WE. Review of muscle wasting associated with chronic kidney disease. *Am J Clin Nutr.* 2010;91(4):1128S–32S.

74. Rossi AP, Burris DD, Lucas FL, Crocker GA, Wasserman JC. Effects of a renal rehabilitation exercise program in patients with CKD: a randomized, controlled trial. *Clin J Am Soc Nephrol.* 2014;9(12):2052–8.

75. Painter PL, Hector L, Ray K, et al. A randomized trial of exercise training after renal transplantation. *Transplantation.* 2002;74(1):42–8.

76. Wilkinson TJ, Shur NF, Smith AC. "Exercise as medicine" in chronic kidney disease. *Scand J Med Sci Sports.* 2016;26(8):985–8.

77. Castaneda C, Gordon PL, Uhlin KL, et al. Resistance training to counteract the catabolism of a low-protein diet in patients with chronic renal insufficiency. A randomized, controlled trial. *Ann Intern Med.* 2001;135(11): 965–76.

78. Gordon BT, Durstine JL, Painter PL, Moore GE. Basic physical activity and exercise recommendations for persons with chronic conditions. In: Moore GE, Durstine JL, Painter PL, editors. *ACSM's Management for Persons with Chronic Diseases and Disabilities.* 4th ed. Champaign (IL): Human Kinetics; 2016. p. 15–32.

79. Billat LV. Interval training for performance: a scientific and empirical practice. Special recommendations for middle-and long-distance running. Part I: aerobic interval training. *Sports Med.* 2001;31(1):13–31.

80. Gibala MJ, Little JP, Macdonald MJ, Hawley JA. Physiological adaptations to low-volume, high-intensity interval training in health and disease. *J Physiol.* 2012;590(5):1077–84.

81. Laursen PB, Jenkins DG. The scientific basis for high-intensity interval training: optimising training programmes and maximising performance in highly trained endurance athletes. *Sports Med.* 2002;32(1):53–73.

82. Ross LM, Porter RR, Durstine JL. High-intensity interval training (HIIT) for patients with chronic diseases. *J Sport Health Sci.* 2016;5(2):139–44.

83. Durstine JL, Gordon BT, Wang Z, Luo X. Chronic disease and the link to physical activity. *J Sport Health Sci.* 2013;2(1):3–11.

84. Cornish AK, Broadbent S, Cheema BS. Interval training for patients with coronary artery disease: a systematic review. *Eur J Appl Physiol.* 2011;111(4):579–89.

85. Guiraud T, Nigam A, Gremeaux V, Meyer P, Juneau M, Bosquet L. High-intensity interval training in cardiac rehabilitation. *Sports Med.* 2012;42(7):587–605.

86. Beauchamp MK, Nonoyama M, Goldstein RS, et al. Interval versus continuous training in individuals with chronic obstructive pulmonary disease — a systematic review. *Thorax.* 2010;65(2):157–64.

87. Ehrman J. *ACSM's Resource Manual for Guidelines for Exercise Testing and Prescription.* 6th ed. Philadelphia (PA): Lippincott Williams & Wilkins; 2010. 868 p.

88. Bird SR, Hawley JA. Exercise and type 2 diabetes: new prescription for an old problem. *Maturitas.* 2012;72(4):311–6.

89. Jelleyman C, Yates T, O'Donovan G, et al. The effects of high-intensity interval training on glucose regulation and insulin resistance: a meta-analysis. *Obes Rev.* 2015;16(11):942–61.

90. Balady GJ, Williams MA, Ades PA, et al. Core components of cardiac rehabilitation/secondary prevention programs: 2007 update: a scientific statement from the American Heart Association Exercise, Cardiac Rehabilitation, and Prevention Committee, the Council on Clinical Cardiology; the Councils on Cardiovascular Nursing, Epidemiology and Prevention, and Nutrition, Physical Activity, and Metabolism; and the American Association of Cardiovascular and Pulmonary Rehabilitation. *Circulation.* 2007;115(20):2675–82.

91. Jaacks LM, Siegel KR, Gujral UP, Narayan KM. Type 2 diabetes: a 21st century epidemic. *Best Pract Res Clin Endocrinol Metab.* 2016;30(3):331–43.

92. Boule NG, Haddad E, Kenny GP, Wells GA, Sigal RJ. Effects of exercise on glycemic control and body mass in type 2 diabetes mellitus: a meta-analysis of controlled clinical trials. *JAMA.* 2001;286(10):1218–27.

93. Davis EA, Keating B, Byrne GC, Russell M, Jones TW. Hypoglycemia: incidence and clinical predictors in a large population-based sample of children and adolescents with IDDM. *Diabetes Care.* 1997;20(1):22–5.

94. Rabe KF, Hurd S, Anzueto A, et al. Global strategy for the diagnosis, management, and prevention of chronic obstructive pulmonary disease: GOLD executive summary. *Am J Respir Crit Care Med.* 2007;176(6):532–55.

95. Tremblay MS, Aubert S, Barnes JD, et al. Sedentary Behavior Research Network (SBRN) — terminology consensus project process and outcome. *Int J Behav Nutr Phys Act.* 2017;14(1):75.

96. Murphy SL, Xu J, Kochanek KD, Curtin SC, Arias E. Deaths: final data for 2015. *Natl Vital Stat Rep.* 2017;66(6):1–75.

97. GBD Mortality, Causes of Death Collaborators. Global, regional, and national life expectancy, all-cause mortality, and cause-specific mortality for 249 causes of death, 1980–2015: a systematic analysis for the Global Burden of Disease Study 2015. *Lancet.* 2016;388(10053):1459–544.

98. Heron M. Deaths: leading causes for 2017. *Natl Vital Stat Rep.* 2019;68(6):1–77.

99. Hunt SA. ACC/AHA 2005 guideline update for the diagnosis and management of chronic heart failure in the adult: a report of the American College of Cardiology/ American Heart Association Task Force on Practice Guidelines (writing committee to update the 2001 guidelines for the evaluation and management of heart failure). *J Am Coll Cardiol.* 2005;46(6):e1–82.

100. Giannuzzi P, Saner H, Bjornstad H, et al. Secondary prevention through cardiac rehabilitation: position paper of the Working Group on Cardiac Rehabilitation and Exercise Physiology of the European Society of Cardiology. *Eur Heart J.* 2003;24(13):1273–1278.

101. Pescatello LS, Franklin BA, Fagard R, et al. American College of Sports Medicine position stand. Exercise and hypertension. *Med Sci Sports Exerc.* 2004;36(3):533–53.

102. Keteyian SJ. Exercise rehabilitation in chronic heart failure. *Coron Artery Dis.* 2006;17(3):233–7.

103. Vongpatanasin W, Wang Z, Arbique D, et al. Functional sympatholysis is impaired in hypertensive humans. *J Physiol.* 2011;589(Pt 5):1209–20.

104. Kokkinos P. Cardiorespiratory fitness, exercise, and blood pressure. *Hypertension.* 2014;64(6):1160–4.

105. Juneau M, Roy N, Nigam A, Tardif JC, Larivee L. Exercise above the ischemic threshold and serum markers of myocardial injury. *Can J Cardiol.* 2009;25(10):e338–41.

106. Regensteiner JG, Bauer TA, Reusch JE. Rosiglitazone improves exercise capacity in individuals with type 2 diabetes. *Diabetes Care.* 2005;28(12):2877–83.

107. Williams B, Poulter NR, Brown MJ, et al. British Hypertension Society guidelines for hypertension management 2004 (BHS-IV): summary. *BMJ.* 2004;328(7440):634–40.

108. Womack L, Peters D, Barrett EJ, Kaul S, Price W, Lindner JR. Abnormal skeletal muscle capillary recruitment during exercise in patients with type 2 diabetes mellitus and microvascular complications. *J Am Coll Cardiol.* 2009;53(23):2175–83.

109. Castellani JW, Young AJ, Ducharme MB, et al. American College of Sports Medicine position stand: prevention of cold injuries during exercise. *Med Sci Sports Exerc.* 2006;38(11):2012–29.

110. Sigal RJ, Kenny GP, Wasserman DH, Castaneda-Sceppa C. Physical activity/exercise and type 2 diabetes. *Diabetes Care.* 2004;27(10):2518–39.

111. Genest J, McPerson R, Frohlich J, et al. 2009 Canadian Cardiovascular Society/Canadian guidelines for the diagnosis and treatment of dyslipidemia and prevention of cardiovascular disease in the adult — 2009 recommendations. *Can J Cardiol.* 2009;25(10):567–79.

112. Naghavi M, Abajobir AA, Abbafati C, et al. Global, regional, and national age-sex specific mortality for 264 causes of death, 1980-2016: a systematic analysis for the Global Burden of Disease Study 2016. *Lancet.* 2017;390(10100):1151–210.

113. Chooi YC, Ding C, Magkos F. The epidemiology of obesity. *Metabolism.* 2019;92:6–10.

114. Shah K, Villareal DT. Combination treatment to CONQUER obesity? *Lancet.* 2011;377(9774):1295–7.

115. Cooper CB. Exercise in chronic pulmonary disease: aerobic exercise prescription. *Med Sci Sports Exerc.* 2001;33(7 Suppl):S671–9.

116. Johansen KL. Exercise and chronic kidney disease: current recommendations. *Sports Med.* 2005;35(6):485–99.

117. Painter PL. Exercise after renal transplantation. *Adv Ren Replace Ther.* 1999;6(2):159–64.

118. Palmer R, Weiss R, Zusman RM, Haig A, Flavin S, MacDonald B. Effects of nabumetone, celecoxib, and ibuprofen on blood pressure control in hypertensive patients on angiotensin converting enzyme inhibitors. *Am J Hypertens.* 2003;16(2):135–9.

119. Sheridan R, Montgomery AA, Fahey T. NSAID use and BP in treated hypertensives: a retrospective controlled observational study. *J Hum Hypertens.* 2005;19(6):445–50.

120. Li J, Zhang N, Ye B, Ju W, Orser B, Fox JE, et al. Non-steroidal anti-inflammatory drugs increase insulin release from beta cells by inhibiting ATP-sensitive potassium channels. *Br J Pharmacol.* 2007;151(4):483–93.

121. Lindenauer PK, Pekow P, Wang K, Mamidi DK, Gutierrez B, Benjamin EM. Perioperative beta-blocker therapy and mortality after major noncardiac surgery. *N Engl J Med.* 2005;353(4):349–61.

122. Shekelle PG, Rich MW, Morton SC, et al. Efficacy of angiotensin-converting enzyme inhibitors and beta-blockers in the management of left ventricular systolic dysfunction according to race, gender, and diabetic status: a meta-analysis of major clinical trials. *J Am Coll Cardiol.* 2003;41(9):1529–38.

123. Everly MJ, Heaton PC, Cluxton RJ Jr. Beta-blocker underuse in secondary prevention of myocardial infarction. *Ann Pharmacother.* 2004;38(2):286–93.

124. Fonarow GC. Beta-blockers for the post-myocardial infarction patient: current clinical evidence and practical considerations. *Rev Cardiovasc Med.* 2006;7(1):1–9.

125. Kleiner SA, Vogt WB, Gladowski P, et al. Beta-blocker compliance, mortality, and reinfarction: validation of clinical trial association using insurer claims data. *Am J Med Qual.* 2009;24(6):512–9.

126. Ladage D, Schwinger RH, Brixius K. Cardio-selective beta-blocker: pharmacological evidence and their influence on exercise capacity. *Cardiovasc Ther.* 2013;31(2):76–83.

127. Omar MA, Wilson JP, Cox TS. Rhabdomyolysis and HMG-CoA reductase inhibitors. *Ann Pharmacother.* 2001;35(9):1096–107.

128. Skogestad J, Aronsen JM. Hypokalemia-induced arrhythmias and heart failure: new insights and implications for therapy. *Front Physiol.* 2018;9:1500.

129. McGuire DK, Abdullah SM, See R, et al. Randomized comparison of the effects of rosiglitazone vs. placebo on peak integrated cardiovascular performance, cardiac structure, and function. *Eur Heart J.* 2010;31(18):2262–70.

130. Persinger R, Foster C, Gibson M, Fater DC, Porcari JP. Consistency of the talk test for exercise prescription. *Med Sci Sports Exerc.* 2004;36(9):1632–6.

131. Kraemer WJ, Ratamess NA. Fundamentals of resistance training: progression and exercise prescription. *Med Sci Sports Exerc.* 2004;36(4):674–88.

132. Fleck SJ KW. *Designing Resistance Training Programs.* 4th ed. Champaign (IL): Human Kinetics; 2014. 520 p.

Exercise Programming for Individuals with Musculoskeletal Limitations

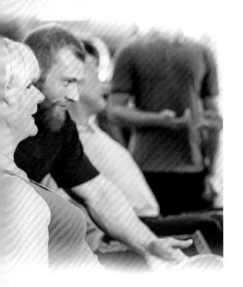

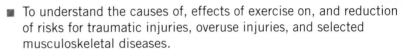

OBJECTIVES

- To understand the causes of, effects of exercise on, and reduction of risks for traumatic injuries, overuse injuries, and selected musculoskeletal diseases.
- To apply appropriate exercise guidelines for traumatic injuries, overuse injuries, and selected musculoskeletal diseases.
- To modify exercise prescription appropriately for traumatic injuries, overuse injuries, and selected musculoskeletal diseases.
- To understand how risk varies between genders and ages for traumatic injuries, overuse injuries, and musculoskeletal diseases.

INTRODUCTION

In previous chapters, exercise prescriptions for individuals without limitations were discussed. In this chapter, selected musculoskeletal injuries and pathologies are discussed as well as causes, effects of exercise, and strategies to reduce risks associated with these conditions. This chapter builds on the basic principles of exercise prescription and is divided into three sections: traumatic injuries, overuse injuries, and chronic conditions. When reading these sections, be reminded that client safety is first and foremost. Risks to client safety may compromise long-term health and is counterproductive to recovery. Therefore, working closely with qualified health care professionals and understanding relevant contraindications is most important in the development and implementation of exercise programs for clients with musculoskeletal limitations. Prior to addressing the three types of injuries, addressing the scope of practice for an exercise physiologist (EP) and the development of relationships with others is important in the continuum of proper client care. Because guidelines vary within each type of injury, specifics on what a client can and cannot do is addressed.

If a condition has resulted in significant pain or limits function, the EP can usually work safely with individuals who have been cleared by a health care provider (*e.g.*, physician, physician's assistant, or therapist). If a client notes he or she is independent with normal activity or the pain is not significant, medical clearance is not usually necessary for activity prior to initiation of a program. Changes in the health care system have resulted in less coverage for therapies (such as physical therapy). Thus, many clients are discharged before they have become fully functional. These patients can greatly benefit from working with an EP to further improve their physical functions. However, a Physical Activity Readiness Questionnaire for Everyone (PAR-Q+) should still always be administered to evaluate readiness and safety to begin an exercise program.

Developing a relationship with local therapists may help the EP obtain referrals of clients who are being discharged. Creating a handout to be taken to area clinics, identifying experience, opportunities, and types of training provided is beneficial. Survey results from previous clients regarding satisfaction might be a good marketing tool. Perhaps having a short meeting with the therapists to discuss potential programs for their clients who need to be discharged would be beneficial. Willingness to collaborate with the therapist regarding recommended activity restrictions is key to whether they will feel comfortable giving patients your contact information when they are discharged from therapy.

Traumatic Movement–Related Injuries

Traumatic injuries, also called "macrotraumatic injuries" generally occur abruptly and include fractures, strains, sprains, and contusions. A few indicators exist suggesting the need for medical referral if a client reports a lower extremity injury for which has not been seen by a physician. These indicators include if the client cannot bear weight for more than two steps, the client has point tenderness to any bony prominence, the pain has progressed since the injury, and/or the patient reports a weakness, loss of function or range of motion (ROM). Females are at a greater risk for specific types of sprains and strains. Several factors appear to contribute to this increase in risk, including poor landing biomechanics, specific muscle weakness, and changes in ligamentous laxity during the menstrual cycle. Risks can be partially mediated by preventive training (1).

Fractures of a traumatic origin associated with a fall or a result of overuse or mechanical breakdown are included in this category. Traumatic fractures will usually present differently than those from overuse, and the injury history is a key factor that will help the physician in diagnosis.

Fractures

Although presence of a fracture may seem obvious and EPs usually will not see patients who have not pursued medical treatment, falls may have seemed so minor that an individual has not sought an assessment without considering the potential of a fracture. Because the foot and ankle are weight-bearing points, pain for the first two to three steps and point tenderness over a bone are indicators that medical follow-up is needed (2–5). If the client fell on an outstretched hand and reports significant pain in the hand or wrist, medical care and evaluation is needed. Some risk factors for overuse fractures include low bone mineral density (BMD), high-impact repetitive activities (such as distance running), and improper progression of training. Females who are at risk for the "female athlete triad" should be screened, following recommended guidelines (6). Females who have several positive risk factors should be referred to a health care provider. Males in some sports (especially distance running) have been shown to have similar changes in energy intake, hormonal deficits, and low BMD (7). If cleared for activity, the primary recommendation is to protect the joint and limit physical activity, so pain does not increase.

Injury to a muscle or tendon is called a *strain*, whereas injury to a ligament, or tissue that connects bones, is called a *sprain*. Both strains and sprains occur in response to unaccustomed stress on the tissue or in response to repeated lower level stress over time because of repetitive motion. In either case, an acute strain or sprain occurs most often during an eccentric contraction and/or when tissue is in an excessively stretched state (2–5,8,9).

Strains

The muscle-tendon unit (MTU) serves to generate force either by concentric contraction to create movement or by eccentric contraction to resist a load (2–5). Injury to the MTU can occur at any point along the MTU continuum, and the location of injury usually depends on the nature of the rate and magnitude of the applied force and type of stress (intrinsic or extrinsic). Acute pain generally accompanies a muscle strain; however, muscle pain and dysfunction often progress and becomes more apparent 1–2 days after the injury. Similarly, with exercise-induced muscle damage (EIMD), muscle pain and dysfunction usually become more apparent 1–2 days after the injury. However, EIMD is due to muscle fiber damage and inflammation that accompanies unaccustomed high-intensity eccentric contractions and is more appropriately classified as a microtrauma, as compared to a sudden muscle-tendon overload (2–5,9–11). Although muscle strains can occur in any MTU, strains are most common in muscles of the calf (gastrocnemius, soleus) and thigh (rectus femoris, biceps femoris, semimembranosus, semitendinosus) (2–5). The degree of MTU strain (not EIMD) is classified from first to third (complete rupture) and is described in Table 9.1. Assessment of strain severity is completed by a trained health

Table 9.1	Grading and Characteristics of Muscle-Tendon Unit Strains	
Classification	**Symptoms**	**Treatment**
First degree: **few torn fibers**	Inflammation, edema, and/or hemorrhage usually near muscle-tendon junction; painful on contraction but strong muscle activity	**PRICE** (**P**rotect, **R**estrict activity, **I**ce, **C**ompression, **E**levation) followed by therapeutic exercise for strength/early gentle ROM
Second degree: **almost one-half of fibers torn**	Moderate to severe muscle pain on contraction and loss of ROM and strength, edema, and/or hemorrhage	PRICE, early gentle ROM and possibly immobilization followed by therapeutic exercise for strength/ROM
Third degree: **all fibers torn (rupture)**	Painless joint instability, moderate to severe edema	PRICE, immobilization, and/or surgical repair referral

Data from Dutton M. *Dutton's Orthopaedic Examination, Evaluation and Intervention.* 4th ed. New York (NY): McGraw-Hill; 2017. p. 37; and Anderson MK, Parr GP, Hall SJ, editors. *Foundations of Athletic Training: Prevention, Assessment, and Management.* 5th ed. Philadelphia (PA): Lippincott Williams & Wilkins; 2013. p. 163.

care professional to ascertain the degree of strain and appropriate treatment. In the case of a severe strain, imaging technology (magnetic resonance imaging [MRI] or x-ray) may be required to determine the degree of MTU damage and determination of possible medical intervention if a complete rupture has occurred. Females are at a greater risk for specific acute ligamentous injury. The risk of anterior cruciate ligament injury in females is more than twofold that of male athletes and is partially related to phase of the menstrual cycle, landing biomechanics, and strength (1,12).

Sprains

Ligaments are collagenous fibrous structures that connect bone to bone and provide passive soft-tissue restraint of bone-to-bone contact. Like muscle strains, ligament sprains are graded according to severity as shown in Table 9.2. The most common site of a sprain is the lateral collateral ligaments in the ankle, caused by ankle inversion (bottom surface of the foot turns inward) versus eversion. An inversion sprain typically occurs, for example, when a basketball player lands from a jump on another player's foot, causing the lateral ankle to roll outward while the foot falls inward (8). Diagnosis of a suspected moderate to serious ligament injury should be left to a trained health care professional who will obtain a detailed history, complete a physical examination, and perform special tests to assess joint stability.

Contusions

In sport, a common type of injury to the muscle is caused by direct impact often causing a *contusion*. A contusion is a soft-tissue hemorrhage and/or hematoma occurring after disruption of the muscle fibers with subsequent inflammation and edema. Contusions are graded by degree (1–6). A first-degree contusion is characterized by superficial tissue damage, no weakness or muscle spasm, mild loss of function, and ecchymosis (discoloration) and swelling and presents no restriction on ROM. A second-degree contusion is characterized by superficial and some deep tissue damage, mild to moderate weakness with no muscle spasm, moderate loss of function, and

Table 9.2	Grading and Characteristics of Ligament Sprains		
Classification	**Symptoms**	**Imaging Evidence**	**Treatment**
First degree: **few torn ligamentous fibers**	Pain with stretching, mild instability, decreased ROM	MRI of microscopic fiber disruption, although not required for diagnosis	**PRICE**, early partial ROM, followed by therapeutic exercise for strength/ROM
Second degree: **almost one-half of ligamentous fibers torn**	Pain with stretching, mild to moderate instability, moderate swelling, decreased ROM	MRI of partial macroscopic tear of ligament; may not be required for diagnosis	PRICE and immobilization to ensure correct healing of torn fibers, early partial ROM for circulation, followed by therapeutic exercise for strength/ROM
Third degree: **all ligamentous fibers torn (rupture)**	Joint instability, moderate to severe swelling, severe loss of function	MRI/x-ray image of malalignment and detect possible avulsion of bone	PRICE, immobilization, and/or surgical repair referral

Data from Dutton M. *Dutton's Orthopaedic Examination, Evaluation and Intervention.* 4th ed. New York (NY): McGraw-Hill; 2017. p. 43; and Anderson MK, Parr GP, Hall SJ, editors. *Foundations of Athletic Training: Prevention, Assessment, and Management.* 5th ed. Philadelphia (PA): Lippincott Williams & Wilkins; 2013. p. 165.

ecchymosis and swelling. This level of damage presents with decreased ROM. Finally, a third-degree contusion is severe and characterized by deep tissue damage, moderate to severe weakness with possible muscle spasm, severe loss of function, and ecchymosis and swelling. Substantial loss of ROM occurs due to swelling (2–5,8).

Immediate Care

If a client experiences an acute musculoskeletal injury during supervised sessions, the EP provides immediate care by **P**rotecting the injured joint/area, having the injured person **R**est or restrict activity, apply **I**ce with **C**ompression, and **E**levate the injured joint (PRICE) (2–5,8). Support and maintain the joint in a position to prevent discomfort, thus protecting from further injury. Following the acronym "PRICE" will serve as a reminder of all steps for immediate care. Also, assist the client, as needed, in seeking medical attention. If there is a potential head or neck injury, the client should not be moved, and emergency personnel should be contacted.

Understanding the process of tissue healing is essential for providing safe and effective exercise guidance to the injured client. The rate and length of each phase of healing varies depending on the type of tissue and degree of tissue damage following injury/surgery. The initial *inflammatory* phase is about 2–3 days or longer. Inflammation occurs in response to acute tissue damage and is mediated chemically (*e.g.*, histamine and bradykinin) causing increased blood flow and capillary permeability with edema resulting. Edema is an accumulation of fluid in surrounding tissues acting as a brace or immobilizer protecting the damaged tissue. Edema inhibits contractile tissue activity and stimulates sensory nerves that cause pain to further inhibit activity. The inflammatory phase is important to prepare for the subsequent phase of tissue repair and, therefore, should be accompanied by relative rest and passive modalities. Relative rest means the individual can do gentle ROM, protected weight bearing, and limited resistance activities for the injured extremity if the diagnosis is a grade I or II sprain or strain, or EIMD. Exercise for more severe injuries during this phase should be limited to non–weight bearing (such as deep end of the pool) and is guided by the medical findings and restrictions (8).

The *repair* phase begins within 3–5 days after injury and varies in length depending on the type of tissue and extent of damage but could last up to 2 months. During this phase, damaged tissue is replaced with scar tissue. The quality of scar tissue development relies on proper management of the injury during this phase. As the scar tissue develops, exercise programming is designed to prevent muscle atrophy and maintain joint integrity at the site of injury and promote synthesis and optimum organization of new collagen fibers. Exercise training progression is gradual and of low-load stress with pain-free ROM muscle setting (low-intensity isometric contraction). During this early phase, low resistance exercise is gradually introduced, again with a focus on pain-free activities. Exercise training is administered under the direction of a rehabilitative health care professional (*e.g.*, physical therapist, certified/licensed athletic trainer, or physician).

The final *remodeling* phase is characterized by weakened, repaired tissue. Exercise principles used during this phase are to promote hypertrophy and strength of the newly repaired tissue. Tissue remodeling can take up to 2–4 months, and exercise should progressively move toward activity-specific exercises. Early-stage progressive loading of tissue is important for collagen fiber alignment and muscle fiber hypertrophy, whereas later stage exercise should transition to activity-specific to prepare for return to activity (2–5,8,9,13). As mentioned earlier, the progression of each phase is highly variable depending on the degree of injury as well as several other factors including, but not limited to, prior fitness, age, nutritional factors, sleep quality, etc. The three phases of tissue healing are summarized in Table 9.3.

Medications for Musculoskeletal Pain and Inflammation

The goal of medical therapy is to reduce pain and inflammation during the acute phase of recovery and to stabilize the joint, if necessary. Oral medications commonly used to manage pain and

Table 9.3	Phases and Goals of Tissue Repair		
Phase	**Duration**	**Characteristics**	**Exercise Goals**
Inflammation	2–3+ d	Pain, edema, redness, ↑ inflammatory cell activity	**PRICE** for 20 min, 3–4 times a day
Repair	Up to 2 mo	Collagen fiber production, ↓ collagen fiber organization, ↓ inflammatory cell number	Progressive low-load stress isometric to ↓ muscle atrophy, ↑ joint integrity; low-level stretching to recover ROM and heat to ↑ blood flow to damaged tissue
Remodeling	2–4 mo	Optimum collagen fiber alignment, ↑ tissue strength	Initial progressive loading exercises followed by transition to activity-specific exercises for return to activity

↑, increase; ↓, decrease.

Adapted from Dutton M. *Dutton's Orthopaedic Examination, Evaluation and Intervention.* 4th ed. New York (NY): McGraw-Hill; 2017. p. 44–5; and Anderson MK, Parr GP, Hall SJ, editors. *Foundations of Athletic Training: Prevention, Assessment, and Management.* 5th ed. Philadelphia (PA): Lippincott Williams & Wilkins; 2013. p. 165–9.

inflammation after acute injury are listed in Table 9.4. Be advised that all medications are accompanied by a risk of toxicity and side effects. Knowledge of such risks should be fully understood prior to use. Recommendation for over-the-counter medications is best made by qualified health care providers, including medical doctors, nurse practitioners, physician, and assistants.

Exercise to Reduce Risk of Strains and Sprains

Appropriate exercises can lessen the risks of strains and sprains. With regard to connective tissue, physiological adaptations to resistance training increase ligament and tendon strength, and collagen content, to enhance the overall integrity of connective tissue (14). Similarly, muscle fiber size,

Table 9.4	Common Medications for Treatment of Musculoskeletal Injuries			
Class	**Generic Name**	**Brand Name**	**Effect**	**Potential Side Effects**
NSAIDs	Ibuprofen	Motrin, Advil	Analgesic, anti-inflammatory, antipyretic	GI bleeding
	Naproxen	Naprosyn, Aleve, Naprelan		
Analgesic	Acetaminophen	Tylenol, FeverAll, Tempra	Pain control	GI bleeding; liver damage
	Hydrocodone + acetaminophen	Vicodin, Lorcet-HD, Lortab	Pain control with sedating properties	Nausea, vomiting, dizziness
	Acetaminophen + codeine	Tylenol with Codeine		Nausea, vomiting, dizziness, confusion

GI, gastrointestinal.

Adapted from Liguori G, editor. American College of Sports Medicine. *ACSM's Guidelines for Exercise Testing and Prescription.* 11th ed. Philadelphia (PA): Wolters Kluwer; 2022. 548 p.; and American College of Sports Medicine. *ACSM's Resource Manual for Guidelines for Exercise Testing and Prescription.* 7th ed. Philadelphia (PA): Lippincott Williams & Wilkins; 2014. p. 717.

fast-twitch fibers, and rate of force production increase with resistance training as well, for an overall increase in muscle and connective tissue durability. Limited research is available showing a decreased risk of some types of muscle strain or sprain based on specific practices. A combination of focused resistance training and biomechanical training has been shown to reduce the incidence of traumatic ligamentous injuries in females (1). However, current practice encourages the client to apply the following strategies:

1. Warm up 5–7 minutes prior to vigorous exercise using large muscle group activities such as walking, jogging, cycling, or rowing ergometry.
2. Dynamic stretching may be performed following warm-up, just prior to a competition or event if the individual reports feeling stiff.
3. Neuromuscular training (balance) and resistance exercises as part of a regular training program have been shown to decrease some risks, such as for sprains (15). Neuromuscular training specific to landing biomechanics may also help reduce ligamentous injuries, especially in females (1).
4. Fatigue can increase injury risk (2–5). Therefore, the client should avoid exercise/sport when fatigued and increase training volume gradually. For optimal performance, a balance between exercise training and sport participation is important. During certain phases of an athlete's training program, fatigue due to overload is a desired outcome to induce specific adaptations, but excessive fatigue just before a significant sports event is detrimental.

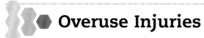# Overuse Injuries

Injuries are generally categorized as acute or overuse. Acute injuries typically occur with a single traumatic event such as joint sprains, muscle strains, or fracture. Overuse injuries result from repetitive microtrauma and occur over time. Periodization implemented into micro-, meso-, and macrocycles is vital to help prevent overuse injuries. Examples of overuse injuries include stress fractures, tendinopathies, and plantar fasciitis (PF).

Tendinopathy

Tendinopathy is a pathological change in the tendon resulting from repeated stress or microtraumas. The most common tendinopathies include tendinitis and tendinosis. Tendinitis is an acute inflammatory tendinopathy (2–5,8). Tendinosis describes a tendon with significant degenerative changes in the absence of an inflammatory response. Tendinosis is the more common of the two as most individuals seek treatment only after the acute inflammatory process has resolved (2–5). Common sites for tendinopathies include rotator cuff, common wrist flexor and extensor tendons, patellar tendon, and Achilles tendon.

Clinical Presentation/Assessment

Tendinopathies often result from repetitive overload injuries that disrupt the MTU. This overload usually occurs with too rapid of an increase in activity or load, such as increased training mileage in the case of runners or increased repetitive motions in the case of those engaged in racquet sports. These specific examples of overload are some of the most common mechanisms for tendinopathies. Other causes include premature return to occupational and/or sport and leisure activities after an injury. Individuals with tendinopathies often present with pain, particularly with contraction or stretch of the involved muscle (2–5,8). Assessment of tendinopathy by a qualified health professional includes evaluating strength and extensibility of the muscle and palpation of the involved tendon to determine tenderness (2–5).

Safe and Effective Exercise

For exercises that do not involve the affected joint/extremity, refer to Chapter 4 for exercise guidelines. For the affected area, the following considerations are important. Until pain has subsided, individuals should reduce activity of the affected muscle to decrease repetitive loading of the damaged tendon. Most individuals improve with conservative treatment that includes relative rest, ice, stretching, and/or use of analgesics (15). For some of the tendinopathies, the health care professional may recommend, for example, per week a counterforce forearm strap or other type of splinting, which reduces pain during activity. Once symptoms have decreased, and cleared by the clinician, strengthening of the affected area is appropriate. Considerable evidence exists supporting the use of appropriately graded concentric and eccentric exercise as a safe and effective means for strengthening the MTU across the affected joint (16,17).

Exercise Considerations for Tendinopathies

The frequency, intensity, time, and type of exercise (FITT) is somewhat variable in the literature. A review of multiple studies yields reports of decreased pain and return to activity with eccentric exercise (18). In addition, decreased weight-bearing activities, such as exercise in chest deep water, is a good option for lower extremity tendinopathies during the early, most acute phase. Refer to Table 9.5 for specific guidelines. Blood flow restriction exercises have also been shown to be effective in the rehabilitation process when implemented properly for specific client needs (19).

Table 9.5	Exercise Guidelines for Tendinopathies and Plantar Fasciitis	
Condition		**Exercise Type**
	Resistance	**Flexibility/Stretching**
Tendinosis		
Type	Eccentric until pain free; then add concentric and plyometrics as tolerated	Passive elongation of the muscle/tendon
Frequency	3–4 sessions per week	Daily
Intensity	6–15 reps	3 reps
	3–4 sets — use body weight with progressive loading as tolerated	■ Gradual force to provide gentle stretch
Time	Completion of reps/sets or until pain level reaches threshold to stop exercise	Hold each rep 30 s
Special considerations	Concentric exercise should be avoided early in the healing process until nonsport activities are pain free (9–11).	
Plantar Fasciitis		
Type		■ Gentle stretch of the fascia to the point of tension ■ Stretching: great toe flexors and gastrocnemius-soleus
Frequency		3 times a day
Intensity		10 reps (hold 10 s)
Time		To completion of reps
Special considerations	Pain determines exercise intensity and duration.	

Bursitis

Bursitis is an inflammation of a small fluid-filled sac called the bursa. The bursa acts as a cushion to reduce friction between muscles, tendons, and joints. Common areas for bursitis are the shoulders, hips, knees, and elbows (2–5). Bursitis can sometimes be a response to an acute injury.

Clinical Presentation/Assessment

Classic symptoms of bursitis include sharp pain, tenderness, and swelling at the site of the bursa. A health professional's assessment of bursitis includes a thorough examination via palpation, mobility, and strength measures. Bursitis is managed conservatively with rest, thermal or low-level shock wave modalities, nonsteroidal anti-inflammatory drugs (NSAIDs), and often corticosteroid injections (8).

Safe and Effective Exercise

Once the clinician has cleared the client for activity, stretching and strengthening exercises can be done within a pain-free ROM. Strengthening follows guidelines for resistance training as identified by the American College of Sports Medicine (ACSM) guidelines for healthy adults (10,13,20). However, starting with one set of light-intensity exercise with the involved extremity will allow the EP to determine the client's response to increased movement of the bursa. Importantly, if the client has had a corticosteroid injection, follow the health care providers' postinjection restrictions. Physician guidelines often restrict activity for 24–48 hours postinjection.

Plantar Fasciitis

PF is relatively common, affecting upward of 10% of the U.S. population (21,22). PF commonly occurs with repeated trauma (overuse) to the origin of the plantar fascia on the medial calcaneal tubercle and is progressive in nature. Although most common in middle-aged individuals, particularly females, PF can also be presented among individuals with other risk factors such as a high body mass index (BMI), abnormal foot biomechanics, gastrocnemius/soleus tightness, or consistent running. Present beliefs are that abnormal stresses to the plantar fascia result in a type of microtrauma, with inflammation and resultant pain (2–5,8).

Clinical Presentation/Assessment

Classic symptoms for PF include pain with first weight-bearing steps in the morning or after sitting as well as during the first few minutes of running. Barefoot walking may exacerbate pain as well (21). Pain usually subsides with activity and increases after prolonged rest. Tight plantarflexor muscles along with either pes planus (flat foot) or pes cavus (high arch) may predispose an individual to PF (2–5).

Health care provider assessment of PF includes palpation along the plantar fascia, evaluating extensibility of the gastrocnemius, and a thorough client history. During the acute stage, PF is best managed with control of pain and minimal or non–weight-bearing exercise. Pain management is often accomplished with ice massage, minimizing excess stress on the fascia (*i.e.*, avoiding barefoot walking), and NSAIDs (2–5). However, a lack of scientific evidence exists supporting NSAID use for PF, although these medications may work for some individuals (15). For many individuals, an orthosis may help reduce the abnormal stress to the plantar fascia. Night splints can reduce pain and shorten recovery time. In addition, qualified professionals may provide orthotic intervention or taping to support the involved structures during weight-bearing exercises (23).

Safe and Effective Exercise

Once the client is cleared for activity by the clinician, the EP can develop a fitness program. One important consideration is to introduce stretching of the plantar fascia as well as the plantarflexors and toe flexors (7,14,23). Individuals experiencing pain during stretching and other activities are to be completed as tolerated by the client. Functional weight-bearing exercises relieve stress on the plantar fascia by supporting the medial longitudinal arch and strengthening the extrinsic (anterior and posterior tibialis and the peroneus longus) and the intrinsic (abductor hallucis, flexor hallucis brevis, flexor digitorum brevis, abductor digiti minimi, and dorsal interossei) musculature of the foot (2–5,24). Examples of appropriate functional weight-bearing exercises include toe and heel raises (extrinsic) and exercises that focus on the small muscles on the bottom of the foot (intrinsic) (25).

Examples of Safe and Effective Exercises for Overuse Injuries

As previously noted, tendinopathies and PF should be addressed using exercises focusing initially on eccentric loading and stretching. Examples of these exercises are shown for calf, wrist, and foot in Figures 9.1 through 9.4. Once cleared for activity by the clinician, the EP can follow ACSM guidelines for exercise prescription for healthy adults. The primary recommendations include modifications of intensity or duration based on the client's response during the activity. A reduction in weight-bearing activities such as pool activities is perhaps a good way to progress the client who has reported significant limitations due to his or her injury. Continued emphasis on a proper warm-up and stretching at the beginning of a session combined with mobility and possibly ice at the end of each session should always be prioritized within the exercise program. Tracking pain, irritability, and tightness in the foot and calf must be monitored.

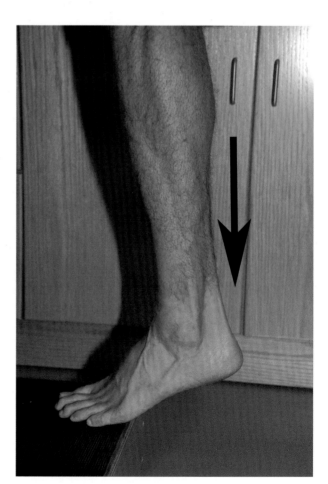

FIGURE 9.1. Eccentric loading of the gastrocnemius. Stand on the edge of a step. Using the uninvolved leg, raise up on toes (plantarflexed position), shift weight to involved leg, and slowly lower to start position. To avoid concentric contractions during the painful stage of healing, ensure that uninvolved limb is used to lift body weight.

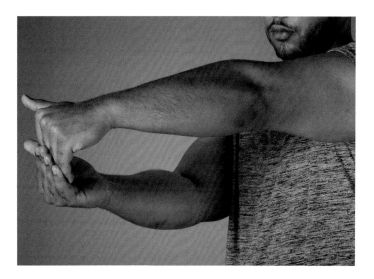

FIGURE 9.2. Stretching exercise for lateral epicondylitis. While sitting or standing, flex the wrist with opposite hand while elbow is extended. Apply pressure until a gentle stretch is felt at the elbow or forearm (wrist extensor) muscles.

Table 9.5 includes exercise guidelines for tendinopathies and PF. As indicated at the bottom of the table, pain is the limiting factor in the exercise intensity and duration and the degree of stretch.

Low Back Pain

Low back pain (LBP) can be traumatic, acute, or chronic. LBP is estimated to affect 60%–80% of the adult population at some point in their lives with an 80% recovery rate within 4–6 weeks, regardless of treatment (26). LBP is also the leading cause of years lived with disability and accounts for more lost workdays than any other musculoskeletal disorder; yet, only 58% of people with LBP seek care (27–29). Many causes of LBP exist that result in including disc compression, degenerative changes in

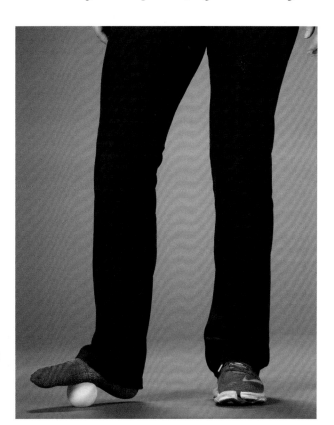

FIGURE 9.3. Stretching exercise for PF. Sitting with involved foot resting on opposite knee, apply stretch by extending great toe and massage arch with opposite hand. Or use a tennis or other ball by placing the ball on a flat surface and use the pressure of the ball to massage the tight arch.

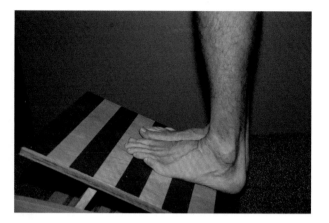

FIGURE 9.4. Stretching exercise for gastrocnemius and soleus. Stand on slanted surface, lean body forward keeping heels in contact with surface until a gentle stretch is felt in the posterior calf. Bend knees slightly to isolate the soleus muscle.

the lumbar spine, various joint and bone pathologies, and muscle imbalances, leading to LBP (26,30). The focus centers on general or idiopathic LBP resulting from issues of muscle imbalance or weakness. Unfortunately, unless the underlying cause of the pain is treated, the recurrence of LBP is quite high. Causes may include improper biomechanics from another body part (*e.g.,* foot, knees, hips) that put stress on the lower back over time. Although sitting for long periods of time, such as in many occupations or leisure activities, has not been shown to be related to LBP, extended sitting time may lead to loss of flexibility in the hip muscles, which may contribute to LBP (26,31). Any individual presenting with significant LBP is evaluated by a qualified health care provider prior to participation in an exercise program. The need for medical evaluation is especially true if the pain radiates beyond the low back, or if the client reports loss of strength or changes in sensation in a lower extremity. Individuals with chronic LBP but without the complications previously noted may safely participate in exercise without health care evaluation. Most individuals will have some pain/discomfort at the onset of exercise. However, pain should not worsen or start to radiate into the lower extremity during exercise.

Clinical Presentation/Assessment

Muscle groups commonly referred to as the core are important to the function of the spine/trunk and consist of multiple layers of muscles acting to stabilize the spine, pelvis, and kinetic chain during functional movements (26,32). Core muscles are thought to provide a stable base of support to allow for optimal performance of the spine and extremities and help prevent injury. Endurance of core musculature seems to be more critical than strength to overall low back health (Table 9.6) (33).

Research indicates that core muscle activity is different in clients with LBP. The pain can be due to holding prolonged postures and the inability of core muscles to adequately stabilize the spine, usually intensified with movement especially toward end of the ROM. Clients may actually present with a stiff posture in an attempt to reduce movement of the back. However, this action will result in further stiffness and pain. Once cleared for activity by a health care practitioner, the client can safely participate in exercise. Assessment of the client includes core muscle activity and ability to perform basic movement. Core muscle assessments should focus on the stabilization of the transverse abdominals, mobility in the psoas/hip flexor complex, and activation of the gluteal muscles. Pain questionnaires and other outcome measures are often used to subjectively quantify pain and functional impairment. Examples are the Oswestry Low Back Pain Scale (34) and the McGill Pain Scale (35).

Safe and Effective Exercise

Core stabilization exercises do not fit the normal FITT template but should be incorporated into daily activities as with any general exercise program (26,36). Many clients respond better to exercise training if the initial training is core stabilization plus aerobic exercise (moderate intensity) even if the underlying cause is not instability. Core stabilization programs progress through various stages

Table 9.6	Core Musculature	
Classification	**Muscle**	**Action**
Global stabilizers	Erector spinae	Extension of vertebral column
	External obliques	Flexion of vertebral column with bilateral contraction, same side lateral flexion, and opposite side rotation of vertebral column with unilateral contraction
	Quadratus lumborum	Assists with extension, lateral flexion of lumbar vertebral column
	Rectus abdominis	Flexes vertebral column
Local stabilizers	Internal obliques	Flexion of vertebral column with bilateral contraction, same side lateral flexion, and same side rotation of vertebral column with unilateral contraction
	Multifidus	Extension of vertebral column with bilateral contraction and rotation of vertebral column with unilateral contraction
	Transversus abdominis	Draws abdominal wall toward spine; helps maintain abdominal pressure

Adapted with permission from Kolber M, Beekhuizen K. Lumbar stabilization: an evidence-based approach for the athlete with low back pain. *Strength Cond J.* 2007;29(2):26–37.

of increasing difficulty or exercise intensity. The first therapy objective is to train the muscles of the trunk to control proximal core stability, which is accomplished during stage I, and is referred to as abdominal bracing (26,36), which requires the client to engage the small, deep stabilizing muscles (transversus abdominis, multifidi, etc.), primarily in a supine position (26,36). The second therapy objective is to challenge core stability by adding extremity and whole-body movements, which will create enough core stability to maintain movement (32,33). During this phase of training, cocontraction of the deep core muscles is required while adding more challenging positions such as quadruped or bird dog into the therapy plan. Other movements activating core muscles include the side plank for the oblique and quadratus lumborum muscles and the front plank for the rectus abdominis and oblique muscles. The third objective focuses on maintaining appropriate cocontraction of these supporting muscles while performing exercises designed to enhance skill transference to performing more functional exercises including pushes, pulls, carries, lifts, lowers, lunges, and squats. Regardless of the stage, the client must maintain core stability. When stabilization is no longer maintained, the exercise is stopped. In some case, adding deep breaths to these exercises assists in transference — clients should not hold breaths. See Table 9.7 for a discussion regarding safe and effective lumbar LBP stabilization exercises (22). Progressions of core exercises are illustrated elsewhere (32,33,36), and examples of selected core exercises are shown in Figures 9.5 through 9.7. In stage I (see Fig. 9.5), develop the abdominal drawing-in maneuver sometimes referred to as "connecting your abdominals," a critical component of all core stabilization exercises (30,36). Table 9.7 includes exercise guidelines for clients who suffer from LBP. Often, but not always, LBP may be alleviated through systematically strengthening the core muscles and posture training. Performing all exercises correctly provides the best opportunity for optimal improvement. For additional information regarding properly performing LBP exercises, please see Chapman and DeFranca (26) and McGill (33).

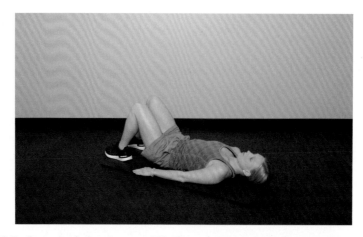

FIGURE 9.5. Example of stage I core stabilization exercise: isolating the transversus abdominis.

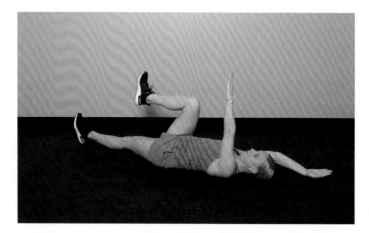

FIGURE 9.6. Example of stage II core stabilization exercise: opposing arm and leg.

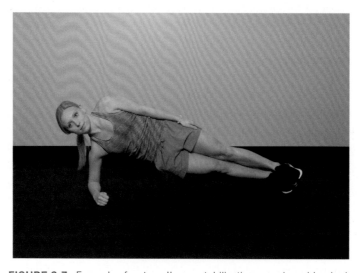

FIGURE 9.7. Example of a stage II core stabilization exercise: side plank.

Visit ⊙ Lippincott® Connect to watch videos 9.1 and 9.2, which demonstrate side plank, front plank, bird dog, farmer's walk, and lunge.

Table 9.7	Exercise Guidelines for Low Back Pain		
	Type		
	Weight-Bearing Aerobic	**Resistance**	**Flexibility/Stretching**
	Fast walking	Bridging, bird dog, curl-ups (body resistance initially)	Limit back exercises to unloaded spinal flexion/extension; full hip flexibility/stretching
Frequency	Daily	Initial — daily; 2–3 times a week for resisted exercises	Daily
Intensity	Prescribed percentage of maximum HR as tolerated below pain threshold	High reps and low loads for initial resistance training	Stretch within pain-free ROM.
Time	Build up to 30 min · d⁻¹.		Hold for 10–30+ s. Repeat for 2–3 reps.
Special considerations	Exercise during the first or second hour after rising from bed should be avoided because of disc hydration and subsequent loading. Any exercise that increases the intensity or frequency of pain should be discontinued, and the client should be referred for further evaluation. Exercises resulting in high-impact loading should be avoided.		

Adapted with permission from McGill S. *Ultimate Back Fitness and Performance.* 6th ed. Waterloo (Canada): Backfitpro; 2017. 331 p.

The first exercise shown in Figure 9.5 is used when teaching the client to isolate the transversus abdominis, a key muscle of the core. The client performs the exercise in supine position, with knees bent and arms relaxed. Instructions to the client are very specific when teaching the activity, as incorrect performance of this seemingly simple maneuver is common. Thus, an example of instructions to the client would be as follows: *Tighten your pelvic floor muscles (as if you were stopping the flow of urine); then, draw in your lower abdomen as if pulling belly button away from waistband. Think about pulling the muscles in the pelvic floor "up and in" like a zipper zipping up from your pelvis to your ribs (rather than down toward the mat).* Have the client hold the contraction for a count of 6–10; repeat four to five times. Some clients find tactile feedback useful; thus, have clients place their fingers just above the iliac crest for physical feedback. This activity is progressed by holding for 30 counts during the contraction or by slowing lifting one foot a few inches off of the ground, alternating and lifting the opposite foot off the ground. Maintaining the contraction while implementing small, slow movements is a way of progressing the activity toward stage II. The client is instructed to avoid holding his or her breath or flattening the back (posterior pelvic tilt).

Stage II exercises shown in Figure 9.6 requires first a contraction of the transversus abdominis (initiated from the starting position — supine with knees bent and feet on the ground), progressing to simultaneously raising the diagonal arm and leg. The arm is raised to a vertical position and the leg to 45°. After returning to the starting position, the client will repeat with the other diagonal pair, alternating in a rhythmic fashion. An important focus during this exercise is to maintain contact between the lumbar spine and the floor while moving arms and legs. Two other exercises which are appropriate during stage II are side planks (see Fig. 9.7) and an exercise in quadruped (on hands and knees; Fig. 9.8), sometimes called the "bird-dog exercise." The side plank is a good exercise for

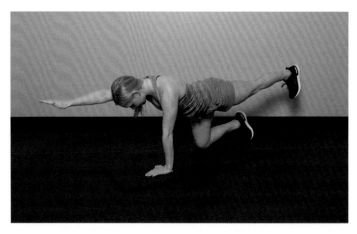

FIGURE 9.8. Example of a stage II core stabilization exercise: quadruped ("bird-dog exercise").

strengthening the multifidus, a strong stabilizer of the back. While partially lying on one side, the client places the forearm on the mat, directly under the shoulder (upper arm perpendicular to the ground). The client raises the hips off of the ground, with the knees acting as a fulcrum, and maintaining a straight trunk. Initially, the client can use his or her knees as the lower base and eventually progress to using the feet as a fulcrum. The "bird-dog exercise" is performed in quadruped form with the client extending the right leg backward and the left arm forward. These exercises are initially safe and are held for 10 seconds. The client proceeds to extends the left leg backward and the right arm forward. These exercises are repeated three to five times.

Stage III exercises provide a challenge to the core muscles by incorporating unstable surfaces or movement while maintaining the pelvis and spine in a neutral (vertical) position. Physioball or tubing exercises provide a means of introducing increased activation and control of the core muscles without requiring movement. The lunge is illustrated in Figure 9.9 and requires contraction of the abdominals followed by a lunge forward. As with other exercises, the client returns to the starting standing position with both feet together and repeats with the other leg. The client must strive to maintain a vertical torso without side-to-side movement during the lunge. The EP must closely supervise this exercise to ensure proper position and control of the movement.

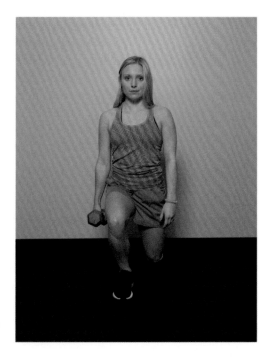

FIGURE 9.9. Example of stage III core stabilization exercise: lunge with hand weight.

The exercise guidelines found in Table 9.7 are for clients who suffer from LBP. Often, but not always, LBP may be alleviated through systematically strengthening the core muscles and posture training. Performing all exercises correctly provides the best opportunity for optimal improvement (36–38). As noted earlier, resistance training follows ACSM guidelines for a healthy individual (20). Clients respond better if the stabilization exercises are started during the first week. Dependent on symptoms, resistance training is incorporated when appropriate (36–38). If back pain increases or if the symptoms start to radiate, exercise training is stopped, and the client sent back to his or her physician. Scientific evidence suggests participation in regular physical activity is essential in LBP management (26,39). For additional information regarding properly performing LBP exercises, please see Chapman and DeFranca (26) and McGill (33).

EPs should emphasize to the client that basic appropriate posture throughout his or her everyday activities is crucial in helping to prevent or treat LBP. The exercises in stages I, II, and III are important, but more impact will be made if the client can implement back exercises throughout the day as well as maintain posture in everyday activities (*e.g.*, sedentary occupation or leisure activities). Poor posture outside of the exercise session will work against the improvements made during an exercise session. Appropriate posture throughout the day will reinforce the improvements made during the exercise sessions and help lead to long-term relief from LBP and prevention.

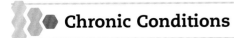

Chronic Conditions

Chronic conditions are prolonged in duration, do not resolve spontaneously, and are rarely resolved completely. More than 75% of health care costs are estimated to be due to treating chronic conditions (40). Discussions in this section pertain to two progressive chronic conditions: arthritis and osteoporosis. Arthritis is the leading cause of functional impairments and activity limitations (41).

Arthritis

Arthritis is typified as inflammation of a joint and often surrounding tissues. The two most common types of arthritis are rheumatoid arthritis (RA) and osteoarthritis (OA) (41). Recommendation for treatment of arthritis includes exercise as an important component of therapy (42).

Rheumatoid Arthritis

RA is an autoimmune, chronic inflammatory disease affecting the synovial lining of joints and other connective tissues. RA is a slow-progressing disease that affects 1 in 12 adult women and 1 in 20 adult men in the United States with symptoms that cycle through periods of exacerbation and remission (43).

Clinical Presentation/Assessment

Individuals with RA typically present with severe joint pain and inflammation, reduced muscle mass, decreased muscular strength and endurance, decreased mobility, and impaired physical activity. Onset of RA is typically after 40 years of age. Loss of initial muscle strength is related to decreased activity; however, over time, the disease causes cytokine-driven hypermetabolism, resulting in protein degradation, and loss of muscle mass, which is termed *rheumatic cachexia*. RA is also associated with increased cardiovascular disease risk, independent of normal cardiovascular risk factors (44,45). Interestingly, cardiovascular risk is similar to cohorts without RA with early use of specific medications that mediate the immune system response (46).

Prior to participating in an exercise training program, a physician completes an RA assessment of the client to include a thorough history, ROM and strength tests, and appropriate outcome measures to determine the stage of the disease and the client's functional status. In addition, the physician determines if a joint is unstable and needs splinting to safely perform activities. Importantly, early pharmacological intervention slows joint deterioration and allows the individual to participate in physical activity.

Safe and Effective Exercise

Once cleared for activity, regular dynamic exercises are effective for improving muscular strength, cardiorespiratory function, and cardiovascular health in individuals with RA (47). Exercise training can reduce pain, joint stiffness, and fatigue. After a period of exercise training, an individual with RA can perform moderate-intensity exercises with little or no joint damage (48,49). In fact, if the individual has mild or moderate RA, exercise training can progress to higher intensity exercise. Clients with severe joint pain and stiffness may prefer aquatic activities during periods of exacerbation, as the weight-reduced environment puts less stress through the joints in the lower extremity. Individuals with RA are encouraged to pursue activities of daily living requiring movement, as the benefits of an exercise program are lost when no longer continued (44,50). If clients have been prescribed a splint or brace, the individual should wear that during all activities (refer to Table 9.8 for specific exercise guidelines). In addition to aerobic,

Table 9.8	Exercise Guidelines for Rheumatoid Arthritis and Osteoarthritis		
	Type		
	Weight-Bearing Aerobic	**Resistance**	**Flexibility/Stretching**
Type	Walking, cycling, rowing, swimming	Weight machines, free weights, elastic bands, or body weight for initial program	Combination of dynamic and static stretching focused on joints with decreased ROM
Frequency	$3–5\ d \cdot wk^{-1}$	$2–3\ d \cdot wk^{-1}$	Daily
Intensity	Moderate to vigorous; 40%–50% to 60%–80% of maximum HRR, RPE = 11–16	Initial: 50%–60% 1-RM; progress to 60%–80% 1-RM	
Time	$150\ min \cdot wk^{-1}$ of moderate intensity; $75\ min \cdot wk^{-1}$ of vigorous intensity or a combination	8–12 reps; 2–4 sets	10–30+ s per static stretch × 3 reps
Special considerations for RA	With acute exacerbation, avoid high-intensity resistance exercises to minimize pain. Those with significant damage of large joints (assessed radiographically) should limit high-intensity weight-bearing exercise to avoid further damage (36).		
Special considerations for OA	Avoid overstretching unstable joints. Pain should not increase with activity. No strenuous exercise during acute flare-ups of OA and during periods of inflammation.		

HRR, heart rate reserve; RPE, rating of perceived exertion; 1-RM, one repetition maximum.

Adapted from Foxworth J, Millar AL, White E. Musculoskeletal concerns. In: Thompson WR, editor. *ACSM's Clinical Exercise Physiology*. Philadelphia (PA): Wolters Kluwer; 2018. p. 475–530; and American College of Sports Medicine. *ACSM's Guidelines for Exercise Testing and Prescription*. 11th ed. Philadelphia (PA): Wolters Kluwer; 2021. 548 p.

resistance, and flexibility training, balance training is an important component of a training program for someone with arthritis (20).

Osteoarthritis

OA is a relatively common chronic degenerative joint disease that becomes more prevalent with age (42). OA first presents as stiffness and pain during physical activity. The x-rays show deficits in articular cartilage of synovial joints, although the relationship between pain or functional changes and the amount of damage reflected on an x-ray is very low (51). As OA progresses, bone remodeling and overgrowth at the joint margins also occurs. Although originally thought to be limited to the joint, evidence shows inflammation as a component of OA. Previous joint injury, resulting from excessive loading (such as overweight) or repeated low-force stressors, is predictive of OA development (42). The most common anatomical locations for OA are the large weight-bearing joints, including the hips, knees, the cervical and lumbar spine, the distal interphalangeal joints of the fingers, and carpometacarpal joint of the thumb.

Obesity and Osteoarthritis

Obesity is associated with OA development. For each kilogram of increased body mass, risk of OA genesis is increased by 14% (51,52). Increased body mass seems to affect the large, weight-bearing joints more than the smaller, non–weight-bearing joints. Regardless of the mechanism, individuals must maintain an optimal BMI to minimize the effect of body mass on OA. Additionally, weight loss has been shown to decrease the associated symptoms of OA (53). Exercise training remains an important component to long-term management of obesity (20,47).

Clinical Presentation/Assessment

Individuals with OA often present with pain, joint stiffness, decreased strength, decreased flexibility, and decreased cardiovascular fitness. Prior to participation in an exercise training program, an assessment of the client is completed by a health care provider if the client has severe pain or movement limitations. However, individuals often self-diagnose during the early stages of OA without seeing a physician. In general, clients with OA can safely participate in exercise as long as the pain is not worse after physical activity, or "giving way" of a joint or joints is reported. Similar to RA, progression of OA can lead to joint instability and the client may need a splint or brace. Assessments for OA include a thorough client history, ROM and strength testing, and evaluation of cardiovascular fitness. As part of the client history, pain is evaluated using a variety of pain questionnaires including the Western Ontario and McMaster Universities Osteoarthritis Index (54).

Safe and Effective Exercise

Scientific evidence supports initiation or continuation of exercise for individuals with OA (37,47,55–58). Exercise improves overall function and prevents disability. Benefits include improved flexibility, muscular strength, cardiovascular fitness, and quality of life as well as decreased pain. Similar to research findings with RA, individuals with OA can safely participate in high-intensity exercise (57). However, starting with low-intensity exercise and progress slowly is important so that symptoms and response are monitored (35,46). Exercise may include land-based or aquatic-based programs. Aquatic programs provide an alternative environment benefitting clients who do not tolerate land-based exercise because of pain or obesity (59). Health care providers may prescribe a brace if the client has evidence of joint instability. If the individual has been prescribed a brace for weight-bearing activities, the brace should be worn regularly. Evidence suggests pain and stiffness often decrease during exercise. However, if joint pain persists or increases beyond preexercise level, duration and/or intensity should be reduced (20,36,47).

Medication Effects for Rheumatoid Arthritis and Osteoarthritis

Pharmacological management is commonly used to reduce pain and inflammation and, in the case of RA, to control the immune system. Clients should be aware that prolonged and/or excessive use of NSAIDs can cause GI bleeding and may reduce kidney function (47). Also, RA-remitting drugs may cause secondary organ disease, including myopathy. Steroids may predispose individuals to stress fractures. Finally, oral corticosteroids cause skeletal myopathy, truncal obesity, osteoporosis, and GI bleeding (47). On the positive side and as noted earlier, scientific evidence suggests some disease-modifying drugs used for RA may actually reduce cardiovascular risk (43). Aside from pharmacological management, other dietary changes have shown to be effective for some individuals to naturally reduce pain and inflammatory symptoms.

Exercise Guidelines for Rheumatoid Arthritis and Osteoarthritis

Examples of safe and effective aerobic and resistance exercises for RA and OA are shown in Figure 9.10. Additional details regarding exercise guidelines are supplied in Table 9.8. An exercise program should follow ACSM recommendations for individuals who are otherwise healthy adults with modifications for pain or evidence of inflammation such as swelling. Exercise training is reduced during periods of symptom flare-ups. However, regular, systematic exercise is effective for preserving and improving physical function and independence in those with RA and OA (42). Home exercise programs are known to be effective with proper instruction (60). Neuromotor activities for balance are an important component of a prescription as arthritis negatively affects proprioception, reducing overall balance (20,61). In addition, clients should be encouraged to

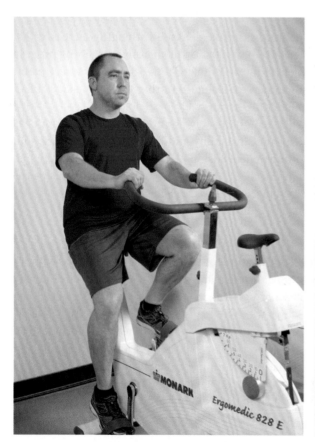
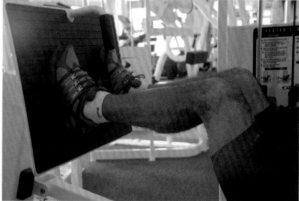
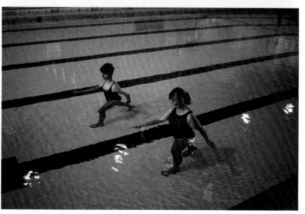

FIGURE 9.10. Types of aerobic and resistance exercises for persons with RA and OA.

reduce their sedentary behavior throughout the day, particularly long periods of sitting because this is also related to pain and joint stiffness.

Osteoporosis

Osteoporosis, or the "silent disease," is characterized by low BMD or bone mass and deterioration of the bone microarchitecture and/or geometry that increases skeletal fragility and fracture risk (62,63). This condition often goes undetected because early stages lack clear or overt symptoms. Current research indicates that as much as 80% of low trauma fractures occur in individuals who are not diagnosed with osteoporosis but have normal or osteopenia bone density based on dual-energy x-ray absorptiometry (DEXA) assessment, thus highlighting the limitations of DEXA to accurately assess bone strength (64). Thus, anyone working with older individuals who have multiple risk factors should incorporate balance activities and progressive resistance early in the training process.

Osteoporosis is largely preventable yet is a serious public health concern afflicting 1 in 2 women and 1 in 5 men older than 50 years (63,64). Women are 3 times more likely to suffer from osteoporosis (62,65). In the United States, approximately 10 million women and men have osteoporosis, and another 34 million are at risk for developing osteoporosis. Globally, the number of those with osteoporosis is greater than 200 million (66). More than 2 million osteoporotic fractures were identified in 2005 with a predicted increase to more than 3 million fractures by 2025 (66). Because osteoporosis often leads to fracture, the potential exists for loss of workdays or employment and increased hospitalizations. The economic burden of osteoporotic fractures, including loss of work, loss of independence, and cost of treatment, is substantial and projected to reach $25.3 billion in the United States for treatment-related costs alone (66). More significantly, the loss of function in older adults is a risk factor for loss of independence due to osteoporotic fractures or related pain. The most prevalent types of osteoporotic fracture in later life are of the hip, spine, and forearm (63). Treatment and rehabilitation often translate into a long hospital visit and subsequent physical therapy before one can manage on his or her own. However, disuse atrophy after surgical repair compounds a potentially long, arduous recovery, and the osteoporotic fracture often develops to a life-threatening event for an older adult (67). More than 70% of osteoporotic fractures occur in individuals older than 70 years and present a direct threat to aging independently — a goal of older adults. In fact, more than 25% of older adults with an osteoporotic fracture die within 5 years (68). However, even in older women with normal BMD, the risk of falling and reduced quadriceps strength contributes to subsequent fracture risk (68). Therefore, activity programs for older adults should focus on bone growth and maintenance as well as lower body strength and reducing risk of falls.

Risk Factors for Osteoporosis

In addition to individuals having osteoporosis, many other individuals have low bone density or osteopenia, which predisposes one to osteoporosis. Much work is needed to determine the cause(s) of osteoporosis and osteopenia; however, research suggests a number of risk factors for developing low bone density, particularly pertaining to nutritional imbalances or deficiencies. Both modifiable and nonmodifiable risk factors increase the chances of developing osteoporosis and are found in Table 9.9. Modifiable risk factors are influenced by lifestyle choices indicating that we do have some control and influence over bone health.

Osteoporosis is classified as primary or secondary. Primary osteoporosis is age related, and secondary osteoporosis is due to other factors such as medication regimens that decrease bone mass at any time during the lifespan (69). The female athlete triad is an example of secondary osteoporosis and begins with disordered eating followed by amenorrhea resulting in early-onset osteoporosis (20,36). In addition to medications, some research has shown increased risk of osteoporosis

Table 9.9	Risk Factors for Bone Loss, Osteoporosis, and Fracture

Nonmodifiable Risk Factors	Modifiable Risk Factors	Disorders Associated with Osteoporosis
Female	Physical inactivity	Previous low body weight
Aging	Low calcium intake ($<$500–850 mg $\cdot$ d^{-1}), vitamin D, Mg, Ph deficiency	RA
Family history of osteoporosis or hip fracture	Smoker (current)	Malabsorption syndromes (including chronic liver disease, inflammatory bowel disease)
White or Asian ethnicity	Excessive alcohol consumption	Primary hyperparathyroidism
	Excessive caffeine intake	
	Prescription medicine side effects	
Loss of height and thoracic kyphosis	Excessive soda and sugar consumption	Long-term immobilization
Small body frame	Low strength/physical capability	
Natural or surgical menopause before age 45 yr	Low body weight (BMI $<$19)	
	Amenorrhea, including female athlete triad	
Previous fracture after low-energy trauma	Low testosterone in males	
	Impaired vision	
	Impaired hearing	
	Postural hypotension	
	Unstable/risky environment (low light, uneven floor, unsecured carpets)	
	Poorly fitting footwear, need for assistive devices	
	Multiple medications	

Mg, magnesium; Ph, phosphorus.

Data from Finigan J, Greenfield DM, Blumsohn A, et al. Risk factors for vertebral and nonvertebral fracture over 10 years: a population-based study in women. *J Bone Miner Res.* 2008;23(1):75–85; Iacono MV. Osteoporosis: a national public health priority. *J Perianesth Nurs.* 2007;22(3):175–82; and Holroyd C, Cooper C, Dennison E. Epidemiology of osteoporosis. *Best Prac Res Clin Endocrin Metab.* 2008;22(5):671–85.

and related fractures with specific comorbidities — specifically hypertension and arthritis (70). Consideration is given to all comorbidities when screening a client.

Peak bone density, or highest lifetime bone density, is achieved in the age range of 20–25 years, and loss of bone density begins around the age of 25–30 years (71,72). Men and women lose bone at about the same rate until women approach menopause, which occurs around the age of 52 years. Bone loss accelerates in women in late perimenopause (40–50 yr) and continues at an increased rate through early postmenopausal years (72–74). The increased rate of loss after menopause and overall lower peak bone mass in women likely contribute to the higher incidence of osteoporosis and fragility fractures in women (74). However, men are also at risk for developing osteoporosis with an increased fracture risk after age 65 years (75).

Most bone growth occurs by the end of the second decade of life with the achievement of peak bone mass and density in the 20s. Because all individuals will lose bone density and mass after the peak bone growth years, the goal for healthy aging of bone is to maximize the development of peak bone mass, achieve a high lifetime peak bone mass level, and minimize the rate of bone loss throughout the lifespan. In doing so, the lowest lifetime bone density, usually occurring later in life, will still be high enough to protect from osteoporotic fracture. The age range around puberty (13–15 yr) is the time of peak bone velocity when bone growth occurs at the fastest lifetime rate. Bone growth occurring during this critical period is inversely related with the amount of bone loss during the last four decades of life (76). Although genetics play an important role in overall bone mass, nutrition and physical activity are equally important influences on the bone development. Therefore, particular attention is paid to these lifestyle behaviors during the critical prepubertal (10–12 yr) and pubertal years when bone is most responsive to the exercise stimulus. Maximizing bone growth during puberty will confer important benefits to bone health in later life (76).

Clinical Presentation/Assessment

Individuals with osteoporosis may not initially present differently than other clients. However, health care providers generally start to do risk assessment for osteoporosis for individuals over 40 years of age, or if there are other risk factors such as amenorrhea. A widely used risk assessment tool is the Fracture Risk Assessment Tool (FRAX) (77). Diagnosis of osteoporosis is based on bone densitometry measured by a DEXA (or DXA) scan. Scan results are compared with those of an ethnicity- and gender-matched, 30-year-old reference. Bone density within +1.0 and −1.0 standard deviation (*SD*) unit (or *T* score) of the reference density is considered normal. A density score of −2.5 *SD* units or lower is deemed osteoporosis. *Osteopenia* is defined as bone density between normal and osteoporosis and describes those at risk for osteoporosis, with a density *SD* between −1.0 and −2.5 (78,79).

In addition to bone density, a clinician will assess hormone levels, general muscular strength, and balance. Once cleared for activity, the EP should assess all components of fitness, including balance. Typically, the client with osteoporosis has reduced muscle mass, decreased muscular strength and endurance, decreased mobility, poor balance, and impaired physical activity. If an older client has some apparent risk factors for osteoporosis, such as female, postmenopausal, or slight build, the EP is encouraged to recommend that the client be cleared by a physician prior to activity. If the EP suspects decreased bone density in a younger client, particularly female, the EP should encourage the client to seek medical consultation. Females participating in distance running, swimming, and gymnastics are reported to be at the greatest risk for presenting with the "Female Athlete Triad," which includes low BMD. As noted earlier, they and some males should be screened following recommended guidelines and referred to a health care professional for follow-up (6,7).

Dietary and Pharmacological Support for Bone Health

Nutritional support for bone growth and maintenance requires adequate amounts of calcium and vitamin D. The Institute of Medicine recommendations for calcium and vitamin D intake are shown in Table 9.10 (80). Magnesium, phosphorus, and vitamin C are also key nutrients for bone growth. The client should be advised to consult with his or her health care provider regarding supplementation. Furthermore, other whole foods, such as dried plum, are shown to also support bone growth and should take an individual's diet as a whole into account when considering dietary changes.

Several pharmacological agents increase or preserve bone or reduce bone loss. The common categories of agents to combat osteoporosis are shown in Table 9.11. Most older adults use medications and in particularly postmenopausal women. The recommended guidelines for premenopausal women not regularly menstruating and have not responded to more conservative care

Table 9.10	Dietary Reference Intakes for Calcium and Vitamin D					
Age Group	**Calcium**			**Vitamin D**		
	Estimated Average Requirement $(mg \cdot d^{-1})$	Recommended Dietary Allowance $(mg \cdot d^{-1})$	Upper Level Intake $(mg \cdot d^{-1})$	Estimated Average Requirement $(mg \cdot d^{-1})$	Recommended Dietary Allowance $(mg \cdot d^{-1})$	Upper Level Intake $(mg \cdot d^{-1})$
0–6 mo	200	200	1,000	400	400	1,000
6–12 mo	260	260	1,500	400	400	1,500
1–3 yr	500	700	2,500	400	600	2,500
4–8 yr	800	1,000	2,500	400	600	3,000
9–13 yr	1,100	1,300	3,000	400	600	4,000
14–18 yr	1,100	1,300	3,000	400	600	4,000
19–30 yr	800	1,000	2,500	400	600	4,000
31–50 yr	800	1,000	2,500	400	600	4,000
51–70 yr males	800	1,000	2,000	400	600	4,000
51–70 yr females	1,000	1,200	2,000	400	600	4,000
>70 yr	1,000	1,200	2,000	400	800	4,000
14–18 yr pregnant/lactating	1,100	1,300	3,000	400	600	4,000
19–50 yr pregnant/lactating	800	1,000	2,500	400	600	4,000

Adapted from Institute of Medicine. Dietary reference intakes for calcium and vitamin D [Internet]. Washington (DC): National Academies Press; [cited 2015 Nov 11]. Available from: http://www.iom.edu/Reports/2010/Dietary-Reference-Intakes-for-Calcium-and-Vitamin-D.aspx.

(energy management and reduced training) include hormonal supplementation. Hormonal supplementation will be determined by the medical professional (6). Becoming educated on risks associated with each drug should be considered before a drug is chosen. The EP must be aware of drug side effects, and counsel clients to see a health care provider to determine if symptoms their experiencing are due to medications.

Safe and Effective Exercise

Physical activity decreases the risk of osteoporosis by increasing bone-forming osteoblast cell activity and reducing the bone-resorbing osteoclast activity for an overall osteogenic effect of bone growth or slowing of bone loss. Bone adapts positively to sufficient and appropriate levels of stress balanced with adequate rest between stress sessions (81). Bone adaptation to stressors is site- and load-specific, meaning that only the stressed bone will adapt favorably. Thus, activities such as jogging confer little benefit to appendicular bones of the upper body but do improve lower extremity bone density. Furthermore, greater physical stress does not always add more BMD. Research suggests that frequency and impact are most important and a "few loading cycles" will stimulate the needed bone growth (82). Therefore, development of an appropriate and effective exercise program should consider the following: current state of bone health, site of adaptation, inclusion of activities that provide stress and strain, safety of exercise for the individual, and likelihood of compliance.

Table 9.11	Pharmacological Agents for Treatment of Osteoporosis		
Agent	**Indication/Effect**	**Potential Side Effects**	**Comments**
Calcium and vitamin D	Low BMD and/or high risk of fractures/development and maintenance of bone	Calcium — gas, constipation; vitamin D — generally none unless taking too much	As an adjunct to other osteoporosis therapies — efficacy is questionable in those with already normal calcium and vitamin D levels.
Selective estrogen receptor modulators (SERM)	For those with high risk of fracture Estrogen agonist in bone and fat; antagonist in breast and endometrium	Hot flashes, leg cramps, and blood clots	For those with low risk of deep vein thrombosis, if other therapies not appropriate; may not be effective for nonvertebral fractures; decreased risk for breast cancer
Hormone replacement therapy (HRT)	Prevention only for those at high risk for fractures/ decreased risk for vertebral and nonvertebral fracture	Cancer, myocardial infarction, stroke, blood clot	Usually considered for short-term use for menopausal symptoms
Bisphosphonate	For those with high risk of fracture; decreased bone resorption by osteoclast inhibition	GI disturbance (can use intravenous alternative); heartburn, esophageal irritation, headache, constipation, gas, diarrhea	Generally effective at all clinical bone sites; long-term use may increase the risk of femur fracture (53).
Strontium ranelate	High risk of fractures/ decreased bone resorption	GI disturbance, blood clot	**Approved in Europe, not in United States**
Parathyroid hormone (PTH)	High risk of fractures/ increased bone deposition	Bone cancer in rat studies	Injection only; continuous exposure to PTH causes bone resorption.
Calcitonin	High risk of fracture/modest reduction in the risk of vertebral fractures	Stomach upset and flushing	Indicated when other therapies not tolerated; may relieve pain associated with bone fractures
Denosumab	High risk of fractures; bone remodeling	Low calcium levels, back and muscle pain	Alternative to other initial treatments

GI, gastrointestinal.

Data from Eastell R, Rosen CJ, Black DM, Cheung AM, Murad MH, Shoback D. Pharmacological management of osteoporosis in postmenopausal women: an Endocrine Society* clinical practice guideline. *J Clin Endocrinol Metab.* 2019;104(5):1595–622; and Keen R. Osteoporosis: strategies for prevention and management. *Best Pract Res Clin Rheumatol.* 2007;21(1):109–22.

Appropriate forms of resistance-type exercise are necessary to stimulate bone (81,83). Research has shown that participation in only aerobic exercise will not help retard bone loss (84). Exercise training does lead to increased bone density, but the increased bone density reverts back to near preexercise training levels when exercise training is discontinued (85,86). Thus, continued exercise is most important for older adults seeking to maintain bone density or minimize bone loss with age.

As with other musculoskeletal issues, the exercise program should follow ACSM guidelines for all program components (20). The information found in Table 9.12 includes guidelines that

Table 9.12   Exercise Guidelines for Prevention and Treatment of Osteoporosis

Condition	Type		
	Weight-Bearing Aerobic	**Resistance**	**Balance/Posture/ Fall Prevention**
Healthy Skeletal Status			
Frequency	3–5 d · wk^{-1}	2–3 d · wk^{-1}	Daily
Intensity	Moderate to high	Moderate to high	To point of tightness
		60%–80% estimated 1-RM, 8–12 reps, progress to 80%–90% estimated 1-RM, 5–6 reps	
		Impact jumps from floor, height of 1–2 in	
		Multidirectional	
Time	30–60 min · d^{-1} — total exercise time (aerobic + resistance)		10–30+ s per static stretch × 2–4 reps
At Risk for Osteoporosis			
Frequency	3–5 d · wk^{-1}	2–3 d · wk^{-1}	Daily
Intensity	Moderate to high	Moderate to high	To point of tightness
		60%–80% 1-RM, 8–12 reps progress slower to 80%–90% 1-RM, 5–6 reps	
		Impact jumps from floor, height of 1–2 in	
Time	30–60 min · d^{-1} — total exercise time (aerobic + resistance)		10–30+ s per static stretch × 2–4 reps
Osteoporosis			
Frequency	4–5 d · wk^{-1}	2–3 d · wk^{-1}	Daily
Intensity	40%–<60%	Moderate to high	To point of tightness
		Begin with 1 set, increase to 2 sets after several weeks	
	Heart rate reserve or $\dot{V}O_{2max}$	Same as earlier but consider individual circumstances	10–30+ s per static stretch × 2–4 reps
Time	30–60 min · d^{-1} — total exercise time (aerobic + resistance + balance)		

Special Considerations

Avoid explosive, high-impact exercises. Dynamic abdominal exercises (*e.g.*, sit-ups), exercises that involve twisting (*e.g.*, golf swing), bending, compression, excessive flexion should be done with caution. Avoid **unsupported forward flexion** of spine. Provide posture education, fall prevention education, and movement education for lifting, bending, and carrying tasks to reduce fracture risk when doing activities of daily living.

1-RM, one repetition maximum; $\dot{V}O_{2max}$, maximal oxygen consumption.

Data from Hughes JM. Exercise prescription for patients with osteoporosis. In: American College of Sports Medicine. *ACSM's Resource Manual for Guidelines for Exercise Testing and Prescription*. 7th ed. Philadelphia (PA): Lippincott Williams & Wilkins; 2014. p. 699–712; Nikander R, Sievänen H, Heinonen A, Daly RM, Uusi-Rasi K, Kannus P. Targeted exercise against osteoporosis: a systematic review and meta-analysis for optimising bone strength throughout life. *BMC Med*. 2010;8:47; Giangregorio LM, Papaioannou A, Macintyre NJ, et al. Too fit to fracture: exercise recommendations for individuals with osteoporosis or osteoporotic vertebral fracture. *Osteoporos Int*. 2014;25(3):821–35; Perry SB, Downey PA. Fracture risk and prevention: a multidimensional approach. *Phys Ther*. 2012;92(1):164–78; and Liguori G, editor. American College of Sports Medicine. *ACSM's Guidelines for Exercise Testing and Prescription*. 11th ed. Philadelphia (PA): Wolters Kluwer; 2021. 548 p.

incorporate characteristics of exercise important for improving or maintaining overall bone health. A wide variance in bone status among individuals with osteopenia and osteoporosis exists, and for this reason, prescribing exercise with particular attention to exercise intensity must be individualized and appropriate for each client. Pain-free moderate- to high-impact weight-bearing exercise when combined with progressive resistance exercise and agility training is most effective for preserving or improving spine and hip bone density as well as improving overall physical function (81–84,86,87). If the individual is sedentary or is diagnosed with severe osteoporosis (one or more fractures), the initial exercise prescription must follow guidelines for sedentary individuals (20).

Other needs of the client with respect to physical function and select exercises are considered, satisfying more than one objective such as exercises to improve balance and coordination and to reduce the risk of falls in older adults. Because falls often result in fractures in older adults, an exercise strategy to reduce fall risk and improve posture could indirectly benefit bone health as well as overall physical function and independence (83). Likewise, back-strengthening exercises for older adults to reduce thoracic hyperkyphosis (dowager's hump) can reduce back pain and risk of falls (83,88).

Research in animals and humans indicate whole-body vibration (WBV; standing on a special, gently oscillating mechanical plate) for 10–20 minutes a day can reduce bone loss in the hip, although the information is less clear for the spine (89). In addition, WBV can also increase lower limb muscle function to reduce fall risk. Further research is still needed to better understand short- and long-term retention of WBV effects on bone and the dose-response relationship. Likewise, WBV is a higher risk type of exercise that must be administered under supervision and may not be appropriate for all older adults (89–92).

Specific modifications or precautions are considered for the individual with osteoporosis, especially if a history of a previous fracture is present. Activities related to risk of fracture involve loaded trunk flexion or twisting when transitioning from one position to another. Examples of such activities include bowling or golf. However, the benefits of physical activity outweigh the risk of fractures for individuals with osteoporosis. Activities requiring a quick change of direction might increase the risk of falling, thus agility training should progress from slower, more controlled movements to more rapid direction changes. Agility training as part of an exercise program is recommended by the National Osteoporosis Foundation to help decrease risk of falls (84).

In summary, once a client has been cleared by the appropriate health care professional, most clients can safely participate in an exercise program, which follows the ACSM guidelines for a healthy adult (20). Modifications typically are made based on acuity of the injury or pain, motion restrictions, and risk of falls. Recognizing a client's joint ROM is crucial for averting injury when using machines or weights allowing movement that may exceed the client's ROM (93). The proper exercise training dose (repetitions, resistance, sets) and form are based on the individuals' limitations as well as his or her previous and current level of physical activity. Before selecting an exercise for a client, consider the value and risk of the exercise for the individual. If the value outweighs the risk, determine the client's ability and willingness to perform the exercise correctly and within the constraints deemed to be appropriate. Counteracting chronic postural habits and daily movements with appropriate exercises is a good goal for most nonathlete clients. This line of reasoning will enable the identification of appropriate and effective exercises so the client will adapt positively and with limited risk.

The Case of Mrs. Williams

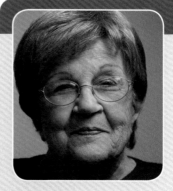

A 75-year-old woman was recommended for exercise programming by her primary care physician to improve mobility and function and to decrease pain of OA symptoms. Mrs. Williams's exercise program for the past year was aquatic classes 45 minutes, 2 days a week. She came to her first appointment with symptom-limited ambulation and a walker but a willingness to further her exercise program.

Narrative

A 75-year-old woman was recommended for exercise programming by her primary care physician to improve mobility and function and to decrease pain of OA symptoms. Mrs. Williams reports that her knee pain is "aching" and is 2–3/10 at rest. Notes from primary care physician indicate that Mrs. Williams has moderately severe OA in bilateral knees. She is symptom limited in walking more than 50 yards with pain of 5–6/10 and needing assistance with walking. Mrs. Williams reports for hospital visits, holding on to side rails of the walls and stopping every 50 yards. Mrs. Williams's current exercise program for the past year is aquatic classes 45 minutes, 2 days a week. She came to her first appointment at the fitness center with symptom-limited ambulation and a walker but a willingness to further her exercise program.

Physical Information

Height: 64 in
Weight: 171.7 lb
BMI: 29.5 kg · m^{-2}
Body fat percentage (measured by direct segmental bioelectrical impedance InBody 520 by Biospace, Inc.): 51.4

Medical History from Primary Care Physician

OA
Type 2 diabetes
Hypertension
High cholesterol

Physical Assessments

Strength: dynamometer
Hip flexion: right, 20 lb; left, 18 lb
Leg extension: right, 15 lb; left, 10 lb
Physical activity limited by knee pain, lower body weakness

Activity Plan

Add progressive muscular and functional conditioning plan 2 days a week with aquatic aerobics.

Goals

Goal 1: Increase strength in lower extremities.
Goal 2: Increase mobility and function for quality of life.
Goal 3: Decrease pain at rest and during activity.

Exercise Program

Aerobic

Frequency: 4 days a week
Intensity: 65%–75% target heart rate (THR)
Time: 10–45 minutes
Types: aquatic aerobics, 45 minutes, 2 days a week
Stationary recumbent bike: level 1, speed 60–80 rpm, start with 2-minute increments work/rest ratio to 10 minutes before muscular conditioning exercises
Progression: increase to 30 minutes continuous exercise in 3–6 months

Muscular Conditioning

2 d · wk^{-1}, supervised
Exercise leg band light to start two to three sets low repetitions to start
Short-term progress to medium leg band and 10–12 reps in 2–3 months
In 3–6 months, progress to exercise circuit machines.
Incorporate upper body bands medium to start for overall conditioning two to three sets of 12–15 reps.
Types: exercise leg band (cuffs) intensity light, two to three sets of 5- to 8-rep exercises:
Lower body exercises: leg extension, hip flexion, partial squat, hip abduction and adduction, hamstring curl, isometric hold for 20 seconds × 3 sets
Upper body exercises: medium band: lateral raise, chest fly, row, bicep curl, and triceps extension

Progression Updates

At 4 Weeks

Mrs. Williams progressed to lower body light bands: three sets of 10 reps, and reported able to ambulate better, pain reported with walking 5/10 and rest 2–3/10. Upper body exercises: three sets of 12–15 reps medium remained the same.

At 8 Weeks

Mrs. Williams progressed to medium lower body cuffs: three sets of 8–10 reps; patient reported able to walk with rest periods of approximately 100 yards and intermittently having to hold on to the handrails for support in fitness center to exercise appointments. She reported pain with walking 4–5/10 and rest 2/10. Upper body exercises: three sets of 15 reps, medium intensity remained for lateral raise, chest fly; hard intensity was increased for row, bicep curl, and triceps extension for three sets of 8–10 reps.

At 3 Months

Mrs. Williams progressed to circuit training machines: two to three sets of 8–10 reps. Lower body: hamstring curl: 10 lb, leg press: 65 lb, hip abduction: 60 lb, hip adduction: 50 lb, assisted (holding on to upper bar) Reebok step up two sets of 8 reps. Upper body: lat pull-down: 35 lb, chest press: 20 lb, incline chest press: 10 lb, lateral raise: 15 lb, bicep curl: 10 lb, triceps extension: 25 lb. She reported able to walk approximately 200 yards, one-third of way to fitness center to exercise appointment, and still intermittently holding to handrails for support. The patient reported pain with activity 4/10 and rest 2/10.

At 6 Months

Mrs. Williams progressed to circuit training machines: three sets of 10 reps (upper three sets of 12 reps). Lower body: hamstring curl: 20 lb, leg press: 80 lb, hip abduction: 75 lb, hip adduction: 60 lb, assisted (holding on to upper bar) Reebok step up three sets of 10 reps. Upper body: lat pull-down: 45 lb, chest press: 27.5 lb, incline chest press: 20 lb, bicep curl: 15 lb, lateral raise: 22.5 lb, triceps extension: 32.5 lb. Aerobic: Mrs. Williams maintained aquatic aerobics 45 minutes, 2 days a week, stationary bike increased to level 2, and she was able to perform 10 minutes without stopping, and the following 10 minutes were work/rest ratios of 2 minutes. Mrs. Williams reported able to walk approximately 600 yards to fitness center to exercise appointment and rarely need handrails for support. The patient reported pain with activity 3–4/10 and rest 1–2/10.

At 1 Year

Lower body: hamstring curl: 35 lb, leg press: 100 lb, hip abduction: 100 lb, hip adduction: 90 lb, no assistance needed Reebok step up three sets of 10 reps. Upper body: lat pull-down: 55 lb, chest press: 40 lb, incline chest press: 37.5 lb, bicep curl: 30 lb, lateral raise 35 lb, triceps extension: 40 lb. Aerobic: She maintained aquatic aerobics 45 minutes, 2 days a week, stationary bike increased to level 3 speed 60–80 rpm, and she was able to perform 20 minutes without stopping, and the following 10 minutes were work/rest ratios of 2 minutes. Mrs. Williams reported ability to walk approximately 600 yards to fitness center to exercise appointment and did not need handrails for support. She reports pain with activity 2–3/10 and rest 0/10. She was able to participate in community outings walking in mall with friends, walked with friends to visit museums in Washington, DC, and was able to stand entire choir practice for 1 hour.

3-Year Assessment

Physical Data

Height: 64 in
Weight: 160 lb
BMI: 27.5
Body composition: body fat percentage: 48.1 kg · m^{-2}, InBody 520 DSM-BIA

Fitness Data

Muscular strength: strength: dynamometer; hip flexion: R: 35 lb, L: 35 lb; leg extension: R: 30 lb, L: 30 lb
Lower body: three sets of 10 reps: hamstring curl: 50 lb, leg press: 135 lb, hip abduction: 115 lb, hip adduction: 110 lb, no assistance needed Reebok step up with 5-lb medicine ball, three sets of 10 reps, ball squat against the wall with 5-lb dumbbells
Upper body: three sets of 15 reps: lat pull-down: 60 lb, chest press: 50 lb, incline chest press: 40 lb, bicep curl: 35 lb, lateral raise: 42.5 lb, triceps extension: 60 lb
Aerobic: Mrs. Williams maintained aquatic aerobics 2 days a week for 45 minutes, stationary bike increased to level 3 speed 60–80 rpm, and was able to perform 30 minutes without stopping. Mrs. Williams reports ability to perform exercise 3 days a week, recumbent bike, and muscular conditioning by herself. Instructed on proper progression from American College of Sports Medicine and National Strength and Conditioning Association guidelines for muscular conditioning exercises and gave patient handout. Mrs. Williams reported pain in knees with walking after 2 miles 2/10, 0/10 at rest.

Conclusion

Mrs. Williams was able to progress to increase quality of life with managing OA by incorporating muscular and aerobic conditioning to routine. She was able to maintain 5 days a week for 45–60 minutes for more than 2 years, and pain was managed well. This client was motivated to increase ambulation and quality of life and was consistent with exercise programming over time. Such results may not be reflective of all clients but gives an example for exercise programming if a client is consistent that this will help long-term exercise prescription goals.

> **QUESTIONS**
>
> - What is a good starting muscular conditioning program for a client who has OA in terms of days per week, number of sets, and repetitions?
> - How often each week should muscular conditioning or resistance exercises be completed for a client who has OA?

References

1. American College of Sports Medicine. *ACSM's Guidelines for Exercise Testing and Prescription*. 11th ed. Philadelphia (MD): Wolters Kluwer; 2022. 548 p.
2. Haff GG, Triplett NT, editors. *National Strength and Conditioning Association: Essentials of Strength Training and Conditioning*. 4th ed. Champaign (IL): Human Kinetics; 2016. 752 p.
3. Wallace JP, Ray S. Obesity. In: Moore GE, Durstine JL, Painter PL, editors. *ACSM's Exercise Management for Persons with Chronic Diseases and Disabilities*. 4th ed. Champaign (IL): Human Kinetics; 2016. p. 80–84.

SUMMARY

This chapter examined and provided guidelines for the exercise professional to effectively address common traumatic and overuse musculoskeletal injuries and selected chronic musculoskeletal conditions related to physical activity or inactivity. Common causes of, role of exercise on, and strategies for reducing the risk of traumatic and overuse injuries and selected chronic conditions were discussed. When applicable and within the scope of practice for the exercise professional, appropriate and current exercise guidelines were discussed with particular focus on modifying the exercise prescription to address special circumstances for these conditions.

STUDY QUESTIONS

1. What recommendations would you make for maximizing bone health and reducing risk of osteoporosis to a client who is 55 years old? 25 years old? 12 years old? How would this differ between genders at each age?

2. Explain resistance exercise recommendations for a 70-year-old female client diagnosed with osteoporosis of the spine who has physician clearance to exercise with appropriate limitations. What types of resistance exercises are appropriate and safe? How frequently should these exercises be performed and at what intensity?

3. A young female client who is an athlete sprained her ankle (inversion) during soccer practice a day earlier but did not want to miss a personal training session with you, nor has she seen a physician. She can walk, but the ankle is swollen and sore. What recommendations would you give this client regarding the injury and exercise?

4. Using the general guidelines presented, explain the progression of exercises for tendinopathies, including examples of types of exercise, frequency, and intensity.

5. Explain the difference between RA and OA, and taking into account special considerations for both, provide exercise recommendations.

REFERENCES

1. Petushek EJ, Sugimoto D, Stoolmiller M, Smith G, Myer GD. Evidence-based best-practice guidelines for preventing anterior cruciate ligament injuries in young female athletes: a systematic review and meta-analysis. *Am J Sports Med.* 2019;47(7):1744–53.

2. Dutton M. Tissue behavior, injury, healing and treatment. In: Dutton M, editor. *Dutton's Orthopaedic Examination, Evaluation and Intervention.* 4th ed. New York (NY); McGraw-Hill; 2017. p. 29–63.

3. Dutton M. Improving muscle performance. In: Dutton M, editor. *Dutton's Orthopaedic Examination, Evaluation and Intervention.* 4th ed. New York (NY); McGraw-Hill; 2017. p. 463–520.

4. Dutton M. Elbow. In: Dutton M, editor. *Dutton's Orthopaedic Examination, Evaluation and Intervention.* 4th ed. New York (NY); McGraw-Hill; 2017. p. 711–2.

5. Dutton M. Lower leg, ankle and foot. In: Dutton M, editor. *Dutton's Orthopaedic Examination, Evaluation and Intervention.* 4th ed. New York (NY); McGraw-Hill; 2017. p. 1081–190.

6. De Souza MJ, Aurelia Nattiv A, Joy E, et al. 2014 Female athlete triad coalition consensus statement on treatment and return to play of the female athlete triad. *Br J Sports Med.* 2014;48:289. doi:10.1136/bjsports-2013-093218.

7. Tenforde TS, Barrack, M Nattiv, A, Fredericson M. Parallels with the female athlete triad in male athletes. *Sports Med.* 2016;46:171–82.

8. Anderson MK, Parr GP, Hall SJ, editors. *Foundations of Athletic Training: Prevention, Assessment, and Management.* 5th ed. Philadelphia (PA): Lippincott Williams & Wilkins; 2013. p. 85–222.

9. Lewis J, Thompson DL. Anatomy and kinesiology. In: Battista RA, editor. *ACSM's Resources for the Personal Trainer.* 5th ed. Philadelphia (PA): Wolters Kluwer; 2018. p. 44–110.

10. Alvar BA. Resistance training. In: Battista RA, editor. *ACSM's Resources for the Personal Trainer.* 5th ed. Philadelphia (PA): Wolters Kluwer; 2018. p. 375–412.

11. Feito Y, Goslin. Exercise physiology. In: Battista RA, editor. *ACSM's Resources for the Personal Trainer*. 5th ed. Philadelphia (PA): Wolters Kluwer; 2018. p. 133–61.

12. Wojtys EM, Huston LJ, Lindenfeld TN, Hewett TE, Greenfield MLVH. Association between the menstrual cycle and anterior cruciate ligament injuries in female athletes. *Am J Sports Med*. 1998;26(5):614–9.

13. Hayes A, Bushman B. Comprehensive program design. In: Battista RA, editor. *ACSM's Resources for the Personal Trainer*. 5th ed. Philadelphia (PA): Wolters Kluwer; 2018. p. 354–74.

14. Kubo K, Ikebukuor T, Yata H, Tsundoa N, Kanehisa H. Time course of changes in muscle and tendon properties during strength training and detraining. *J Strength Cond Res*. 2010;24(2):322–31.

15. Verhagen E, van der Beek A, Twisk J, et al. The effect of a proprioceptive balance board training program for the prevention of ankle sprains: a prospective controlled trial. *Am J Sports Med*. 2004;32(6):1385–93.

16. Wilson J, Best T. Common overuse tendon problems: a review and recommendations for treatment. *Am Fam Physician*. 2005;72(5):811–8.

17. Lorenz D, Reiman M. The role and implementation of eccentric training in athletic rehabilitation: tendinopathy, hamstring strains, and ACL reconstruction. *Int J Sports Phys Ther*. 2011;6(1):27–44.

18. Wasielewski NJ, Kotsko KM. Does eccentric exercise reduce pain and improve strength in physically active adults with symptomatic lower extremity tendinosis? A systematic review. *J Athletic Training*. 2007;42(3):409–21.9.

19. Hughes L, Paton B, Rosenblatt B, Gissane C, Patterson SD. Blood flow restriction training in clinical musculoskeletal rehabilitation: a systematic review and meta-analysis. *Br J Sports Med*. 2017;51:1003–1011.

20. American College of Sports Medicine. *ACSM's Guidelines for Exercise Testing and Prescription*. 11th ed. Philadelphia (PA): Wolters Kluwer; 2022. 548 p.

21. Covey CJ, Mulder MD. Plantar fasciitis: how best to treat? *J Fam Practice*. 2013;62(9):466–71.

22. Nahin RL. Prevalence and pharmaceutical treatment of plantar fasciitis in United States adults. *J Pain*. 2018;19(8):885–96.

23. Landorf KB. Plantar heel pain and plantar fasciitis. *BMJ Clin Evid*. 2015;11:1–46.

24. Headlee D, Leonard J, Hart J, Ingersoll C, Hertel J. Fatigue of the plantar intrinsic foot muscles increases navicular drop. *J Electromyogr Kinesiol*. 2007;18(3):420–5.

25. Jung D-Y, Kim M-H, Koh E-K, Kwon O-Y. A comparison in the muscle activity of the abductor hallucis and the medial longitudinal arch angle during toe curl and short foot exercises. *Phys Ther Sport*. 2011;12(1):30–5.

26. Chapman SA, DeFranca CL. Rehabilitation of the low back. In: Cox JM, editor. *Low Back Pain — Mechanism, Diagnosis, and Treatment*. 7th ed. Philadelphia (PA): Wolters Kluwer; 2011. p. 621–44.

27. GBD 2015 Disease and Injury Incidence and Prevalence Collaborators. Global, regional, and national incidence, prevalence, and years lived with disability for 310 diseases and injuries, 1990–2015: a systematic analysis for the Global Burden of Disease Study 2015. *Lancet*. 2016;388:1545–602.

28. GBD 2015 DALYs and HALE Collaborators. Global, regional, and national disability-adjusted life-years (DALYs) for 315 diseases and injuries and healthy life expectancy (HALE), 1990–2015: a systematic analysis for the Global Burden of Disease Study 2015. *Lancet*. 2016;388:1603–58.

29. Ferreira ML, Machado G, Latimer J, Maher C, Ferreira PH, Smeets RJ. Factors defining care-seeking in low back pain — a meta-analysis of population based surveys. *Euro J Pain*. 2010;14:747.e1–7.

30. Kolber M, Beekhuizen K. Lumbar stabilization: an evidence-based approach for the athlete with low back pain. *Strength Cond J*. 2007;29(2):26–37.

31. Korshøj M, Hallman DM, Mathiassen SE, Aadahl M, Holtermann A, Jørgensen MB. Is objectively measured sitting at work associated with low-back pain? A cross sectional study in the DPhacto cohort. *Scand J Work Environ Health*. 2018;44(1):96–105.

32. Faries M, Greenwood M. Core training: stabilizing the confusion. *Strength Cond J*. 2007;29(2):10–25.

33. McGill S. *Ultimate Back Fitness and Performance*. 6th ed. Waterloo (Canada): Backfitpro; 2017. 331p.

34. Fairbank J, Pynsent P. The Oswestry Disability Index. *Spine*. 2000;25(22):2940–53.

35. Melzack R. The McGill Pain Questionnaire: major properties and scoring methods. *Pain*. 1975;1(3):277–99.

36. Foxworth J, Millar AL, White E. Musculoskeletal concerns. In: Thompson WR, editor. *ACSM's Clinical Exercise Physiology*. Philadelphia (PA): Wolters Kluwer; 2018. p. 475–530.

37. McGill S. Opinions on the links between back pain and motor control: the disconnect between clinical practice and research. In: Hodges PW, Cholewicki J, vanDieen JH, editors. *Spinal Control: The Rehabilitation of Back Pain: State of the Art and Science*. New York (NY): Churchill Livingstone; 2013. p. 75–87.

38. Mayer J, Mooney V, Dagenais S. Lumbar strengthening exercise. In: Dagenais S, Haldeman S, editors. *Evidence-Based Management of Low Back Pain*. St. Louis (MO): Elsevier Mosby; 2012. p. 104–21.

39. Colby LA, Kisner C, Rose J, Borstad J. The ankle and foot. In: Kisner C, Colby LA, Borstad J, editors. *Therapeutic Exercise — Foundations and Techniques*. 7th ed. Philadelphia (PA): F.A. Davis; 2018. p. 894–904.

40. Centers for Disease Control and Prevention. Cost-effectiveness of chronic disease interventions [Internet]. Atlanta [GA]: Centers for Disease Control and Prevention; [cited 2021 Mar 25]. Available from: https://www.cdc.gov/chronicdisease/programs-impact/pop/index.htm.

41. Barbour KE, Helmick CG, Boring M, Brady TJ. Vital signs: prevalence of doctor-diagnosed arthritis and arthritis-attributable activity limitation — United States, 2013–2015. *Morb Mortal Wkly Rep*. 2017;66:246–53.

42. Hochberg MC, Altman RD, April KT, et al. American College of Rheumatology 2012 recommendations for the use of nonpharmacologic and pharmacologic therapies in

osteoarthritis of the hand, hip, and knee. *Arthritis Care Res.* 2012;64(4):465–74.

43. Crowson C, Matteson E, Myasoedova E, et al. The lifetime risk of adult-onset rheumatoid arthritis and other inflammatory autoimmune rheumatic diseases. *Arthritis Rheum.* 2011;63(3):633–9.

44. Cooney JK, Law RJ, Matschke V, et al. Benefits of exercise in rheumatoid arthritis. *J Aging Res.* 2011;2011:681640.

45. Naranjo A, Sokka T, Descalzo MO. Cardiovascular disease in patients with rheumatoid arthritis: results from the QUEST-RA study. *Arth Res Ther.* 2008;10:1–10.

46. Peters MJL, Symmons DPM, McCarey D, et al. EULAR evidence-based recommendations for cardiovascular risk management in patients with rheumatoid arthritis and other forms of inflammatory arthritis. *Ann Rheum Dis.* 2010;69:325–331.

47. Swain DP, editor. *ACSM's Resource Manual for Guidelines for Exercise Testing and Prescription.* 7th ed. Philadelphia (PA): Lippincott Williams & Wilkins; 2014. 896 p.

48. van den Ende CH, Breedveld FC, le Cessie S, Dijkmans BA, de Mug AW, Hazes JM. Effect of intensive exercise on patients with active rheumatoid arthritis: a randomised clinical trial. *Ann Rheum Dis.* 2000;59:615–21.

49. de Jong Z, Munneke M, Kroon HM, et al. Long-term follow-up of a high-intensity exercise program in patients with rheumatoid arthritis. *Clin Rheumatol.* 2009;28(6):663–71.

50. Plasqui G. The role of physical activity in rheumatoid arthritis. *Physiol Behav.* 2007;94(2):270–5.

51. Denning WM, Winward JG, Pardo MB, Hopkins JT, Seeley MK. Body weight independently affects articular cartilage catabolism. *J Sport Sci Med.* 2013;14:290–6.

52. Jiang L, Rong J, Wang Y, et al. The relationship between body mass index and hip osteoarthritis: a systematic review and meta-analysis. *Joint Bone Surg.* 2011;78(2):150–5.

53. Messier SP, Loeser RF, Miller GD, et al. Exercise and dietary weight loss in overweight and obese older adults with knee osteoarthritis: the Arthritis, Diet, and Activity Promotion trial. *Arthritis Rheum.* 2004;50:1501–10.

54. Ehrich EW, Davies GM, Watson DJ, Bolognese JA, Seidenberg BC, Bellamy N. Minimal perceptible clinical improvement with the Western Ontario and McMaster Universities osteoarthritis index questionnaire and global assessments in patients with osteoarthritis. *J Rheumatology.* 2000;27(11):2635–41.

55. Fransen M, McConnell S, Harmer AR, Van der Esch M, Simic M, Bennell KL. Exercise for osteoarthritis of the knee. *Cochrane Database Syst Rev.* 2015;(1):CD004376.

56. Fransen M, McConnell S, Hernandez-Molina G, Reichenbach S. Exercise for osteoarthritis of the hip. *Cochrane Database Syst Rev.* 2014;(4):CD007912.

57. Fitzgerald GK, Piva SR, Gill AB, Wisniewski SR, Oddis CV, Irrgang JJ. Agility and perturbation training techniques in exercise therapy for reducing pain and improving function in people with knee osteoarthritis: a randomized clinical trial. *Phys Ther.* 2011;91:452–69.

58. Regnaux JP, Lefevre-Colau MH, Trinquart L, et al. High-intensity versus low-intensity physical activity or exercise in people with hip or knee osteoarthritis. *Cochrane Database Syst Rev.* 2015;(10):CD010203.

59. Hinman R, Heywood S, Day A. Aquatic physical therapy for hip and knee osteoarthritis: results of a single-blind randomized controlled trial. *Phys Ther.* 2007;87:32–43.

60. Goksel Karatepe A, Gunaydin R, Turkmen G, Kaya T. Effects of home-based exercise program on the functional status and the quality of life in patients with rheumatoid arthritis: 1-year follow-up study. *Rheumatol Int.* 2011;31(2):171–6.

61. Vlieland TPMV, van den Ende CH. Nonpharmacological treatment of rheumatoid arthritis. *Curr Opin Rheumatol.* 2011;23:259–64.

62. Holroyd C, Cooper C, Dennison E. Epidemiology of osteoporosis. *Best Prac Res Clin Endocrin Metab.* 2008;22(5):671–85.

63. Looker AC, Borrud LG, Dawson-Hughes B, Shepherd JA, Wright NC. Osteoporosis or low bone mass at the femur neck or lumbar spine in older adults: United States, 2005-2008. *NCNS Data Brief.* 2012;(93):1–8.

64. Neviaser AS, Lane JM, Lenart BA, Edobor-Osula F, Lorich DG. Low-energy femoral shaft fractures associated with alendronate use. *J Orthop Trauma.* 2008;22(5):346–50.

65. Sambrook P, Cooper C. Osteoporosis. *Lancet.* 2006;367(9527):2010–8.

66. Burge R, Dawson-Huges B, Solomon DH, Wong JB, King A, Tosteson A. Incidence and economic burden of osteoporosis-related fractures in the United States, 2005-2025. *J Bone Mineral Res.* 2007;22(3):465–75.

67. Mosely K, Jan de Beur S. Osteoporosis in men and women. In: Legato M, editor. *Principles of Gender-Specific Medicine.* 2nd ed. Cambridge (MA): Elsevier; 2010. p. 716–36.

68. Bliuc D, Nguyen ND, Nguyen TV, Eisman JA, Center JR. Compound risk of high mortality following osteoporotic fracture and refracture in elderly women and men. *J Bone Miner Res.* 2013;28(11):2317–24.

69. Mazziotti G, Canalis E, Giustina A. Drug-induced osteoporosis: mechanisms and clinical implications. *Am J Med.* 2010;123(10):877–84.

70. Yang S, Nguyen ND, Center JR, Eisman JA, Nguyen TV. Association between hypertension and fragility fracture: a longitudinal study. *Osteoporos Inter.* 2014;25:97–103.

71. Firooznia H, Golimbu C, Rafii M, Schwartz MS, Alterman ER. Quantitative computed tomography assessment of spinal trabecular bone. I. Age-related regression in normal men and women. *J Comput Tomogr.* 1984;8(2):91–7.

72. Lang TF. The bone-muscle relationship in men and women. *J Osteoporosis.* 2011;2011:1–4.

73. Finkelstein JS, Brockwell SE, Mehta V, et al. Bone mineral density changes during the menopause transition in a multiethnic cohort of women. *J Clin Endocrinol Metab.* 2008;93(3):861–8.

74. O'Flaherty EJ. Modeling normal aging bone loss, with consideration of bone loss in osteoporosis. *Toxicol Sci.* 2000;55(1):171–88.

75. Berger C, Langsetmo L, Joseph L, et al. Change in bone mineral density as a function of age in women and men and association with the use of antiresorptive agents. *Can Med Assoc J.* 2008;178(13):1660–8.

76. Lloyd T, Petit MA, Lin HM, Beck TJ. Lifestyle factors and the development of bone mass and bone strength in young women. *J Pediatr*. 2004;144(6):776–82.

77. Kanis J, Johnell O, Oden A. FRAX and the assessment of fracture probability in men and women from the UK. *Osteoporos Int*. 2008;19;385–97.

78. Kanis JA. Assessment of fracture risk and its application to screening for postmenopausal osteoporosis: synopsis of a WHO report. WHO Study Group. *Osteoporos Int*. 1994;4(6):368–81.

79. World Health Organization. *WHO Scientific Group on the Assessment of Osteoporosis at Primary Health Care Level. Summary Meeting Report*. Brussels (Belgium): World Health Organization; 2004. Available from: https://www.who.int/chp/topics/Osteoporosis.pdf.

80. Institute of Medicine. *Dietary Reference Intakes for Calcium and Vitamin D*. Washington (DC): National Academies Press; 2011.

81. Howe TE, Shea B, Dawson LJ, et al. Exercise for preventing and treating osteoporosis in postmenopausal women. *Cochrane Database Syst Rev*. 2011;(7):CD000333.

82. Morseth B, Emaus N, Jørgensen L. Physical activity and bone: the importance of the various mechanical stimuli for bone mineral density. A review. *Norsk Epidemiologi* 2011;20(2):173–8.

83. Cosman F, de Beur S J, LeBoff MS, et al. Clinician's guide to prevention and treatment of osteoporosis. *Osteoporos Int*. 2014;25:2359–81.

84. Giangregorio LM, Papaioannou A, MacIntyre NJ, et al. Too fit to fracture: exercise recommendations for individuals with osteoporosis or osteoporotic vertebral fracture. *Osteoporos Int*. 2014;25:821–35.

85. Iwamoto J, Takeda T, Ichimura S. Effect of exercise training and detraining on bone mineral density in postmenopausal women with osteoporosis. *J Orthop Sci*. 2001;6(2):128–32.

86. Winters KM, Snow CM. Detraining reverses positive effects of exercise on the musculoskeletal system in premenopausal women. *J Bone Miner Res*. 2000;15(12):2495–503.

87. Watson SL, Weeks BK, Weis LJ, Harding AT, Horan SA. High-intensity resistance and impact training improves bone mineral density and physical function in postmenopausal women with osteopenia and osteoporosis: the LIFTMOR randomized controlled trial. *J Bone Miner Res*. 2018;33(2):211–20.

88. Pfeifer M, Sinaki M, Geusens P, Boonen S, Preisinger E, Minne HW. Musculoskeletal rehabilitation in osteoporosis: a review. *J Bone Miner Res*. 2004;19(8):1208–14.

89. Beck BR, Norling TL. The effect of 8 mos of twice-weekly low-or higher intensity whole body vibration on risk factors for postmenopausal hip fracture. *Am J Phys Med Rehabil*. 2010;89(12):997–1009.

90. Liu P-Y, Brummel-Smith K, Ilich JZ. Aerobic exercise and whole-body vibration in offsetting bone loss in older adults. *J Aging Res*. 2011;2011:1–9.

91. Merriman H, Jackson K. The effects of whole-body vibration training in aging adults: a systematic review. *J Geriatr Phys Ther*. 2009;32(3):134–45.

92. Mikhael M, Orr R, Fiatarone Singh MA. The effect of whole-body vibration exposure on muscle or bone morphology and function in older adults: a systematic review of the literature. *Maturitas*. 2010;66(2):150–7.

93. Colado JC, Garcia-Masso X. Technique and safety aspects of resistance exercises: a systematic review of the literature. *Phys Sports Med*. 2009;37(2):104–11.

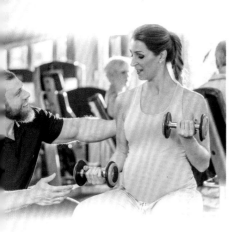

10

Exercise Programming across the Lifespan: Children and Adolescents, Pregnant Women, and Older Adults

OBJECTIVES

- To understand the physical and selected physiological changes during the aging process (childhood to older adult).
- To understand the adaptations to training for children, adolescents, older adults, and pregnant women.
- To understand the differences in exercise prescriptions between children, adolescents, older adults, and pregnant women.
- To apply the American College of Sports Medicine (ACSM), American Heart Association (AHA), and U.S. Department of Health and Human Services (USDHHS) guidelines to exercise prescriptions for children, adolescents, older adults, and pregnant women.

INTRODUCTION

Individuals at any phase in life can have beneficial adaptations to exercise training assuming the stimulus is appropriate and when adequate time for recovery between exercise sessions is provided. However, placing an inappropriate load on a developing, frail, or compromised system is ineffective or even contraindicated. Therefore, the goal of this chapter is to describe the changes with development, aging, and pregnancy on selected physiological systems as well as the effect of exercise training on these systems. This chapter summarizes the practical applications of exercising programming across the lifespan.

To achieve this goal, this chapter focuses on three separate populations: children and adolescents, pregnant women, and older adults. Discussion of each population will address physical and physiological changes, the impact of chronic exercise, and relevant exercise programming (*e.g.*, including specific exercise considerations and meeting physical activity recommendations). In accordance with American College of Sports Medicine's (*ACSM*) *Guidelines for Exercise Testing and Prescription* (1), "children" are classified as younger than 13 years, "adolescents" are 13–17 years, and "older adults" are 65 years and older and 50–64 years with significant physical or physiological limitations that affect physical movement or capacity.

An understanding of physical and physiological changes across the lifespan is important when prescribing exercise for children, adolescents, pregnant women, and older adults. However, the purpose of this chapter is not to provide a comprehensive discussion of growth, development, and aging. For a complete description of these topics, see Malina et al. (2) for youth, Skinner (3) and Chodzko-Zajko et al. (4) for aging, and Mottola et al. (5,6) for pregnancy. Instead, this chapter focuses on those areas that are pertinent to the safe and effective prescription of exercise by the certified exercise physiologist (EP) for children, adolescents, older adults, and pregnant women. Pertinent discussion areas include musculoskeletal system status and function, alterations in body composition, the function of the cardiorespiratory system during rest and exercise, endocrine system alterations, thermoregulation, and motor performance.

Children and Adolescents

Children and adolescents quite simply are not miniature adults. In fact, children and adolescent physiological systems are very different from adults, and these differences directly impact exercise prescription. In addition, many exercise measurement methods originally designed for adults are not scalable to children solely on the basis of body size. Social, behavioral, and psychological issues are important considerations when prescribing exercise for children and adolescents in order to ensure maximal participation and benefit.

Physical and Physiological Changes

Body Size and Composition

The obvious physical change observed during childhood and adolescence is the increase in body size. Besides weight and height increasing with age, growth occurs across the lifespan with rapid growth in infancy, steady increases in early childhood, an accelerated period at puberty (about 12 yr for girls and 14 yr for boys), and slow gains until adult height and weight are attained (7). In general, girls stop growing in stature by 15 years of age, and boys reach their adult height by about 17 years of age (7). Boy's longer growth period results in a gender difference, which makes adult males about 10–12 cm, or 4–5 in, taller than average adult females (7). The increase in height during childhood is achieved by long bone growth, in which a layer of cartilage called the growth plate undergoes proliferation and subsequent ossification, resulting in the lengthening of the bone. This process eventually ceases once the growth plates have completely ossified and adult height is achieved (8).

Also, noticeable and important tissue changes that constitute body weight are bone mass, fat mass, and fat-free mass (8). Bone mass of the lower and upper extremities increase in childhood with accelerated growth in adolescence, whereas head and trunk bone mass remain fairly constant during these same periods (8). Increases in bone mass are parallel to height increases with age; for males, this increase continues until 20 years of age (8). Fat-free mass (primarily skeletal muscle) and height increase in parallel in both boys and girls. As a result of females' shorter stature, adult females have about 30% less skeletal muscle mass than males (9). Similar absolute increases in fat mass exist for boys and girls, but because boys accumulate more fat-free mass, the body fat percentage increases in girls but decreases in boys (10). It is well established how greater muscle mass will have increasing effects on metabolism.

Cardiorespiratory Function

As children grow, their cardiorespiratory system continues to develop. At birth, children have high respiration and heart rates, which decline with age as the nervous system matures. The resting heart rate of young children ranges between 100 and 110 bpm, and maximal heart rate (HR_{max}) is higher than adults. Respiratory frequency is not only elevated in children relative to adults but also decreases throughout childhood and adolescence until adulthood (11). Lung function measures increase with age, mainly as a function of height (12). Due to increased metabolism, children recover faster from a single exercise session compared to adults; thus, heart rate, volume of oxygen consumption per unit of time ($\dot{V}O_2$), and minute ventilation return to resting values more quickly than adults (13).

Although heart rate is higher in children, stroke volume is lower, resulting in lower cardiac output values (13). Systolic blood pressure and, to a lesser extent, diastolic blood pressure at rest and during exercise are lower in children than in adults. As children age, resting blood pressure (especially systolic) increases mainly due to changes in compliance of vessel walls (11). Hemoglobin concentration and red blood cell count increase during childhood with an accelerated increase at puberty, and values for boys are greater than girls. However, children have greater blood flow and oxygen extraction during exercise (13). Despite this discrepancy, children and adolescents have a greater oxygen cost during exercise than adults even after accounting for size differences. The relative inefficiency may be due to immature motor patterns, nervous system, and hormone responses, which improve with age. Peak volume of oxygen consumed per unit of time ($\dot{V}O_{2peak}$) is lower in children than in adults but increases with age once size, adiposity, and gender are considered (13). A gender difference exists in oxygen measures with girls demonstrating lower $\dot{V}O_{2peak}$ measures, most likely due to body composition and blood hemoglobin differences, and more sedentary behaviors especially around puberty (13).

Muscular Strength, Flexibility, and Motor Performance

In boys and girls, muscular strength increases with age and is related to the increases in body weight, height, fat-free mass, and muscle mass (9). This size increase is accelerated in boys during puberty but plateaus in girls in proportion to the fat-free mass and muscle mass (10). Motor performance measures tend to follow the same pattern of improving with physical maturation (14). The smaller increases in girls, especially for weight-dependent performance measures such as vertical jump and long jump, are likely due to increases fat mass at puberty. The decrease in physical activity among girls at puberty also contributes to this trend. However, girls tend to outperform boys in flexibility measures and some measures of balance (14).

Rating of Perceived Exertion

Children and adolescents are able to distinguish between different levels of effort. However, children tend to rate exertion lower than adolescents and adults. Adolescents also rate exertion lower than adults (13). Children may not be as able to reproduce an exercise intensity that corresponds to a particular rating of perceived exertion (RPE), although some studies have shown that children can do so during a cycling exercise using the child-friendly OMNI scale (13). This scale is a 0–10 rating scale with pictures corresponding to different levels of effort for walking/jogging and for cycling. A scale also exists for the perceived exertion of resistance exercise (15). However, an RPE scale without illustrations is less useful for children.

Thermoregulation

During exercise in hot environments, sweat evaporation in humans is the main avenue for heat dissipation. However, children are less efficient at producing sweat compared to adults (13). Although children have more sweat glands, the output of each gland is lower than adults, and the temperature of sweating initiation is higher (13). Children cannot sustain exercise for as long as adults when temperatures exceed 40°C, or 104°F. Inability to thermoregulate is exacerbated when children are not well hydrated, thus further limiting the children's ability to produce sweat (13). Children and adolescents are at risk for heat-related illnesses usually when proper hydration is not maintained. Staying well hydrated, particularly in warm conditions, must always be emphasized and encouraged by the EP.

Obese children tend to acclimatize to heat stress more slowly and have a lower threshold for core temperature regulation. Although lean and obese children do not show a difference in heat tolerance, obese children exercising in the heat have increased core temperatures and higher heart rates at submaximal work rates (16). Mechanisms for lower heat tolerance in obese children have not fully been examined, but adiposity is known to decrease abdominal heat transfer in adults and therefore may contribute to increased core temperature in children as well.

Motor Skills and Physical Activity

Researchers, using different methodologies, have investigated the relationship between motor skills and physical activity in children, with studies reporting an association between low motor skills performance and low levels of participation in physical activity (17–19). Others have reported that physical activity and sport competence perceptions are also related to the child's level of mastery of motor skills such as throwing and catching a ball (20,21), which in turn may contribute to the child's willingness to engage in physical activity.

It seems that as early as the preschool years, the level of motor and physical literacy could be a predictor to physical activity participation later in life (22). Levels of motor skills during childhood not only could predict physical activity participation during adulthood but also as early into adolescence (23,24), making motor skills an important factor to be considered when prescribing exercise to children and adolescents.

The Impact of Chronic Exercise

Physically active youth have improved cardiorespiratory and muscular fitness, metabolic health, cardiometabolic profiles, body composition, and, for some, mental health (25,26). Children performing exercise training for certain sports can improve motor performance and efficiency and increase muscular strength and endurance, and children who complete more intense aerobic activity improve cardiorespiratory fitness and aerobic performance (26,27). Chronic exercise participation and physical activity combined with reduced sedentary time and healthy eating is important for the prevention and treatment of childhood obesity (28,29). As with adults, a dose-response effect exists for the health benefits of exercise. Increases in the exercise quantity and quality will result in more health-related improvements, especially for all individuals older than 6 years of age (26,27). Recent guidelines (26) recognize the same health benefits of exercise for children younger than the age of 6 years, including the reduced risk for excessive increases in body weight and favorable indicators of bone health. Insufficient evidence was reported for the positive effect of exercise on cardiometabolic risks on this younger group of children.

No evidence exists that exercise, including resistance training, weightlifting, and plyometric training, has any adverse effects on children and adolescents when exercises are performed properly and are supervised by qualified adults (26,27,30,31). In fact, resistance training and sports conditioning are known to reduce the rate of sports-related injuries (27). The possibility is always present that, as with any physical activity, an injury of the epiphyseal or growth plate may occur, which could negatively impact growth. A few children with undetected medical conditions may suffer adverse reactions, even sudden cardiac death, during physical activity. However, most evidence suggests exercise is safe and the benefits outweigh the risks. Precautions should be taken, especially for children who have cardiometabolic risk factors, who cannot adequately follow directions, or who are exercising in hot environments, to reduce the risk of injury or sudden death. Finally, growing concern exists that a lack of aerobic activity, a lack of muscular activity (causing pediatric dynapenia), and a decrease in the confidence and competence to exercise (physical illiteracy) are a complex dynamic interaction not just affecting children and youth but that may have lasting effects into adulthood (32).

Exercise Programming and Specific Exercise Considerations

To experience health benefits, the recommended amount of physical activity for children and adolescents is described in detail in the *Physical Activity Guidelines for Americans* (26). The *Guidelines* report that children and adolescents should perform at least 60 minutes of moderate- to vigorous-intensity activity daily, with vigorous activity included at least 3 d · wk^{-1}. In addition, sedentary activities such as watching television, using a computer, or playing video games should be limited to less than 2 h · d^{-1} (33). Examples of moderate aerobic activity are brisk walking, hiking, casual biking, or activities that result in an effort of 5–6 on an RPE scale of 0–10. Vigorous aerobic activities receive an RPE score of 7–8 and include activities such as running, skipping, and jumping; chasing games such as tag; jump rope; or playing sports such as soccer or field hockey. Active video games provide another option for obtaining the recommended amount of exercise. A literature review found that most active video games provide light or moderate activity; however, not enough evidence is available to draw conclusions concerning the long-term role of video games for increasing physical activity and exercise in youth (28). Youth not meeting the guidelines for physical activity and exercise should follow a gradual progression of increasing the intensity and duration of activities until minimum levels are achieved (26,34).

Muscle- and bone-strengthening activities are recommended at least 3 d · wk^{-1} as part of the daily 60 minutes of physical activity (26). Muscle-strengthening exercises require moving against resistance, which can include body weight (push-ups, pull-ups, squats), free weights (dumbbells and barbells), or properly sized weight machines. Other examples of resistance training are playing on jungle gyms, using climbing walls, tree climbing, and playing tug of war. Bone-strengthening exercises are those that result in a physical impact on the skeletal system, such as jumping, running, hopping, jumping rope, or gymnastics. Guidelines and recommendations exist for resistance training and plyometric training for youth (26,27,31).

In general, a muscle-strengthening program should target large muscles of the whole body and include a 5- to 10-minute warm-up and end with a cool-down. These exercises are body weight exercises or machine-based exercises, depending on the child's ability to safely perform the exercises with proper form. For each exercise, 6–15 repetitions to fatigue are performed in one to three sets on nonconsecutive days (27). One to three sets of power exercises are performed for 3–6 repetitions (27). The EP should monitor proper form, start with light weights, and gradually increase intensity by 5%–10%. One repetition maximum (1-RM) testing is performed under direct supervision by an EP, ensuring all recommended procedures are followed (35). For all exercises, proper form with light weight should be emphasized first, followed by a progression to heavier weights as tolerated by the child or adolescent. If a child consistently fails to perform resistance exercises safely, the child may not be emotionally or physically mature enough to safely engage in these activities.

Children

Parents and the EP should encourage physical activities that are age appropriate and enjoyable for children. Families are encouraged to engage in active and fun activities together to establish positive lifelong physical activity habits. To this end, the EP should realize that physical activity for children ought to be fun and intermittent in order for a child to continue participation. Physical activity programs for children should emphasize games, fun activities, and unstructured play rather than using an adult prescription paradigm. For best results, children are allowed to self-regulate the intensity and the duration of their activity (31). With this concept in mind, games and activities should have intermittent rest opportunities as part of the game. Games that eliminate children from participation based on poor performance are to be avoided. High-intensity games are often alternated with low-intensity games, or safe zones can be included for children to have recovery time and still be included in the game. This strategy is especially important for obese children whose cost of locomotion is higher than a nonobese child. Another important point is to focus on limiting sedentary behavior among children. Insufficient data is available for children younger than 6 years of age to establish a dose response between exercise and health benefits (26). However, children in this age group should be active throughout the day, engaging in active play and in activities such as jumping, leaping, and landing, aiming for at least $3 \text{ h} \cdot \text{d}^{-1}$ (26).

Adolescents

As children become adolescents, the physical activity paradigm becomes more structured but still emphasizes enjoyment (31). More complex games and activities requiring maturity ought to be included. Rather than play-based strengthening activities used for very young children, older children and adolescents prefer a more structured resistance training program. Incorporation of child-sized resistance equipment and dumbbells is recommended on the basis of how well children follow directions. Children as young as 7 or 8 years can be successful in a structured resistance training program (27). Incorporation of medicine balls and resistance bands are meaningful as long as the child respects the rules given by the EP. Again, use of these options varies depending on the child's ability to follow directions. Most adolescents are mature enough to participate in a resistance training program that includes free weights, medicine balls, resistance bands, and weight machines. Because adolescents of the same chronological age have different biological ages, consideration given to the biological age is important when determining appropriate exercises for this population.

Many children, their parents, or pediatricians are increasingly concerned about weight status during childhood and adolescence. The Summary Report from the American Academy of Pediatrics Expert Committee on the Prevention, Assessment, and Treatment of Child and Adolescent Overweight and Obesity is a good resource for the EP and other professionals who work with youth (36). This Expert Committee recommends encouraging all children to engage in specific healthy eating behaviors, reduce screen time, and increase physical activity. The recommendations stress the importance of children being taught to self-regulate these behaviors with the help of their parents. For those who are overweight or obese, strategies are presented depending on the age of the child and his or her body weight status. Generally, older and more obese youth are candidates for aggressive weight loss strategies such as caloric restriction and higher levels of physical activity. Younger children, even obese children, should not restrict calories in an effort to lose weight but are encouraged to develop healthy behaviors to improve body weight status (36). In all cases, the parents, the family, and the pediatricians are all active participants in promoting behaviors that produce a healthy body weight.

Overall, physical activity and exercise interventions for children aged 3–12 years and adolescents aged 13–17 years should include school-based programs, community-based programs, and family-based programs (37). Interventions should be designed to be fun and age appropriate, should aim to reduce sedentary behavior, and should increase physical activity at a variety of intensities, which includes aerobic and muscle and bone strengthening (26).

 ## Pregnant Women

Physical and Physiological Changes

The U.S. Department of Health and Human Services (USDHHS) and the American College of Obstetricians and Gynecologists (ACOG) have issued exercise recommendations for pregnant and postpartum women (26,38). Furthermore, the World Health Organization and the ACSM support that the exercise benefits far outweigh the risks (39,40). Currently, a systematic review of 675 randomized control trials (41) indicates exercise during pregnancy decreases the incidence of most adverse conditions during pregnancy (*e.g.*, gestational diabetes mellitus [GDM], hypertensive disorders, preeclampsia, preterm delivery, excessive weight gain, macrosomia) (41,42). Thus, exercise training is safe and recommended for most pregnant women (38). Women should receive approval by an obstetric provider in order to start or continue exercising throughout pregnancy (38). As an EP, documenting this approval is essential before exercise programming starts. Women's bodies undergo many changes during pregnancy. These changes involve adaptations in multiple systems, including cardiorespiratory, endocrine, thermoregulation, neuromuscular, and metabolic, in order to provide an optimal environment for fetal growth. Knowledge of the normal pregnancy changes as well as those changes that occur with acute and chronic exercise are essential for safe exercise prescription throughout pregnancy.

The female cardiovascular system changes during pregnancy to accommodate the demands of the placenta, growing fetus, and her physical changes (*e.g.*, mammary glands). In order to meet physical needs as well as those of the fetus and placenta, pregnancy induces an increased blood volume. Furthermore, heart rate and stroke volume are increased at rest, thus leading to increased cardiac output. Additionally, vascular resistance decreases at rest, thus leading to a slight drop in blood pressure (43). As a result of these physiological cardiovascular changes, exercising during pregnancy is associated with higher heart rates at lower intensities but lower HR_{max} when compared to the nonpregnant state (44,45). Therefore, heart rate reserve, or the range of exercise heart rate response, is smaller during pregnancy (44). Importantly, during exercise, the uterus, placenta, and fetus continue to receive adequate blood and oxygen levels (46–48). Maternal exercise responses are similar regardless of exercise type (*e.g.*, aerobic, resistance, or combination training) (43,49).

Due to slight flaring of the lower ribs during pregnancy, an increase in tidal volume with normal respiratory rate occurs (50). Ultimately, these changes lead to increased oxygen consumption at rest and during submaximal exercise, more than is expected from the increase in body weight. Most likely, these changes are to maintain fetal and placental growth (51–53). In late pregnancy, regardless of fitness level (54), women may experience pregnancy-induced increases in exertional breathlessness associated with increased respiratory effort, which limits some individual's exercise tolerance in late gestation (55). Women are allowed to change intensity in order to accommodate the need to catch their breath and continue exercising.

Metabolism is altered during pregnancy in order to accommodate the needs of the growing fetus, especially in the third trimester. The Institute of Medicine recommends healthy body weight gains during pregnancy that depend on prepregnancy body mass index (BMI): underweight BMI gains of 28–40 lb, normal weight BMI gains of 25–35 lb, overweight BMI gains of 15–25 lb, and obese BMI gains of 11–20 lb (56,57). Exercise is used to help maintain appropriate glucose control and weight gain during pregnancy, especially in overweight, obese, and diabetic women. The majority of scientific evidence involves aerobic exercise or a combination of aerobic with resistance exercise in the normalizing of maternal weight gain (5,58,59). The EP must know that although exercise training improves glucose tolerance during pregnancy (60), a moderate-intensity exercise session is associated with blood glucose decreasing at a faster rate and to a lower level postexercise, especially in the third trimester, compared to the nonpregnant state (61,62).

As pregnancy progresses, an enlargement of the breasts and the growth of the fetus occur, causing an expansion of the uterus into the abdominal cavity. Altogether, these physical changes and anterior distribution of body weight cause (a) a shift in the center of gravity, (b) potentially increased lumbar lordosis, (c) joint laxity, and (d) core muscle changes relative to the nonpregnant state (63). Practitioners believe this shift of a pregnant woman's center of gravity may lead to balance problems and increased falls during pregnancy (63). However, to date, exercise is associated with a decreased likelihood of falling while pregnant (64) similar to the research reported in the elderly, people with Parkinson disease, and other populations. Many pregnant women have increased lumbar lordosis and suffer with low back and pelvic pain (65,66). However, exercise during pregnancy, especially involving core muscle exercises and stretching of posterior body segments, is associated with decreased pain even in late pregnancy (67,68). Furthermore, the hormonal changes during pregnancy often lead to increased joint laxity (69) increasing the likelihood of joint sprains (70). Therefore, the EP is mindful of proper form during exercises and stretching in order to protect joints. Lastly, the expansion of the abdomen during pregnancy is associated with diastasis recti and/or pelvic floor dysfunction during pregnancy (12,71). Regarding diastasis recti abdominis, this condition is not associated with exercise while pregnant (72). However, research shows that abdominal crunches decreased the separation of the rectus abdominis muscle, while drawing-in exercises (*e.g.*, engaging the transverse abdominal muscle) increased the separation and should be avoided during pregnancy (73,74). The EP should recommend pelvic floor muscle training (*e.g.*, 30 near-maximum contractions per day) as part of a regular exercise program during pregnancy to avoid weakening and eventually urinary incontinence (75).

In order to prevent neural tube defects from an elevated core temperature (>103°F), a woman's core temperature and threshold for sweating decreases while pregnant (76,77). The EP should know that even exercise at vigorous intensity (60%–70% of maximal volume of oxygen consumption per unit of time [$\dot{V}O_{2max}$]) in a controlled environment for up to 60 minutes does not raise temperature to this level (78). However, in order to avoid potential congenital defects, women should exercise in a cool environment to ensure body heat dissipates externally rather than toward the fetus. Thus, popular practices such as hot yoga or exercising in hot, humid environments should be avoided during pregnancy (79). Besides environmental conditions, temperature status is associated with hydration status. Therefore, pregnant women must stay hydrated and cool.

The Impact of Chronic Exercise

Exercise training during pregnancy is beneficial for those who exercised prior to pregnancy and for those who begin after conception (80). Although most of the research related to chronic exercise adaptations during pregnancy has focused on aerobic exercise, other forms of exercise (resistance training, stretching, etc.) and similar physical activities are safe as well.

Chronic aerobic exercise participation confers similar cardiovascular, metabolic, and psychological benefits for pregnant women as found in the general population. Similar to the nongravid state, exercise participation throughout pregnancy improves a woman's overall cardiovascular function and attenuates the natural increase in resting heart rate that occurs with progressing gestation (81–83). Consistent exercise training maintains blood pressure levels, thus helping to reduce the risk of developing high blood pressure conditions (*e.g.*, preeclampsia, gestational hypertension) during pregnancy (84). Similarly, exercise improves circulation and decreases pregnancy-related edema often occurring in the extremities (84). In addition to normalized body weight gain, women gain less body fat with regular exercise during pregnancy (33,85). This effect on maternal weight gain is also associated with delivering normal size (*e.g.*, birth weight) infants and experiencing less delivery complications (59). Regular exercise participation throughout pregnancy also improves mood and helps alleviate discomforts associated with pregnancy (80). In addition to the benefits women experience by regular aerobic exercise participation during pregnancy, decreased birth weight (86), improved heart (87–90) and nervous system function (87–90), and motor skill maturation (91) in the offspring exposed to aerobic exercise throughout pregnancy compared to offspring of women who were not physically active have been reported.

Resistance training has grown in popularity among women, and recent research is focusing on exercise during pregnancy including resistance exercises. Similar to aerobic training, pregnant women participating in resistance training have similar exercise responses, normal body weight gain, and decreased fat gain (92–94) with the added benefit of increased lean mass and strength (94,95), an important benefit especially for overweight, obese, and diabetic women. Due to the nature of resistance training and an increased likelihood of postural hypotension during pregnancy, the EP must educate pregnant clientele on proper breathing and lifting techniques to avoid dizziness (96). Resistance training while pregnant is also associated with increased fetal heart and nervous system maturation (97), decreased likelihood of fetal or pregnancy complications (98), and no differences in type of delivery (*e.g.*, cesarean section, vaginal delivery) (93).

Combining aerobic and resistance training during pregnancy is popular and of increased research interest. Participation in combination exercise programming has similar benefits as aerobic or resistance alone: improved cardiorespiratory fitness, decreased incidence of gestation conditions (*e.g.*, hypertension, diabetes), less complications with delivery, increased maternal strength, but no differences in birth weight of offspring when compared to nonexercising mothers (59,99–101). Lastly, improved heart and nervous system maturation (67) are associated with combined resistance and aerobic exercise programming (97). All types of exercise are encouraged during pregnancy due to the benefits for improved maternal health, delivery outcomes, and possible benefits for the child.

Aquatic or water exercise is increasingly used during pregnancy because water provides buoyancy and provides body weight support. Moderate-intensity water exercise at recommended levels (150 min · wk^{-1}) is not associated with adverse outcomes, and women report improved quality of life (102,103). Aquatic physical activity is also beneficial for decreasing edema that often occurs in late pregnancy, regulating body temperature, decreasing joint pain, and improving mood and sleep (58,104–109). Additionally, aquatic exercise throughout pregnancy is associated with promoting healthy gestational weight gain as well as birth weight (110).

Lastly, other forms of physical activity are also safe during pregnancy and recommended for overall health. Although regular stretching is recommended by ACSM as part of exercise routines, current U.S. recommendations for exercise during pregnancy do not include recommendations related to stretching (1,38,111,112). To date, exercising pregnant women have improved heart function, normalized resting heart rate and blood pressure, and decreased low back pain associated with a regular stretching routine of 20–40 minutes, 5 d · wk^{-1} (113–116). Similarly, yoga and Pilates, focused on stretching and strengthening moves, are safe during pregnancy and are associated with decreased disorders of pregnancy and decreased pain and stress levels of pregnant women (117,118). Because some pregnant women have postural hypotension, frequent and abrupt body position changes should be completed with caution (43,44). However, an area for future research focus is on the influence of yoga throughout pregnancy on women and child health. Another form of physical activity termed *qigong*, consisting of gently repeated movements to strengthen and stretch the body, enhance balance, and improve body awareness, is associated with decreased pain and depression symptoms in pregnant women (119). Further research is needed to determine recommended levels of other physical activities, such as stretching, yoga, and qigong during pregnancy.

Exercise Programming and Specific Exercise Considerations

Pregnancy is a special time in women's life where they are likely to increase activity levels if they are educated on the different benefits for both mother and child (120,121). The EP should know the similarities of exercise prescription principles for pregnant women compared to the general population. The exercise prescription described in this chapter applies to all pregnant women who have no absolute or relative exercise contraindications for exercise (38). With this in mind, the EP should keep on file a clearance letter or PARmed-X for Pregnancy (122) completed by an obstetric provider prior to a woman's exercise participation. The USDHHS, ACOG, ACSM, and American Heart Association (AHA) agree that pregnant women should aim to achieve 150 minutes of moderate-intensity exercise every week during pregnancy (26,38,40,111).

In order to achieve the recommended level of 150 minutes of exercise per week, an individual exercise prescription should provide details for the frequency, intensity, time, and type of exercise acceptable for the pregnant population. The recommended exercise frequency and time include three to five times per week for 30–50 minutes each session (1,38). Each exercise session should include a 5-minute warm-up and a 30- to 50-minute exercise session at moderate intensity and end with core exercises, pelvic floor muscle training, a cool-down, and stretching (1). Women previously sedentary before conception should start with 5- to 20-minute low-intensity exercise sessions and gradually increase the exercise intensity and duration (*e.g.*, 5 min) until recommended levels are met (38,42). Exercise benefits reported for pregnant mother and child are dose related, such that a small amount of physical activity provides small changes for mother and fetus. Increased amounts of exercise duration provide greater health benefits for both mother and child (95,123). Keep in mind, the ceiling for physical activity during pregnancy is not well defined. Pregnant women exercising at an elite or competitive level should be closely followed by an obstetric provider to ensure adequate caloric intake (124). Although benefits are seen with lighter intensity exercise, the current recommendations are moderate intensity, or 40%–59% of heart rate reserve to achieve health benefits for mother and child (38,42). A guide for moderate heart rate ranges are <29 years old 125–146 bpm and 30+ years old 121–141 bpm (1,42). Because pregnancy alters the exercise heart rate response, exercise intensity is monitored with RPE or the "talk test" (38). Moderate intensity is the equivalent of 5–6 RPE on a 0–10 scale or having the ability to converse while exercising (5,38,125).

The types of exercise during pregnancy is an important topic to discuss with pregnant women. In general, exercise modes found safe during pregnancy are aerobic exercises, resistance exercise, combination exercises (including aerobic and strength components), aquatic/water exercises, and light-intensity physical activities such as stretching, yoga, Pilates, and qigong during pregnancy. During all exercises, the EP must instruct pregnant clients to breathe appropriately and avoid the Valsalva maneuver that could cause hypotension/dizziness. Women who experience nausea or light-headedness while lying supine during pregnancy should modify their exercise position to avoid this event and maintain venous return (44). If resistance training is conducted, exercises should be dynamic in nature and focus on the large muscle groups. A resistance training program producing moderate levels of muscular fatigue within 12–15 repetitions is recommended, as is maintaining an RPE between 5 and 6 (0–10 scale), achieving a heart rate within the target heart rate range, maintaining the ability to converse while exercising, and providing appropriate rests between exercises (1,45).

Although these exercise modes are safe during pregnancy, the EP must start an exercise program at an appropriate level, progress the individual properly, and make modifications when necessary. For instance, pregnant women should avoid extended periods of motionless standing and any activity that is conducted in a supine position, especially after the first trimester when venous return can become compromised (38). Furthermore, ACOG recommends avoiding activities that cause trauma to the abdomen (*i.e.*, ice hockey, soccer, and basketball) or have a high risk of falling (horseback riding, downhill skiing, gymnastics, or vigorous racquet sports) (1,38). Scuba diving or exercise at altitudes higher than 6,000 feet are avoided to ensure appropriate fetal oxygen supply, unless she already lives at high altitude (1,38). A woman's ability to dissipate heat is vital during pregnancy (77,126), and the EP should ensure exercises are performed in a cool comfortable environment to prevent fetal harm from hyperthermia (38). Moreover, proper hydration is maintained by ingesting 16 oz or 500 mL of water prior to exercise and a cup every 20 minutes during exercise to replace fluid lost during exercise (45,63) in order to ensure appropriate thermoregulation.

In addition to the frequency, intensity, time, and type of exercise, another consideration is the timing of exercise initiation during pregnancy. Exercise started after the 20th week of pregnancy had a smaller effect on birth weight than exercise beginning before the 20th week of pregnancy (13). The EP must understand that fatigue and nausea are common occurrences especially during the first trimester making exercise more challenging (84). Beginning in the second trimester, women usually feel better, more energetic, and ready to exercise. Even though exercise often diminishes in the third trimester (127,128), health outcomes are dose related and improved for mother and child if exercise is maintained until delivery (76). Therefore, the EP needs to encourage women to maintain their physical activity levels throughout their pregnancy as much as possible.

Pregnant women who develop a medical condition or other contraindications to exercise should stop exercising immediately and consult their obstetric provider to determine if exercise can continue. Under these circumstances, the EP waits until the pregnant client receives reapproval from her health care provider before further engaging in physical activity. The EP must know the warning signs for terminating exercise and when to consult a physician (38): vaginal bleeding, shortness of breath prior to exertion, dizziness, headache, chest pain, muscle weakness, calf pain or swelling, preterm labor, decreased fetal movement, or a leaking of amniotic fluid.

Overall, research has found that exercise is beneficial for women; however, numerous studies have found exercise during pregnancy benefits the fetus during and after pregnancy. A few studies have evaluated fetal outcomes related to chronic maternal exercise throughout pregnancy. Similar to adult exercise training, regular prenatal exercise was associated with improved fetal cardiac autonomic nervous system (80,89) and heart function (129) which recovered more quickly to baseline values (130) and was more prominent based on amount of regular exercise throughout gestation (123). Additionally, fetal cardiac and autonomic benefits may differ based on type of maternal exercise (97). Additionally, there are trends (131) of decreased body fat in the third trimester of fetuses exposed to maternal aerobic exercise compared to fetuses of nonexercisers. The most common measures for pregnancy studies, due to its availability, are measures from the birth record (*e.g.,* birth weight and length). Overall, a meta-analysis of 73 randomized control trials concludes that exercise during pregnancy is associated with decreased birth weight and decreased odds of macrosomia (132). This effect is most likely due to the effect exercise has on maternal glucose control, an important determinant of fetal growth. Exercise is not associated with neonatal hypoglycemia, metabolic acidosis, hyperbilirubinemia, and Apgar scores (132). Importantly, birth measures are predicted by maternal exercise as well as her lipid levels (86); thus, healthy nutrition is essential during pregnancy for better offspring outcomes. Numerous studies have evaluated the influence maternal prenatal exercise on infant health. Similar to fetal findings and adult exercise training, regular maternal exercise is associated with lower heart rate and improve cardiac autonomic system (90). A systematic review of neonatal body composition suggests prenatal exercise decreases neonatal weight (132). This is predominantly explained by decreased body fat (133). A few studies have shown improved measures of neurodevelopment in response to maternal exercise (134). These benefits may differ by maternal exercise type (135), but this is a current area of research interest in the field of exercise and pregnancy.

Special Considerations during Pregnancy

Overweight or obese pregnant women are encouraged to make healthy lifestyle modifications to include physical activity (136). When initiating an exercise program, overweight and obese women should start with short low-intensity periods of exercise and gradually progress as able. Overweight or obese pregnant women who start exercising during pregnancy may have modest reductions in weight gain without adverse outcomes (137,138). Pregnant women diagnosed with GDM follow a multifaceted approach in order to improve maternal and child health during pregnancy maternal education, diet modification, exercise, pharmacology, and fetal surveillance (62). The combination of aerobic with resistance exercise is most effective in blood glucose management (61). Women with GDM are recommended to do aerobic exercise 5–7 d · wk^{-1} and resistance exercise three times per week and include 5–10 exercises involving the major muscle groups (upper body, lower body, and core) and 10–15 repetitions for each set. A minimum of one set is performed for strength gains, but up to three sets total is optimal for glucose uptake and strength gains (138,139). Similarly, competitive pregnant athletes require frequent and closer supervision because they tend to maintain a more strenuous exercise training schedule throughout pregnancy. Such athletes should pay particular attention to avoiding hyperthermia, maintaining proper hydration, and sustaining adequate caloric intake to prevent weight loss, which may adversely affect fetal growth. Lastly, pregnant women with physically active occupations requiring physical labor and/or extended periods of time on their feet are cautioned to consult with their obstetric providers. Occupational physical activity of this nature is not similar to all previous activities mentioned and is often associated with adverse pregnancy outcomes (38).

In conclusion, maternal physiology demonstrates the unique capability to adapt to various anatomical, physiological, and hormonal changes as a result of pregnancy, and understanding this normal process is important for the EP when initiating an exercise program during pregnancy. To date, exercise during pregnancy is beneficial for maternal health, pregnancy outcome, and the developing fetus. Although the recommended level of exercise during pregnancy is 150 min · wk^{-1} of moderate-intensity exercise, exercise adaptations are dose related and every minute counts. EP professionals must understand the normal and the abnormal changes associated with pregnancy in order to understand the physiological responses during a single acute exercise session and with chronic exercise. Furthermore, EP professionals must know (a) a process for obtaining health care provider approval prior to training, (b) current guidelines for exercise and pregnancy, (c) contraindications for exercise, and (d) overall adaptations of exercise and pregnancy in order to properly write a prescription and (e) the necessary information needed to educate a pregnant client about the safety and exercise benefits during pregnancy.

Older Adults

Older adults and those who are younger but severely deconditioned present fitness professionals with unique challenges. The process of aging affects every system, and these changes are inevitable. Of course, a healthy lifestyle in most people alters the rate of these changes resulting in increased longevity and better physical functioning (4). However, the older adult population tends to have more diseases and also tends to be further progressed in those conditions. The AHA has identified core health behaviors (smoking, physical activity, diet, and weight) and health factors (cholesterol, blood pressure, and glucose control) that contribute to cardiovascular disease. The percentage of U.S. adults 40–59 years old who had ideal levels of five or more of these factors was 13.3% (140). Only 5% of U.S. adults older than 60 years had ideal levels of five or more of these factors (140). This means that a large percentage of older Americans have multiple health behaviors and factors that place them at risk for cardiovascular disease. Currently, 77.2% of males and 78.2% of females between 60 and 79 years have a cardiovascular disease (coronary heart disease, heart failure, or stroke) with hypertension (140). For those older than 80 years, the prevalence increases to 89.3% and 91.8%, for males and females, respectively (140). Therefore, it is quite likely that an older adult seeking the help of an EP will present with at least one, if not more, health conditions or diseases. Several disease states are discussed elsewhere in this book. The discussion here focuses on the relatively healthy older adult who is free from the advanced stages of disease but is sedentary and generally deconditioned.

Physical and Physiological Changes

Body Composition and Musculoskeletal Function

During adulthood up until the age of 70 years, individuals tend to gain body weight and fat mass and tend to lose fat-free mass, height, and bone (3,4). During this time, an accumulation of visceral fat, which is linked to metabolic and cardiovascular diseases, is especially predominant in men (4). However, the increases in percentage fat and body weight in older adults are largely lifestyle related rather than a natural consequence of aging (3). The weight increases seen in older adults are driven by the increases in fat mass because fat-free mass decreases about 2%–3% per decade between 30 and 70 years of age (4). Therefore, the actual changes in body composition will be undetected by a weight or BMI measurement (4). The loss of fat-free mass comes largely from muscle mass and mainly reflects the loss of muscle from the legs (4). Mirroring the loss of muscle mass is a loss of muscular strength, endurance, and the associated decreases in physical function (4). The numbers and size of muscle fibers are reduced, especially type II fibers leading to a loss in the speed of contraction and power output (4). The loss of strength, muscle mass, and bone density are larger in women than in men, especially for bone density during the postmenopausal years (4). Fracture risk is elevated in those with osteopenia, which is a bone density 1–2.5 standard deviations below young controls (4).

In adults older than 70 years, the loss of body weight, body fat, and body cell mass occurs (3), and this loss of weight is associated with a higher mortality rate (121). A rapid loss of weight can indicate the presence of a disease process. Although the loss of fat-free mass occurs during adulthood, more rapid loss occurs after 65–70 years with limbs losing at a more rapid rate than other sites (4). Neuromotor function also deteriorates with age because of a reduction in the number of neurons resulting in reduced coordination, slower walking speed, shorter stride length, slower reaction time, poorer balance, and lower agility (3,4). The nervous system changes combined with the loss of muscle mass and strength result in reduced physical function and an increased risk and fear of falling. Mobility becomes impaired, the caloric cost of walking increases, and activities of daily living become more difficult (4).

As the total body water content decreases with age, so does the elasticity and pliability of tissues such as cartilage and connective tissues found within joints among other places (4). Range of motion becomes reduced by 20%–30% or more in some cases, the effects of which are compounded by the low levels of physical activity in many older adults (3,4). The reduced flexibility may contribute to the risk of falling or injury and to back pain (4).

EXERCISE IS MEDICINE CONNECTION

Exe℞ciseisMedicine®

Gianoudis and colleagues (141) tested a 12-month multimodal high-speed power training program on older adults in a community-based randomized controlled trial to determine the effects on muscular strength, functional muscle power, functional muscle performance, and falls. Body composition including bone density was also measured. One hundred sixty-two men and women 60 years and older were recruited and randomized into either a standard care group or a multimodal, diverse loading, weight-bearing, and moderate-impact training program. The program included balance, functional exercises, and rapid power movements. It was periodized and included a combination of weight machines and free weights. Both strength and weight-bearing exercises were progressively adjusted to account for improvements. Strength, functional muscle power, and functional muscle performance improved in exercisers at 6 months compared to the control group. These improvements were maintained at the 12-month mark. Exercisers also experienced a small but significant improvement in bone density after 12 months compared to the control group. Lean mass, fat mass, and falls were not different between groups. The authors concluded that a multimodal exercise program is effective for improving musculoskeletal and functional outcomes in older adults in community settings.

Cardiorespiratory Function and Thermoregulation

The cardiorespiratory system is affected by aging and a sedentary lifestyle resulting in a 9% decline in maximal $\dot{V}O_2$ per decade in healthy sedentary adults (4). Vessels become stiffer and elasticity is lost in cardiac tissue, including the heart valves. Blood pressure at rest is increased, especially systolic blood pressure, and higher resistance to blood flow develops, which creates more work for the heart (3,4). During submaximal exercise, aging tends to result in higher ventilation and blood pressure; lower cardiac output and stroke volume; and little change in heart rate, oxygen extraction, and $\dot{V}O_2$ (3,4). The heart rate response at the start of exercise is slowed, and heart rate variability during exercise is also reduced (4). At maximal levels of exercise, oxygen uptake, ventilation, cardiac output, heart rate, stroke volume, oxygen extraction, and lactic acid concentrations are lower, whereas total peripheral resistance and blood pressure is higher than in a younger person (3,4). Older individuals have a reduced ability to vasoconstrict in the renal and splanchnic areas, which corresponds with a reduced blood flow to the legs at rest, during submaximal and maximal exercise (4). This reduced blood flow may influence functional ability, exercise, and blood pressure regulation as individual age. The reduced HR_{max} is the major determinant of the reduced exercise capacity (4). Because collagen fibers in the lungs also lose elasticity and bronchioles lose their tone, less air can be moved per minute in an older adult (3,4). Alveoli are lost with aging and the remaining alveoli are larger in size, which results in a reduced surface area for gas exchange; however, arterial blood gases are not affected even at maximal exercise (4). Pulmonary aging does not limit exercise capacity in sedentary older adults (4). EPs need to recognize that older individuals have a lower overall exercise capacity and that any given absolute submaximal exercise intensity represents a higher percentage of their maximum.

Thermoregulatory ability also declines with aging (4). The number and activity of sweat glands and capillary density decrease with age. The thirst sensation declines, the ability to conserve water and sodium are diminished, and total body water decreases with aging (4). These changes result in a lower ability for the body to benefit from evaporative or radiant cooling, a lower tolerance for heat, and may predispose an older adult to dehydration. Older adults also cannot withstand the cold compared to younger adults because of a reduced ability to divert blood flow toward deeper tissues (4). In individuals older than 70 years, this inability is exacerbated by the loss of body fat (4,142).

The Impact of Chronic Exercise

This discussion is not meant to provide a comprehensive literature review on the benefits of chronic exercise because this topic is well documented elsewhere (4,26,40,143,144). However, strong evidence exists that an adequate amount and type of exercise lowers the risks of several cancers, cardiovascular disease, some metabolic diseases, and premature death in older adults (4,26,40,143,144). Exercise results in a more favorable cardiovascular risk profile, increases physical function, helps in the management of back pain, lowers the risk for falls and fall related injuries, improves some mental health outcomes (such as a reduction in anxiety, a reduced risk of depression, and a lowered risk of dementia), improves fitness, improves sleep, improves quality of life, and helps with achieving a healthy weight (4,26,40,143,144). Habitual exercise also improves executive function, attention, memory, crystallized intelligence, and processing speed (26). In fact, many of the age-related declines in fat-free mass, strength, and motor performance are at least partially reversible with the onset of a regular exercise program (4,26,40,143,144). Evidence is available that these benefits are reaped even in sedentary older adults who initiate an exercise program later in life (4,26,40,143,144).

Exercise Programming and Specific Exercise Considerations

As is the case for all adults, the EP should perform proper baseline assessments, health screenings, and risk factor stratification for an older adult to determine whether contraindications for exercise exist as well as to determine the type, intensity, and quantity of exercise to safely be performed. Individualized approaches to designing programs are based on this risk. This process is discussed elsewhere in this book and is described in the *ACSM's Guidelines for Exercise Testing and Prescription* (1). These following general guidelines are recommended for older adults who are healthy but may be deconditioned.

Exercise testing is not required for most older adults to start an exercise program, but the EP may perform exercise testing for other purposes (such as determining the cardiovascular response to exercise) or for those where a physician requests such a test (1). Testing procedures do not differ materially from that which is performed for other healthy adult populations; however, the EP should make special consideration for physical limitations or medical conditions that exist, which would require procedures to be altered (1). For example, for those with balance and coordination issues, a cycle ergometer might be preferable over a treadmill or a treadmill with handrails over a treadmill without handrails (1,3). For deconditioned older adults, the EP should choose a protocol that provides a lower initial workload such as the Naughton treadmill protocol (1,3). Given that older adults are likely to have multiple chronic health conditions, the EP should be aware of medications that may affect the cardiovascular responses to exercise or which may require alterations in the cool-down phase of the test (1). The EP should also be aware that older adults will more often meet the early test termination criteria (presented in an earlier Chapter 3) than younger healthy populations (1).

Given that maximal exercise tests may not be feasible in many situations or may not be well tolerated by some older adults, simple physical function tests are currently in use to quantify baseline status and progress over time. The best physical performance tests are those that have been validated and have normative tables or identified cut points that are associated with poorer health (1). The EP should choose tests that meet these criteria and that are appropriate for the person being measured. For example, a test should be used if it was developed for the age range and the health status of the person being measured (1). Also, many physical performance tests are subject to ceiling and floor effects (1). A ceiling effect is when someone scores in the highest category and therefore will not be able to show further improvement on the test even though their physical status is actually improving. A floor effect is when someone scores in the lowest category or below the lowest category and their small improvements over time are not captured because they remain in the lowest category. Although physical performance testing is easy to perform under a variety of conditions, the EP must be aware of these limitations in his or her application.

A variety of testing batteries are available and are described elsewhere (1). The two most common tests are the Senior Fitness Test (145) and the Short Physical Performance Battery (146). The Senior Fitness Test includes seven items representing different areas of fitness. They are a 30-second chair stand test, a 30-second arm curl test, an 8-foot up-and-go test, a 6-minute walk test, a 2-minute step test, a sit-and-reach test, and a back scratch test (145). There are normative tables for each test (145). This test was developed for older adults 60–94 years and have thresholds identified that predict functional independence through age 90 years (for those 65–85 yr who are taking the test) (147). The Short Physical Performance Battery contains balance tests, chair stand tests, and gait speed tests with results scored on a point system (146). This test is more prone to ceiling and floor effects due to its point system of scoring but is predictive of disability, institutionalization, and death. Other testing batteries exist that are more oriented toward the ability to perform activities of daily living, such as the Continuous-Scale Physical Performance Test (148). The EP should assess the needs of the client and the purpose of testing in determining the most appropriate testing battery.

In exercise programming for all components of fitness, the EP should ensure that the choice of exercise is appropriate for the older adult while considering any prior injuries, orthopedic concerns, vision concerns, or deficits in balance and agility (1). Exercise in water or using a weight-supported machine such as a cycle are more appropriate than walking and running for individuals with poor balance. Treadmills with handrails offer more stability than other modes of exercise for someone who is visually impaired or who has balance issues. Exercises that provide support such as weight training machines are more appropriate for the very deconditioned than exercises that require more balance and skill such as free weights.

Exercises should be individualized and tailored for each older adult to allow for successful completion before progressing to more challenging exercises. To start, a conservative approach is recommended for those who are deconditioned, have functional limitations, or have chronic health conditions until the person's response to exercise is understood (1). The EP should also understand the health conditions, risk factors, and medications his or her clients have or are taking while these factors may affect the response to exercise, how exercise is monitored, and whether an extended cool-down is beneficial (such as for those with cardiovascular disease) (1). A more cautious approach and closer monitoring is essential until the exercise response is understood for that individual. Some healthy, disease-free older individuals may have an underlying undiagnosed condition that could be exacerbated by exercise. For these reasons, the EP must refer to the resources available to them (1) to anticipate, and prevent if possible, potential negative outcomes. A more thorough discussion of specific health conditions is in Chapter 8.

For every component of fitness, some physical activity is better than none, and the requirement for physical activity to occur in 10-minute bouts has been eliminated (26). The EP must realize that the greatest health benefits occur when a person moves from being sedentary to being physically active and that building the confidence to begin incorporating exercise into a healthy lifestyle is an important goal for an older adult (1,26). Initial sessions may need to focus on behavioral strategies to promote and enhance exercise adoption. In these cases, the initial exercise prescription may not meet ACSM guidelines but nevertheless is an important positive step toward adopting a healthy lifestyle. This positive movement should not be discounted.

Aerobic Activity

Older adults should strive for the same amount of aerobic activity that is recommended for all adults: Accumulate 30–60 minutes of moderate-intensity activity on 5 or more days a week, or 20–30 minutes of vigorous activity for 3 d · wk^{-1}, or a combination of vigorous and moderate activity for 3–5 d · wk^{-1} (1,26). Any mode of exercise that uses the large muscle groups is appropriate, and for those with physical limitations, using a mode of exercise that does not impose an orthopedic stress such as walking, aquatic activity, or cycling is appropriate (1,26). Individuals who are very deconditioned should start with lighter intensity activities and progress to higher intensity activities until the guidelines are met. Also, those individuals who are frail or very deconditioned may need to focus on the development of strength because they lack the physical ability to engage in aerobic exercise (1). Greater levels of physical activity are encouraged in individuals who are able to do so safely. Exceeding these minimal recommendations will result in further health benefits and will improve an older adult's ability to manage existing conditions and further reduce disease risk (144). However, any person having advanced medical conditions should seek advice from their physician regarding physical activity with supervision as appropriate (1).

Because of the heterogeneity of aerobic capacities in the older adult population, a different definition of moderate versus vigorous intensity is required (144). Because the subjective rating of any physical activity is vastly different for an unconditioned person compared to a well-conditioned person, an exercise that is easy for one person may be very difficult for another person. For adults, exercise intensity is defined in absolute terms, but for older adults, a subjective rating system is used to determine the exercise intensity, which accounts for different conditioning levels. Moderate exercise intensity is a 5–6 on a 0–10 scale (where 0 is sitting and 10 is a maximal effort) and represents an exercise intensity, which produces a noticeable change in breathing and heart rate. A vigorous effort would be a 7–8 on the same scale and would produce large increases in heart rate and breathing (1). Considering that any physical activity is beneficial, the EP must emphasize reducing sedentary behaviors and use a gradual approach to progress exercise training. Deconditioned adults may initially aim for light-intensity physical activity (<5 subjective rating of effort) and perform exercise in shorter bouts until more continuous exercise can be sustained (26,144).

Muscle-Strengthening Activity

All adults are recommended to perform one to three sets of muscle-strengthening or power activities (such as weight training programs and weight-bearing calisthenics) on at least 2 nonconsecutive days a week, targeting the major muscle groups in 8–10 exercises (1,4,40,144). Older adults should choose a weight or resistance that can be performed 8–12 times, which requires a level of effort that is moderate to vigorous. An RPE of 5–6 is moderate, and a 7–8 is considered vigorous on a 10-point scale (1). For individuals who are beginners, one set of 10–15 repetitions using a lighter initial starting weight (about 40%–50% of 1-RM) with a focus on proper form followed by progressively increasing loads to moderate to vigorous (60%–80% 1-RM) based on each person's ability is recommended. Achieving more than the minimum recommendations for muscle-strengthening activity will confer proportionally greater health benefits and should be encouraged, if possible, on the basis of how well exercise is tolerated (144). Power training is also beneficial to older adults because this is a known area of loss with aging. Both single-joint and multijoint exercises can be used at a load of 30%–60% of 1-RM for 6–10 repetitions at a high velocity (1). The EP must be certain that the individual has the balance and coordination required to perform power exercises. Supervision should be provided for those who are naive to these exercises.

Flexibility Activity and Neuromotor Exercises

Exercises targeting joint mobility are recommended for all adults. For older adults, flexibility recommendations include stretching exercises held for 30–60 seconds to a point of tightness or slight discomfort for each of the major muscle groups (after a warm-up) and performed at least 2 d · wk^{-1} (1). Neuromotor exercises meant to improve balance, coordination, agility, gait, and proprioception are recommended for older adults to reduce the number and severity of falls, aid in functional tasks, and improve the quality of life (40,144). Balance training should include several aspects designed to challenge the proprioception system. Programs should progressively reduce the base of support, should be dynamic in nature and disturb the center of gravity, should target the postural muscles, should reduce sensory input (standing with eyes closed), and should include tai chi. Exercises such as two-legged stand, semi-tandem stand, tandem stand, one-legged stand, tandem walks, and circle turns are some that can be used to challenge proprioception. Dancing, tai chi, qigong, and yoga have been studied and have been shown to reduce falls, but not enough evidence exists to recommend a frequency, duration, or intensity for these activities (40,144).

Thermoregulation

As with children and other vulnerable populations, the EP should protect against a heat injury in the older adult (4) by conducting exercise in a thermoneutral environment and encouraging clients to avoid exercise in the hottest times of day. Adequate hydration is also important so that evaporative cooling is maximized. Older adults exercising in the cold should also be monitored (4). Older adults should dress in layers for increased warmth and for the ability to add or remove layers as needed.

The Case of Suzie

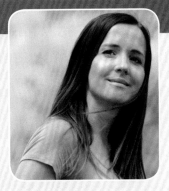

Suzie is a 30-year-old woman, who just found out she is pregnant for the first time. She is interested in doing everything she can to be healthy during her pregnancy. She is not sure if exercise is safe during her pregnancy; if it is, then she also does not know what she can and cannot do while pregnant.

Narrative

Suzie is a 30-year-old woman who is 8 weeks pregnant with her first child. She works full-time at the local university. Her work is stressful and demands a lot of time working on her computer.

Health Appraisal

Age: 30 years old
Family history: none
Cigarette smoking: none
Sedentary lifestyle: She has not really been active besides walking her dog. She still has morning sickness/nausea during the day.
Obesity: none; BMI is 29.8 (overweight) before becoming pregnant
Hypertension: none
Dyslipidemia: none
Diabetes: Her mother had gestational diabetes when she was pregnant with her and family history of diabetes.
Risk classification: low risk

Physical Data

Height: 5 ft 7 in
Weight: 190 lb (before pregnancy); 188 lb (current weight)
% Body fat: NA
BMI: 29.8 kg · m^{-2} before pregnancy (overweight)
Blood pressure: 110/70 mm Hg
Resting heart rate: 90 bpm
Fasting blood sugar: 96
No exercise test was done.

To date, Suzie's pregnancy is uncomplicated. Because her mother had gestational diabetes with her pregnancy and is now diabetic, Katie wants to do what is best to eat right and hopefully exercise. She was not physically active prior to conception and leads a fairly sedentary lifestyle. She has a family history of Type 2 diabetes, and this is her first pregnancy. She is motivated to exercise regularly and eat healthy but does not know what she can do. Nausea and vomiting are less in the afternoon. Suzie is ready to start exercise but is unsure how much or what type of exercise is safe during pregnancy.

Goals

Her main goals include healthy weight gain and to feel healthy.

Goal 1: Begin a moderate-intensity (RPE 12–14) aerobic activity of her choice, such as walking (3 d · wk^{-1}), which includes a 3- to 5-minute low-intensity warm-up and 3- to 5-minute cool-down. Begin at 10 to 15 minutes and progress 5 min · wk^{-1} until 150 minutes each week is achieved.

Goal 2: Begin a muscular strength program, 2 d · wk^{-1} for 10–15 minutes using resistance bands and a stability ball.

Goal 3: Be sure to include pelvic floor and abdominal exercises as well as a whole-body stretching regimen.

QUESTIONS

- Identify exercise precautions that should be taken during pregnancy.
- Identify four symptoms that would require exercise be terminated if a woman is pregnant.
- Identify four appropriate modes of physical activity during pregnancy.

SUMMARY

Exercise is beneficial for all individuals regardless of age or physical activity status; however, the EP must be aware of the unique concerns of older individuals, the young, and pregnant women. Benefits can be achieved for each of these populations once exercise type, quantity, and intensity have been adjusted on the basis of unique individual needs.

STUDY QUESTIONS

1. How is exercise programming different for children than for adults?
2. Describe how exercise is modified for pregnant women.
3. Under what conditions should a pregnant woman stop exercising?
4. What are different ways exercise intensity is gauged for older adults and why?
5. What are some exercise precautions taken when children, pregnant women, or older adults are exercising in the heat?

REFERENCES

1. American College of Sports Medicine. *ACSM's Guidelines for Exercise Testing and Prescription.* 11th ed. Philadelphia (PA): Wolters Kluwer; 2022. 548 p.
2. Malina RM, Bouchard C, Bar-Or O. *Growth, Maturation, and Physical Activity.* 2nd ed. Champaign (IL): Human Kinetics; 2004. 712 p.
3. Skinner JS. Aging for exercise testing and exercise prescription. In: Skinner JS, editor. *Exercise Testing and Exercise Prescription for Special Cases.* 3rd ed. Baltimore (MD): Lippincott Williams & Wilkins; 2005. p. 85–99.
4. Chodzko-Zajko WJ, Proctor DN, Fiatarone Singh MA, et al. American College of Sports Medicine position stand. Exercise and physical activity for older adults. *Med Sci Sports Exerc.* 2009;41(7):1510–30.
5. Mottola MF. Exercise prescription for overweight and obese women: pregnancy and postpartum. *Obstet Gynecol Clin North Am.* 2009;36(2):301–16, viii.
6. Mottola MF, Davenport MH, Brun CR, Inglis SD, Charlesworth S, Sopper MM. $\dot{V}O_{2peak}$ prediction and exercise prescription for pregnant women. *Med Sci Sports Exerc.* 2006;38(8):1389–95.
7. Malina RM, Bouchard C, Bar-Or O. Somatic growth. In: *Growth, Maturation, and Physical Activity.* 2nd ed. Champaign (IL): Human Kinetics; 2004. p. 41–81.

8. Malina RM, Bouchard C, Bar-Or O. Bone tissue in skeletal growth and body composition. In: *Growth, Maturation, and Physical Activity*. 2nd ed. Champaign (IL): Human Kinetics; 2004. p. 121–35.

9. Malina RM, Bouchard C, Bar-Or O. Skeletal muscle tissue. In: *Growth, Maturation, and Physical Activity*. 2nd ed. Champaign (IL): Human Kinetics; 2004. p. 137–57.

10. Malina RM, Bouchard C, Bar-Or O. Body composition. In: *Growth, Maturation, and Physical Activity*. 2nd ed. Champaign (IL): Human Kinetics; 2004. p. 101–19.

11. Malina RM, Bouchard C, Bar-Or O. Heart, blood and lungs. In: *Growth, Maturation, and Physical Activity*. 2nd ed. Champaign (IL): Human Kinetics; 2004. p. 181–93.

12. van Veelen GA, Schweitzer KJ, van der Vaart CH. Ultrasound imaging of the pelvic floor: changes in anatomy during and after first pregnancy. *Ultrasound Obstet Gynecol*. 2014;44(4):476–80.

13. Hebestreit HU, Bar-Or O. Differences between children and adults for exercise testing and prescription. In: Skinner JS, editor. *Exercise Testing and Exercise Prescription for Special Cases*. 3rd ed. Baltimore (MD): Lippincott Williams & Wilkins; 2005. p. 68–84.

14. Malina RM, Bouchard C, Bar-Or O. Strength and motor performance. In: *Growth, Maturation, and Physical Activity*. 2nd ed. Champaign (IL): Human Kinetics; 2004. p. 215–33.

15. Faigenbaum AD, Milliken LA, Cloutier G, Westcott WL. Perceived exertion during resistance exercise by children. *Percept Mot Skills*. 2004;98(2):627–37.

16. Dougherty KA, Chow M, Kenney WL. Critical environmental limits for exercising heat-acclimated lean and obese boys. *Eur J Appl Physiol*. 2010;108(4):779–89.

17. Castelli D. The relationship of physical fitness and motor competence to physical activity. *J Teach Phys Educ*. 2007;26(4):358–74.

18. Erwin HE, Woods AM, Woodard MK, Castelli DM. Children's environmental access in relation to motor competence, physical activity, and fitness. *J Teach Phys Educ*. 2007; 26:404–15.

19. Faught BE, Cairney J, Hay J, Veldhuizen S, Missiuna C, Spironello CA. Screening for motor coordination challenges in children using teacher ratings of physical ability and activity. *Hum Mov Sci*. 2008;27(2):177–89.

20. Cairney J, Hay JA, Faught BE, Wade TJ, Corna L, Flouris A. Developmental coordination disorder, generalized self-efficacy toward physical activity, and participation in organized and free play activities. *J Pediatr*. 2005;147(4): 515–20.

21. Lifshitz F. Obesity in children. *J Clin Res Pediatr Endocrinol*. 2008;1(2):53–60.

22. Ali A, Pigou D, Clarke L, McLachlan C. Literature review on motor skill and physical activity in preschool children in New Zealand. *Adv Phys Educ*. 2017;7:10–26.

23. Barnett LM, van Beurden E, Morgan PJ, Brooks LO, Beard JR. Childhood motor skill proficiency as a predictor of adolescent physical activity. *J Adolesc Health*. 2009;44(3): 252–9.

24. Loprinzi PD, Davis RE, Fu YC. Early motor skill competence as a mediator of child and adult physical activity. *Prev Med Rep*. 2015;2:833–8.

25. Expert Panel on Integrated Guidelines for Cardiovascular Health and Risk Reduction in Children and Adolescents: summary report. *Pediatrics*. 2011;128(Suppl 5):S213–56.

26. U.S. Department of Health and Human Services. *2018 Physical Activity Guidelines for Americans*. 2nd ed. [Internet]. Washington (DC): U.S. Department of Health & Human Services; 2018 [cited 2021 Mar 25]. Available from: https://health.gov/paguidelines/second-edition/pdf/Physical_Activity_Guidelines_2nd_edition.pdf.

27. Faigenbaum AD, Kraemer WJ, Blimkie CJR, et al. Youth resistance training: updated position statement paper from the National Strength and Conditioning Association. *J Strength Cond Res*. 2009;23(5):S60–79.

28. Biddiss E, Irwin J. Active video games to promote physical activity in children and youth: a systematic review. *Arch Pediatr Adolesc Med*. 2010;164(7):664-72.

29. Daniels SR, Hassink SG. The role of the pediatrician in primary prevention of obesity. *Pediatrics*. 2015;136(1): e275–92.

30. Faigenbaum AD, McFarland J. Relative safety of weight-lifting movements for youth. *J Strength Cond Res*. 2008; 30(6):23–5.

31. Johnson BA, Salzberg CL, Stevenson DA. A systematic review: plyometric training programs for young children. *J Strength Cond Res*. 2011;25(9):2623–33.

32. Faigenbaum AD, Rial Rebullido T, MacDonald JP. The unsolved problem of paediatric physical inactivity: it's time for a new perspective. *Acta Paediatr*. 2018;107(11): 1857–9.

33. Strasburger VC, Hogan M. Children, adolescents, and the media. *Pediatrics*. 2013;132(5):958–61.

34. Williamson P. Exercise for youth. In: *Exercise for Special Populations*. Baltimore (MD): Lippincott Williams & Wilkins; 2011. p. 82–120.

35. Faigenbaum AD, Milliken LA, Westcott WL. Maximal strength testing in healthy children. *J Strength Cond Res*. 2003;17(1):162–6.

36. Barlow SE, Expert Committee. Expert Committee recommendations regarding the prevention, assessment, and treatment of child and adolescent overweight and obesity: summary report. *Pediatrics*. 2007;120(Suppl 4):S164–92.

37. Ward DS, Saunders RP, Pate RR. *Physical Activity Interventions in Children and Adolescents*. Champaign (IL): Human Kinetics; 2007. 288 p.

38. ACOG Committee Opinion No. 804: physical activity and exercise during pregnancy and the postpartum period. *Obstet Gynecol*. 2020;135(4):e178–88.

39. World Health Organization. *Global Recommendations on Physical Activity for Health*. Geneva (Switzerland): World Health Organization Press; 2010. 58 p.

40. Garber CE, Blissmer B, Deschenes MR, et al. American College of Sports Medicine position stand. Quantity and quality of exercise for developing and maintaining cardiorespiratory, musculoskeletal, and neuromotor fitness in apparently healthy adults: guidance for prescribing exercise. *Med Sci Sports Exerc*. 2011;43(7):1334–59.

41. Davenport MH, Ruchat S-M, Mottola MF, et al. 2019 Canadian guideline for physical activity throughout pregnancy: methodology. *J Obstet Gynaecol Canada*. 2018;40(11):1468–83.

42. Mottola MF, Davenport MH, Ruchat SM, et al. 2019 Canadian guideline for physical activity throughout pregnancy. *Br J Sports Med.* 2018;52(21):1339–46.

43. May L. Cardiac physiology of pregnancy. *Compr Physiol.* 2015;5(3):1325–44.

44. Goland S, Shimoni S, Zornitzki T, et al. Cardiac abnormalities as a new manifestation of nonalcoholic fatty liver disease: echocardiographic and tissue Doppler imaging assessment. *J Clin Gastroenterol.* 2006;40(10):949–55.

45. Stevenson L. Exercise in pregnancy. Part 2: recommendations for individuals. *Can Fam Physician.* 1997;43:107–11.

46. Bonnin P, Bazzi-Grossin C, Ciraru-Vigneron N, et al. Evidence of fetal cerebral vasodilatation induced by submaximal maternal dynamic exercise in human pregnancy. *J Perinat Med.* 1997;25(1):63–70.

47. Rafla NM, Beazely JM. The effect of maternal exercise on fetal umbilical artery waveforms. *Eur J Obstet Gynecol Reprod Biol.* 1991;40(2):119–22.

48. Szymanski LM, Satin AJ. Strenuous exercise during pregnancy: is there a limit? *Am J Obstet Gynecol.* 2012;207(3):179.e1–6.

49. Petrov F, Glantz KA, Fagevik Olsen M. Hemodynamic responses to single sessions of aerobic exercise and resistance exercise in pregnancy. *Acta Obstet Gynecol Scan.* 2016;95(9):1042–7.

50. Wiswell RA, Artal Mittelmark R. *Exercise in Pregnancy.* Baltimore (MD): Williams & Wilkins; 1986. 241 p.

51. Davies GA, Wolfe LA, Mottola MF, et al. Exercise in pregnancy and the postpartum period. *J Obstet Gynaecol Can.* 2003;25(6):516–29.

52. Melzer K, Schutz Y, Boulvain M, Kayser B. Physical activity and pregnancy: cardiovascular adaptations, recommendations and pregnancy outcomes. *Sports Med.* 2010;40(6):493–507.

53. Wolfe LA, Davies GA. Canadian guidelines for exercise in pregnancy. *Clin Obstet Gynecol.* 2003;46(2):488–95.

54. McAuley SE, Jensen D, McGrath MJ, Wolfe LA. Effects of human pregnancy and aerobic conditioning on alveolar gas exchange during exercise. *Can J Physiol Pharmacol.* 2005;83(7):625–33.

55. Jensen D, Webb KA, Davies GA, O'Donnell DE. Mechanical ventilatory constraints during incremental cycle exercise in human pregnancy: implications for respiratory sensation. *J Physiol.* 2008;586(19):4735–50.

56. Institute of Medicine. *Committee on Nutritional Status During Pregnancy and Lactation. Subcommittee for a Clinical Application Guide.* Washington (DC): National Academy Press; 1992. 133 p.

57. Truong YN, Yee LM, Caughey AB, Cheng YW. Weight gain in pregnancy: does the Institute of Medicine have it right? *Am J Obstet Gynecol.* 2015;212(3):362.e1–8.

58. Lamina S, Agbanusi E. Effect of aerobic exercise training on maternal weight gain in pregnancy: a meta-analysis of randomized controlled trials. *Ethiop J Health Sci.* 2013;23(1):59–64.

59. Perales M, Santos-Lozano A, Ruiz JR, Lucia A, Barakat R. Benefits of aerobic or resistance training during pregnancy on maternal health and perinatal outcomes: a systematic review. *Early Hum Dev.* 2016;94:43–8.

60. Barakat R, Cordero Y, Coteron J, Luaces M, Montejo R. Exercise during pregnancy improves maternal glucose screen at 24-28 weeks: a randomised controlled trial. *Br J Sports Med.* 2012;46(9):656–61.

61. Colberg SR, Sigal RJ, Fernhall B, et al. Exercise and type 2 diabetes: the American College of Sports Medicine and the American Diabetes Association: joint position statement executive summary. *Diabetes Care.* 2010;33(12):2692–6.

62. Padayachee C, Coombes JS. Exercise guidelines for gestational diabetes mellitus. *World J Diabetes.* 2015;6(8):1033–44.

63. Wang TW, Apgar BS. Exercise during pregnancy. *Am Fam Physician.* 1998;57(8):1846–52, 1857.

64. Cakmak B, Ribeiro AP, Inanir A. Postural balance and the risk of falling during pregnancy. *J Matern Fetal Neonatal Med.* 2016;29(10):1623–5.

65. Aldabe D, Milosavljevic S, Bussey MD. Is pregnancy related pelvic girdle pain associated with altered kinematic, kinetic and motor control of the pelvis? A systematic review. *Eur Spine J.* 2012;21(9):1777–87.

66. Aldabe D, Ribeiro DC, Milosavljevic S, Dawn Bussey M. Pregnancy-related pelvic girdle pain and its relationship with relaxin levels during pregnancy: a systematic review. *Eur Spine J.* 2012;21(9):1769–76.

67. Gallo-Padilla D, Gallo-Padilla C, Gallo-Vallejo FJ, Gallo-Vallejo JL. Low back pain during pregnancy. Multidisciplinary approach. *Semergen.* 2016;42(6):e59–64.

68. Marin-Jimenez N, Acosta-Manzano P, Borges-Cosic M, Aparicio VA. Association of self-reported physical fitness with pain during pregnancy. The GESTAFIT Project. *Scand J Med Sci Sports.* 2019;29(7):1022–30.

69. Cherni Y, Desseauve D, Decatoire A, et al. Evaluation of ligament laxity during pregnancy. *J Gynecol Obstet Hum Reprod.* 2019;48(5):351–7.

70. Shephard RJ. Exercise and training in women, part I: influence of gender on exercise and training responses. *Can J Appl Physiol.* 2000;25(1):19–34.

71. Chitra TV, Panicker S. Child birth, pregnancy and pelvic floor dysfunction. *J Obstet Gynecol India.* 2011;61(6):635–7.

72. Davenport MH, Ruchat SM, Sobierajski F, et al. Impact of prenatal exercise on maternal harms, labour and delivery outcomes: a systematic review and meta-analysis. *Br J Sports Med.* 2019;53(2):99–107.

73. Mota P, Pascoal AG, Carita AI, Bo K. The immediate effects on inter-rectus distance of abdominal crunch and drawing-in exercises during pregnancy and the postpartum period. *J Orthop Sports Phys Ther.* 2015;45(10):781–8.

74. Sancho MF, Pascoal AG, Mota P, Bo K. Abdominal exercises affect inter-rectus distance in postpartum women: a two-dimensional ultrasound study. *Physiotherapy.* 2015;101(3):286–91.

75. Morkved S, Bo K. Effect of pelvic floor muscle training during pregnancy and after childbirth on prevention and treatment of urinary incontinence: a systematic review. *Br J Sports Med.* 2014;48(4):299–310.

76. Clapp JF III, Kim H, Burciu B, Schmidt S, Petry K, Lopez B. Continuing regular exercise during pregnancy: effect of exercise volume on fetoplacental growth. *Am J Obstet Gynecol.* 2002;186(1):142–7.

77. Lindqvist PG, Marsal K, Merlo J, Pirhonen JP. Thermal response to submaximal exercise before, during and after pregnancy: a longitudinal study. *J Matern Fetal Neonatal Med.* 2003;13(3):152–6.

78. Stevenson L. Exercise in pregnancy. Part 1: update on pathophysiology. *Can Fam Physician.* 1997;43:97–104.

79. Chan J, Natekar A, Koren G. Hot yoga and pregnancy: fitness and hyperthermia. *Can Fam Physician.* 2014;60(1):41–2.

80. May LE. *Physiology of Prenatal Exercise and Fetal Development.* New York (NY): Springer; 2012. 44 p.

81. Davenport MH, Steinback CD, Mottola MF. Impact of pregnancy and obesity on cardiorespiratory responses during weight-bearing exercise. *Respir Physiol Neurobiol.* 2009;167(3):341–7.

82. May LE, Knowlton J, Hanson J, et al. Effects of exercise during pregnancy on maternal heart rate and heart rate variability. *PM R.* 2016;8(7):611–7.

83. Purdy GM, James MA, Wakefield PK, et al. Maternal cardioautonomic responses during and following exercise throughout pregnancy. *Appl Physiol Nutr Metab.* 2019;44(3):263–70.

84. Williamson P. Exercise during pregnancy. In: *Exercise for Special Populations.* Baltimore (MD): Lippincott Williams & Wilkins; 2011. p. 46–81.

85. Clapp JF III. Long-term outcome after exercising throughout pregnancy: fitness and cardiovascular risk. *Am J Obstet Gynecol.* 2008;199(5):489.e1–6.

86. Clark E, Isler C, Strickland D, et al. Influence of aerobic exercise on maternal lipid levels and offspring morphometrics. *Int J Obes (Lond).* 2019;43(3):594–602.

87. May L, Suminski RS. Amount of physical activity in pregnancy and infant heart outcomes. *J Neonat Biol.* 2014;3(5):1–5.

88. May L, Terry M, Drake WB, Suminski RR. Effects of exercise during pregnancy on childhood heart measures. *J Cardiobiol.* 2014;(Suppl 1):5.

89. May LE, Glaros A, Yeh HW, Clapp JF III, Gustafson KM. Aerobic exercise during pregnancy influences fetal cardiac autonomic control of heart rate and heart rate variability. *Early Hum Dev.* 2010;86(4):213–7.

90. May LE, Scholtz SA, Suminski R, Gustafson KM. Aerobic exercise during pregnancy influences infant heart rate variability at one month of age. *Early Hum Dev.* 2014;90(1):33–8.

91. McMillan AG, May LE, Gaines GG, Isler C, Kuehn D. Effects of aerobic exercise during pregnancy on 1-month infant neuromotor skills. *Med Sci Sports Exerc.* 2019;51(8):1671–6.

92. Barakat R, Lucia A, Ruiz JR. Resistance exercise training during pregnancy and newborn's birth size: a randomised controlled trial. *Int J Obes (Lond).* 2009;33(9):1048–57.

93. Barakat R, Ruiz JR, Stirling JR, Zakynthinaki M, Lucia A. Type of delivery is not affected by light resistance and toning exercise training during pregnancy: a randomized controlled trial. *Am J Obstet Gynecol.* 2009;201(6):590.e1–6.

94. Benton MJ, Swan PD, Whyte M. Progressive resistance training during pregnancy: a case study. *PM R.* 2010;2(7):681–4.

95. Baena-Garcia L, Ocon-Hernandez O, Acosta-Manzano P, et al. Association of sedentary time and physical activity during pregnancy with maternal and neonatal birth outcomes. The GESTAFIT Project. *Scand J Med Sci Sports.* 2019;29(3):407–14.

96. O'Connor PJ, Poudevigne MS, Cress ME, Motl RW, Clapp JF III. Safety and efficacy of supervised strength training adopted in pregnancy. *J Phys Act Health.* 2011;8(3):309–20.

97. May LE, Suminski RR, Berry A, Langaker MD, Gustafson KM. Maternal physical activity mode and fetal heart outcome. *Early Hum Dev.* 2014;90(7):365–9.

98. Beilock SL, Feltz DL, Pivarnik JM. Training patterns of athletes during pregnancy and postpartum. *Res Q Exerc Sport.* 2001;72(1):39–46.

99. Barakat R, Pelaez M, Cordero Y, et al. Exercise during pregnancy protects against hypertension and macrosomia: randomized clinical trial. *Am J Obstet Gynecol.* 2016;214(5):649.e1–8.

100. Hall DC, Kaufmann DA. Effects of aerobic and strength conditioning on pregnancy outcomes. *Am J Obstet Gynecol.* 1987;157(5):1199–203.

101. Price BB, Amini SB, Kappeler K. Exercise in pregnancy: effect on fitness and obstetric outcomes — a randomized trial. *Med Sci Sports Exerc.* 2012;44(12):2263–9.

102. Rodriguez-Blanque R, Sanchez-Garcia JC, Sanchez-Lopez AM, Exposito-Ruiz M, Aguilar-Cordero MJ. Randomized clinical trial of an aquatic physical exercise program during pregnancy. *J Obstet Gynecol Neonatal Nurs.* 2019;48(3):321–31.

103. Vallim AL, Osis MJ, Cecatti JG, Baciuk EP, Silveira C, Cavalcante SR. Water exercises and quality of life during pregnancy [Internet]. *Reproductive Health.* 2011 [cited 2020 Oct 4];8. Available from: https://www.ncbi.nlm.nih.gov/pmc/articles/PMC3113331/pdf/1742-4755-8-14.pdf.

104. Aguilar-Cordero MJ, Sanchez-Garcia JC, Rodriguez-Blanque R, Sanchez-Lopez AM, Mur-Villar N. Moderate physical activity in an aquatic environment during pregnancy (SWEP study) and its influence in preventing postpartum depression. *J Am Psychiatr Nurses Assoc.* 2019;25(2):112–21.

105. Juhl M, Kogevinas M, Andersen PK, Andersen AM, Olsen J. Is swimming during pregnancy a safe exercise? *Epidemiology.* 2010;21(2):253–8.

106. McMurray RG, Katz VL, Berry MJ, Cefalo RC. The effect of pregnancy on metabolic responses during rest, immersion, and aerobic exercise in the water. *Am J Obstet Gynecol.* 1988;158(3 Pt 1):481–6.

107. Rodriguez-Blanque R, Sanchez-Garcia JC, Sanchez-Lopez AM, Mur-Villar N, Aguilar-Cordero MJ. The influence of physical activity in water on sleep quality in pregnant women: a randomised trial. *Women Birth.* 2018;31(1):e51–e8.

108. Vern K. Exercise in water during pregnancy. *Clin Obstet Gynecol.* 2003;46(2):432–41.

109. Katz VL. Water exercise in pregnancy. *Semin Perinatol.* 1996;20(4):285–91.

110. Bacchi M, Mottola MF, Perales M, Refoyo I, Barakat R. Aquatic activities during pregnancy prevent excessive maternal weight gain and preserve birth weight: a randomized clinical trial. *Am J Health Promot.* 2018;32(3): 729–35.

111. American Heart Association. American Heart Association recommendations for physical activity in adults and kids [Internet]. Dallas (TX): American Heart Association; [cited 2021 Mar 25]. Available from: https://www.heart.org/en/healthy-living/fitness/fitness-basics/aha-recs-for-physical-activity-in-adults.

112. American College of Sports Medicine. Exercise during pregnancy [Internet]. Amherst (MA): University of Massachusetts Amherst; [cited 2021 Mar 25]. Available from: https://blogs.umass.edu/bodyshop/files/2009/07/exerciseduringpregnancy.pdf.

113. Logan JG, Kim SS, Lee M, Byon HD, Yeo S. Effects of static stretching exercise on lumbar flexibility and central arterial stiffness. *J Cardiovasc Nurs.* 2018;33(4):322–8.

114. Logan JG, Yeo S. Effects of stretching exercise on heart rate variability during pregnancy. *J Cardiovasc Nurs.* 2017;32(2):107–11.

115. Yeo S. Prenatal stretching exercise and autonomic responses: preliminary data and a model for reducing preeclampsia. *J Nurs Scholarsh.* 2010;42(2):113–21.

116. Yeo S, Davidge S, Ronis DL, Antonakos CL, Hayashi R, O'Leary S. A comparison of walking versus stretching exercises to reduce the incidence of preeclampsia: a randomized clinical trial. *Hypertens Pregnancy.* 2008;27(2):113–30.

117. Jiang Q, Wu Z, Zhou L, Dunlop J, Chen P. Effects of yoga intervention during pregnancy: a review for current status. *Am J Perinatol.* 2015;32(6):503–14.

118. Oktaviani I. Pilates workouts can reduce pain in pregnant women. *Complement Ther Clin Pract.* 2018;31:349–51.

119. Ji ES, Han HR. The effects of Qi exercise on maternal/fetal interaction and maternal well-being during pregnancy. *J Obstet Gynecol Neonatal Nurs.* 2010;39(3):310–8.

120. May LE, Suminski RR, Linklater ER, Jahnke S, Glaros AG. Exercise during pregnancy: the role of obstetric providers. *J Am Osteopath Assoc.* 2013;113(8):612–9.

121. Nawaz H, Adams ML, Katz DL. Physician-patient interactions regarding diet, exercise, and smoking. *Prev Med.* 2000;31(6):652–7.

122. Canadian Society for Exercise Physiology. PARmed-X for pregnancy. Physical activity readiness medical examination [Internet]. Ottawa (Canada): Canadian Society for Exercise Physiology. Available from: https://www.csep.ca/CMFiles/publications/parq/parmed-xpreg.pdf.

123. May LE, Suminski RR, Langaker MD, Yeh HW, Gustafson KM. Regular maternal exercise dose and fetal heart outcome. *Med Sci Sports Exerc.* 2012;44(7):1252–8.

124. Bo K, Artal R, Barakat R, et al. Exercise and pregnancy in recreational and elite athletes: 2016 evidence summary from the IOC expert group meeting, Lausanne. Part 1 — exercise in women planning pregnancy and those who are pregnant. *Br J Sports Med.* 2016;50(10):571–89.

125. Davenport MH, Charlesworth S, Vanderspank D, Sopper MM, Mottola MF. Development and validation of exercise target heart rate zones for overweight and obese pregnant women. *Appl Physiol Nutr Metab.* 2008;33(5):984–9.

126. Clapp JF III. The changing thermal response to endurance exercise during pregnancy. *Am J Obstet Gynecol.* 1991;165(6 Pt 1):1684–9.

127. Borodulin K, Evenson KR, Herring AH. Physical activity patterns during pregnancy through postpartum. *BMC Womens Health.* 2009;9:32.

128. Forczek W, Curylo M, Forczek B. Physical activity assessment during gestation and its outcomes: a review. *Obstet Gynecol Surv.* 2017;72(7):425–44.

129. May LE, McDonald SM, Jones R, et al. Influence of maternal aerobic exercise during pregnancy on fetal cardiac function and outflow. *Am J Obstet Gynecol MFM.* 2020;2(2):100095.

130. Roldan-Reoyo O, Pelaez M, May LE, Barakat R. Influence of maternal physical exercise on fetal and maternal heart rate responses. *German J Exerc Sport Res.* 2019;49:446–53.

131. McDonald SM, Newton ER, Strickland D, et al. Influence of prenatal aerobic exercise on fetal morphometry. *Matern Child Health J.* 2020;24(11):1367–75.

132. Davenport MH, Meah VL, Ruchat SM, et al. Impact of prenatal exercise on neonatal and childhood outcomes: a systematic review and meta-analysis. *Br J Sports Med.* 2018;52(21):1386–96.

133. McDonald SM, Isler C, Haven K, et al. The effects of moderate intensity aerobic exercise during pregnancy on one-month infant morphometry. *Birth Defects Res.* 2021;113(3):238–47.

134. Moyer C, Reoyo OR, May L. The influence of prenatal exercise on offspring health: a review. *Clin Med Insights Womens Health.* 2016;9:37–42.

135. Moyer C, May L. Influence of exercise mode on maternal, fetal, and neonatal health outcomes. *Med J Obstet Gynecol.* 2014;2(2):7.

136. ACOG Practice Bulletin No 156: obesity in pregnancy. *Obstet Gynecol.* 2015;126(6):e112–26.

137. Choi J, Fukuoka Y, Lee JH. The effects of physical activity and physical activity plus diet interventions on body weight in overweight or obese women who are pregnant or in postpartum: a systematic review and meta-analysis of randomized controlled trials. *Prev Med.* 2013;56(6):351–64.

138. Renault KM, Norgaard K, Nilas L, et al. The Treatment of Obese Pregnant Women (TOP) study: a randomized controlled trial of the effect of physical activity intervention assessed by pedometer with or without dietary intervention in obese pregnant women. *Am J Obstet Gynecol.* 2014;210(2):134.e1–9.

139. ACOG Practice Bulletin No. 190: gestational diabetes mellitus. *Obstet Gynecol.* 2018;131(2):e49–64.

140. Benjamin EJ, Muntner P, Alonso A, et al. Heart disease and stroke statistics — 2019 update: a report from the american heart association. *Circulation.* 2019;139(10): e56–528.

141. Gianoudis J, Bailey CA, Ebeling PR, et al. Effects of a targeted multimodal exercise program incorporating

high-speed power training on falls and fracture risk factors in older adults: a community-based randomized controlled trial. *J Bone Miner Res.* 2014;29(1):182–91.

142. Williamson P. Exercise for senior adults. In: *Exercise for Special Populations.* Baltimore (MD): Lippincott Williams & Wilkins; 2011. p. 121–78.

143. Haskell WL, Lee IM, Pate RR, et al. Physical activity and public health: updated recommendation for adults from the American College of Sports Medicine and the American Heart Association. *Med Sci Sports Exerc.* 2007;39(8):1423–34.

144. Nelson ME, Rejeski WJ, Blair SN, et al. Physical activity and public health in older adults: recommendation from the American College of Sports Medicine and the American Heart Association. *Circulation.* 2007;116(9):1094–105.

145. Rikli RE, Jones CJ. Development and validation of criterion-referenced clinically relevant fitness standards for maintaining physical independence in later years. *Gerontologist.* 2013;53(2):255–67.

146. Guralnik JM, Simonsick EM, Ferrucci L, et al. A short physical performance battery assessing lower extremity function: association with self-reported disability and prediction of mortality and nursing home admission. *J Gerontol.* 1994;49(2):M85–94.

147. Rikli RE, Jones CJ. *Senior Fitness Test Manual.* Champaign (IL): Human Kinetics; 2001.

148. Cress ME, Buchner DM, Questad KA, Esselman PC, deLateur BJ, Schwartz RS. Continuous-Scale Physical Functional Performance in healthy older adults: a validation study. *Arch Phys Med Rehabil.* 1996;77(12):1243–50.

ADDITIONAL RESOURCES

Swain DP, editor. *ACSM's Resource Manual for Guidelines for Exercise Testing and Prescription.* 7th ed. Baltimore (MD): Lippincott Williams & Wilkins; 2013. 896 p.

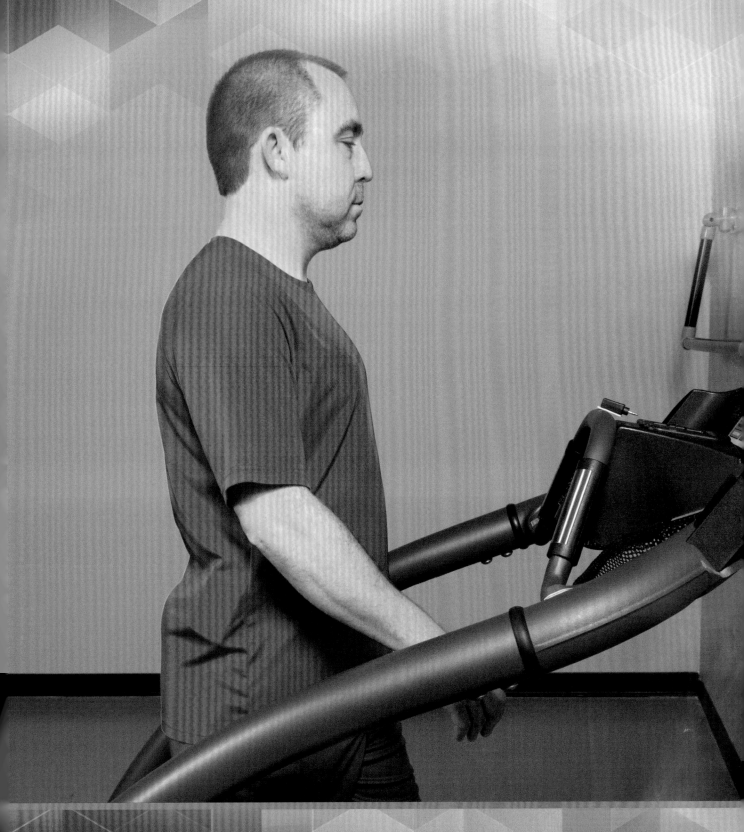

PART **IV** Behavior Changes

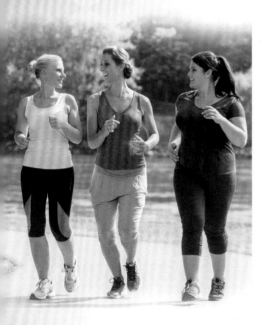

11

Theories of Behavior Change

OBJECTIVES

- To identify and describe the evidence-based theories and models used to explain physical activity behaviors.
- To understand key terminology as it relates to facilitating behavior change.
- To summarize the evidence-based support for the theories and models.
- To understand the practical application of these concepts in facilitating physical activity behavior change.

INTRODUCTION

This chapter summarizes evidence-based theories and models that have been shown to facilitate physical activity behavior change. These include the transtheoretical model (TTM), social cognitive theory (SCT), social ecological model, theory of planned behavior (TPB), self-determination theory (SDT), and hedonic theory. The evidence supporting each of the theories in the context of physical activity behavior and their practical application will be highlighted. Chapter 12 expands on this chapter by describing how concepts from these theories and models are applied to physical activity interventions.

Importance of Theories and Models

A theory refers to a systematic view of a behavior by specifying relationships between variables and predicting specific behaviors and situations (1). For example, an exercise physiologist would be interested in understanding the variables that influence physical activity behavior, how these variables interact with one another, and the circumstances or conditions under which physical activity occurs. There are several reasons why it is important for the exercise physiologist to have a working knowledge of theories and models in the context of physical activity behavior. First, theories and models provide a framework for better understanding the continuum of physical activity behavior, from adoption to maintenance. Second, theories and models can help the exercise physiologist to understand why a client stops physical activity participation or does not achieve physical activity or other health-related goals (*e.g.*, healthy eating, sleep hygiene, stress management). Finally, theories and models allow the exercise physiologist to identify which types of clients respond to which types of physical activity promotion strategies.

Transtheoretical Model

The TTM has been used to explain a variety of health behaviors (2–5), understand physical activity behavior (6), and create physical activity interventions (7–9). According to the TTM, individuals move through a series of stages when making a behavior change which include (10,11) (a) precontemplation, (b) contemplation, (c) preparation, (d) adoption, and (e) maintenance (Table 11.1) (12). The exercise physiologist can use a series of questions to assess a client's stage of change, or readiness for change, for physical activity.

Specific behavioral and cognitive processes occur and are used as individuals move through these stages of change. The various processes are thought to receive differential emphasis during particular stages of change (10,11,13,14). Cognitive processes of change include increasing knowledge, being aware of risks, caring about consequences to others, comprehending benefits, and increasing healthy opportunities. Behavioral processes of change include substituting alternatives, enlisting social support, rewarding yourself, committing yourself, and reminding yourself (15). These processes represent principles of change in behavior and are considered critical for movement through the various stages of the TTM (16). Exercise physiologists can use the processes of change to provide information and learning opportunities for their clients to encourage a client's transition or progression through the stages (17) (Box 11.1).

Research indicates that physical activity interventions based on the TTM are efficacious for increasing physical activity among sedentary adults (18–21) and specialized populations (22–26). Using a TTM-based intervention model, the exercise physiologist can tailor messages to increase physical activity behavior. One study among individuals with Type 2 diabetes found that self-efficacy

Table 11.1	The Transtheoretical Model: Stages of Change	
Stage of Change	**Progression through the Five Stages**	**Application to Physical Activity**
Precontemplation	Individuals in this stage are not intending to take action within the next 6 mo. There may be a variety of reasons why an individual would be in the precontemplation stage. For example, a person may be uninformed about the health effects of a sedentary lifestyle, not motivated to make changes, or frustrated after failed attempts at physical activity.	Stage 1: inactive and not thinking about becoming more active These individuals do not currently engage in physical activity and do not plan on doing so in the near future.
Contemplation	Individuals in this stage are intending to alter their behavior within the next 6 mo. They may be becoming more aware of the pros of engaging in physical activity; however, the costs associated with physical activity may still outweigh the benefits.	Stage 2: inactive and thinking about becoming more active These individuals are thinking about adopting physical activity and are planning to become more physically active within a reasonable time frame.
Preparation	Individuals in this stage are intending to increase their physical activity in the immediate future. These individuals may have a specific plan to change behavior and may be seeking out resources for assistance.	Stage 3: doing some physical activity These individuals are currently doing physical activity but are not meeting the standards and guidelines identified by the ACSM.
Action	Individuals in this stage have made specific, measurable changes in their physical activity in the past 6 mo.	Stage 4: doing enough physical activity These individuals are currently engaging in physical activity 5 d · wk^{-1} for at least 30 min each session. These individuals have participated in regular physical activity for less than 6 mo.
Maintenance	Individuals in this stage are maintaining their physical activity and are working to prevent relapse.	Stage 5: making physical activity a habit These individuals have been participating in regular physical activity at the recommended levels for at least 6 mo.

was increased when more processes of change were used in the intervention (27). Physical activity interventions guided by the TTM typically leads to increases in behavioral strategies, cognitive processes, self-efficacy, and positive changes in decisional balance (*i.e.*, relatively more pros than cons for becoming physically active when moving through the stages) (Table 11.2).

Social Cognitive Theory

SCT (28–30), first known as social learning theory, is one of the most popular theoretical frameworks for understanding physical activity adoption (31,32). SCT emphasizes reciprocal determinism, which is the interaction between individuals and their environments (Fig. 11.1). SCT identifies three main factors that influence behavior: (a) the environment (*e.g.*, neighborhood

HOW TO   Assess a Client's Stage of Change for Physical Activity

According to the TTM, behavior change interventions should be tailored to the individual depending on stage of change. The exercise physiologist can ask the following questions to determine a client's readiness for change for physical activity:

1. Are you currently accumulating at least 150 min of moderate-intensity physical activity each week? (If yes, present stage is action or maintenance and go to question 2; if no, go to question 3.)

2. Have you been regularly physically active over the past 6 mo? (If yes, present stage is maintenance and stop questions; if no, in action stage and stop questions.)

3. Are you doing any physical activity? (If yes, present stage is preparation and stop questions; if no, go to question 4.)

4. Have you made any actions and/or concrete plans for increasing your physical activity (*i.e.*, gym membership, purchasing exercise equipment, and hiring a trainer)? (If yes, present stage is preparation and stop questions; if no, go to question 5.)

5. Do you plan on becoming more physically active over the next 6 mo? (If yes, present stage is contemplation; if no, present stage is precontemplation.)

Answers to these questions can facilitate the development of a more optimal plan of action specific to each client and tailored to the client's current stage or readiness for behavior change. For example, clients in the contemplation or preparation stages will need detailed guidance on starting a physical activity program. Clients in the maintenance stage, on the other hand, may need strategies for implementing new exercises or goals to prevent relapse.

and proximity to gym), (b) individual personality characteristics and/or experience (including cognitions), and (c) behavioral factors. According to SCT, behavior is the product of the interplay between these three factors. In other words, the environment can influence individuals and groups, but individuals and groups can also influence their environments and, in turn, govern their own behaviors. Using SCT for physical activity adoption can be individual-based self-regulation like self-monitoring, goal setting, and feedback, or it can be more complex involving all three factors. For example, an individual intending to be more active may seek out guidance from an exercise physiologist. The exercise physiologist provides education and opportunity for the client that results in increased confidence and an increase in physical activity behavior. The client's coworkers see the improvement in mood of the client and, in turn, begin to increase their physical activity behavior by joining the client at the gym. The client now has a group of coworkers to meet at the gym, which further motivates the client to continue exercise.

Self-Efficacy

A key concept related to SCT is self-efficacy (8,28,29). Self-efficacy refers to a person's belief in his or her ability to successfully engage in and perform a specific behavior. The more confident one feels in his or her capabilities and skills to succeed (*i.e.*, higher self-efficacy), the more likely he or she will engage in that behavior (29). Intervention studies indicate that self-efficacy is likely an important component of physical activity behavior change for healthy adults (33), children, adolescents, older adults (34–37), and adults with medical conditions (31,38–41). Consequently, fitness professionals should create an environment that instills a sense of confidence while educating on

Box 11.1   Example Strategies to Facilitate Stage of Transitions

Precontemplation → Contemplation
- Provide information about the benefits of regular physical activity.
- Discuss how some of their barriers may be misperceived. For example, if time is a barrier, they may not be aware of the benefits of short bouts of physical activity.
- Have them visualize what they would feel like if they were physically active with an emphasis on short-term, easily achievable benefits of activity.
- Explore how their inactivity impacts individuals other than themselves.

Contemplation → Preparation
- Explore potential solutions to their physical activity barriers.
- Assess level of self-efficacy and begin techniques to build efficacy.
- Emphasize the importance of even small steps in progressing toward being regularly active.
- Encourage viewing oneself as a healthy, physically active person.

Preparation → Action
- Help develop an appropriate plan of activity to meet their physical activity goals and use a goal setting worksheet or contract to make it a formal commitment.
- Use reinforcement to reward steps toward being active.
- Teach self-monitoring techniques such as tracking time and distance.
- Continue discussion of how to overcome any obstacles they feel are in their way of being active.
- Encourage them to help create an environment that helps remind them to be active.
- Encourage ways to substitute sedentary behavior with activity.

Action → Maintenance
- Provide positive and contingent feedback on goal progress.
- Explore different types of activities they can do to avoid burnout.
- Encourage them to work with and even help others become more active.
- Discuss relapse prevention strategies.
- Discuss potential rewards that can be used to maintain motivation.

specific skills necessary to facilitate the client's desired behavior change. See Table 11.3 for specific strategies for enhancing self-efficacy as it relates to physical activity behavior.

Self-efficacy is situation-specific confidence influenced by four sources of information including: (a) mastery experience, (b) vicarious experience, (c) verbal persuasion, and (d) physiological or affective states (29). First, mastery experience is the successful performance of the target behavior (in this case, physical activity), which should enhance perceptions of confidence and build self-efficacy. In contrast, failure to perform the behavior as intended or not meeting expectations typically decreases confidence. For example, a previously sedentary individual who is able to successfully maintain a regular physical activity program for 6 weeks would have higher levels of perceived self-efficacy. Similarly, a person who completes an exercise session after a cardiac event would have increased confidence to continue rehabilitation.

Second, vicarious experience refers to seeing a similar individual successfully perform a behavior and comparing one's own performance with the performance of the other individual. For example, the *Instant Recess* program, developed by Dr. Toni Yancey, encourages adults to add short

Table 11.2	Processes of Change	
Processes of Change	**Description**	**Strategy Examples**
Experiential Processes		
Consciousness raising (Become informed.)	Learning new facts, ideas, and tips that support exercise	Read books, magazines, or Web sites that focus on exercise and health.
Dramatic relief (Pay attention to feelings.)	Experiencing negative emotions (fear, anxiety) that go along with the health consequences of not exercising or the positive emotions (e.g., inspiration) that go along with regular exercise	Think about somebody close to you who has had severe health problems that may have been prevented by regularly exercising. Does their inactivity and subsequent health problem upset you?
Environmental reevaluation (Notice your effect on others.)	Realizing the negative impact not exercising has on others and our society — and the positive impact that exercising could have	Consider the example your inactivity sets for your children, family, friends, and coworkers.
Self-reevaluation (Create a new self-image.)	Realizing that regular exercise is an important part of one's identity	Ask yourself, "How do I think and feel about myself as someone who is not exercising regularly? How might I feel differently if I was exercising regularly?"
Social liberation (Notice social trends.)	Realizing that social norms are changing to support exercise	Name some social changes that support exercise (e.g., walking paths).
Behavioral Processes		
Self-liberation (Make a commitment.)	Believing in one's ability to exercise regularly and making a commitment to change based on that belief	Set a date to start exercising regularly and tell your friends, family, and coworkers your plan.
Helping relationships (Get support.)	Seeking and using social support to start and/or continue exercising	Join an adult sports league or ask a friend to walk around the neighborhood with you every evening after dinner.
Counterconditioning (Use substitutes.)	Substituting healthy alternative behaviors and thoughts for unhealthy ones	Ride your bike to work instead of driving your car.
Reinforcement management (Use rewards.)	Increasing the intrinsic and extrinsic rewards for exercise and decreasing the rewards for being sedentary	Buy a new set of workout clothes after you have met an exercise goal.
Stimulus control (Manage your environment.)	Removing reminders or cues to be sedentary and using cues to exercise	Leave your running shoes and clothes in a bag by the door to remind you to run during your lunch break.

From American College of Sports Medicine. *ACSM's Behavioral Aspects of Physical Activity and Exercise*. Philadelphia (PA): Lippincott Williams & Wilkins; 2013. 336 p. Table 4.1.

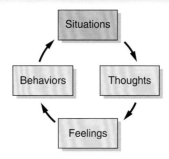

FIGURE 11.1. Thoughts, feelings, and behaviors.

Table 11.3	Strategies for Enhancing Self-Efficacy	
Source of Self-Efficacy Information	**Description**	**Strategies**
Mastery experiences	Have person successfully perform the behavior.	■ Set realistic goals that can be achieved. ■ Progress gradually over time. ■ Provide proper instruction and demonstration. ■ Use physical activity logs to track progress.
Vicarious experiences	Have person watch others with similar background perform tasks.	■ Have appropriate group exercise leaders that the individual can identify with. ■ Use videos to model behavior. ■ Identify "success" stories of individuals with similar backgrounds and characteristics.
Verbal persuasion	Have others tell the person that he or she can be successful.	■ Give frequent feedback (*e.g.*, encouragement, compliments) and express confidence in the individual's abilities. ■ Prompt discussion of previous successful attempts at behavior change. ■ Discuss existing skills and knowledge which can help with behavior change.
Physiological feedback	Communicate the meaning of symptoms associated with the behavior change.	■ Provide appropriate instruction and reassurance. ■ Discuss how physical activity makes the individual feel. ■ Provide education about the possible discomfort associated with physical activity. ■ Encourage using music, scenery, etc., to make physical activity pleasurable.

From American College of Sports Medicine. *ACSM's Guidelines for Exercise Testing and Prescription.* 11th ed. Philadelphia (PA): Wolters Kluwer; 2022. 548 p. Table 12.2.

bouts of physical activity (5–10 min) into their daily routine. The program is designed to attract diverse populations in nontraditional settings by "reengineering" the way physical activity is incorporated into individuals' daily schedules. *Instant Recess* provides vicarious learning opportunities to participants by recruiting program peer leaders and creating teams. The peer leaders and team members serve as mentors and sources of support for participants. This program structure also encourages opportunities for participants to observe team members' and peers' successes (42).

Third, verbal persuasion occurs when others express faith in the individual's capabilities. For example, the exercise physiologist can provide frequent encouragement and emphasize existing skills and knowledge that assist in behavior change. For example, clients may demonstrate skills in time management or organization. The exercise physiologist can then provide verbal feedback on how these skills translate to maintaining physical activity.

Finally, how the client feels about the physiological sensations while engaging in physical activity may influence self-efficacy. Providing appropriate instruction (*e.g.*, safety cues) and using music are tools an exercise physiologist can use to create the presence of an optimal emotional and affective state. See Table 11.2 for additional ideas on how the exercise physiologist can create an environment that promotes and enhances the development of a client's self-efficacy as it relates to physical activity behavior.

Substantial evidence supports SCT as an effective means of influencing human behavior and, consequently, a viable resource for intervention design for behavior change, including physical activity (32,43). Results compiled from multiple studies indicate that the most successful behavioral interventions for enhancing self-efficacy were found when vicarious experiences and feedback techniques (*e.g.*, providing feedback by comparing participants' performance with the performance of others, providing feedback on the participants' past performances) were used in an intervention (44). Some researchers have found that mastery experience, verbal self-persuasion, and reduction in negative affective states as the most important predictors of high self-efficacy for physical activity among older adults (45).

In addition, monitoring an individual's behavior and performance based on task mastery and skill development may also have a positive influence on self-efficacy. Setting a specific detailed plan and encouraging individuals to set a specific intention of how to adopt physical activity are common among successful intervention programs (46). See Chapter 12 for additional techniques on increasing self-efficacy for physical activity.

Relapse Prevention

Emerging literature also supports a focus on relapse prevention to increase self-efficacy for physical activity. Relapse prevention is an ongoing process in which efforts are made to prevent reverting to previous maladaptive behaviors and habits that contradict desired change (47). Relapse prevention has been found to be to be one of the most effective means of improving self-efficacy toward physical activity (44,46,48) and is most effective once the client has established a regular exercise routine. When counseling a client in relapse prevention training, the exercise physiologist should focus on what the individual can do to achieve and sustain the desired behavior change rather than emphasizing what he or she is not able to do. For example, the exercise physiologist can assist the client in creating a relapse prevention plan that includes information about high-risk situations (*e.g.*, inclement weather that interferes with exercise plan), situations associated with relapses in the past (*e.g.*, holidays that interfere with exercise schedule), early signs of a relapse (*e.g.*, progressively cutting exercise time short), and a specific plan for responding to these warning signals. The specific plan can include rehearsal of coping skills (*e.g.*, exercising indoors), relapse-crisis debriefing (*e.g.*, reevaluating effectiveness of techniques), education (*e.g.*, normalizing fitness plateau), and lifestyle modification. Chapter 12 offers additional suggestions on how exercise physiologists can successfully engage clients in relapse prevention training.

Although there are numerous correlates of physical activity, such as attitudes, perceived barriers, enjoyment, and expected benefits, the prevailing evidence supports self-efficacy as an important component of physical activity behavior change (32). In general, there are consistent increases in physical activity (46) even when the improvements in self-efficacy are less significant (49,50). Some techniques that could be used in building physical activity self-efficacy include the following:

- Use verbal persuasion to reinforce task mastery.
- Provide exposure to positive vicarious experiences.
- Explain and reinforce the positive physiological and affective states achieved from exercise.
- Encourage various forms of physical activity, noting what is most enjoyed.
- Encourage client recall of previous successful behavior change.
- Maintain a physical activity log to help track success and progress.
- Encourage reasonable, specific physical activity goals that can be achieved in a short time.
- Encourage perseverance and praise efforts toward goals, not just the attainment of goals.
- Prepare for high-risk situations that interfere with physical activity and plan specific ways to prevent relapse.

EXERCISE IS MEDICINE CONNECTION

Exe℞cise is Medicine®

Putting Theory to Practice
Wilcox S, Dowda M, Leviton LC, et al. Active for life: final results from the translation of two physical activity programs. *Am J Prev Med.* 2008;35:340–51.

Theory-based physical activity interventions have been demonstrated to be effective when translated into real-world settings. Active Choices and Active Living Everyday are two examples. Active Choices is a 6-months, telephone-based physical activity program targeted to adults older than 50 years of age. Active Choices includes a face-to-face intervention and up to eight telephone contacts. Participants are given a physical activity log, a pedometer, and a resource guide at the initial face-to-face visit. Participants set physical activity goals and are provided SCT and TTM-based strategies (*e.g.*, overcoming barriers and self-monitoring) to promote physical activity behavior change. The efficacy of the Active Choices program in increasing physical activity has been tested in a series of well-designed clinical research trials, showing Active Choices as successful method in assisting sedentary older adults in the adoption and maintenance of regular physical activity.

Similarly, Active Living Every Day is a 12-week physical activity program delivered in small groups. Based on a multisite clinical trial, the weekly facilitator-led intervention focuses on behavioral skill building. In addition, the curriculum is available as a publicly available self-directed workbook. Results of a dissemination study involving multiple community organizations indicated that the number of individuals meeting or exceeding the American College of Sports Medicine (ACSM)/Centers for Disease Control and Prevention (CDC) physical activity guidelines increased from pre- to posttest. The researchers reported that the interventions were adapted to meet the needs of the organization while maintaining high treatment fidelity. This study indicated that theory-based efficacious physical activity interventions can be successfully disseminated into real-world settings. Although these protocols do work for the period of time enlisted, there are still questions regarding how to best ensure maintenance of physical activity when the program ends.

For more information on Active Choices and Active Living Every Day visit:
https://www.ncoa.org/resources/program-summary-active-choices/
http://med.stanford.edu/healthyaging/active-choices-program.html
https://www.cdc.gov/arthritis/interventions/programs/aled.htm
https://us.humankinetics.com/blogs/active-living

Social Ecological Model

The social ecological model is a comprehensive approach integrating multiple variables and layers that influence behavior. These layers include intrapersonal and interpersonal factors, community and organizational factors, institutional factors, environmental factors, and public policies (Fig. 11.2). Within this model, each layer has a resulting impact on the next layer. For example, an individual's social environment of family, friends, and workplace is embedded within the physical environment of geography and community facilities. This is then embedded within and influenced

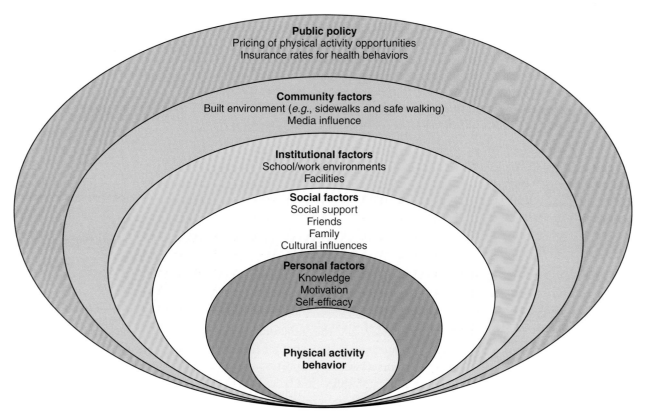

FIGURE 11.2. Social ecological model of physical activity behavior: based on Bronfenbrenner's social ecological model. (Reproduced with permission from Bronfenbrenner U. *The Ecology of Human Development: Experiments by Nature and Design.* Cambridge [MA]: Harvard University Press; 1979. 352 p.)

by the policy environment of government or other official bodies. All levels of the social ecological model influence the behavior of the individual (51,52).

There are many versions of the social ecological model for physical activity, including systems theory, ecological model of health behavior, and social ecology model for health promotion. Each of these applications uses slightly different classifications of environmental influences. For example, systems theory uses the "microsystem" (*e.g.,* personal interactions between family members, work groups), "mesosystem" (physical settings for family, school, and work), and "exosystem" (the larger social influences including economics, policies, culture, and politics) (51). The social ecological model is specific to an individual's health behaviors and includes factors such as intrapersonal, interpersonal processes, institutional influences, community factors, and public policies (53). The social ecology model focuses on the promotion of health behaviors using assumptions related to influencing the physical and social environments; multidimensional environments; interactions between individuals, families, communities; and how individuals influence their surroundings (Box 11.2) (55,56). A number of multidimensional models specific to the physical activity domain have been proposed and empirically supported (57,58).

Uncovering the motivational factors that underlie the successful adoption and maintenance of physical activity programs requires a multidimensional approach that considers not only behavioral change and intrapersonal factors but also social and environmental factors. Many of the traditional ecological models were meant to apply broadly across a variety of behaviors; yet, more recent models have been developed to apply specifically to health behaviors (53,55,56). Many health behaviors, including physical activity, are too complex to be adequately evaluated

Box 11.2	Social Ecological Practical Application Research Example — Trial of Activity for Adolescent Girls

Research specific to adolescent girls described a framework created to promote physical activity behavior (24). This framework guided the intervention known as Trial of Activity for Adolescent Girls (TAAG) and adopted principles from behavioral modification, social cognitive, and organizational change theories to influence physical activity behavior in adolescent girls' intrapersonal, school, and community environments. The TAAG approach has been used to promote positive physical activity behaviors in middle school girls, and when incorporated in a school and community-based environment, girls in the intervention schools demonstrated a trend of increased physical activity in comparison with those in the schools that did not receive the program (24,54).

For more information on TAAG, visit https://www.sc.edu/study/colleges_schools/public_health/research/research _centers/usc_cparg/research_studies/taag/index.php.

and understood by simply addressing the individual. Research suggests that coordinating and planning efforts among the agencies responsible for transportation, urban planning, school zoning, and facilities and programs as well as supporting social environments that encourage activity (*e.g.*, walking and biking trails, sidewalks, and reduction of crime) may help to optimize physical activity behavior (59–64). Strategies the exercise physiologist can use to create an environment that promotes physical activity include the following:

■ Assist clients in identifying the wide variety of physical activity options that exist within proximity to their home. This may include opportunities such as parks, gyms, community centers, clubs, and hiking trails.
■ Discuss with the client the existing potential environmental barriers that deter regular physical activity. See Chapter 12 for additional techniques on addressing environmental barriers.
■ Encourage the client to join a walking, jogging, or training group in the local community.

For the exercise physiologist, the social ecological model provides a useful framework for better understanding the multiple factors and barriers that influence physical activity behavior. Behavior can be difficult to change, especially in an environment that does not support change. To increase physical activity, the exercise physiologist may need to focus efforts on facilitating change for both the behavior choices of the client as well as factors that influence those choices. The social ecological model helps the exercise physiologist identify opportunities to promote participation in physical activity and recognize barriers that may make physical activity difficult.

As advocates of regular physical activity, exercise physiologists may find that they are more successful at influencing an individual's physical activity when multiple levels of influence are addressed at the same time. According to this model, in order for physical activity interventions to be effective, the exercise physiologist must go beyond simple exercise prescriptions. Other factors that influence physical activity behavior choices must also be addressed. For example, the exercise physiologist may help the client choose new exercise equipment for the home, recruit family members to join in physical activity, find ways to decrease sedentary behavior in the home, and assist in identifying and problem solving possible environmental barriers to exercise. This holistic approach may help the exercise physiologist develop more appropriate, sensitive, and effective motivational and intervention strategies.

EXERCISE IS MEDICINE CONNECTION

Physical Activity as a Vital Sign

Recent efforts of ACSM's Exercise is Medicine® (EIM®) have focused on strengthening the connection between evidence-based physical activity resources and health care. Specifically, this global health initiative works to make physical activity assessment and promotion a standard in clinical care and views physical activity as a vital sign assessed like any other vital sign (*e.g.*, pulse rate, temperature, respiration rate, blood pressure) at a health care provider visit to gather information on an individual's general physical condition. EIM encourages the medical community to promote physical activity for disease prevention and management and urges health care providers to assess physical activity during patient visits, prescribe exercise in treatment plans, and refer patients to certified fitness professionals. Considering physical activity as a vital sign can alert the health care provider of inadequate physical activity behavior and prompt exercise counseling and referral to the exercise physiologist. For this reason, it is important for the exercise physiologist to have adequate credentials, education, and familiarity with exercise prescription for populations with medical needs. EIM stresses the importance of exercise physiologists staying current on the science of exercise and its role in the prevention and treatment of disease. Many clients are likely motivated to seek out fitness professionals based on physician referral or a perceived change in health status. Therefore, exercise physiologists must know how to behaviorally and practically support their clients through tailored physical activity programs that consider unique medical needs and motivational factors.

For more information on Exercise is Medicine, visit http://www.exerciseismedicine.org.

Theory of Planned Behavior

The TPB is an intention-based model used to explain physical activity behavior (7,65) and is an extension of the theory of reasoned action which proposes (66) and identifies intention as the primary influence in determining behavior (Fig. 11.3). Intention directly reflects an individual's level of motivation (*i.e.*, willingness and amount of effort exerted) to perform the desired behavior. According to the TPB, one's attitude, subjective norms, and perceived behavioral control influence intention, which then influences actual behavior. Specifically related to physical activity, attitude is defined as a positive or negative evaluation of physical activity. Subjective norm is the individual's perception of social pressure to participate, or not, in physical activity. Perceived behavioral control is the individual's perception of the ease or difficulty for engaging in physical activity. This can be perceived as similar to self-efficacy because it involves an individual's perception that he or she has the ability to execute the desired behavior.

The research literature is mixed in terms of support for intention predicting physical activity behavior (67–69). Although intention appears to be the most influential factor in predicting behavior, perceived behavioral control significantly adds to the prediction of actual behavior (33,70,71). Importantly, TPB predicts that perceived behavioral control may also directly impact behavior itself (68,71). Therefore, each can stand on its own to predict behavior; however, combined, they have a much stronger effect.

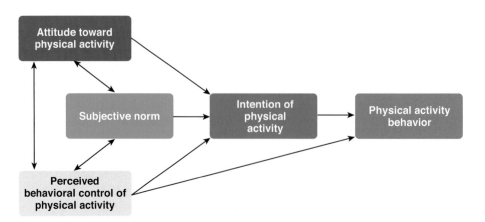

FIGURE 11.3. Theory of planned behavior: based on Ajzen's TPB. (Adapted from Ajzen I. The theory of planned behavior. *Organ Behav Hum Decis Process.* 1991;50[2]: 179–211, and Marcus BH, Forsyth LH. *Motivating People to Be Physically Active.* 2nd ed. Champaign [IL]: Human Kinetics; 2009. 216 p.)

In using the TPB in practice, the exercise physiologist may assist clients in identifying and developing their intentions. These intentions will then be influenced by the individual's attitude, perceived level of behavioral control, and subjective norm. Exercise physiologists can encourage physical activity behavior by assisting in the development of self-efficacy; helping the client create an environment of social support by recruiting coworkers, friends, and family to provide encouragement and reminders for physical activity (subjective norm); and making physical activity easily accessible (perceived behavioral control). With these changes, the client's intention for physical activity behavior will increase, facilitating physical activity behavior change. Although intention is crucial for increasing physical activity behavior, changes in intention alone are often insufficient in successfully changing behavior. Currently, research is being conducted in order to determine how to bridge the "intention-behavior gap" (72).

Self-Determination Theory

SDT is built around the premise that individuals have three basic psychological needs that must be met in order to engage in a behavior: (a) competence, (b) relatedness, and (c) autonomy (66). Competence is the sense of being capable of completing an activity or mastering a task and the perception of being effective in that task. Relatedness is the need to be connected and involved with the social world. Autonomy is characterized by maintaining a perceived internal locus of control and a sense that behaviors are freely chosen. When a behavior is self-determined, an individual perceives that the locus of control is internal to self. However, when an individual feels that a behavior is not under direct personal control, then the locus of control is perceived to be external to self. A perceived internal locus of control increases the likelihood that the individual will continue the desired self-directed behavior long-term. According to SDT, individuals who have greater choice in physical activity (perceived internal locus of control) versus being told specifically which physical activity to engage in (perceived external locus of control) are more likely to adhere to the desired physical activity behavior.

SDT proposes that the extent to which the needs (*i.e.*, competence, relatedness, and autonomy) are met describes how motivated an individual is to complete a task. In other words, when individuals feel competent, related, and autonomous, they will be motivated to participate in physical activity, and the motivation will be based on self-determination rather than external factors.

Motivation is described as a continuum and ranges from amotivation (complete lack of motivation), to extrinsic motivation (motives based on external factors), to intrinsic motivation (motivation based on enjoyment and excitement). According to SDT, motivations more proximal to intrinsic motivation are more likely to promote the desired behavior. An individual who is intrinsically motivated to participate in physical activity would be motivated by a genuine affinity or appreciation of physical activity. An extrinsically motivated individual would engage in physical activity for reasons such as weight control and stress reduction. An amotivated person would not engage in physical activity because he or she has no motivation at all. Motivational interviewing (MI) is a person-centered, autonomy-supportive communication approach that can be used to increase intrinsic motivation and inspire self-directed behavior change (73).

It is important to note that truly intrinsic motivation toward physical activity, or many other health behaviors, may be somewhat rare and should not be considered necessary for successful change and continuation of exercise behavior. Within the motivation continuum exists a threshold of autonomy. Not all extrinsic motives are the same, and there may be a nonlinear prediction along the continuum. For example, a person can exercise to avoid disease or exercise because being healthy is important. These motives may seem similar on the surface, but they are very different from a theoretical perspective. That is, exercising to avoid disease presumes some amount of pressure and coercion, whereas exercising to be healthy presumes free choice and autonomy.

SDT is an approach that can help gain a stronger understanding of exercise behavior and a better understanding of the intrapersonal (*e.g.*, psychological needs) and interpersonal (*e.g.*, influence of exercise environment) factors that influence physical activity. This theory considers the social context in which the individual operates. According to SDT, individuals who are in an autonomy-supportive climate (a climate in which the client plays an active role in choosing behavior) are more likely to feel like their needs of autonomy, relatedness, and competence are being met (74), which promotes greater intrinsic motivation. In addition, events that are interpreted by the individual to be informational, rather than controlling, will result in the endorsement of intrinsic motivating behaviors. According to this theory, sociocontextual variables can be manipulated to create an environment conducive to exercise. Therefore, this theory can provide insight into why individuals intend to adopt and maintain physical activity, as preliminary research supports SDT as a predictor of individual motivation to engage in physical activity (75–79).

Using the foundational principles of SDT, the exercise physiologist may see improved levels of motivation for physical activity if the psychological needs of autonomy, competence, and relatedness are met. Autonomy can be encouraged by allowing the client to have input on the physical activity plan, including choice of activity mode and intensity. Competence can be encouraged by making sure the client is entering a physical activity environment in which he or she will feel challenged but can be successful. Tailoring goals and appropriate progression will help the client feel more capable and confident in behavior change. Finally, the exercise physiologist should encourage clients to find others who have similar health goals or exercise with others to meet the relatedness need component of SDT. For example, a client who is new to running, might find encouragement and support from joining a beginner running group. See Chapter 12 for strategies on how the exercise physiologist can use self-monitoring, self-regulation, goal-setting, and social support to increase clients' competence, relatedness, and autonomy.

Hedonic Theory

Hedonic theory is an evolution of learning theory (80) and refers to individuals becoming accustomed to a positive or negative stimulus (81). This theory is based on the concept of "hedonic psychology," which states that the perceived utility of a behavior or experience is defined by an individual's affective response to the behavior (82). Within the context of physical activity, this means that feeling good in response to physical activity is more likely to lead to adherence. Individuals seeking to enhance or prolong pleasure and avoid or minimize pain are engaging in what is known as "the hedonic principle." Therefore, an individual's decision to engage in physical activity is due to the affective consequences or affective anticipation (*i.e.*, expectations) of the physical activity experience (83). Although it has received somewhat less attention with respect to physical activity than other theories (82,84), it is important for exercise physiologists to consider.

Research suggests that feelings can play an important role in accounting for exercise behavior (85). For example, researchers have found that sedentary participants who reported positive affective responses to a single session of moderate-intensity exercise at baseline reported more minutes of physical activity 6 months and a full year later (86). Additionally, research demonstrates that exercising at or just below the ventilatory threshold produces positive affect and pleasure, whereas intensities above the ventilatory threshold produces less pleasure (54). Other research demonstrates that allowing exercisers to self-select and maintain that intensity report more stable and positive affect in comparison to exercise imposed at a slightly higher intensity. However, participants who were told what intensity to use reported a decrease in positive affect (87). Additionally, research has noted that increases in positive affect during treadmill exercise predicted exercise behavior 3 months later (84). Taken together, these studies suggest that individuals may be more likely to adhere to self-paced exercise than higher intensity prescription-based exercise, especially sedentary adults (88,89).

Affective expectations have also been found to be predictive of physical activity behavior (90). For example, research indicates that participants exposed to a positive affective expectation manipulation prior to 10 minutes of exercise had a better postexercise mood and higher exercise intentions compared to a no-expectation condition (91). This study suggests that postexercise feelings, intentions, and, consequently, physical activity behaviors can be altered by exposure to an affective expectation manipulation. These results support previous research indicating that expecting exercise to improve affect predicts higher levels of exercise (92,93).

In summary, research suggests that exercise may be reinforcing for individuals who experience or expect to feel good as a result of exercise. Consequently, individuals who experience positive affect after exercise may be more likely to adhere to exercise programs. Although some individuals experience improvements in affect during exercise, others may experience no change or even an increase in negative affect (88,94). This may depend on contextual factors (*e.g.*, the setting in which the exercise takes place), stimulus factors (*e.g.*, exercise intensity), and individual differences (*e.g.*, the individual's current exercise level; 95). Exercise physiologist should consider affect while working with clients which may mean allowing the client to self-select intensity or staying below ventilatory threshold. Additional research is needed that examines the application of hedonic theory to exercise behavior, but existing research provides encouragement that this concept can be used by exercise physiologists to improve the efficacy of physical activity interventions.

HOW TO Apply the Hedonic Theory to Physical Activity

The exercise physiologist can use the following strategies based on hedonic theory to help his or her clients adopt and maintain physical activity.

- Work with clients to determine their personal preferences regarding intensity level.
- Brainstorm with the client to create a list of new types of exercise and encourage the client to try these new exercises.
- Discuss ways to make exercise more enjoyable such as listening to music, exercising with a friend, or wearing more comfortable workout clothing.
- Determine the time of day for exercise that elicits the most positive affect for the client.
- Prior to an exercise session, work with the client to generate a list of positive associations with exercise and actively reframe negative associations with exercise.
- Help clients identify positive outcomes that occur immediately after exercise and throughout the day (*e.g.*, more energy, better sleep).

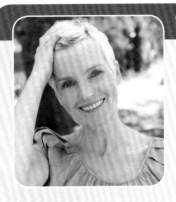

The Case of Anna

Submitted by **Steve McClaran, PhD Associate Professor, Colorado State University-Pueblo, Pueblo, CO**

Anna was an almost 60-year-old woman who could barely walk four blocks before she began a supervised exercise program. Anna had a history of attempting an exercise program in the past but had low adherence to these programs.

Narrative

When I first met Anna, we decided to go for a walk — she barely made it four blocks. Five years later after exercising regularly, she had lost more than 150 lb and walked a half marathon in 4 hours! She was almost 60 years old when we started our project, and we concentrated on the process of behavior change. What were the best practices to stay motivated for exercise? We started with three questions:

1. Where are you now? To help with this question, we did a fitness assessment. As a note, we redid the fitness assessment after the first 3 months, again after 6 months, after a year, and then yearly for the next 5 years.
2. Where do you want to go? To help with this, we felt that first, we wanted to personalize the goal. Anna had tried many times to be successful and had failed a lot. We started off slowly and used short-term goals every month. Of course, we had long-term goals, but we concentrated on the short-term goals to keep building her confidence in the long-term success. We continuously asked what the potential positive outcome was and then molded the goal to optimize the long-term outcome. Lastly, and maybe most importantly, we concentrated on focusing goals on specific and measurable behaviors rather than specific fitness outcomes. There was a strong sense that in Anna's past attempts, she concentrated on the outcomes as opposed to the behaviors that would lead to these positive outcomes. It is the behavior goals that are the important and sustainable pieces of long-term behavior change.
3. How are you going to get there? As someone new to exercise who had been unsuccessful in the past, it was important to help Anna develop strategies that could help her meet her short-term goals as well as continue to be active in the long term. We found that attention to behavior change skills was extremely helpful.

We concentrated on benefits of physical activity, barriers or obstacles to long-term success, goal setting, social support, and monitoring her activities. It started with a commitment: Together, we devised a behavior change contract, and our responsibilities to the cause were delineated and signed. As far as benefits, not only is it the knowledge of what the benefits are, but there was also a discussion of what Anna was feeling toward our original list of benefits during each of our weekly exercise walks. We felt that realizing the benefits during the behavior change process was critical for continued motivation. Social support strategies include practical support (we focused a lot on finding realistic solutions to barriers), technical support (I found a lot of shared experiences on the Internet and would find something each month to discuss during our weekly walks), group support (she joined a gym and did aerobics classes at the senior center), and emotional motivational support (she shared the experience with her sister, daughter, son, and her colleagues at work).

Barriers or obstacles were our next order of business to solve. We started with a list of five obstacles and then came up with creative and workable solutions to each of the issues. We looked on each of the obstacles as a challenge, and we revisited them every 3 months to determine our progress. As obvious and simple as logistics and practical solutions are, any failure to pay attention to logistical details is often a cause of relapse. If plan A didn't work for some reason, having plans B and C ready helped our chances of success. Planning for weather changes was essential for exercise; walking in cold weather means you need either different gear or an inside track. We found that scheduling exercise before work was logistically more effective than planning to do it later, when complications may interfere. Logistical problems were never completely solved, so it was also important for Anna to adopt the mindset of finding a solution to any problem that arises.

We felt that environment control was an important consideration for Anna. First, we discussed removing temptations for physical inactivity and unhealthy eating. Anna owned her own business with four other women. Prior to her starting her journey toward the half-marathon, there was always some form of pastries at the office, so she asked her partners if it was all right to bring in fruit and vegetable platters to replace the pastries, and they all agreed. Maybe more importantly was making the desired behavior easier and more supportive: She joined a gym and signed up for aerobics classes at the senior center. Concentrating on emotional control reduced both the risk of returning to the old behavior and increased the opportunity to engage in the new behavior. Anna also sets up a stationary bike and a Bowflex in the basement, which helped with those times that weather was an issue. As a further note, Anna found music when exercising in her basement. She would often share with me those songs that were the most inspirational. By the end of the third year, she had a library of more than 500 songs she could use and rock out to in her basement.

Reward systems also worked for us. Most of us need a system of reward that includes external incentives followed by internal ones. Anna liked to put stickers on her calendar when she completed a desired behavior, and then she gave herself a reward when she earned a certain number of stickers. Eventually, her continued success brought its own reward, and external rewards became less important. Another idea she came up with was to give her clothes away to charity as she lost weight and waist size. Anna felt that giving the clothes away would close that part of her life and make it more difficult to go back to her old clothes.

Maybe one of the biggest reasons for Anna's success was her continued self-monitoring and reporting. Once she had completed her exercise for the week, she e-mailed me every Sunday evening. She is a pretty competitive person; in the first year and a half, she would sometimes exercise later in the week just so she wouldn't have to send in a low-volume exercise report. This helped the new behavior become a habit and offered accountability and the opportunity for feedback. One interesting part about our monitoring and reporting plan was the first and second yearly summaries. After the first year, I used a computer graphing package to make a picture of how much she exercised every week — I made an average weekly amount of exercise line that went through each of the 52 bars that represented the amount of exercise for that week. Both of us could see her activity ups and downs. We then made some goals and developed strategies that would help in planning ahead and preventing relapse. This helped a lot with motivation. Eventually, we went with pedometers, which helped by reminding and challenging her to achieve success. I crossed that finish line at the end of the half-marathon with Anna and her daughter.

It is difficult to describe how great it was to see how happy Anna was at accomplishing those many goals along her journey. Her daughter took pictures and videos, and many family members were there to help her celebrate her half-marathon. I have since moved halfway across the country, but we still keep in touch. She sends me postcards from Africa, South America, and Europe as she and her sister do many hiking adventures that were essentially unavailable to her before she went on her successful exercise journey. Anna now enjoys being active and incorporates physical activity into other aspects of her life.

QUESTIONS

- What elements of behavior change theory can you identify in the case study?
- How did the application of behavior change theories change as Anna progressed in her health journey?
- How could the behavior change theories be applied to other health behaviors?

SUMMARY

In recent years, an expansion has occurred in the number and type of factors examined as theoretically based correlates and determinates of physical activity behaviors. The TTM, SCT, social ecological model, TPB, and SDT have been used to better understand physical activity behavior. The TTM has been researched most frequently followed by SCT and the TPB (96,97). Self-determination and hedonic theories are newer but have received greater interest recently (97). Exercise physiologists can use strategies and tools from these models to motivate individuals to adopt physical activity and other health behaviors. Understanding theories can help exercise physiologists understand specific client needs, motivations, and behaviors and give an evidence-based framework for tailoring physical activity recommendations. Otherwise, simply providing an exercise prescription without considering the behavioral aspects of why someone may or may not fully engage in physical activity will likely lead to poor adherence and low retention rates.

The purpose of this chapter is to outline the basic tenets of various theories and models that have been applied to physical activity behavior. Chapter 12 explores in more detail how these theories have been specifically applied to exercise interventions and how exercise physiologists can use these theory-based interventions to facilitate physical activity behavior change among their clients.

STUDY QUESTIONS

1. How can knowledge of theories/models in the context of physical activity behavior aid the exercise physiologist in designing physical activity interventions?
2. What are the five stages of change, as identified by the TTM? How would the exercise physiologist use the five stages of change to assess his or her client's readiness to participate in physical activity?
3. What are the four sources of self-efficacy? What techniques would the exercise physiologist use to improve self-efficacy?
4. Briefly describe other models of change and how the exercise physiologist could use them to increase physical activity participation.
5. How does the hedonic theory explain promotion and adherence to physical activity?

REFERENCES

1. Glanz K, Rimer BK, Viswanath K. Theory, research, and practice in health behavior. In: Glanz K, Rimer BK, Viswanath K, editors. *Health Behavior: Theory, Research, and Practice.* 5th ed. San Francisco (CA): Jossey-Bass; 2015. p. 23–42.
2. de Menezes MC, Mingoti SA, Cardoso CS, de Deus Mendonça R, Lopes ACS. Intervention based on transtheoretical model promotes anthropometric and nutritional improvements — a randomized controlled trial. *Eat Behav.* 2015;17:37–44.
3. Prochaska JO, DiClemente CC, Norcross JC. In search of how people change: applications to addictive behaviors. *Am Psychol.* 1992;47(9):1102–14.
4. Yusufov M, Rossi JS, Redding CA, et al. Transtheoretical model constructs' longitudinal prediction of sun protection over 24 months. *Int J Behav Med.* 2016;23(1):71–3.
5. Kim H, Kohl III HW, Pettee Gabriel KK, Han H. Differential use of strategic constructs of the transtheoretical model across accelerometer-determined sedentary time. *Am J Health Behav.* 2020;44(1):18–25.
6. Gourlan M, Bernard P, Bortolon C, et al. Efficacy of theory-based interventions to promote physical activity. A meta-analysis of randomised controlled trials. *Health Psychol Rev.* 2016;10(1):50–66.
7. Ajzen I. The theory of planned behavior. *Organ Behav Hum Decis Process.* 1991;50(2):179–211.
8. Bandura A. Self-efficacy mechanism in psychobiologic functioning. In: Schwarzer R, editor. *Self-efficacy: Thought Control of Action.* Washington (DC): Hemisphere Publishing; 1992. p. 355–94.
9. Romain AJ, Bortolon C, Gourlan M, et al. Matched or nonmatched interventions based on the transtheoretical

model to promote physical activity. A meta-analysis of randomized controlled trials. *J Sport Health Sci.* 2018;7(1): 50–57.

10. DiClemente CC, Prochaska JO, Fairhurst SK, Velicer WF, Velasquez MM, Rossi JS. The process of smoking cessation: an analysis of precontemplation, contemplation, and preparation stages of change. *J Consult Clin Psychol.* 1991;59(2):295–304.

11. Prochaska JO, DiClemente CC. Stages and processes of self-change of smoking: toward an integrative model of change. *J Consult Clin Psychol.* 1983;51(3):390–5.

12. Marcus BH, Forsyth LH. *Motivating People to Be Physically Active.* 2nd ed. Champaign (IL): Human Kinetics; 2009. 216 p.

13. DiClemente CC, Prochaska JO. Self-change and therapy change of smoking behavior: a comparison of processes of change in cessation and maintenance. *Addict Behav.* 1982;7(2):133–42.

14. Prochaska JO, Velicer WF, DiClemente CC, Fava J. Measuring processes of change: applications to the cessation of smoking. *J Consult Clin Psychol.* 1988;56(4):520–8.

15. Romain AJ, Chevance G, Caudroit J, Bernard P. The transtheoretical model: description, interests and application in the motivation to physical activity among population with overweight and obesity. *Obesity.* 2016;11(1):47–55.

16. Nigg CR, Harmon B, Jiang Y, Ginis KAM, Motl RW, Dishman RK. Temporal sequencing of physical activity change constructs within the transtheoretical model. *Psychol Sport Exerc.* 2019;45:101557.

17. Romain AJ, Horwath C, Bernard P. Prediction of physical activity level using processes of change from the transtheoretical model: experiential, behavioral, or an interaction effect? *Am J Health Promot.* 2018;32(1):16–23.

18. Marcus BH, Rossi JS, Selby VC, Niaura RS, Abrams DB. The stages and processes of exercise adoption and maintenance in a worksite sample. *Health Psychol.* 1992;11(6): 386–95.

19. Marshall S, Biddle S. The transtheoretical model of behavior change: a meta-analysis of applications to physical activity and exercise. *Ann Behav Med.* 2001;23(4): 229–46.

20. Nigg CR, Courneya KS. Transtheoretical model: examining adolescent exercise behavior. *J Adolesc Health.* 1998;22(3):214–24.

21. Prochaska JO, Velicer WF, Rossi JS, et al. Stages of change and decisional balance for 12 problem behaviors. *Health Psychol.* 1994;13(1):39–46.

22. Bassilios B, Judd F, Pattison P, Nicholas A, Moeller-Saxone K. Predictors of exercise in individuals with schizophrenia: a test of the transtheoretical model of behavior change. *Clin Schizophr Relat Psychoses.* 2015;8(4):173–82.

23. Carlson J, Sallis J, Ernesto R, Ramirez K, Norman GJ. Physical activity and dietary behavior change in Internet-based weight loss interventions: comparing two multiple-behavior change indices. *Prev Med.* 2012;54(1):50–4.

24. Lewis BA, Gjerdingen DK, Avery MD, et al. A randomized trail examining a physical activity intervention for the prevention of postpartum depression: the healthy mom trial. *Ment Health Phys Act.* 2014;7(1):42–9.

25. Yang HJ, Chen KM, Chen MD, et al. Applying the transtheoretical model to promote functional fitness of community older adults participating in elastic band exercises. *J Adv Nurs.* 2015;71(10):2338–49.

26. Shaver ER, McGlumphy KC, Gill AK, Hasson RE. Application of the transtheoretical model to physical activity and exercise behaviors in African-American adolescents. *Am J Health Behav.* 2019;43(1):119–32.

27. Romain AJ, Bernard P, Galvez M, Caudroit J. Response to an exercise intervention for patients with Type 2 diabetes: a preliminary study of processes of change. *J Appl Biobehav Res.* 2015;20(3):130–6.

28. Bandura A. *Self-Efficacy: The Exercise of Control.* New York (NY): W.H. Freeman; 1997. 604 p.

29. Bandura A. Self-efficacy: toward a unifying theory of behavioral change. *Psychol Rev.* 1977;84(2):191–215.

30. Bandura A. *Social Foundations of Thought and Action: A Social Cognitive Theory.* Englewood Cliffs (NJ): Prentice-Hall; 1986. 544 p.

31. McAuley E, Blissmer B. Self-efficacy determinants and consequences of physical activity. *Exerc Sport Sci Rev.* 2000;28(2):85–8.

32. Beauchamp MR, Crawford KL, Jackson B. Social cognitive theory and physical activity: mechanisms of behavior change, critique, and legacy. *Psychol Sport Exerc.* 2019;42:110–7.

33. Jekauc D, Völkle M, Wagner MO, Mess F, Reiner M, Renner B. Prediction of attendance at fitness center: a comparison between the theory of planned behavior, the social cognitive theory, and the physical activity maintenance theory. *Front Psychol.* 2015;6:121.

34. Dishman RK, Motl RW, Saunders R, et al. Self-efficacy partially mediates the effect of a school-based physical-activity intervention among adolescent girls. *Prev Med.* 2004;38:628–36.

35. Manley D, Cowan P, Graff C, et al. Self-efficacy, physical activity, and aerobic fitness in middle school children: examination of a pedometer intervention program. *J Pediatr Nurs.* 2014;29(3):228–37.

36. White SM, Wójcicki TR, McAuley E. Social cognitive influences on physical activity behavior in middle-aged and older adults. *J Gerontol B Psychol Sci Soc Sci.* 2011;67(1):18–26.

37. Schroeder K, Kubik MY, Lee J, Sirard JR, Fulkerson JA. Self-efficacy, not peer or parent support, is associated with more physical activity and less sedentary time among 8- to 12-year-old youth with elevated body mass index. *J Phys Act Health.* 2020;17(1):74–9.

38. Ginis KA, Latimer AE, Arbour-Nicitopoulos KP, Bassett RL, Wolfe DL, Hanna SE. Determinants of physical activity among people with spinal cord injury: a test of social cognitive theory. *Ann Behav Med.* 2011;42(1):127–33.

39. Haas BK. Fatigue, self-efficacy, physical activity, and quality of life in women with breast cancer. *Cancer Nurs.* 2011;34(4):322–34.

40. McAuley E, White SM, Rogers LQ, Motl RW, Courneya KS. Physical activity and fatigue in breast cancer and multiple sclerosis: psychosocial mechanisms. *Psychosom Med.* 2010;72(1):88–96.

41. Snook EM, Motl RW. Physical activity behaviors in individuals with multiple sclerosis: roles of overall and specific symptoms, and self-efficacy. *J Pain Symptom Manage.* 2008;36(1):46–53.

42. Yancey AK, Yancey T. *Instant Recess: Building a Fit Nation 10 Minutes at a Time.* Oakland (CA): University of California Press; 2010. 280 p.

43. Tougas ME, Hayden JA, McGrath PJ, Huguet A, Rozario S. A systematic review exploring the social cognitive theory of self-regulation as a framework for chronic health condition interventions. *PLoS One.* 2015;10(8): e0134977.

44. Ashford S, Edmunds J, French DP. What is the best way to change self-efficacy to promote lifestyle and recreational physical activity? A systematic review with meta-analysis. *Br J Health Psychol.* 2010;15(2):265–88.

45. Warner LM, Schüz B, Wolff JK, Parschau L, Wurm S, Schwarzer R. Sources of self-efficacy for physical activity. *Health Psych.* 2014;33(11):1298–308.

46. Williams SL, French DP. What are the most effective intervention techniques for changing physical activity self-efficacy and physical activity behaviour — and are they the same? *Health Educ Res.* 2011;26(2):308–22.

47. Marlatt GA, George WH. Relapse prevention: introduction and overview of the model. *Br J Addict.* 1984;79(3): 261–73.

48. Olander EK, Fletcher H, Williams S, Atkinson L, Turner A, French DP. What are the most effective techniques in changing obese individuals' physical activity self-efficacy and behaviour: a systematic review and meta-analysis. *Int J Behav Nutr Phys Act.* 2013;10(29):1–15.

49. Hallam J, Petosa R. A worksite intervention to enhance social cognitive theory constructs to promote exercise adherence. *Am J Health Promot.* 1998;13(1):4–7.

50. Hallam JS, Petosa R. The long-term impact of a four-session work-site intervention on selected social cognitive theory variables linked to adult exercise adherence. *Health Educ Behav.* 2004;31(1):88–100.

51. Bronfenbrenner U. *The Ecology of Human Development: Experiments by Nature and Design.* Cambridge (MA): Harvard University Press; 1979. 352 p.

52. Rhodes RE, Zhang R, Zhang C-Q. Direct and indirect relationships between the built environment and individual-level perceptions of physical activity: a systematic review. *Ann Behav Med.* 2020;54(7):495–509.

53. McLeroy KR, Bibeau D, Steckler A, Glanz K. An ecological perspective on health promotion programs. *Health Educ Behav.* 1988;15(4):351–77.

54. Ekkekakis P, Hall EE, Petruzzello SJ. Practical markers of the transition from aerobic to anaerobic metabolism during exercise: rationale and a case for affect-based exercise prescription. *Prev Med.* 2004;38(2):149–59.

55. Stokols D. Establishing and maintaining healthy environments: toward a social ecology of health promotion. *Am Psychol.* 1992;47(1):6–22.

56. Miller JM, Wolfson J, Laska MN, Nelson TF, Pereira MA, Neumark-Sztainer D. Factor analysis test of an ecological model of physical activity correlates. *Am J Health Behav.* 2019;43(1):57–75.

57. Elder JP, Lytle L, Sallis JF, et al. A description of the social-ecological framework used in the trial of activity for adolescent girls (TAAG). *Health Educ Res.* 2007;22(2): 155–65.

58. Saelens B, Sallis J, Frank L. Environmental correlates of walking and cycling: findings from the transportation, urban design, and planning literatures. *Ann Behav Med.* 2003;25(2):80–91.

59. Ewing R, Schmid T, Killingsworth R, Zlot A, Raudenbush S. Relationship between urban sprawl and physical activity, obesity, and morbidity. *Am J Health Promot.* 2003;18(1):47–57.

60. Heath GW, Brownson RC, Kruger J, et al. The effectiveness of urban design and land use and transport policies and practices to increase physical activity: a systematic review. *J Phys Act Health.* 2006;3(Suppl 1):S55–76.

61. Sallis JF, Floyd MF, Rodríguez DA, Saelens BE. Role of built environments in physical activity, obesity, and cardiovascular disease. *Circulation.* 2012;125(5):729–37.

62. Rundle AG, Chen Y, Quinn JW, et al. Development of a neighborhood walkability index for studying neighborhood physical activity contexts in communities across the US over the past three decades. *J Urban Health.* 2019;96(4): 583–90.

63. Cheval B, Rebar AL, Miller MW, et al. Cognitive resources moderate the adverse impact of poor perceived neighborhood conditions on self-reported physical activity of older adults. *Prev Med.* 2019;126:105741.

64. Cohen DA, Han B, Kraus L, Young DR. The contribution of the built environment to physical activity among young women. *Environ Behav.* 2019;51(7): 811–27.

65. Hagger MS, Chatzisarantis NLD, Biddle SJH. A meta-analytic review of the theories of reasoned action and planned behavior in physical activity: predictive validity and the contribution of additional variables. *J Sport Exerc Psychol.* 2002;24(1):3–32.

66. Fishbein M, Ajzen I. *Belief, Attitude, Intention, and Behavior: An Introduction to Theory and Research.* Reading (MA): Addison-Wesley; 1975. 480 p.

67. Armitage C. Can the theory of planned behavior predict the maintenance of physical activity? *Health Psychol.* 2005;24(3):235–45.

68. Duncan MJ, Rivis A, Jordan C. Understanding intention to be physically active and physical activity behaviour in adolescents from a low socio-economic status background: an application of the theory of planned behaviour. *J Adolesc.* 2011;35(3):761–4.

69. Kwan MYW, Bray SR, Ginis KA. Predicting physical activity of first-year university students: an application of the theory of planned behavior. *J Am Coll Health.* 2009;58(1):45–52.

70. Cheng OY, Yam CLY, Cheung NS, Lee PLP, Ngai MC, Lin CY. Extended theory of planned behavior on eating and physical activity. *Am J Health Behav.* 2019;43(3): 569–581.

71. Plotnikoff RC, Lubans DR, Costigan SA, et al. A test of the theory of planned behavior to explain physical activity in a large population sample of adolescents from Alberta, Canada. *J Adolesc Health.* 2011;49(5):547–9.

72. Rebar AL, Rhodes RE, Gardner B. How we are misinterpreting physical activity intention–behavior relations and what to do about it. *Int J Behav Nutr Phys Act.* 2019;16(1):71.

73. Miller WR, Rollnick S. *Motivational Interviewing: Preparing People for Change.* New York (NY): Guilford Press; 2002. 428 p.

74. Ryan RM, Deci EL. Self-determination theory and the facilitation of intrinsic motivation, social development, and well-being. *Am Psychol.* 2000;55(1):68–78.

75. Edmunds J, Ntoumanis N, Duda JL. Testing a self-determination theory-based teaching style intervention in the exercise domain. *Eur J Soc Psychol.* 2008;38(2):375–88.

76. Wilson PM, Rodgers WM. The relationship between perceived autonomy support, exercise regulations and behavioral intentions in women. *Psychol Sport Exerc.* 2004;5(3):229–42.

77. Ntoumanis N, Ng JY, Prestwich A, et al. A meta-analysis of self-determination theory-informed intervention studies in the health domain: effects on motivation, health behavior, physical, and psychological health. *Health Psychol Rev.* 2020;3:1–31.

78. Gillison FB, Rouse P, Standage M, Sebire SJ, Ryan RM. A meta-analysis of techniques to promote motivation for health behaviour change from a self-determination theory perspective. *Health Psychol Rev.* 2019;13:110–30.

79. Teixeira PJ, Carraça EV, Markland D, Silva MN, Ryan RM. Exercise, physical activity, and self-determination theory: a systematic review. *Int J Behav Nutr Phys Act.* 2012;9(1):78.

80. Thorndike EL. The law of effect. *Am J Psychol.* 1927;39:212–22.

81. Young PT. The role of hedonic processes in the organization of behavior. *Psych Rev.* 1952;59(4):249.

82. Kahneman D, Diener E, Schwarz N, editors. *Well-Being: Foundations of Hedonic Psychology.* New York (NY): Russell Sage Foundation; 1999. 605 p.

83. Ekkekakis P. People have feelings! Exercise psychology in paradigmatic transition. *Curr Opin Psychol.* 2017;16:84–8.

84. Kwan BM, Bryan AD. Affective response to exercise as a component of exercise motivation: attitudes, norms, self-efficacy, and temporal stability of intentions. *Psychol Sport Exer.* 2010;11(1):71–9.

85. Kerrigan SG, Schumacher L, Manasse SM, Loyka C, Butryn ML, Forman EM. The association between negative affect and physical activity among adults in a behavioral weight loss treatment. *Psychol Sport Exerc.* 2019;101507.

86. Williams DM, Dunsiger S, Ciccolo JT, Lewis BA, Albrecht AE, Marcus BH. Acute affective response to a moderate-intensity exercise stimulus predicts physical activity participation 6 and 12 months later. *Psychol Sport Exer.* 2008;9(3):231–45.

87. Lind E, Ekkekakis P, Vazou S. The affective impact of exercise intensity that slightly exceeds the preferred level 'pain' for no additional 'gain.' *J Health Psychol.* 2008;13(4):464–8.

88. Ekkekakis P, Parfitt G, Petruzzello SJ. The pleasure and displeasure people feel when they exercise at different intensities. *Sports Med.* 2011;41(8):641–71.

89. Williams DM, Dunsiger S, Emerson JA, Gwaltney CJ, Monti PM, Miranda R. Self-paced exercise, affective response, and exercise adherence: a preliminary investigation using ecological momentary assessment. *J Sport Exerc Psychol.* 2016;38(3):282–91.

90. Lewis BA, Williams DM, Frayeh A, Marcus BH. Self-efficacy versus perceived enjoyment as predictors of physical activity behaviour. *Psychol Health.* 2016;31(4):456–69.

91. Helfer SG, Elhai JD, Geers AL. Affect and exercise: positive affective expectations can increase post-exercise mood and exercise intentions. *Ann Behav Med.* 2015;49(2):269–79.

92. Dunton GF, Vaughan E. Anticipated affective consequences of physical activity adoption and maintenance. *Health Psychol.* 2008;27(6):703–10.

93. Gellert P, Ziegelmann JP, Schwarzer R. Affective and health-related outcome expectancies for physical activity in older adults. *Psychol Health.* 2012;27(7):816–28.

94. Decker ES, Ekkekakis P. More efficient, perhaps, but at what price? Pleasure and enjoyment responses to high-intensity interval exercise in low-active women with obesity. *Psychol Sport Exerc.* 2017;28:1–10.

95. Da Silva DF, Peixoto EM, Ferraro ZM, Adamo KB, Machado FA. Changes in mood state and recovery-stress perception after an HRV-guided running program in untrained women. *J Sport Psychol.* 2020;29(1):83–94.

96. Rhodes RE, Pfaeffli LA. Mediators of physical activity behavior change among adult non-clinical populations: a review update. *Int J Behav Nutr Phys Act.* 2010;7:37.

97. Rhodes RE, McEwan D, Rebar AL. Theories of physical activity behaviour change: a history and synthesis of approaches. *Psychol Sport Exerc.* 2019;42:100–9.

12 Facilitating Health Behavior Change

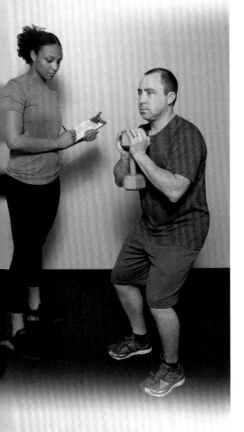

INTRODUCTION

Research indicates that the majority of Americans are not meeting minimal physical activity guidelines (1). Exercise physiologists must examine ways to facilitate exercise adoption and maintenance to help individuals reap the health benefits of physical activity. These efforts are especially important in light of the difficulties many people face in changing their exercise and physical activity behavior. Theory-based interventions can provide the exercise physiologist with a framework for helping clients adopt a new exercise program or adhere to an existing exercise program. More specifically, theory-based interventions can inform behavioral skills and approaches tailored to each individual's specific interests, preferences, and readiness for change to help individuals incorporate more physical activity into their daily routines. The purpose of this chapter is to expand on Chapter 11, which discussed various theories related to exercise promotion, by applying theory to practice. This chapter summarizes several intervention strategies, including using self-regulation strategies (*e.g.*, self-monitoring, goal setting, self-control); overcoming barriers to exercise; increasing social support; identifying outcome expectancies; and engaging in motivational interviewing (MI), relapse prevention, and effective communication.

Exercise physiologists must have the knowledge and understanding to help facilitate behavior change in their clients. This includes an appreciation of the evidence-based framework for behavior change and an ability to apply the appropriate strategies based on their clients' current lifestyle, physical activity and health goals, and the barriers and facilitators in their lives.

 ## Practical Strategies for Behavior Change

A key role of the exercise physiologist is helping clients learn skills and strategies to support long-term behavior change. These strategies are derived from theory (see Chapter 11) to provide an evidence-based approach to increase physical activity and promote the adoption and maintenance of exercise throughout the lifespan and across populations. Although not an exhaustive list, the following behavior change approaches can be readily incorporated into physical activity interventions and tailored to clients' individual needs.

Identifying Benefits of Physical Activity

A key feature in behavior change is the outcome expectation associated with performing the behavior. This concept is linked to social cognitive theory and health belief model and has significant relevance to exercise behavior as research involving a wide range of individuals indicates that outcome expectations are linked to exercise behavior (2,3). Individuals typically choose to do behaviors in which they see a desirable outcome as likely. For example, individuals who would like to have an improved mood after exercising are more inclined to initiate physical activity if they hold a firm expectation that exercise can make them feel better. In contrast, overweight individuals seeking weight loss who do not believe that exercise is an important part of losing weight are not likely to start a training program. An important consideration is that expectations of outcomes are the stimulus for motivating the initiation of the activity, although actual outcomes are key to long-term maintenance of the behavior. Key roles of the exercise physiologist include ensuring that clients are fully aware of the benefits that can be reasonably expected in response to exercise participation and designing an appropriate program to help clients achieve those desired benefits. Given the numerous benefits of exercise, there is a great likelihood that an exercise physiologist can help his or her clients identify one or more of those outcomes, which would be highly valued and could therefore help initiate the adoption of regular exercise.

Setting Goals

Goals have a significant impact on a person's thoughts and behavioral choices, and helping clients create and achieve new, healthy goals is an important task of the exercise physiologist. Goal setting has long been established as an effective strategy for exercise adherence (4) and is a critical component of the overall exercise prescription plan. Goals should direct effort and attention toward activities that are goal relevant and away from those that are irrelevant (5). Goals also increase persistence, knowledge, and skill attainment. Thus, there are some key features of goals that can enhance the effectiveness of facilitating behavior change and maintenance.

The strategies and tools used to set health behavior goals vary; however, most goals should include key components to ensure that goals are SMART. The exercise physiologist and client can work together to make sure that goals are

- *Specific*: carefully identify the what, where, and how aspects of the goal
- *Measurable*: ensure that change and progress are clearly noted
- *Attainable*: set up goals that are challenging but within reach with good effort
- *Relevant*: focus energy toward goals that help achieve outcomes that are highly valued
- *Time-bound*: explicitly state dates for goal completion

Explicit goals that state the desired outcome reduce the ambiguity of the task, which makes the achievement of the goal more likely. In contrast, setting goals that are too vague, complex, or difficult can limit success and negatively impact confidence. Furthermore, repeatedly creating unobtainable goals of this nature enforces a belief that any goal is unreachable and, therefore, goal setting is unnecessary (6). Setting specific short-term goals in the context of a long-term goal is a more successful approach to behavior change than setting a single long-term goal (7). Creating specific action plans, or implementation intentions, can enhance goal achievement by specifying exactly what, when, where, and with whom clients plan to exercise. Effective goal setting also requires clients to monitor progress and assess capabilities, identify skills and strategies to support progress, and adjust or set a new goal as needed. It is important for the exercise physiologist to provide regular feedback and encouragement regarding the individual's progress and work with the client to create new goals when the previous goals are attained (5). There are tools such as goal setting worksheets, which can be used to help guide the development of goals, timelines, and action plans and serve as a platform for feedback.

Using Self-Monitoring Tools

Self-monitoring involves observing and recording behavior and has been shown to be important in exercise behavior change (7,8). The process of self-monitoring brings about awareness of positive and negative behaviors and cognitions through "paying attention on purpose" and creates opportunity for change. For example, regular self-monitoring of weight by weighing oneself on a schedule is associated with weight loss and the prevention of weight gain (9,10). Self-monitoring of exercise can be in the form of a paper-and-pencil log, a heart rate monitor, pedometer, or wearables such as a smartwatch. Technology devices and apps can provide the individual with detailed feedback that includes minutes of exercise, exercise intensity, distance travelled, or step counts. Visual documentation (*e.g.*, workout log) can be useful for tracking progress toward goals, identifying barriers to changing behavior, and as a reminder to exercise. Self-monitoring of physical activity can be an effective facilitator of behavior change and serve as a tool for collaboration between the client and exercise physiologist. However, there are some key features to self-monitoring that can optimize its effectiveness (11).

Self-Monitoring Recommendations

1. Select a method of self-monitoring that fits the client's needs and preferences.
2. Encourage commitment by having clients form intentions and make plans (*e.g.*, help client complete a goal setting worksheet).
3. Provide timely and meaningful feedback on behavior (*e.g.*, provide regular reports with information about progress).
4. Select simple self-monitoring tasks that do not require a lot of time and effort to reduce burden and increase the likelihood of use (*e.g.*, encourage passive or automated monitoring via devices).
5. Ensure use of a variety of short-term, or even daily, behavioral goals (*e.g.*, the target number of steps to engage in each day).
6. Encourage consistent self-monitoring, which is better than intermittent self-monitoring (12).

Self-monitoring also requires use of behavior change strategies. An exercise physiologist can help clients recognize the perceived benefits, barriers, facilitators, and consequences of self-monitoring. Consider physical activity monitoring as an example. *Perceived benefits* of monitoring physical activity might be feedback that activity goals are being met or providing accountability. *Perceived barriers* of monitoring physical activity might be time burden or not knowing how to self-monitor. *Facilitators* enhance the use of self-monitoring such as providing instructions on self-monitoring or encouraging the client through positive messages and feedback to the client. *Consequences* of self-monitoring can be either positive (*e.g.*, improved behavior or clinical outcomes) or negative (*e.g.*, dislike of the monitoring process). Awareness of these key factors can help clients' use of self-monitoring be more effective in facilitating behavior change.

EXERCISE IS MEDICINE CONNECTION

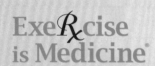

Turner-McGrievy GM, Beets MW, Moore JB, Kaczynski AT, Barr-Anderson, Tate DF. Comparison of traditional versus mobile app self-monitoring of physical activity and dietary intake among overweight adults participating in an mHealth weight loss program. *J Am Med Inform Assoc.* 2013;20(3):513–8.

There exists an old idea that one of the best ways to improve a behavior is to monitor that behavior. Paying close attention to and recording the things we do tends to produce desirable behavior changes. This principle has been demonstrated in a variety of contexts including diet and physical activity. The clear message from this research is that tracking and monitoring activity produces notable increases in total exercise. Importantly, this old idea has been applied to new technologies such as smartphones. A recent study of overweight adults enrolled in a 6-month weight loss intervention indicates that participants were more likely to report exercise when assigned to the mobile app monitoring group compared to the group using a paper journal. Mobile app participants reported more than twice as much exercise and concluded the study with a lower body mass index than their paper journal counterparts. It seems the convenience provided by the mobile phone method combined with our insatiable appetite to use technology made a meaningful difference on outcomes. Although excessive use of media and screens can negatively impact physical activity, the results of this study make clear that technology can be leveraged in a positive manner and encourage the utilization of exercise as medicine for healthful living.

Physical Activity Monitors

As new activity monitoring technology continues to emerge, activity monitors have become a common tool for self-monitoring and prompting physical activity. The most common activity monitor individuals are likely to use include smartwatches paired with their phones but may also include pedometers or other accelerometers. Of the more popular consumer-grade monitors, Fitbit and other watch-based accelerometers are showing promise as a valid measure of steps and energy expenditure (13,14). Like the Fitbit and other similar wearable monitors, smartphones use accelerometer technology to measure movement, and research evidence is providing support that phone-based monitoring tools can provide valid and reliable physical activity information (15,16). Pedometers and accelerometers are effective in facilitating behavior change, especially when a step goal is provided (17). These devices can be a simple, convenient, and cost-efficient method of physical activity monitoring. Evidence-based guidelines include recommendations for adult physical activity ($\geq$7,500 steps per day), exercise (3,000 of total daily steps at 100 steps per minute), and limiting sitting time ($>$5,000 steps per day) (18,19). Guidelines have also been established for older adults (20) and children/adolescents (21). In addition, 3 days of self-monitoring with a pedometer can provide a reasonable estimate of the number of steps one gets per day, thus useful in physical activity assessment of clients (22). Step goals can be adjusted based on the client's baseline activity, fitness, health status, and other factors.

As the market for physical activity monitors and wearable devices expands, the research cannot keep up with the number of devices and new technology. With this growth, exercise physiologists should be wary of product claims and help clients evaluate the evidence supporting new devices. That is, not every monitor is valid or accurately assesses activity amounts. It is important for the exercise physiologist to have good familiarity with the various products and technology used in monitoring and to stay current on the research that evaluates the scientific validity of these tools. Similarly, the exercise professional should be comfortable discussing complimentary self-monitoring approaches, such as heart rate values or ratings of perceived exertion (RPE) during exercise. An exercise physiologist must be prepared to help clients correctly interpret the data, which the clients will now have access to from their devices and use the information in the context of behavior change. Scheduling a time to discuss the data and what it means in the context of the client's goals is an important way to provide feedback and prevent potentially harmful misinterpretation.

Increasing Social Support

Behavior change efforts are challenging, but the support of others can enhance the opportunity for success. This support from significant others, such as family and friends, is referred to as social support and is described as the perceived and actual caring and assistance received by the individual engaging in behavior change efforts. Four primary types of social support have been identified (23):

- Instrumental: providing tangible, practical assistance for goal achievement (*e.g.*, driving a spouse to a cardiac rehabilitation appointment, providing childcare for a mother)
- Emotional: expressing encouragement, empathy, and concern (*e.g.*, praising an exerciser for his or her efforts, demonstrating compassion for sore muscles)
- Informational: giving instructions, advice, and feedback (*e.g.*, providing exercise tips, giving valuable health-related information)
- Companionship: providing a sense of belonging and connectedness (*e.g.*, making oneself available as an exercise partner or group)

These types of support can be provided by a variety of sources, including family, significant others, and exercise physiologists, with each source of social support having the potential to provide benefit. One other important consideration within social support is whether the support is actually received or is instead perceived. Although support that is real and tangible is valuable in the promotion of health behavior change, research demonstrates that perceptions of support or nonsupport are also critical elements in health behavior (24). That is, perceptions of support can be more important than actual or received support. Thus, it is important to consider what a client perceives about the support provided by his or her available resources.

A critical aspect of social support is that the relative importance of the type and source of support varies from person to person. Providing social support in the form of guidance is most common for exercise physiologists working with clients. Individuals beginning an exercise program need to feel supported in times of stress or times when continuing to exercise is difficult (25,26). Moreover, individuals beginning an exercise program may have low confidence or feelings of incompetence. Increasing clients' beliefs about their capabilities can be done through mastery experiences, social modeling, and providing praise (27). The characteristics of social support most beneficial for a busy single mother employed full-time might be tangible and instrumental such as childcare or transportation. In contrast, perceived emotional support from a spouse might be of greatest value to a newly enrolled cardiac rehabilitation patient. It is important not to assume what a client needs. In addition, many individuals may find it hard to identify and ask for help, and role-playing such scenarios can be a practical behavioral strategy.

Implementing ways to increase an individual's attachment and feelings of being part of a group is also important to adoption and maintenance of exercise. The exerciser needs to feel competent in his or her workouts, and one method to accomplish this is to establish buddy groups. In group settings, exercisers can benefit from watching others complete their exercise routines and from instructors and fellow exercisers giving input on proper technique and execution. In addition, groups can increase enjoyment of exercise and offer peer accountability. Creating supportive exercise groups within communities has been linked with greater levels of exercise behavior (28).

Regulating Emotions

Emotions play a key role in one's level of motivation, effort, and behavioral choice (29). First, positive emotions can be generally related to continued motivation to keep going, whereas negative emotions might promote motivation to change, try harder, or give up. Interestingly, specific emotions, especially around awareness to not meeting up to a self-held standard, can lead to quite different levels of effort. For example, frustration and anger appear to be effort-enhancing type emotions, whereas feelings of sadness, depression, or despondency might be related to less effort (30). Thus, the exercise physiologist must be attentive to how clients feel, especially when they did not reach a highly valued goal. The professional can then help the client reach an emotional state that is more productive for behavior change, thus helping the clients maintain their behavioral efforts.

The positive feelings experienced from a single bout of exercise can predict physical activity levels a year later (31,32). Importantly, research indicates each unit of increase in positive feelings translates to significantly more physical activity over time. The exercise physiologist's goal should be to maximize positive feeling states associated with exercise and understand the complexity of such responses. The fitness professional should encourage clients to pick exercise activities that they enjoy, as people are more likely to both try, and continue to maintain an activity that they find pleasant or enjoyable.

Additional steps the exercise physiologist can take to promote positive feelings associated with exercise include assessing whether the client views the exercise experience as pleasant or unpleasant during the exercise itself. The self-reported feelings of pleasantness/unpleasantness can be used when prescribing exercise in part by helping to identify the transition from aerobic to anaerobic metabolism. If clients report increasing feelings of displeasure, this may be a good indication that the exercise intensity may be too high and that intensity should be reduced to reduce feelings of displeasure (33).

Exercise provides an array of physiological feedback to be interpreted by the brain, and individuals can vary in their interpretations. For example, a new exerciser or postrehabilitation client might interpret feelings of rapid heart rate, hyperventilation, sweat, and muscle fatigue in a negative or even fearful way, thus resulting in a negative feeling state associated with exercise. Past feeling states associated with behavior tend to shape attitudes toward future behavior, so it is important to reduce these negative feeling states. In contrast, an avid exerciser may feel all of the same stimuli but think, "Wow, that was a great workout!" The exercise physiologist should check in with the clients about how they are interpreting their physiological feedback to better understand emotional responses.

A strategy the exercise physiologist can use to help clients who are new to exercise to start and maintain a program of exercise is to encourage them to self-select the intensity of their exercise and choose an intensity that feels good. This can be a particularly useful strategy for those who are overweight or obese (34–36). When self-selecting intensities for exercise that feel good, individuals tend to still exercise at a moderate intensity (37). Other strategies that can help promote positive feelings associated with exercise include exercising in a context that is enjoyable, trying new activities, introducing variety into the types of exercises performed (38), and establishing a reward system for exercise (39). Lastly, it is important that clients understand that health behavior change can be an emotional journey, and proper understanding and handling of these emotions can facilitate goal-directed behaviors.

Enhancing Self-Efficacy

Self-efficacy describes the confidence a person has in his or her ability to carry out the actions needed to perform a specific behavior (27). Increasing exercise self-efficacy is associated with increases in physical activity behavior (40); therefore, the exercise physiologist should work with client to enhance self-efficacy. Sources of information that drive a person's overall feeling of self-efficacy include mastery experience, vicarious experience, verbal persuasion, physiological feedback, and emotional states (Table 12.1).

Promoting mastery experience requires that a person successfully perform the behavior. The exercise physiologist can help clients by providing proper instruction and demonstration of exercises and using tailored progression in physical activity plans. Additional strategies include having clients set realistic goals and encouraging clients to use physical activity logs to monitor their progress so that they can recognize accomplishments.

To promote vicarious experience, a person needs to be able to observe others performing a similar task. Strategies the exercise physiologist can use to promote vicarious experiences include using videos that model behavior, sharing success stories about other individuals with similar backgrounds, and having the client exercise in group environments where they can identify with others. For example, interventions that use peer mentors or facilitators have shown success in various health behaviors such as weight loss and physical activity (41).

Verbally encouraging the client that he or she can be successful is an important strategy to enhance self-efficacy. The exercise physiologist should give frequent feedback and express confidence in the client's ability to exercise and remind the client about any previous successful attempts to exercise.

Physical activity provides a number of physiological cues that can positively and negatively impact exercise self-efficacy. It is important for an exercise physiologist to spend time discussing how physical activity makes the client feel physically and emotionally and use this information to guide physical activity choices and exercise progression. As part of this discussion, the possible discomforts associated with physical activity should be addressed, in addition to providing instruction about physical activity and the associated physical symptoms that arise when exercising. The exercise physiologist can help clients learn to use physical cues to monitor activity and reframe maladaptive thoughts and emotions. This can be particularly useful for professionals working with clinical populations who have medical risk factors.

Table 12.1	Strategies for Increasing Physical Activity Self-Efficacy
Information Sources for Self-Efficacy	**Strategies**
Mastery experiences	■ Assess physical activity history and behavioral goals; use positive experiences and successes to build confidence. ■ Set small goals and rehearse activity behaviors. ■ Use self-monitoring tools to track success.
Vicarious experiences	■ Arrange workout/accountability partners tailored to client needs. ■ Use videos and success stories of active peer role models. ■ Have peer role models lead group physical activity sessions.
Verbal persuasion	■ Praise and encourage progress. ■ Encourage family and friends to support and reinforce the activity behavior. ■ Enlist additional support from other health professionals.
Physiological cues	■ Help clients anticipate and positively interpret physical signs and discomforts related to physical activity (*e.g.*, fatigue, increased breathing, muscle soreness). ■ Use relaxation training to decrease stress and anxiety. ■ Use an incremental exercise prescription matched to client fitness.
Emotional states	■ Help clients identify positive feelings associated with physical activity such as accomplishment, pride, and enjoyment. ■ Address and reframe negative emotions (*e.g.*, frustration, dislike, doubt).

Data from Pekmezi D, Jennings E, Marcus B. Evaluating and enhancing self-efficacy for physical activity. *ACSMs Health Fit J.* 2009;13(2):16–21; ACSM 2013.

Problem-Solving Barriers to Physical Activity

The most common barriers to exercise across populations include lack of time, lack of energy, and a lack of motivation (42,43). Barriers differ from person to person and change over time. A first step in problem solving is to identify the barrier and understand the impact on behavior. Barriers to physical activity can be actual or perceived. Actual barriers are those that are objectively manifested, such as a client not having a ride to the gym or lack of childcare. Perceived barriers are those that are subjectively manifested from the client's perspective; however, perceived barriers are powerful and hinder behavior change as much as actual barriers. For example, researchers have found that actual time commitments did not predict lack of time for physical activity in women (44). In other words, the barrier does not have to be real or objectively manifested to be a hindrance to the client. Rather, if the client *perceives* it to be a barrier, then that perceived barrier can negatively affect behavior change.

It is also important to consider how much control a person has over barriers. The environment is another potential barrier to exercise. However, people tend to have less control over environmental factors such bad weather, lack of exercise facilities, cost, and safety issues. In addition, living in rural, suburban, and urban areas brings about specific barriers. For example, a more prominent barrier for an older adult in a rural area might be lack of sidewalks, inadequate lighting, lack of access to facilities, or unattended dogs, whereas concerns related to safety might be a prominent barrier in an urban area (45). The role of the exercise physiologist is to help troubleshoot problems with his or her clients. For example, together they might identify a safe, public space to walk such as a mall or high school track. Or, the exercise physiologist could develop an exercise prescription that includes home-based exercise that can be done regardless of weather or safety concerns. One key to helping overcome environmental barriers is ensuring that clients perceive that they have a variety of ways in which they can meet their exercise goals. This might mean being more creative with solutions or working to enhance other behavioral strategies such as increasing social support or enhancing self-efficacy and positive emotions.

Clients commonly will have psychosocial barriers to exercise that decrease self-efficacy. Past negative experiences with exercise, anxiety, and intimidating exercise environments can limit the desire to engage in activities (46). Exercise physiologists should be aware that certain environmental variables may create challenges for some clients. Examples include unclear social norms, lack of instructions for exercise equipment, the use of mirrors, aggressive colors or loud noise within the gym setting, intimidating group exercise environments, and revealing clothing by instructors or gym members. Exercise physiologists can help create an environment that limits these concerns by providing adequate orientation and instruction, helping ensure greater privacy, modeling less revealing clothing, and engaging in positive, nonshaming feedback. Also, navigating social norms of a fitness facility can be an intimidating barrier to exercising, especially if the client is disrupted by the lack of knowledge, comfort, and confidence to navigate these norms. For example, clinical environments have been found to intensify self-presentational concerns in women due to inadequate views of their physical appearance, the presence of men or younger women in the clinic, perceived inability to perform exercise as well as expected, and mirrors/windows in the clinic (47). Thus, the exercise physiologist should ensure that the client is not placed in a situation or environment that could exacerbate any perceived feelings of physique anxiety or self-presentational concerns and work to create a nonintimidating and safe exercise environment.

Health-related barriers associated with exercise are common in clinical populations. Symptoms such as difficulty breathing, low back or knee pain, arthritis, or weakness can be challenging for both the client and the exercise physiologist. First, medical conditions and symptoms can make specific exercises difficult or even contraindicated. Second, such barriers can negatively affect the client's motivation to be active, especially in light of the discomfort they expect to experience or anxiety over the anticipation of symptoms. Modifying the exercise prescription can help clients maintain motivation and positive perceptions of exercise.

HOW TO   Use the IDEA Method

The IDEA method can provide a practical framework to help exercise physiologists facilitate an action plan for problem solving barriers to physical activity. The steps include the following:

1. Identify the barrier. Be specific and thoroughly describe the challenge and the effect it has on physical activity.
2. Develop a list of potential solutions. Brainstorm creatively — you never know what might help.
3. Evaluate the solutions. Select one that seems to work best. You can always come back to this list later and try another option.
4. Act on the solution and assess how well the plan worked. If it helped, great! If not, think about what can be done differently or if another solution might work better.

It is important to allow the clients to direct the process. It is tempting to want to provide a solution for the client, especially if the answer seems obvious. However, giving advice often backfires and increases resistance. Further, by learning the skill of problem solving, clients will be able to apply the approach to future barriers as they arise.

Increasing Options for Physical Activity

Suppose a client has been walking around the neighborhood three times a week for the last 2 weeks. Today is a day to walk, but it is raining. What does the client do? Unfortunately, for many clients, a common response might be to do nothing. One major reason might be the perceived lack of other options to be physically active. To facilitate behavior change, clients need to perceive additional options to be active. In this example, other physical activity opportunities would have helped the client meet daily physical activity goal. With options, the client might have walked at the mall, used a gym membership, or enjoyed a favorite exercise video. Thus, the perception of options for physical activity could increase the odds that clients will be active. Research supports this suggestion, as having four places for physical activity was related to 1,000% increase in the odds of adult women *meeting* physical activity guidelines of 150 min · wk^{-1} compared to those with no perceived options (48).

Options for physical activity can also facilitate autonomy, or the belief that the client is the origin of his or her own actions and has the power to choose. Autonomy is a key innate need that all humans possess and is crucial in helping facilitate more self-determined forms of motivation (see Chapter 11). In seeking ways to encourage, support, and enhance autonomy, the exercise physiologist can provide more physical activity options for the client to choose from. This could be as simple as letting a client choose from a list of exercises during a training session instead of dictating what exercises must be completed.

Options also allow clients to tap into another important source of intrinsic motivation — to experience stimulation, fun, and pleasure. For example, the exercise physiologist could provide the client with a large list of moderate-intensity physical activities. The client could then highlight the physical activities that are enjoyable, alongside others he or she would like to try. A choice can be then be made from options that are self-determined, rather than those forced on the client by the professional or someone else, while providing an ample list of activities to choose from when difficult times arise.

The exercise physiologist should also be aware of clients' perceptions of access to physical activity and healthy eating opportunities, which can vary across urban, suburban, and rural environments. The professional can help the client assess perceptions and consider how supportive a rural environment is perceived to be for physical activity (49). Similarly, there are ways to assess the perceived nutritional environment (50), which could greatly vary between urban or suburban areas where clients might have more access compared to a rural setting with limited access to a single convenience store and fast-food outlet (51).

Preventing Relapse

Although initial health behavior change is not easy, maintaining behavior change over time is perhaps more difficult because it requires ongoing commitment and effort. Although the timeline varies according to different theories and types of behavior, 6 months is often used as a threshold of transition from starting to maintaining behavior change (52). *Relapse prevention* is an ongoing process in which efforts are made by the individual engaging in behavior change to prevent a return to an undesirable behavior, which is a sedentary lifestyle in this case (53). Although full relapse is undesirable and highly problematic, individuals engaging in behavior change are encouraged to plan for brief lapses in behavior. Maintaining a perfect exercise plan is almost impossible. Therefore, a healthy approach is to expect lapses to occur and to have a plan in place to restart the desired behavior change immediately (8). A significant challenge to long-term behavior change is the common perspective that a single lapse in behavior means that all hope is lost and that returning to prior unhealthy behaviors is the natural next step. The primary goal is preventing a relapse, but an important secondary goal is being ready to respond when lapses occur. Relapse prevention incorporates various techniques, many of which are also used during the initial behavior change process. For example, goal setting, self-monitoring, and rewards are often used in both the initiation of behavior change and relapse prevention processes. Exercise physiologists should encourage their clients to develop specific plans for how they will prevent relapse and how they will handle lapses when they occur (Box 12.1).

> **Box 12.1** **Skills and Strategies for Physical Activity Behavior Change**
>
> - Identify benefits that have personal meaning.
> - Set SMART goals tailored to individual needs and abilities.
> - Use self-monitoring strategies to track progress and prompt physical activity.
> - Identify and enlist different types of social support.
> - Promote positive feelings toward physical activity and reframe negative emotions.
> - Enhance self-efficacy for physical activity and exercise.
> - Identify and problem solve barriers.
> - Increase opportunities for physical activity and encourage autonomy to enhance motivation.
> - Identify high-risk situations and plan for lapses to prevent relapse.

Facilitating Behavior Change: The Role of the Exercise Physiologist

The exercise physiologist plays a multifaceted role in helping clients achieve a physically active lifestyle. For many individuals, the choice to make a lifestyle change can be daunting as it presents new challenges and barriers that the client must navigate. The client may not be anticipating the effort that it takes to overcome these barriers beyond the physical work that he or she is asked to do in the gym or at a fitness class (54). It is important for the exercise physiologist to recognize that a person's choice to engage or not engage in healthy lifestyle behaviors throughout the lifespan is underscored by interactions between the body, mind, and environment.

The theories presented in Chapter 11 demonstrate key constructs to focus on when working to promote and sustain a physically active lifestyle. Exercise physiologists can make an impact by using these constructs to guide discovery of individual needs and differences in their clients. By training, exercise physiologists are experts in changing the body from a physiological perspective and understand the methods, guidelines, and principles (overload, progression, specificity of training) for achieving this. Although evidence-based exercise prescriptions impact the physiology, these are only effective if the exercise physiologist is able to get the client to continuously engage in the work. Thus, the key to be an effective fitness professional may lie in the ability to blend strong exercise prescription with individual-level interpersonal and behavioral factors. The intersection of biological response with these behavioral factors may enhance the professional–client relationship and create a positive atmosphere for behavior change.

The next sections assist the exercise physiologist with practical strategies and tools for incorporating behavior changing into practice.

Incorporating Behavior Change into Practice

Motivation is described in Chapter 11 as being on a continuum spanning from being amotivated (having a lack of motivation) to being extrinsically motivated (based on external factors) and then being intrinsically motivated (based on enjoyment and excitement). Most often, when a client approaches the exercise physiologist, according to the stages of change from the transtheoretical model, the participant is likely somewhere between the contemplation, preparation, and action stages. In contemplation, the client may be weighing his or her choice to act based on an interaction with an exercise physiologist; this may be a transitioning factor that shifts the potential client's awareness into preparation then action. In the preparation and action stages, the client may be looking for a fitness professional that has the expertise to help him or her realize and/or reach his or her goals. However, consider that a client may not just come to the exercise physiologist for his or her expertise in exercise but instead because the exercise physiologist is the external motivator that will provide the client with accountability and encouragement (verbal persuasion from social cognitive theory). The client may be relying on the exercise physiologist for his or her continued source of external motivation rather than having his or her own ownership over changing the behavior. This is a unique opportunity for the exercise physiologist to partner with the client to facilitate moving the client from solely relying on the exercise physiologist to developing intrinsic motivation and self-efficacy for a physically active lifestyle.

Although the theories of behavior change provide us with guidelines and targets for intervention, it can be difficult for the exercise physiologist to know where to start. Facilitating behavior change can be an individualized process, and each client will have different responses to increasing exercise influenced by many intrinsic and extrinsic factors; a one-theory approach or strategy may not work for all clients.

Interactions with clients can serve as the cornerstone of incorporating behavior change into our practice. It cannot always be about the work that happens in our fitness and health settings. These important interactions with clients need to be a part of the work. For example, preparticipation screening is a well-accepted method employed to learn more about a clients' health history and often includes questions about exercise goals. This is a great area to add questions related to learning more about a client's engagement state. Consider the following questions to get started.

Why is the client coming to you to exercise?

- *Did their doctor tell them to start exercising (extrinsic) or do they have an intrinsic reason or motivation for getting moving? This important information may guide which strategy the exercise physiologist uses next to target behavior change.*

What is relevant to your client?

- *Is it really because the client wants to lose weight, or is it because they want to lose weight, so they have more energy to keep up with their young kids? Knowing this deeper layer of information will help the exercise physiologist understand what the client may value (i.e., their family). Consider that the client may not have the same intrinsic passion or appreciation for exercise compared to the exercise physiologist, and linking exercise in a relevant way may help the client find a personal connection to the work accompanied with being more physically active.*

What does your client enjoy and not enjoy related to exercise?

- *What previous fitness- or health-related experiences may be shaping a client's attitudes and intentions? Knowing this information will help the exercise physiologist's prescribing approaches linked to enjoyment. Even though the exercise physiologist may know that an exercise and/or particular training method may be optimal for physiological adaptations, it is key to use this information to make appropriate adaptations and connect back to what the client will enjoy to facilitate adherence. This approach can also support autonomy promotion.*

What does your client feel comfortable doing related to changing his or her exercise?

- *Does your client actually want to come to the gym 3 times per week, and is that really feasible? Is the client comfortable doing exercises on their own in front of other people? Knowing this information can help the exercise physiologist get a sense of the client's self-efficacy plus the reality of what they are feasibly able to do and potential barriers that may inhibit engagement.*

These questions are entry-level engagement opportunities that an exercise physiologist can use to learn and engage at a deeper behavioral level with his or her clients. These interactions are not just limited to initial discussions but can also be useful to promote reevaluation of goals and motivation to

| Box 12.2 | **Practical Resources for Physical Activity Behavior Change** |

ACSM's Behavioral Aspects of Physical Activity and Exercise available from https://shop.lww.com
/ACSM-s-Behavioral-Aspects-of-Physical-Activity-and-Exercise/p/9781451132113
Active Living Every Day available from https://us.humankinetics.com/blogs/active-living
Exercise is Medicine Rx for Health Series available from http://www.exerciseismedicine.org
We Can! Ways to Enhance Children's Activity & Nutrition available from https://www.nhlbi.nih.gov
/health/educational/wecan/
Go4Life available from https://www.nia.nih.gov/health/exercise-physical-activity
Physical Activity Guidelines for Americans, 2nd edition, available from https://health.gov/our-work
/physical-activity

assist with long-term engagement and adherence. Behavior-driven conversations can occur monthly, weekly, or daily during training sessions (before, after, and during exercises; *i.e.*, rest breaks between sets) or with communications outside of the gym (motivational e-mails and text reminders).

Strategies such as improving communication, MI, and recognizing facilitators and barriers to exercise when working the diverse populations can further assist the exercise physiologist with having the most impact during these key interactions. "The Case of Linda" presented later provides an in-depth example of an interaction with a client illustrating how an exercise physiologist can incorporate behavior change into practice. Box 12.2 provides some practical resources to support physical activity behavior change.

Improving Communication

Communication skills, as they relate to behavior change, are extremely important for a number of reasons. First, the exercise physiologist is faced with a challenging task of extracting a client's thoughts and experiences and then being able to take the client's words and applying them back to psychological and behavioral concepts that can aid in developing interventions to facilitate behavior change. For example, Chapter 11 introduced self-efficacy and ways to improve it. However, a client is unlikely to state, "I do not feel very *efficacious* in doing those exercises on my own; thus, I need more mastery experience to enhance my feelings of efficacy." Rather, the client might say something like "I am not too sure I can exercise this week with how busy I am" or "I do not feel very confident when I am at the gym." The exercise physiologist must then discern that the client is actually talking about self-efficacy, and knowing this information, the professional can then develop interventions and communicate with the client to enhance perceptions of self-efficacy using one of several different strategies.

This important dynamic of communication between exercise physiologist and client is vital in the behavior change process. Although the natural tendency is to presume that verbal communication is far and away the most important channel for communication, nonverbal factors are key in the overall interpretation of interpersonal communication. The exercise physiologist should look for facial cues and body language that can give insight into how the client is feeling. Listening is also of great importance within the communication process. Active listening is a specific type of listening that demonstrates understanding of the message by listening with attention and repeating back to the speaker a meaningful summary of the message that was heard, which enhances accuracy of interpretation. Effective listening provides assurance that the message is receiving appropriate attention and consideration, which helps to build rapport between the exercise physiologist and the client. Facilitation of quality communication is key to developing trust and promoting change. The exercise physiologist should strive to convey messages in a manner that encourages, inspires, and motivates. Additionally, no single communication style should be used exclusively. Exercise physiologists should adapt and tailor their communication styles to the needs of the individual client.

Using Motivational Interviewing

One effective approach to motivating change involves MI, which is person centered, and intends to facilitate autonomy and strengthen motivation for change (55). This is an important approach that an exercise physiologist should engage in with the client as they begin to work together to establish a strong rapport and build an understanding and appreciation for the client's goals, concerns, and life situation. A basic premise of MI is that behavior change is more successful when the client takes the lead in discovering and fully considering all the factors that impact action and inaction toward a specific behavior. This is more participatory and autonomy-supportive than most traditional counseling orientations that focus on the expert or professional directing and instructing the client toward change. The strategies associated with MI have been shown to be effective for promoting a variety of healthy behaviors, including exercise (56,57).

HOW TO   Perform a Motivational Interview

First: Complete the readiness ruler.

On the following scale, indicate your readiness to increase your physical activity level.
0   1   2   3   4   5   6   7   8   9   10
Not Ready   Fully Ready

Second: Complete the change grid.
Use the grid below to list and describe your thoughts and feelings about changing and increasing your level of exercise. The grid should be completed in numerical order.

	Pros	Cons
Maintaining Current Activity	1	2
Increasing Activity	4	3

Instructions and Tips
Readiness and motivation for change is dynamic and will vary over time. The readiness ruler can be completed at different points in time to allow for measurement of change over time. Alternatively, a single measurement time point could ask the client to rate his or her level of readiness at some point in the past and compare that value to readiness today. Changes toward lesser or greater readiness can be used to initiate conversation about what is behind the change and what factors led to the change and/or what could impact readiness in the future.

The change grid provides an opportunity for the client to explore his or her motivations and ambivalence toward change. Clients should be encouraged to provide thoughtful entries that can be used as talking points. Completing the sections in order allows the client to flow away from a position that does not support change behavior toward a final position that can provide a launch point for further communication and potential commitment to change.

A key feature within MI is helping clients overcome their feelings of ambivalence or uncertainty for change. That is, many inactive individuals have contemplated increasing their activity but are unsure if they really want to make a commitment to change. MI helps clients explore and work through their ambivalence about change (58). Four general principles underlie MI, and each is important in facilitating behavior change:

- Express empathy: Reflect an attitude of acceptance, use skillful listening, demonstrate understanding.
- Develop discrepancies: Clarify the difference between current and preferred behavior, encourage exploration of likely outcomes in life with and without change.
- Roll with resistance: Avoid arguing, offer new perspectives, demonstrate patience and flexibility.
- Support self-efficacy: Instill confidence in ability to change, limit and redirect negativity, affirm appropriate goals.

As individuals discuss their ambivalence about behavior change, they typically produce two types of talk regarding their behavior: sustain talk and change talk. Sustain talk refers to talking about the costs of changing and the benefits of not changing. Sustain talk is used as a way for the client to not feel obligated to adopt any change. Change talk refers to talk about the benefits of behavior change and the costs of not changing. The goal of MI is to generate change talk, as this indicates movement toward readiness to adopt change. This is accomplished by asking open-ended questions, summarizing, and skillfully using reflective listening to express empathy, with the goal of guiding the conversation toward more change talk. Change talk is facilitated by communication that focuses on observations made by the exercise physiologist and is hindered when the focus shifts toward judgment, interpretation, and evaluation, which inhibits open and relaxed communication. Use of good MI technique provides a pathway for change that is directed by the individual, which enhances the likelihood of success.

The Case of Linda

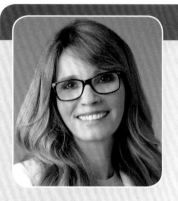

Submitted by **Renee J. Rogers, PhD; and Audrey M. Collins, MS**

This case describes how MI is used to effect change with a 48-year-old client wanting to reenter an active lifestyle.

Background

Linda is a 48-year-old married woman who has three children in middle and high school and is busy with her family's activities (parent–teacher association [PTA] meetings, sports practices). She has worked as an administrative assistant for 20 years. Linda has noticed a decrease in stamina and reports extreme tiredness or fatigue. She has noticed a change in her body weight of approximately 15 lb in the last few years. With her role as an involved parent and with her demanding job, she found it increasingly difficult to "find" the time to exercise and to consider her health needs. Linda was active in high school where she was a cheerleader. Linda has not performed structured exercise since her kids were young.

Linda is meeting with a certified exercise physiologist who is working with her in a consult format to discuss her goals and barriers and to develop a plan for physical activity.

Weight History

Height: 5 ft 8 in
Heaviest weight: 165 lb
Current weight: 165 lb
Goal weight: 150 lb
Lowest weight: 138 lb

Medical History

Postmenopausal
No history of coronary artery disease, hypertension, diabetes mellitus, cancer, smoking, thyroid disorders, or chronic fatigue
No surgeries
Bone density — NA
Labs: complete blood count and lipid profile: all values within normal ranges
Medications/supplements: daily multivitamin
Physical complaints: upper back pain due to tension and being at a computer all day; changes in posture; noticeable fatigue when climbing stairs and carrying heavy objects
Sleep: approximately 7 hours a night, reports sleeping well throughout the night
Social support: serves on multiple committees related to her children's activities at school; regular weekend dinners with family

Objective

Using MI strategies, the coach guides, listens, and elicits information from the client to encourage the process of change. (Please note that this was a conversation that took place as a part of a consult.)

Conversation 1

Linda: I feel tired all of the time.
Coach: I'm sorry to hear that, Linda. Why do you feel this way?

Linda: Each day, I'm always running between home, work, and my kid's school and sport events. I feel as though I just don't have the energy for all of that!

Coach: I appreciate you sharing this information with me. Tell me about your current activity levels.

Linda: I don't perform regular exercise anymore. Since my evenings are consumed with family events, getting dinner on the table and then helping the kids prepare for the next day, I haven't had the time. While I'm at work, I feel like I'm glued to my computer and feel pressure to always be at the office. If I'm not at my desk, I'm in a meeting. I support many people at work, and they rely on my ability to stay productive.

Coach: Wow! Based on what you've told me, it sounds like you are quite busy.

Linda: I'll say! I feel like I can't find time for anything anymore.

Coach: I understand that you have a lot going on, both inside and outside of work. Finding time to be active can feel impossible when facing a busy schedule. How do you think you can be more active throughout the day? Maybe tell me a little about what a typical day looks like for you.

Linda: Before work, I spend time caring for my family, as most of my daytime is spent at the office. While at work, I am usually sitting in my office or meetings. After work, I go right home, organize the kids, and transport them to practice or whatever school event they have on most nights of the week. I really don't know how I can fit activity in, but I know I should do it. I feel like I already don't have enough energy for all of this!

Coach: I can understand why you feel that way. This may be surprising, but being active can provide you with the energy needed to conquer your busy day! How would you feel about performing activity while at work?

Linda: Activity during the workday? I won't be able to leave the office for an exercise class.

Coach: What if I told you that you could perform activity without leaving your office for an extended period?

Linda: While in my suit and heels? I don't think so!

Coach: I hear what you're saying. It may seem as though movements can be restricted by the professional dress that is seen within the workplace. What other challenges may be presented by being active in the workplace?

Linda: Well, I've had neck and upper back pain while working that makes any movement uncomfortable. In addition, there are college students that just began interning at our office. I can't imagine doing exercise in front of them or other colleagues that I work with, but I am lucky to have my own space. I could maybe do exercises in my office.

Coach: Let's talk about strategies that we can use to overcome these challenges. You proposed a fantastic suggestion by performing exercises in your office. You also expressed neck and upper back pain while working. When do you experience this pain?

Linda: I usually feel it while working at my desk. I have noticed the pain when working at my computer or reading e-mail and documents.

Coach: I have felt these feelings while working at my own desk at times. I understand how you feel. One way that I combatted this pain is by performing a few exercises. Let me show you! [Demonstrates exercise that can be done in a small workspace.]

Linda: Now, I don't know if I can do that!

Coach: I understand that this exercise may look difficult, but I know that you can do it. There are many versions of this exercise. Let's try a few together! [Perform exercise together.]

Linda: I think I may have done a version of this exercise during high school when I used to cheer!

Coach: I am glad to hear that! How did you feel about this movement when you used to do it?

Linda: Surprisingly, I enjoyed it! I can't believe that I can still perform this same exercise.

Coach: You did a fantastic job. How would you feel about performing this same exercise, and similar movements, during your workday?

Linda: I don't know where I would fit this time into my day.

Coach: It seems hard while getting started, but I am confident that you can do it. A strategy that can help is to schedule these activities on your calendar and treat them as an appointment, just as if you had a meeting.

Linda: I think I would be able to do that.

Coach: That's great. Let's look at your calendar together. [Linda opens calendar.] What times each day are you most likely to perform an activity break?

Linda: Every day, I have a 10-minute window in my schedule from 12:00 to 12:10 p.m. I think that I could try these exercises on Monday, Wednesday, and Friday at that time.

Coach: Those times sound great. Earlier in our conversation, I heard you say that you felt out of your routine. These scheduled activity breaks may assist in adding this sense of routine back into your day. Please write them into your calendar to make these scheduled appointments with yourself official.

Linda: [Writes in calendar.]

Coach: Next, let's work together to determine some activities that can help break up your sitting during the day and build up your stamina. It may be a good idea to consider activities that are aerobic or those that increase your heart rate. Given your time constraints and the fact that we are working on developing a plan during the workday — getting on a piece of cardio equipment does not seem realistic. However, there are definitely other ways to get aerobic activity in. Do you enjoy any aerobic activities?

Linda: I feel disconnected from the most active time in my life, which was before I had a family, maybe even as far back as high school when I was a cheerleader. I can't imagine busting out cheers in the office, even though I bet it would feel good to release energy in that manner.

Coach: That's very interesting, what do you mean by releasing energy?

Linda: Well, when you cheer you sometimes dance or perform very rhythmic movements and you yell out calls and cheers. I know it sounds funny, but when I was a stressed-out teenager, cheering made me feel better — I always felt better after practice even though I was tired.

Coach: It is interesting that you found a connection between stress and activity — that's really great! Based on what you have already shared, it seems like your busy family schedule and high demands at work may be causing you stress. Do you agree?

Linda: Absolutely.

Coach: Okay, so I am wondering if together we can think about a way to use activity during the workday to help relieve your stress just like cheering used to help you in high school.

Linda: You aren't going to make me cheer in front of my colleagues at work, are you?

Coach: Is that something that you want to do? [Says jokingly] No, there are many ways to increase activity. Can you think of a strategy to get your body moving move that might be feasible for you?

Linda: I have noticed that when I have been sitting at my desk for a while, when I get up and walk to the printer or bathroom, I tend to feel better when I sit back down. Does walking count?

Coach: Yes! It absolutely can. Why would you think that it wouldn't count?

Linda: I figured that I wouldn't be working hard enough for it to be beneficial.

Coach: I can understand why you may feel that way; however, walking can be a great form of physical activity. How can you incorporate more walking breaks into your workday — when do you find that you are the most stressed?

Linda: I spend a large portion of my day sending and responding to e-mails. This is a definite source of stress for me. Although recently, I have limited myself to only answering e-mails a few times per day so I don't get distracted — I do this first thing in the morning, again between 1:00 and 2:00 p.m. depending on my meetings, and at the end of my workday.

Coach: That's such a smart approach to planning out your day — have you noticed that this helps with your stress related to e-mail?

Linda: Yes and no — yes because it is not constantly causing me stress because I am not constantly looking at it but also no because when I am answering it, I still feel stressed after.

Coach: It sounds like e-mail is a definite source of stress, but I still think that it is impressive that you found a way to control your exposure to the stress by scheduling e-mail time. Do you think that taking a brisk walk may help with your stress as well?

Linda: Actually, I think that I would like to take a walk after finishing my e-mail each time. I tend to get up anyway because I am so tired of looking at my computer. Taking a walk might actually feel like a reward!

Coach: I like that idea and you also just developed a structured plan for walking. This can serve multiple goals — it gets you up and out of your chair, may help reduce your stress, and brisk walking can improve your stamina. Let's take a 2-minute walk together. [Linda and coach take a brisk walk around the room together.]

Coach: How do you feel, Linda?

Linda: Great — I am looking forward to seeing how this activity can help me with my stress but also my stamina. I want to get back to having more energy.

Coach: I think the strategies that we came up with today are a great starting point and together we will evaluate your progress and decide when it is appropriate for you to increase your activity. When is the best time for me to check in with you on your progress?

Linda: [Looks at calendar] I have time at 12:30 p.m. on Monday, 2 weeks from now.

Coach: Thank you for making time for our check in, as I know that your schedule is busy. We have started to create a plan/goal for next week. What do you hope to achieve by our phone call?

Linda: I have scheduled 10 minutes into my day on Monday, Wednesday, and Friday at 12:00 p.m. to perform exercises in my office. Beyond that, I plan to take at minimum a 2- to 5-minute brisk walk after I finish my daily e-mail sessions. I am not sure if I will get three walking breaks in, but I would like to start with a goal of two per day.

Coach: This is wonderful goal to start with, Linda. I am confident that you will have success. I plan to call you in 2 weeks on Monday at 12:30 p.m. That time will be right after your exercises that are scheduled at noon. We can talk about how your plan is going and to check in on how your activity went!

Conversation 2 (Two Weeks Later)

Coach: How did your goal of performing 10 minutes of office exercises on Monday, Wednesday, and Friday go this past week?

Linda: I was able to do these exercises at my desk on Monday, Wednesday, and Friday of last week. I even did them today at 12:00 p.m., right before our call.

Coach: Nice job! How did you feel after performing these exercises in the middle of your day?

Linda: Some days, I honestly found it to be a little challenging, but I am noticing that I have a little more energy. I think it may be the walking breaks.

Coach: That is awesome to hear, Linda. It sounds like you have more energy, despite your busy schedule. Tell me more about the walking breaks.

Linda: At first, it was skeptical and felt like I had to do it, but after I got up and moved — I did feel better. I was surprised that 2 minutes made me feel less stressed. I was able to get in two walking breaks after e-mailing every day except for Thursday. I got pulled into a meeting early, and I wasn't able to take my first walking break. I actually think that this was a good thing because I realized that I missed my break! I actually found time at lunch to sneak in a walk, and I was proud of myself.

Coach: You should be! Nice job! I am glad to hear that you found value in taking a walking break. You are really committed to making changes that make a difference in how you feel!

Coach: Let me summarize where we are at after the past 2 weeks. Last time we met, we talked about the challenges to performing activity in your busy schedule and at the workplace. We determined that it was not feasible to leave the office for an exercise class but were able to schedule three 10-minute activity breaks throughout your week at work along with some stress-relieving walking breaks. From our conversation, it sounds like you were successful in working on your initial goals. Does that sound correct?

Linda: Yes, that's right.

Coach: How can we continue this progress?

Linda: I really like focusing on my activity during the workday and avoiding the evenings for now, so I don't have to worry about it interfering with my family's needs. Is it okay to continue what we are already doing?

Coach: Absolutely. You already indicated that you feel like you have more energy, and healthy patterns and habits can take time to develop. If you are comfortable with continuing with this plan, I am supportive as well. I am impressed that you overcame one barrier already and made time for walking during another part of your day. Do you think that there are other barriers that could potentially get in the way of your walking and 12:00 p.m. activity breaks?

Linda: Yes, unfortunately, as much as I plan — I cannot control when my supervisors will pull me into a meeting. Every day, my schedule is different.

Coach: I can understand how difficult that can be when trying to develop a plan, but it is good that you realize this potential barrier. Have you thought about a strategy to get your walking in when your workday agenda suddenly changes?

Linda: I can always try and squeeze it in at lunch, but as a backup, I think I will try and increase how long I walk during my other breaks to make up the time.

Coach: That sounds like a really great strategy! I appreciate that you are willing to maintain how many minutes of activity you get each day. In time, we can work on increasing your exercise minutes, but for now — we have a plan!

Follow-Up

Linda continued to have biweekly contact with her coach. One time per month, they met in person and then 2 weeks later completed a follow-up call similar to the preceding text to review progress. Linda was slow to dive into a typical structured pattern of activity but after 2 months increased to three 5-minute walking breaks per day for a total of 75 minutes per week. This slow but steady change that focused on developing a routine that Linda was comfortable with helped to increase her self-efficacy for exercise and motivated her to continually develop new goals.

A Message from the Case Authors

This conversation with Linda highlights the need to make a connection to what is relevant to a client. It would be easy to simply read Linda's history and determine that she needs to do a structured plan of aerobic activity to improve her fitness and fatigue levels, optimally getting to 150 $min \cdot wk^{-1}$. However, in conversation with Linda, the coach learned that she is genuinely busy with her job and her family and that there is little flexibility to change these priorities. The coach also learned that Linda experiences stress at work and used this information to help Linda make a connection between the benefits of being active and stress reduction. This was something that was relevant to Linda. Of importance, the coach was careful to not "push" recommendations on Linda but instead gave Linda the choice in many situations to express what she was comfortable with and what was feasible — the coach made Linda a partner in planning and promoted her autonomy. Many aspects of the initial consult and follow-up were designed to promote an increase in self-efficacy. For example, verbal persuasion was used to reinforce behaviors, the coach and Linda performed activities together, positive physiological responses to activity were highlighted, activities that Linda enjoyed were promoted, reasonable goals were developed, and relapse prevention was discussed to help the client recognize and prepare for high-risk situations.

Working with Diverse Populations

Meeting the needs of diverse clients requires the careful consideration of the broader contextual factors that influence physical activity. During the first meeting with a new client, the exercise physiologist should reflect on how dimensions of diversity may impact a client's barriers and facilitators to exercise. Clients will differ in many ways including age, race/ethnicity, place of residence (*e.g.*, urban, suburban, and rural), stage in the life course, health status/conditions, ability/disability, and level of experience with physical activity. Whereas many barriers and facilitators associated with physical activity may be similar across diverse populations, others may be more salient for specific populations. The following examples, although not an extensive review of any diverse group, provide guidance of how exercise physiologists might begin to think about best serving clients and supporting their efforts to become more physically active.

Older Adults

Regular physical activity has many health benefits for older adults including improved physical health, mental health, and longevity. Despite the many benefits of physical activity, older adults present with barriers and concerns related to their stage of life. Concerns about exercise safety, interest in guidance on how to perform physical activities, exercise motivation, fear and risk of falling, social isolation, and mental health concerns may present as barriers (59,60). Constructs important in other populations play a role for older adults, but how they are manifested may differ. For example, although social support for activity was important to older adults, this was especially true when the support was from family members (61). The built environment is also associated with activity in this demographic. Access to green space, land use mix, and access to public transit are important determinants of physical activity in older adults (62). In working with older adults, it is important to understand how constructs key to physical activity behavior play a role for their specific life stage. For example, older adults may be more willing to walk in their neighborhood if there are benches along the way that they can use to rest during their journey. This consideration may be especially essential for an older adult with mobility limitations or reduced exercise capacity. Although the presence of local recreational centers may be viewed as a resource of physical activity, for the older adult who may no longer drive or avoids driving during specific times (*e.g.*, nighttime), this resource may not be accessible.

Race/Ethnicity

Although there is significant heterogeneity among members of a racial/ethnic group, racial and ethnic minorities may share values, traditions, and beliefs within their specific cultures that play a role in their participation in physical activity. In one review, barriers to physical activity among African American women included a lack of social support, lack of African American role models, fatigue, and caregiving responsibilities (63). In an examination of factors relating to recruiting older Latinos to physical activity programs, issues of childcare, transportation problems, and challenges attending daytime sessions were reported (64). Among Arab Muslim mothers with young children, barriers were varied but included stress, lack of motivation, responsibilities, the negative perception of women who were physically active, and a dress code that served as a barrier to physical activity participation (65).

SUMMARY

The adoption and maintenance of healthful behaviors, such as exercise, is no easy task. The use of behavioral skills and strategies is critical to assist clients in achieving individual physical activity and health goals. The intervention ideas provided within this chapter are based on sound health behavior change theories and evidence made available through scientific research. When tailored to the client and applied appropriately, these strategies can be effective in facilitating long-term behavior change for a wide array of clients.

STUDY QUESTIONS

1. What is self-monitoring? Provide two examples.
2. What does the acronym SMART stand for in the context of goal setting?
3. What are the four types of social support? Provide examples of each.
4. What is MI? Describe its four guiding principles.
5. What is relapse prevention? Provide physical activity examples.

REFERENCES

1. 2018 Physical Activity Guidelines Advisory Committee. *2018 Physical Activity Guidelines Advisory Committee Scientific Report.* Washington (DC): U.S. Department of Health and Human Services; 2018. 779 p.

2. Rodgers WM, Brawley LR. The influence of outcome expectancy and self-efficacy on the behavioral intentions of novice exercisers. *J Appl Soc Psychol.* 1996;26(7):618–34.

3. Sears SR, Stanton AL. Expectancy-value constructs and expectancy violation as predictors of exercise adherence in previously sedentary women. *Health Psychol.* 2001;20(5):326–33.

4. Shilts MK, Horowitz M, Townsend MS. Goal setting as a strategy for dietary and physical activity behavior change: a review of the literature. *Am J Health Promot.* 2004;19(2):81–93.

5. Locke EA, Latham GP. Building a practically useful theory of goal setting and task motivation: a 35-year odyssey. *Am Psychol.* 2002;57(7):705–17.

6. Strecher VJ, Seijts GH, Kok GJ, et al. Goal setting as a strategy for health behavior change. *Health Educ Q.* 1995;22(2):190–200.

7. Kyllo LB, Landers DM. Goal setting in sport and exercise: a research synthesis to resolve the controversy. *J Sport Exerc Psychol.* 1995;17(2):117–37.

8. Knapp DN. Behavioral management techniques and exercise promotion. In: Dishman RK, editor. *Exercise Adherence: Its Impact on Public Health.* Champaign (IL): Human Kinetics; 1988. p. 203–35.

9. Wing RR, Tate D, LaRose JG, et al. Frequent self-weighing as part of a constellation of healthy weight control practices in young adults. *Obesity.* 2015;23:943–9.

10. Zheng Y, Klem ML, Sereika SM, Danford CA, Ewing LJ, Burke LE. Self-weighing in weight management: a systematic literature review. *Obesity.* 2015;23(2):256–65.

11. Michie S, Abraham C, Whittington C, McAteer J, Gupta S. Effective techniques in healthy eating and physical activity interventions: a meta-regression. *Health Psychol.* 2009;28(6):690–701.

12. Polzien KM, Jakicic JM, Tate DF, Otto AD. The efficacy of a technology-based system in a short-term behavioral weight loss intervention. *Obesity.* 2007;15(4):825–30.

13. Case MA, Burwick HA, Volpp KG, Patel MS. Accuracy of smartphone applications and wearable devices for tracking physical activity data. *JAMA.* 2015;313(6):625–6.

14. Kooiman TJ, Dontje ML, Sprenger SR, Krijnen WP, van der Schans CP, de Groot M. Reliability and validity of ten consumer activity trackers. *BMC Sports Sci Med Rehabil.* 2015;7(1):24.

15. Hekler EB, Buman MP, Grieco L, et al. Validation of physical activity tracking via android smartphones compared to ActiGraph accelerometer: laboratory-based and free-living validation studies. *J Med Internet Res.* 2015;3(2):e36.

16. Nolan M, Mitchell JR, Doyle-Baker PK. Validity of the Apple iPhone®/iPod Touch® as an accelerometer-based physical activity monitor: a proof-of-concept study. *J Phys Act Health.* 2014;11(4):759–69.

17. Kang M, Marshall SJ, Barreira TV, Lee JO. Effect of pedometer-based physical activity interventions: a meta-analysis. *Res Q Exerc Sport.* 2009;80(3):648–55.

18. Tudor-Locke C, Craig CL, Brown WJ, et al. How many steps/day are enough? For adults. *Int J Behav Nutr Phys Act.* 2011;8:79.

19. Tudor-Locke C, Schuna JM. Steps to preventing type 2 diabetes: exercise, walk more, or sit less? *Front Endocrinol.* 2012;3:142.

20. Tudor-Locke C, Craig CL, Aoyagi Y, et al. How many steps/day are enough? For older adults and special populations. *Int J Behav Nutr Phys Act.* 2011;8:80.

21. Tudor-Locke C, Craig CL, Beets MW, et al. How many steps/day are enough? For children and adolescents. *Int J Behav Nutr Phys Act.* 2011;8:78.

22. Tudor-Locke C, Burkett L, Reis JP, Ainsworth BE, Macera CA, Wilson DK. How many days of pedometer monitoring predict weekly physical activity in adults? *Prev Med.* 2005;40(3):293–8.

23. Uchino B. *Social Support and Physical Health: Understanding the Health Consequences of Relationships.* New Haven (CT): Yale University Press; 2004. 234 p.

24. Haber MG, Cohen JL, Lucas T, Baltes BB. The relationship between self-reported received and perceived social support: a meta-analytic review. *Am J Community Psychol.* 2007;39(1–2):133–44.

25. Estabrooks PA. Sustaining exercise participation through group cohesion. *Exerc Sport Sci Rev.* 2000;28(2):63–7.

26. Estabrooks PA, Munroe KJ, Fox EH, et al. Leadership in physical activity groups for older adults: a qualitative analysis. *J Aging Phys Act.* 2004;12(3):232–45.

27. Bandura A. *Self-Efficacy: The Exercise of Control.* New York (NY): Freeman; 1997. 604 p.

28. Kahn EB, Ramsey LT, Brownson R, et al. The effectiveness of interventions to increase physical activity: a systematic review. *Am J Prev Med.* 2002;22(4 Suppl):73–107.

29. Carver CS, Scheier MF. *On the Self-Regulation of Behavior.* New York (NY): Cambridge University Press; 2001. 460 p.

30. Carver CS, Harmon-Jones E. Anger is an approach-related affect: evidence and implications. *Psychol Bull.* 2009;135(2):183–204.

31. Rhodes RE, Kates A. Can the affective response to exercise predict future motives and physical activity behavior? A systematic review of published evidence. *Ann Behav Med.* 2015;49(5):715–31.

32. Williams DM, Dunsiger S, Ciccolo JT, Lewis BA, Albrecht AE, Marcus BH. Acute affective response to a moderate-intensity exercise stimulus predicts physical activity participation 6 and 12 months later. *Psychol Sport Exerc.* 2008;9(3):231–45.

33. Ekkekakis P, Parfitt G, Petruzzello SJ. The pleasure and displeasure people feel when they exercise at different intensities. *Sports Med.* 2011;41(8):641–71.

34. Oliveira B, Deslandes A, Santos T. Differences in exercise intensity seems to influence the affective responses in self-selected and imposed exercise: a meta-analysis. *Front Psychol.* 2015;6:1105.

35. Williams DM, Dunsiger S, Miranda R Jr, et al. Recommending self-paced exercise among overweight and obese adults: a randomized pilot study. *Ann Behav Med.* 2014;49(2);280–5.

36. Freitas LAG, dos Santos Ferreira S, Freitas RQ, de Souza CH, de Abreu Garcia EDS, da Silva SG. Effect of a 12-week aerobic training program on perceptual and affective responses in obese women. *J Phys Ther Sci.* 2015;27(7);2221–4.

37. Baldwin AS, Kangas JL, Denman DC, Smits JA, Yamada T, Otto MW. Cardiorespiratory fitness moderates the effect of an affect-guided physical activity prescription: a pilot randomized controlled trial. *Cogn Behav Ther.* 2016;45(6):445–57.

38. Stevens CJ, Smith JE, Bryan AD. A pilot study of women's affective responses to common and uncommon forms of aerobic exercise. *Psychol Health.* 2016;31(2):239–57.

39. Mitchell M, White L, Lau E, Leahey T, Adams MA, Faulkner G. Evaluating the carrot rewards app, a population-level incentive-based intervention promoting step counts across two Canadian provinces: quasi-experimental study. *JMIR Mhealth Uhealth.* 2018;6(9):e178.

40. Artinian NT, Fletcher GF, Mozaffarian D, et al. Interventions to promote physical activity and dietary lifestyle changes for cardiovascular risk factor reduction in adults: a scientific statement from the American Heart Association. *Circulation.* 2010;122(4):406–41.

41. Martin Ginis KA, Nigg CR, Smith AL. Peer-delivered physical activity interventions: an overlooked opportunity for physical activity promotion. *Transl Behav Med.* 2013;3(4):434–43.

42. Canadian Fitness and Lifestyle Research Institute. Progress in prevention [Internet]. Ottawa, Ontario (Canada): Canadian Fitness and Lifestyle Institute; [cited 2015 Aug 28]. Available from: http://www.cflri.ca/document/bulletin-04 -barriers-physical-activity.

43. Netz Y, Zeev A, Arnon M, Tenenbaum G. Reasons attributed to omitting exercising: a population-based study. *Int J Sport Exerc Psych.* 2008;6:9–23.

44. Heesch KC, Mâsse LC. Lack of time for physical activity: perception or reality for African American and Hispanic women? *Women Health.* 2004;39(3):45–62.

45. Wilcox S, Castro C, King AC, Housemann R, Brownson RC. Determinants of leisure time physical activity in rural compared with urban older and ethnically diverse women in the United States. *J Epidemiol Community Health.* 2000;54(9):667–72.

46. Sabiston CM, Pila E, Pinsonnault-Bilodeau G, Cox AE. Social physique anxiety experiences in physical activity: a comprehensive synthesis of research studies focused on measurement, theory, and predictors and outcomes. *Int Rev Sport Exerc Psychol.* 2014;7(1):158–83.

47. Driediger MV, McKay CD, Hall CR, Echlin PS. A qualitative examination of women's self-presentation and social physique anxiety during injury rehabilitation. *Physiotherapy.* 2015;102(4):371–76.

48. Parks SE, Housemann RA, Brownson RC. Differential correlates of physical activity in urban and rural adults of various socioeconomic backgrounds in the United States. *J Epidemiol Community Health.* 2003;57(1):29–35.

49. Umstattd MR, Baller SL, Hennessy E, et al. Development of the Rural Active Living Perceived Environmental Support Scale (RALPESS). *J Phys Act Health.* 2012;9(5):724–30.

50. Green SH, Glanz K. Development of the perceived nutrition environment measures survey. *Am J Prev Med.* 2015;49(1):50–61.

51. Sharkey JR, Johnson CM, Dean WR, Horel SA. Association between proximity to and coverage of traditional fast-food restaurants and non-traditional fast-food outlets and fast-food consumption among rural adults. *Int J Health Geogr.* 2011;10:37.

52. Prochaska JO. *Systems of Psychotherapy: A Transtheoretical Analysis.* Homewood (IL): Dorsey Press; 1979. 407 p.

53. Marlatt GA, George WH. Relapse prevention: introduction and overview of the model. *Br J Addict.* 1984;79(3):261–73.

54. Dibonaventura MD, Chapman GB. The effect of barrier underestimation on weight management and exercise change. *Psychol Health Med* 2018;13(1):111–22.

55. Miller WR, Rollnick S. *Motivational Interviewing: Preparing People for Change.* New York (NY): Guilford Press; 2002. 428 p.

56. Martins RK, McNeil DW. Review of motivational interviewing in promoting health behaviors. *Clin Psychol Rev.* 2009;29(4):283–93.

57. Rubak S, Sandbaek A, Lauritzen T, Christensen B. Motivational interviewing: a systematic review and meta-analysis. *Br J Gen Pract.* 2005;55(513):305–12.

58. Rollnick S, Miller WR, Butler CC. *Motivational Interviewing in Health Care: Helping Patients Change Behavior.* New York (NY): Guilford Press; 2008. 210 p.

59. Mehra S, Dadema T, Krose BJA, et al. Attitudes of older adults in a group-based exercise program toward a blended intervention: a focus-group study. *Front Psychol* [Internet]. 2016 [cited 2021 Apr 15];7. Available from: https://www .frontiersin.org/articles/10.3389/fpsyg.2016.01827/full.

60. VanRavenstein K, Davis BH. When more than exercise is needed to increase chances of aging in place: qualitative analysis of a telehealth physical activity program to improve mobility in low-income older adults. *JMIR Publications* [Internet]. 2018;1(2). Available from: https://aging.jmir.org/2018/2 /e11955/?utm_source=TrendMD&utm_medium=cpc&utm _campaign=JMIR_Aging_TrendMD_1. doi:10.2196/11955.

61. Smith LG, Banting L, Eime R, O'Sullivan G, van Uffelen JGZ. The association between social support and physical activity in older adults: a systematic review. *Int J Behav Nutr Phys Act.* 2017;14(1):56.

62. Ward M, Gibney S, O'Callaghan D, Shannon S. Age-friendly environments, active lives? Associations between the local physical and social environment and physical activity among adults aged 55 and older in Ireland. *J Aging Phys Act.* 2019;28(1):140–8.

63. Joseph RP, Ainsworth BE, Keller C, Dodgson JE. Barriers to physical activity among African American women: an integrative review of the literature. *Women Health.* 2015;55(6):679–99.

64. Marquez DX, Aguinaga S, Castillo A, Hughes SL, Der Ananian C, Whitt-Glover MC. Ojo! What to expect in recruiting and retaining older Latinos in physical activity programs. *Transl Behav Med* [Internet]. 2020;10(6). Available from: https://academic.oup.com/tbm /article-abstract/10/6/1566/5551322?redirectedFrom= fulltext. doi:10.1093/tbm/ibz127.

65. Benjamin K, Troung Donnelly T. Barriers and facilitators influencing the physical activity of Arabic adults: a literature review. *Avicenna* [Internet]. 2013;2013(1). Available from: https://www.qscience.com/content/journals/10.5339 /avi.2013.8. doi:10.5339/avi.2013.8.

13 Healthy Stress Management

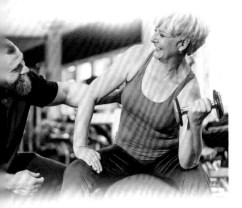

INTRODUCTION

Psychological stress is an enduring and relevant issue for the health/fitness professional. According to the report *Stress in America*, published annually by the American Psychological Association, many U.S. adults report moderate to high levels of stress from a variety of sources (1). This report also corroborates a large literature that has generally found stress to negatively impact emotional and physical health. Specifically, stress has been linked with the common cold; development of chronic illness, including cardiovascular disease and stroke; worsening of autonomic diseases, such as multiple sclerosis (MS); premature death (2); and the development of mental health disorders (3). The connection between stress and health is complex but likely involves physiological influences as well as motivational effects on health behaviors both positive (*e.g.*, exercise and physical activity) and negative (*e.g.*, illicit drug use). A growing literature indicates that exercise has a positive impact on perceptions of stress and also helps to protect people against future episodes of stress (*i.e.*, biological protection) (4). Other stress management techniques have also been successfully used, such as mindfulness meditation, biofeedback, and massage, and can be incorporated into a comprehensive mind–body program.

The Stress Response

Stress is widely used in regular, everyday language. People often use the word *stress* to express uncomfortable situations in life, with phrases such as "I feel stressed out" or "my job is stressful," and the word is often used to refer to pressure or tension (5). From a scientific perspective, stress is defined as the *process* by which one responds to an environmental demand that is perceived as threatening (5). Essentially, stress occurs whenever a stimulus or demand (stressor) taxes one's resources and ability to cope (6). This discrepancy between demands and resources elicits a set of responses to compensate for the threat and restore balance (homeostasis). Responses to stress may be physical (*e.g.*, increased heart rate or blood pressure), behavioral (*e.g.*, increased movement, such as pacing), psychological (*e.g.*, emotional distress), or a combination of these reactions (5).

The classic response to stress is called "fight or flight" (or freeze), which refers to the fact that stress energizes a rapid behavioral response designed to protect the human organism from danger. For example, an encounter with a lion could result in quickly fleeing away, putting up strong efforts to fend off an attack or — if neither of those are good options — perhaps hiding in total stillness. Physical changes that occur with this type of stressor are similar to exercise: rapid increases in heart rate, blood pressure, and a general activation of the sympathetic nervous system. A primitive stressor of this type would likely quickly start and end; however, modern stressors rarely exhibit such qualities. Modern humans experience a number of demands on their time and resources, such as being overextended on commitments and having little support to help. If demands exceed resources over a long period of time, the inability to cope can result in physical or psychological damage (7). Stress encompasses this full process — from demand to response and recovery.

Sources of Stress

Stressors have a diverse set of sources and characteristics. The source of a stressor can come from within the person (*e.g.*, a health problem), the family (*e.g.*, divorce), the community (*e.g.*, crime, traffic), or the society (*e.g.*, civil unrest). Stressors vary in intensity, from mild (*e.g.*, waiting in a long line) to severe (*e.g.*, witnessing the 9/11 tragedy). Stressors differ in their time course, from infrequently to very often. For example, chronic stress is often thought of as the steady accumulation of minor, everyday challenges, such as daily demands from clients or patients at work (8).

Chronic stress could also be described as the long-term grinding kind of stress. Some examples of this might be poverty, demanding jobs with long work hours, or poor relationships (9). The duration of the stressor is not always easy to determine. For example, a major life event may in itself only last seconds, but the repercussions may be long-lasting.

Stressors that are severe, frequent, and of longer duration are considered to be the most impactful and potentially damaging. However, even small incidents in everyday life (*i.e.*, daily hassles) can be perceived as stressful and possibly have a larger effect as they occur consistently over time. That is, recent minor life events, major life events, and traumatic events can add up to form *cumulative adversity*. Thus, any single stressor or event may not be considered a significant disturbance in isolation, but the additive effect of these may be damaging (10).

Importantly, not all stressors are perceived as negative; indeed, some stress is considered favorable and adaptive. Good stress, or eustress, is considered to be a pleasant and stimulating experience that promotes growth, development, and improvement in performance (11). An example of this type of stress might be a marriage, addition to the family, or a job promotion (5). Conversely, bad stress or distress is negative and more likely to be disruptive. An example of this type of stress could include being diagnosed with a chronic illness or loss of employment. However, the perception that an event is stressful depends entirely on the individual and his or her appraisal process and coping resources available to meet the demand.

Appraisal of Stress

According to the transactional model of stress and coping, the impact of a stressor is largely based on one's cognitive appraisal of two components: (a) the event's threat (primary appraisal) and (b) availability of resources (secondary appraisal) (6,12,13). In primary appraisal, individuals gauge both their susceptibility to and the severity of the threat by asking questions such as "What does this mean to me?" and "Will I be in trouble?" These appraisals may, therefore, result in perceptions of positive challenge instead of negative threat (14). For example, a sedentary person starting a new training program may perceive a bout of exercise as unpleasant or unsafe, or he may think of it as a new challenge. With secondary appraisal, one evaluates available resources to control and cope with the stressor to either alter the situation or at least manage the reaction. This includes evaluating (a) resources available to cope with the stressor (perceived control over the threat), (b) emotional reaction (perceived control over feelings), and (c) the ability to identify and use resources to manage stress (coping self-efficacy) (15). For example, exercise may be less threatening if a new exerciser perceives that she has adequate resources to deal with the experience (*e.g.*, plenty of water, time to take breaks), the ability to manage emotions (*e.g.*, minimize anxiety or discomfort), and the ability to manage these resources (*e.g.*, use of a smartphone application, ability to approach someone for guidance). Each of these is a part of the coping process — a process that is critical for understanding the impact of a given demand on each person's response.

Coping

Coping is what people do to alleviate, eliminate, or manage stress. Coping is an ongoing, dynamic process that involves continuous appraisals and reappraisals of the shifting person–environment relationship (6). In general, to neutralize or reduce stress, a person will attempt to change the demands, their perception of it, or the meaning of the stressor. The transactional model of stress and coping suggests that appraisals influence and predict the specific coping processes used (6). According to the original model, coping efforts were conceptualized in two dimensions: problem management (*i.e.*, problem-focused coping) and emotional regulation (*i.e.*, emotion-focused coping).

Problem-Focused Coping

In problem-focused coping, the person attempts to modify the stressor by either reducing the demands or expanding his or her resources to deal with it (14). This type of coping may include actively seeking out information, talking with a professional or friend to get advice, or drawing from previous experience and knowledge to brainstorm, weigh alternatives, and make plans — all in an attempt to resolve the problem (15). Using an example of a person who is stressed due to lack of time, examples of problem-focused coping might include negotiating work hours to get out early for the gym, learning new life skills (*e.g.*, time management, assertiveness training) and exercise skills (high-intensity interval training [HIIT] to shorten the workout), identifying someone who has expertise in the problem area (*e.g.*, personal trainer), or seeking out a job that is less draining on time and energy (14). This type of coping is most often used when people believe that either the personal resources or the demands of the situation are changeable (6), thereby resulting in the perception of control and self-efficacy (15).

Emotion-Focused Coping

Emotional regulation is a more passive coping effort where the person attempts to control or manage the emotional response to a stressful event, particularly one that is difficult to change. In the 2017 *Stress in America* report, more than one-half of respondents reported exercise/walking to deal with stress. Respondents also endorsed listening to music, praying, smoking, and meditating to manage stress (in that order). The key difference from problem-focused coping is that the person is trying to modify his or her emotional response rather than attempting to change the stressor or challenge. People tend to use emotion-focused coping when they believe that the circumstances they are facing are fixed and they cannot change their stressful condition (6). When a stressor is appraised as uncontrollable and highly threatening, individuals often adopt disengaging or passive coping strategies (16). One may attempt to alter thoughts about the stressful situation by denying, distancing, and avoiding the situation (15). Unfortunately, escape-avoidance behavior (*e.g.*, hiding feelings, refusing to think about the situation) has been associated with higher levels of psychological distress and poorer quality of life (17,18). Accepting responsibility (which involves acknowledging the role one has played in the situation and trying to make things right) and positive reappraisal (which involves choosing to create a positive meaning from the situation rather than a negative meaning) are more effective techniques. Recent evidence indicates that suppressing thoughts about the stressful event and the experience of the event have no positive impact on coping with feelings (19). Conversely, reappraising the emotional stimulus and using cognitive techniques like perspective taking are the most effective (19).

Depending on the individual and the situation, a person may be more inclined to engage either in problem-focused or in emotion-focused coping (20,21). However, both may be necessary and can be used in combination to manage emotions and engage in active problem solving.

The Physiological and Psychological Response to Stress

Stress has a variety of interrelated effects on physical, mental, emotional, and behavioral function. Physiological and psychological strain, if severe or prolonged, can negatively affect health, increase illness vulnerability, and worsen disease progression and morbidity (8).

General Adaptation Syndrome and Allostasis

The physiological stress response of the body was first theorized by Hans Selye (24), who later became known as the father of stress research. His research identified a response pattern of stress

HOW TO | **Help Clients Manage Stress Caused by Fitness Testing**

One common stressor in the health/fitness setting is a fitness or body composition assessment. For some, this may be a time of excitement about starting (or completing) a training program. Others may experience feelings of threat and dread. In a study investigating the response to body composition testing with dual-energy x-ray absorptiometry (DXA), all participants had a decline in positive affect (*e.g.*, enthusiasm, high energy, alertness) (22). Seeing an image that depicts body fat may create a sense of displeasure for anyone. However, an increase in negative affect (*e.g.*, distress, anger, guilt) was only observed for overweight and obese individuals, for whom feedback about body fat may have been a particularly threatening experience. Later research (23) suggests that this negative emotional response may actually undermine future motivation for exercise and diet. Specifically, those with a negative response reported eating significantly greater amounts of calorie dense and highly palatable foods in the week following testing (23). This suggests that exercise physiologists must be aware of the potential of their feedback to increase a client's stress and undermine health goals. It is important to help the client cope with health-related feedback through both problem-focused (*e.g.*, choosing an appropriate exercise program) and emotion-focused (*e.g.*, encouragement) efforts.

common across all species known as the general adaptation syndrome (GAS). This concept refers to the rapid activation of bodily systems to cope with a stressor and restore homeostasis as effectively and efficiently as possible. The GAS consists of three broad stages: alarm, resistance, and exhaustion, although the specific response depends on individual characteristics (*e.g.*, fitness, personality) and appraisal of the stressor characteristics. Selye (24) proposed the first stage called the *alarm reaction*, where the stressor is first recognized by the system and a fight-or-flight response is initiated. The second stage is that of *resistance*, where a cascade of cardiovascular, metabolic, hormonal, and immune changes is generated as a compensatory stress reaction (14). During this stage, some compensatory reactions may include the release of glucocorticoids (*e.g.*, cortisol), the activation of the hypothalamic–pituitary–adrenal (HPA) axis, and changes in autonomic neurotransmitters and inflammatory cytokines (25). The last stage is that of *exhaustion*, when the organism has depleted all biochemical substrates and additional resources and is no longer able to mount a defense to the stressor (24). If the stressor continues and activation of these systems is extended for a long period, the bodily systems can eventually break down and result in dysfunction of major organs (*e.g.*, heart or brain). In extreme situations, stress-related exhaustion has the capacity to result in serious illness or death (24).

The impact of repeated stress exposure can be problematic because individuals who remain in the resistance phase often have difficulty withstanding additional challenges (24). Unfortunately, GAS does not adequately explain chronic effects of stress and their consequences. A new concept, called allostasis, describes the ability to achieve stability through changing conditions (8). The concept of allostasis recognizes that all of the systems in the body are involved in the stress response and work to achieve homeostasis, including the autonomic nervous system and HPA axis along with the cardiovascular, immune, and metabolic systems (8). If stressors begin to accumulate, overstimulating allostatic systems without adequate rest and recovery, a person may begin to experience excessive wear and tear (*allostatic load*) where stress responses become dysregulated and ineffective (25), increasing the risk of the development of physical ailments such as cardiovascular disease (CVD) (26–28). Sometimes, the body is unable to stop or shut off the stress response even after the stressor has ended. When this occurs, the systems can be driven to exhaustion resulting in the breakdown of feedback mechanisms and overexposure to stress hormones such as cortisol (26). For example, there is evidence that those experiencing higher levels of chronic, unremitting stress have difficulty recovering from strenuous resistance exercise, taking two to four times as long

EXERCISE IS MEDICINE CONNECTION

Exe℞cise is Medicine®

Stress and Recovery, Implications for Exercise and Adaptation

How people respond to a bout of exercise is also impacted by the experience of stress in their lives. The stress response can essentially be divided into two phases, reactivity and recovery (return to homeostasis). The physical and metabolic stress of exercise results in decrements of function initially. For instance, after completing a vigorous bout of resistance training, muscles that have been exercised will be fatigued and unable to generate high force. Such a response is typically followed by quick rebound and adaptation. However, these processes and the speed of recovery can vary greatly between individuals, from 24 to 96 hours for recovery. Chronic psychological stress includes things navigating the challenges of the coronavirus disease 2019 (COVID-19) pandemic, difficulty managing school and personal responsibilities, and an unhealthy relationship. College students who reported higher chronic stress also had much slower recovery from heavy resistance training (29,30). That is, even though they did the same challenging bout of exercise (multiple repetitions on a leg press machine), they needed almost 4 days to fully recover from the activity. In contrast, a person reporting lower stress recovered in about 1 day. Such an effect may help to account for why some individuals respond to exercise with positive adaptations, whereas others have little to no change (31). Indeed, those reporting higher chronic stress have been shown to gain less strength over a multimonth resistance training program (32). Some of this may be due to interference from the stress response. That is, higher cortisol levels may undermine recovery. It may also be due to how these people cope with stress (*e.g.*, problems with sleep, or change in diet). Regardless, it is important for exercise physiologists to be aware of the stress of their clients and how this might impact their training.

to recover as those reporting lower levels of chronic stress (see "Exercise is Medicine Connection" box) (29,30). Repeated training bouts when in a state of inadequate recovery can easily lead to overreaching, overtraining, and burnout — ultimately resulting in a lack of optimal performance. This also may explain the link between stress and health outcomes.

The Effects of Stress on Health

Stress has consistently been related to poor physical and mental health (10,11). The physical changes in response to chronic or intense stress can lead to, contribute to, or worsen life-threatening and life-altering conditions such as myocardial infarction, stroke, cancer, or autonomic diseases. The American Institute of Stress (33) has compiled a list of signs and symptoms of excessive stress (Table 13.1), including physical, emotional, and behavioral responses and conditions. Some of these symptoms are relatively mild, such as blushing and headaches, whereas others are serious, such as social isolation and excessive drug use. The following sections describe some of the most common stress-related health problems.

Digestive Issues

Ulcers, inflammatory bowel disease, and irritable bowel syndrome are all disorders in the digestive tract that are influenced by stress (14). Ulcers are due to an increase in gastric juices and erosion of the

Table 13.1 Signs and Symptoms of Excessive Stress

1. Frequent headaches, jaw clenching, or pain	26. Insomnia, nightmares, disturbing dreams
2. Gritting, grinding teeth	27. Difficulty concentrating, racing thoughts
3. Stuttering or stammering	28. Trouble learning new information
4. Tremors, trembling of lips, hands	29. Forgetfulness, disorganization, confusion
5. Neck ache, back pain, muscle spasms	30. Difficulty in making decisions
6. Light-headedness, faintness, dizziness	31. Feeling overloaded or overwhelmed
7. Ringing, buzzing, or popping sounds	32. Frequent crying spells or suicidal thoughts
8. Frequent blushing, sweating	33. Feelings of loneliness or worthlessness
9. Cold or sweaty hands, feet	34. Little interest in appearance, punctuality
10. Dry mouth, problems swallowing	35. Nervous habits, fidgeting, feet tapping
11. Frequent colds, infections, herpes sores	36. Increased frustration, irritability, edginess
12. Rashes, itching, hives, "goose bumps"	37. Overreaction to petty annoyances
13. Unexplained or frequent "allergy" attacks	38. Increased number of minor accidents
14. Heartburn, stomach pain, nausea	39. Obsessive or compulsive behavior
15. Excess belching, flatulence	40. Reduced work efficiency or productivity
16. Constipation, diarrhea	41. Lies or excuses to cover up poor work
17. Difficulty breathing, sighing	42. Rapid or mumbled speech
18. Sudden attacks of panic	43. Excessive defensiveness or suspiciousness
19. Chest pain, palpitations	44. Problems in communication, sharing
20. Frequent urination	45. Social withdrawal and isolation
21. Poor sexual desire or performance	46. Constant tiredness, weakness, fatigue
22. Excess anxiety, worry, guilt, nervousness	47. Frequent use of over-the-counter drugs
23. Increased anger, frustration, hostility	48. Weight gain or loss without diet
24. Depression, frequent, or wild mood swings	49. Increased smoking, alcohol, or drug use
25. Increased or decreased appetite	50. Excessive gambling or impulse buying

Source: Adapted with permission from The American Institute of Stress. Stress effects [Internet]. Weatherford (TX): The American Institute of Stress. Available from: http://www.stress.org/stress-effects/.

lining of the stomach or upper small intestine. Inflammatory bowel disease may involve inflammation of the colon and small intestine, whereas irritable bowel syndrome may involve diarrhea, constipation, and abdominal pain (14). The connection between stress and digestive tract problems has been linked to alternations in bacterial growth in the gut, but many other mechanisms likely play a role (34).

Headaches

Intense headaches can also be a physical disorder that results from exposure to chronic stress. The two most common recurrent headaches are migraines and tension-type headaches (35,36). Migraines are typified by intense throbbing and pulsating sensations in the head, often accompanied by sensations of nausea and sensitivity to stimuli. Stress is the most common trigger for the development of migraines but may also magnify the effects of migraines (37). Tension-type headaches are the result of the contraction and tightening of muscles in the neck and head, which is a common reaction of persons under stress (14). In both cases, the strain of the headache itself becomes a stressor, necessitating a coping response, the selection of which may have effects on choices to be physically active or sedentary (38).

Cardiovascular and Metabolic Diseases and the Role of Cortisol

Unresolved chronic stress profoundly affects the cardiovascular system, including the heart, blood vessels, and blood itself (39). High levels of stress have been associated with abnormally enlarged hearts and hypertension (40). These changes in the heart and blood vessels can increase cardiovascular reactivity to a stressor, which is considered a risk factor for the development of coronary heart disease (41,42). Persons under stress have higher concentrations of activated platelets (43,44) and more triglycerides, free fatty acids, and lipoproteins in the blood (45–47), which promote the development of plaques in the arteries or atherosclerosis leading to increased blood pressure and increased likelihood of myocardial infarction and stroke (14). High concentrations of cortisol in the blood over time can increase the risks of cardiovascular disease (26,45). In addition, by blocking the uptake of glucose from the cells, high levels of cortisol increase insulin resistance and can lead to the development of Type 2 diabetes (45). Cortisol also contributes to the accumulation of fat in the abdominal region, and this visceral fat is readily released into the bloodstream. Overall, stress can have a major impact on the functioning of the cardiovascular and metabolic systems and can lead to the development and progression of cardiovascular pathologies.

Immune Suppression, Cancer, and Multiple Sclerosis

The immune systems of persons exposed to chronic, severe stress are often suppressed, rendering a person more vulnerable to infections and susceptible to disease (48). Sympathetic nervous system activity and the release of cortisol after a stressful event suppress the immune system, which limits the number of lymphocytes that are activated in response to a viral challenge (49). For example, people who were exposed to the common cold virus and also reported high stress developed cold symptoms at nearly twice the rate of who had low stress (50). Similarly, psychological stress has been correlated with a reduction in and activity of natural killer (NK) cells, which combat cancerous tumor cells and monitor neoplastic (new and abnormal) growth (51–53). Specific stressors — such as loss of social support — have been found to influence the course of cancer (9). Depression, stress, and trauma have all adversely affected disease progression in patients with HIV (54,55), and recent stressful life events are associated with relapse incidence of MS (56,57). Overall, the functioning of the immune system in fighting off viruses, infections, cancer, and autonomic diseases can be severely compromised because of stress.

Stress and Psychological Functioning

The impact of stress is not limited to the physical body. Stress can affect psychological well-being, cognitive function, emotion (*e.g.*, distress, negative moods), social involvement, and behavior, such as physical activity and sedentarism (58). There are several psychological conditions that can be influenced by chronic stress such as anxiety, depression, fatigue, insomnia, and burnout, and these conditions can have a profound negative impact on quality of life.

Psychological Distress, Anxiety, and Depression

Chronic stress has been shown to promote psychological distress and the development of psychological disorders (9,59). Research studies have shown that people who report exposure to chronic stress in their marriage, household functioning, parenting, or jobs have an increased likelihood of being psychologically distressed (60). Chronic stress is a greater predictor of depressive symptoms than acute stress, and if it is experienced over 2 years or more, it may lead to the development of depression (61). In addition, chronic stress of any type can magnify the impact of even minimal life events on clinical depression (62). Early life event stressors, such as childhood trauma, may lead to the development of anxiety disorders that last a lifetime because of changes in the brain's circuitry (3).

Fatigue and Burnout

Chronic stress is associated with lower levels of energy, greater levels of fatigue, and general dysregulation of energy systems (30). Persons who continually deal with exposure to high levels of occupational, academic, and/or sport-related stress can develop a psychological response called burnout. Burnout is characterized by physical, mental, and emotional exhaustion (5). Burnout is defined as a debilitating psychological condition brought about by unrelieved work stress, which results in (a) depleted energy reserves, (b) lowered resistance to illness, (c) increased dissatisfactions and pessimism, and (d) increased absenteeism and inefficiency at work (5). Employees who experience burnout may develop a variety of symptoms, including overall work dissatisfaction, lack of energy, insomnia and other sleep problems, tension headaches, ulcers, and dysregulated cortisol responses (5,63).

Cognitive Deficits

High levels of cortisol associated with long or extreme exposure to stress have been related to cognitive impairment, specifically in spatial memory tasks (45,64,65). This may be because the elevated levels of glucocorticoids (*i.e.*, cortisol) are associated with shrinkage and toxic degeneration of the brain's memory center, the hippocampus, in which loss of neurons and their connectivity occurs (59,66–69). Burnout symptoms (described earlier) have been associated with cognitive deficits in everyday life, increased inhibition errors, and variability in performance on attention tasks (70). Fortunately, exercise has the opposite effect, promoting memory, attention, and cognitive performance and delaying the onset of dementia (71,72).

 ## Healthy Stress Management

Although stressful events are unavoidable in daily life, there are several strategies for coping and managing stress. Both cognitive and behavioral approaches can help decrease the negative impact of stress. Not all strategies work for everyone, but exercise physiologists can play an important role in helping clients identify strategies that work best for them.

Exercise

Physical exercise is one of the most cited means of managing stress (73). This recommendation is found in any number of news reports, magazine articles, and blogs. Why would exercise be so effective at managing stress? As was illustrated in the earlier discussion of the GAS and the alarm reaction, the stress response is a set of physiological changes that disrupt homeostasis as it readies the body for action — fight or flight. Unfortunately, most stress is psychological in nature (*e.g.*, exams, relationship problems). Not only are these stressors generally not reduced through physical action — they can be made worse if the action is misplaced. This mismatch between the form of stress and the body's reaction can lead to ongoing disruption of homeostasis that undermines physical and mental health. Thus, one way to think about coping with stress is to find a physical action that can make use of the alarm reaction.

Acute bouts of exercise have been shown to effectively serve this role and reduce the stress response. In addition to reducing stress, single bouts of exercise have also been shown to reduce feelings of anxiety and other negative moods. Although these issues are not the same as stress, they do experience similar improvements in response to exercise. The benefit of exercise for state anxiety is very consistent and occurs with nearly all forms of activity — especially those of moderate to low intensity (74,75). The benefit of exercise to improve mood and reduce stress also applies to resistance exercise (76). Continuous exercise above lactate threshold has consistently been shown to reduce negative moods during exercise (77) because high-intensity exercise may increase somatic components of anxiety during exercise. However, cognitive aspects of anxiety remain unaltered, and both kinds reduce during recovery (78).

What is especially interesting is that exercise may also be of benefit to those who are living with chronic mental health conditions. For example, exercise is effective in helping manage anxiety and mood in those who are clinically depressed (79). In fact, for those with a history of depression, as little as 15 minutes of self-selected cycle exercise was enough to improve mood (80). In addition, exercise training has been associated with reductions in clinical levels of ongoing stress (81). Studies have shown a significant reduction in stress across a range of conditions, from panic disorder (82) to posttraumatic stress disorder (PTSD) (83), and in a variety of populations, including methadone-maintained drug abusers (84). Chronic occupational stress (85) and perceived stress (86) also improve with several months of aerobic training.

Moreover, a bout of exercise, especially higher doses of activity (either high intensity or long duration) can actually reduce a person's physiological response to a later stressor (87). That is, on the days that a person completes a bout of exercise, he or she can expect to have less physiological response to stress for the next hour or two than if he or she had been sedentary.

Despite the benefits of exercise in stress management, the experience of stressors can be a significant barrier to physical activity (58). For example, those reporting high levels of chronic stress experience higher ratings of perceived exertion (RPEs) and pain (88,89). Not surprisingly, those who are less habitual in their exercise routines respond to periods of stress with less physical activity (88). In contrast, those who have strong exercise habits appear to be resilient in the face of stress and maintain their levels of activity (88). This may be due to the use of exercise as a form of coping. Regardless, those who are inconsistently active — and are likely to need help from an exercise professional the most — appear to be the least likely to adhere to an exercise program. This may impact how the exercise prescription should be presented to these individuals. For example, among highly active individuals, enjoyment is the primary motive behind exercise, whereas only a small percentage of highly active individuals report stress management as a reason they exercise (90). Branding exercise for its ability to enhance fun, enjoyment, and challenge may be more important than advocating its therapeutic effects on mental and physical health (91).

Enhancing Social Support

Stress is typically perceived when demands outweigh resources. A key resource is social support. Evidence indicates that social support buffers the harmful physical and mental effects of stress (95). It also enhances well-being and health, regardless of stress levels. Increasing social support can lead to more participation in physical activity and health promoting behaviors. (96).

Four types or functions of social support exist (97):

- *Emotional support* — empathy, love, trust, and caring (*e.g.*, actively listening to concerns; offering encouragement)
- *Instrumental support* — tangible aid and services that directly meet a need (*e.g.*, providing services at no additional cost to client when they are experiencing a traumatic stressor, offering childcare options)

HOW TO Use the Perceived Stress Scale

The most common instrument used to assess perception of chronic stress is the 10-item version of the *Perceived Stress Scale* (PSS-10), which measures stress perceptions over the previous month (92–94).

Brief Instructions and Tips

1. The questions in this scale ask you about your feelings and thoughts during the last month.

2. Beside each item, indicate the frequency of these feelings and thoughts (0 = never, 1 = almost never, 2 = sometimes, 3 = fairly often, and 4 = very often).

3. The best approach is to answer fairly quickly. That is, don't try to count up the number of times you felt a particular way that month but rather choose the option that seems like a reasonable estimate.

4. After completing the questions, use the table called "Perceived Stress Scale Scoring" to determine your score.

Question	Never	Almost Never	Sometimes	Fairly Often	Very Often
1. How often have you been upset because of something that happened unexpectedly?	0	1	2	3	4
2. How often have you felt that you were unable to control the important things in your life?	0	1	2	3	4
3. How often have you felt nervous and "stressed"?	0	1	2	3	4
4. How often have you felt confident about your ability to handle your personal problems?	0	1	2	3	4
5. How often have you felt that things were going your way?	0	1	2	3	4
6. How often have you found that you could not cope with all the things that you had to do?	0	1	2	3	4
7. How often have you been able to control irritations in your life?	0	1	2	3	4
8. How often have you felt that you were on top of things?	0	1	2	3	4
9. How often have you been angered because of things that happened that were outside of your control?	0	1	2	3	4
10. How often have you felt difficulties were piling up so high that you could not overcome them?	0	1	2	3	4

Perceived Stress Scale Scoring

PSS scores are obtained by reversing responses (*e.g.*, 0 = 4, 1 = 3, 2 = 2, 3 = 1, and 4 = 0) to the four positively stated items (items 4, 5, 7, and 8) and then summing across all scale items.

Item	Your Response (0–4)	Reverse Score Needed?	Final Item Score
1		No	
2		No	
3		No	
4		Yes	
5		Yes	
6		No	
7		Yes	
8		Yes	
9		No	
10		No	
		Grand total score →	

Interpretation and Normative Values

The scores can range from 0 to 40, and higher scores reflect a higher level of perceived stress. High scores on the PSS-10 questionnaire have been associated with increased difficulty in making lifestyle changes, such as adopting physical activity, and increased susceptibility to stress-induced illness (58). Men in the United States have an average score of about 12, and women have an average of about 14, but scores significantly vary by race or ethnicity, age, and education (92,94).

- *Informational support* — advice and information concerning the problem (*e.g.*, understanding why an issue is causing significant stress, providing a referral to a mental health professional)
- *Appraisal support* — information useful for self-evaluation purposes such as constructive feedback and affirmation (*e.g.*, helping client brainstorm possible solutions to a problem, providing feedback for problem-solving)

All types of support may be offered by a fitness professional. However, the matching hypothesis suggests that social support is most beneficial when it meets the needs caused by a stressful event (98). See "Exercise is Medicine" box for a real-life example.

The mechanisms for how social support improves health and well-being are not clear. Social support may improve coping responses by reducing uncertainty and unpredictability about a stressful situation. This can, in turn, promote a greater sense of personal control and the use of problem-focused coping methods (99). Social support may also relieve some of the stressor-related demands through a sharing of the burden, prompting more adaptive thoughts and emotions. Regardless, the many forms of social support are an important contributor to the ability of people to cope with stress.

Improving Personal Control and Self-Efficacy

There is evidence that people who have a strong sense of personal control experience less of a negative response, or strain, with stressors compared with those who feel they have no control over their lives (101,102). Individuals who believe that they personally have control over their lives are considered to have an internal locus of control. On the other hand, individuals who believe that

EXERCISE IS MEDICINE CONNECTION

Exe℞ciseisMedicine®

Social Support in Action

Consider this scenario. A client of a certified clinical exercise physiologist (CEP) experienced traumatic flooding of his home midway through a 12-week training phase, forcing the client out of his house with only a small bag of clothing saved. The CEP provided an ideal amount of social support: expressing empathy and genuine concern, placing the training sessions on hold (with no penalty), and providing tips on maintaining fitness when staying out of town. Social aspects of exercise (*e.g.*, walking with a friend) were emphasized to him relieve stress and keep a base level of fitness. Later, the CEP provided feedback on how to reinitiate a serious routine once the client was ready. A referral was also made to a social worker, who provided additional assistance, helped the client to strengthen existing relationships, expand his social network and develop new relationships, and get involved in a self-help group. All of these actions improved social support resources (14,97,99,100) and helped the client to manage his experience of a stressful event without sacrificing his health goals.

their lives are dictated by forces outside of themselves, such as destiny, or fate, have an external locus of control (103,104).

Based on how it may impact health, sense of personal control may be further divided into four different types (14):

1. *Informational control* — when a person can glean knowledge about the stressful event and the potential consequences of the situation
2. *Cognitive control* — when a person can use thought processes and strategies to manipulate and modify the impact of the stressor
3. *Decisional control* — when a person can choose between different courses of action
4. *Behavioral control* — when a person can take concrete action to reduce the impact of stress

These two areas of control have a major impact on health and health practices. For instance, those with a more internal sense of control are more persistent in their exercise behavior (104). When people have a good sense of control, they feel like they are able to effectively make decisions and execute a plan of action to produce the outcome desired (14,105). This points to another aspect of personal control, self-efficacy, which is the belief or conviction that one can successfully execute the specific behavior required to produce the outcomes desired in the current situation (106). When encountering challenging situations, people will actively evaluate their ability (*i.e.*, efficacy) to properly execute behaviors and determine if they think that they can be successful (107). Generally speaking, people who are highly efficacious show less psychological and physiological strain in the face of a stressor than those who are less efficacious (63,108,109). Goal setting and preplanning for stressors are useful strategies help to boost self-efficacy in the face of demanding situations (110).

Mind–Body Techniques for Reducing Stress

Although it is critical for the exercise physiologist to understand the role of exercise as a stress management tool, there are numerous nonexercise techniques that are also successful in helping people cope with stress, reduce arousal, and promote relaxation (111). (See here for a list of up-to-date resources: https://nccih.nih.gov/health/stress.) These mind–body exercises include progressive muscle relaxation, deep breathing, biofeedback, meditation, mindfulness, and massage (among many others). Each of these methods takes practice to master, and several, such as massage, have their own certifications and credentialing. However, aspects of each technique may be learned and integrated into exercise programming. Various techniques may also be combined to suit different people and needs (112). These activities can be readily incorporated during the cool-down and stretching period after exercise when the focus is on relaxation and recovery (39,113) or even performed at home on rest days.

Diaphragmatic Breathing and Body Scans

Breathing exercises are the easiest and fastest methods to induce the relaxation response, with capability to relieve symptoms of stress and anxiety, including headaches, muscle tension, irritability, and fatigue (114). Diaphragmatic breathing, or breathing from the stomach (as opposed to the chest), consists of deep breaths into the lungs and exhaling as the diaphragm contracts and relaxes. A first step is to become aware of normal breathing habits, often while lying down with one hand on the abdomen and another on the chest. A *body scan* may also be employed, where a person consciously examines the entire body, usually starting at the toes and upward toward the scalp. Once awareness has been achieved, the practitioner can assume a "dead man" pose, lying with arms and legs spread and palms facing upward, scanning the body for tension, and relaxing. Then, one may focus the attention on the breath, breathing in through the nose and out through the mouth slowly and in a rhythmic fashion. Even short bouts of diaphragmatic breathing can provide immediately stress relief. Practice over a longer period (*i.e.*, 30–60 min) in the recovery period of exercise has even been shown to decrease free radical production and cortisol (113).

Progressive Muscle Relaxation

Progressive muscle relaxation is a technique that teaches people how to focus on certain muscle groups and alternatively contract and relax these muscles, focusing on the sensation of relaxation (114,115). This helps the individual to identify areas of the body that tighten and hold tension when they are under stress (*e.g.*, jaw clenches, shoulders tighten, and fingers cramp). Once identified, feelings of tension can be targeted and neutralized. With practice, whenever a person feels tension rising in these areas, he or she can stop what he or she is doing for 5–10 minutes, breathe deeply, tighten (5–7 s) and relax the affected muscles (20–30 s), repeat systematically, and then return to his or her work (9,114). Researchers have postulated that progressive muscle relaxation may additionally promote feelings of calmness and generate pleasant thoughts in the individual, which counteract negative feelings and thoughts associated with stress (111).

Biofeedback

Biofeedback is a method of increasing control over bodily processes, such as heart rate, muscle tension, or sweating, in response to a stressor (9,116). Biofeedback has been useful in treating stress-related health problems, such as chronic muscle tension headaches (117). The procedure involves attaching sensors to the body that provide immediate biophysiological feedback on how a person's body is responding to a stressor (*i.e.*, seeing fluctuations in heart rate or electrodermal activity). Individuals are then encouraged to modify their bodily response to the stressor. For instance, one may be asked to slow heart rate by blocking out all sounds and breathing deeply until heart rate returns to normal. This practice helps individuals gain awareness of and attain voluntary control over their stress response. Phone apps may be used to help client learn and practice biofeedback.

Massage

Massage is the external application of pressure to muscles and tendons (see https://nccih.nih.gov /health/massage/massageintroduction.htm). This can range from smooth, light pressure to deep kneading motion, depending on technique (*e.g.*, Swedish, Shiatsu, sports), the purpose of the massage (*e.g.*, relaxation, pain relief, circulation), and individual's preference and pain tolerance. Deep tissue massage is the application of forceful, penetrating pressure that is applied to the muscles and joints by a trained massage therapist. This form of massage is an effective method for reducing stress, anxiety, depression, muscle tension, pain, and asthma symptoms and has been shown to boost immune function (14,118,119). Patients with breast cancer in the earlier stages of the disease have shown positive results after 3 weeks of massage therapy, such as a decrease in anxiety, depression, and anger and an improvement in mood (52). These patients also showed a boost in their dopamine and serotonin levels and number of NK immune cells and lymphocytes, which could potentially promote a better and faster recovery (52). Lastly, an added benefit of massage postexercise is that it may help to reduce delayed-onset muscle soreness (120), but it is still not clear if the combination of exercise and massage produces even greater stress reduction benefits.

Meditation and Prayer

Meditation is an exercise of the mind in which the individual actively focuses on calming and quieting the body while keeping the mind alert (5). There are several forms of meditation: (a) Mantra meditation focuses on sounds and phrases, and the same word or verse is repeated over and over again to promote concentration; (b) yantra meditation uses focus on a visual image to eradicate distracting thoughts from the mind; and (c) transcendental meditation incorporates breathing, visualization, relaxation, and repetition (5). Transcendental meditation has been shown to reduce stress and improve mental and physical health by decreasing blood pressure, heart rate, respiratory response, and stress hormone production (121,122). Use of meditation has also been associated with improved lactate recovery after exercise (123). An alternative to meditation is the practice of prayer, which has been associated with facets of recovery from illness and improved health outcomes (124).

Mindfulness

Mindfulness is the discipline of paying attention to the present moment in a deliberate (purposeful) and nonjudgmental manner (125). It is especially useful during periods of stress, when the mind often dwells on past experiences, current frustrations and hurts, and potential negative consequences. The practice of mindfulness can help restore the mind–body connection, support emotional balance, and enhance functioning at work and in relationships (126). By being in the present moment, without worry about the future or preoccupation with the past, one may observe automatic emotions and behaviors with greater clarity and perspective. This permits deeper awareness about thoughts and feelings, body sensations, and habitual stress reactions, which in turn encourages more healthy choices about health behaviors (125). Mindfulness is more effective than relaxation practices for reducing ruminations and distracting thoughts, enhancing positive states of mind (112), and increasing sense of control (127). To facilitate these changes, practitioners practice acceptance, trust, patience, nonjudgment, having a beginner's mind (*i.e.*, curiosity), nonstriving, and letting go (125). Mindfulness can be performed during daily tasks or during physical exercise by focusing more on (a) the present-moment experience of moving, (b) bodily sensations (such as sweating, the heart rate, breathing), and (c) emotional reactions to such perceptions (such as excitement, fear, pain) (128). In the context of physical activity, some of these exercise sensations and emotions are uncomfortable, but these would be observed and approached with openness and self-compassion and not judged or avoided. Furthermore, attention is not paid to goals, striving, and competition, which can detract from the experience and render exercise less enjoyable.

Yoga and Martial Arts

Some individuals may experience greater stress management with exercise programs that incorporate breath control, mindful movements, and meditative practices. Yoga and martial arts, such as tai chi and qigong, incorporate all these elements. Mindful exercise practices have been shown to promote numerous health benefits, such as increases in positive emotions, dampened cortisol and cardiovascular reactivity, and lower inflammatory responses to stress (129–132). Research indicates that those who regularly practice yoga have substantially reduced serum interleukin 6 levels (one of the primary inflammatory cytokines) compared with novice yoga attendees (66). Sessions of yoga, tai chi, or other martial arts performed routinely are effective for reducing symptoms of stress and improving sense of well-being (129,131,132).

Referring a Client or Patient to a Psychologist

Exercise professionals, such as personal trainers, often find themselves as confidants to their clientele. Consequently, conversations about stressful experiences are quite common. Although these are to be expected, occasionally, clients may deal with stress poorly or in an inappropriate manner. They may (a) display several symptoms, such as those in Table 13.1; (b) communicate feelings of distress, worry, anxiety, or other mental health problems; or (c) verbally expresses a need for support. Under such conditions, referral to a mental health professional may be advisable. When referring a client, make sure to be empathetic. Consider using language outlined in Table 13.2. The American Psychological Association provides a number of resources, including a mental health professional locator (http://locator.apa.org/), if a referral is accepted. Additional resources for stress management are listed in Table 13.3. Most importantly, if a person is suicidal or discusses hurting himself or herself in any way, get professional help immediately.

Table 13.2	Suggested Remarks When Making a Referral to a Mental Health Professional	
Step	**Action**	**Suggested Remark**
1	Start by broaching the topic with a general observation.	"You seem to have a lot of stress."
2	Normalize the context.	"I see a lot of people who are dealing with _____ [fill in the blank]."
3	Emphasize strengths.	"It's good that you are doing some healthy things, such as exercising [and anything else you know they are doing] to help you manage this situation."
4	Suggest that they seek out additional support.	"I know some of my clients have found that getting some extra support to help with [stress, sadness, anxiety, grief, etc.] has been helpful."
5	Obtain permission to make a referral.	"Would you like me to make a recommendation?"
6	If they deny needing additional help, keep the option available for future need.	"I am happy to be a resource for you. You can always contact me later for the information."

Created by Lydia R. Malcolm, PhD.

Table 13.3	Resources for Stress Management	
Organization	**Web Site**	**Description**
NIMH — National Institute of Mental Health	https://www.nimh.nih.gov /health/find-help/index.shtml	Information on mental health disorders, how to locate a treatment provider, and what to do in a crisis
SAMHSA — Substance Abuse and Mental Health Services Administration	https://www.samhsa.gov /find-help/national-helpline	Confidential and free treatment, referral, and information service offered 24/7, 365 d a year
USDHHS — U.S. Department of Health and Human Services	https://www.mentalhealth.gov/	Offers information on suicide prevention, mental health resources for U.S. military veterans, and a consumer guide for government mental health benefits

The Case of Terry

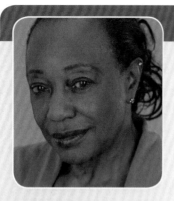

Submitted by **Matthew Stults-Kolehmainen, PhD, FACSM, ACSM-EP, Yale-New Haven Hospital, New Haven, CT, Teachers College Columbia University, New York, NY; and Lydia Malcolm, PhD, Nova Southeastern University, Davie, FL**

Terry is a middle-aged woman attempting to lose weight. Her chief complaint is chronic stress, and she has a history of mild depression. She was referred to an integrated health center by her primary care physician to meet with a licensed psychologist and an American College of Sports Medicine (ACSM) Certified Exercise Physiologist® (ACSM-EP®).

Narrative

Terry is a 55-year-old African American woman was referred to an integrated health center in a midsized urban city by her primary care physician. She is in the obese category for body mass index (BMI) even after numerous attempts to lose weight. She also continues to smoke five to six times a day despite repeated warnings from her doctor. She works full-time and teaches elementary students at a local urban magnet school. Her job requires long hours at work and grading on the weekends and can be very stressful. She suffers from mild depression (diagnosis is "depressive disorder not otherwise specified"), which began after her husband died 3 years ago. In particular, she reports that she has difficulty experiencing pleasure from things she used to enjoy. She has a good relationship with her adult daughter, who lives locally.

Before her husband became sick, she reported that she and her husband were very active hikers and walked daily for exercise at a leisurely pace, which was her preference. During her last attempt to be physically active, she maintained a personal training program (mostly resistance training, 2 times a week) for 8 weeks until her apartment was broken into, disrupting her routine. She finished a 12-week program but with great struggle — citing a crash in motivation. Subsequently, she cancelled her gym membership, and she has been inactive for about a year. However, she averages about 7,500 steps a day (Monday to Friday) because of her occupational work. On weekends, she averages about 4,000 steps a day. Her wrist-worn activity tracker indicates that she sleeps about 5 hours per night on weeknights and 7 hours on weekends. Fortunately, she is metabolically healthy (*e.g.*, normal cholesterol and blood sugar), and her only other complaint is some mild symptoms of arthritis. She has no family history of cardiovascular disease.

Based on her clinical intake and interest to lose weight and increase fitness, she was assigned to a licensed psychologist and exercise physiologist (ACSM-EP) for further evaluation, risk stratification, and treatment. The psychologist screened for mental health problems and shared the results with the exercise physiologist. At intake, she reported that her goals were to lose 15 lb (returning to weight 3 yr ago; approximately 165 lb), increase fitness, improve her mental well-being, and maintain independence going into retirement.

Health/Fitness Examination

PSS-10: Terry scored 20 (see box earlier for an interpretation).

Centers for Epidemiology Depression Scale (Revised): Terry scored 19 and did not meet or exceed the cutoff for major depression based on other criteria.

Exercise Risk Stratification: moderate (*i.e.*, obesity, smoking, sedentarism, age)

Vitals

Age: 55 years; resting HR: 64 bpm, 66 bpm (second visit); resting BP: 119/63 mm Hg, 124/64 mm Hg (second visit); height: 64 in; weight: 178.5 lb, 180.8 lb (second visit); BMI: 30.6, 31.0 (second visit)

Cardiorespiratory Fitness and Body Composition

YMCA Submaximal Cycle Ergometer Test predicted aerobic capacity = 29 mL · kg^{-1} · min^{-1}, 45th percentile for age and gender

Body fat estimated with bioelectrical impedance (Tanita model TBF-300 WA) = 40.0%, 39.8% (second visit)

Waist circumference = 99.5 cm, 99.0 cm (second visit)

Hip circumference = 110.4 cm, 109.5 cm (second visit)

Exercise Recommendations

First, it would be appropriate to reinforce good habits that Terry already has. She is tracking her steps, and she gets a moderate amount of occupational activity. This is a good place to start. Building on her knowledge of steps as they relate to physical activity and exercise is appropriate. She is inactive on the weekends, but not terribly busy, so these days could be targeted first. A good goal might be to increase steadily from 4,000 a day to 4,500 a day and then to 5,000, 6,000, and higher over the next 4+ weeks. These steps can be accumulated from a variety of sources and not just exercise. However, because she is willing to engage in a new formal exercise routine, it is recommended that Terry start with a light- to moderate-exercise program (her preference for intensity) that also increases in volume and intensity progressively, focusing on activities that she enjoys. Going to the gym every day is not likely, so adding some days (*e.g.*, 3 d · wk^{-1}) where she walks outside and 2 days at the gym for resistance training might be a good combination. Consequently, encouraging her to reactivate her old gym membership is a good idea because she can probably more easily navigate the logistics of returning to her old gym. Alternatively, she might want to find a new program that she finds motivating. Perhaps, she can contact her former trainer for a reasonably priced training package to get started. This would help to take advantage of social support as well. Recruiting her daughter to go on walks with her would be a good idea. On days that she struggles, she should be advised not to give up on her exercise routine. Even short walks of 5- to 10-minute duration can help lower feelings of stress and boost mood. Such walks can be done mindfully for an even more powerful stress reduction effect.

QUESTIONS

- What testing and outcome measures may be appropriate in this case besides health/fitness testing?
- Are there indications for use of exercise in clients with chronic stress and mild depression?
- Suggest an alternative exercise program to the one recommended earlier. How might this program be structured, and what additional resources may be needed for a client such as Terry?

References

1. American College of Sports Medicine. *ACSM's Guidelines for Exercise Testing and Prescription.* 11th ed. Philadelphia (PA): Wolters Kluwer; 2022. 548 p.
2. Carek PJ, Laibstain SE, Carek SM. Exercise for the treatment of depression and anxiety. *Int J Psychiatry Med.* 2011;41(1):15–28.
3. Lavie CJ, Milani RV, O'Keefe JH, Lavie TJ. Impact of exercise training on psychological risk factors. *Prog Cardiovasc Dis.* 2011;53(6):464–70.
4. Stults-Kolehmainen M, Malcolm LR, DiLoreto J, Gunnet-Shoval K, Rathbun EI. Psychological interventions for weight management: a primer for the allied health professional. *ACSMs Health Fit J.* 2015;19(5):16–22.

SUMMARY

Stress is an everyday facet of life that must be managed. The perception of an event as stressful greatly depends on the person and his or her perceived resources to deal with the stressors. Situations that are perceived to be stressful may result in a variety of physical and mental symptoms, including burnout, fatigue, headaches, gastrointestinal problems, muscular pain, and greater risk for infections. Long-term chronic stressors can increase the risk of cardiovascular disease, heart attacks, stroke, and cancer. Contrary to popular belief, stress is not always negative. Stress can act as a positive challenge that encourages individuals to rise to the occasion and possibly even face their fears or anxieties. The health/fitness professional can assist clients in identifying a variety of methods for buffering and decreasing the negative impact of stress on the individual. Some tactics and strategies focus on changing the psychological perception of a stressor and others on decreasing the physiological response to a stressor. Research has demonstrated exercise to be an effective stress management strategy, and only 10–15 minutes of moderate aerobic activity, such as a brisk walk, may provide stress-relieving benefits (133). A challenge for the exercise physiologist is to minimize the psychological toll of exercise itself, which may be perceived as yet another task added to an already full plate. Indeed psychological stress is associated with impaired efforts to be physically active (58). A multifaceted approach is important for successful stress management but does require the exercise physiologist to be more mindful of the complexity of the stress experience.

STUDY QUESTIONS

1. Understanding stress: What is stress? How is stress different from *stressors*? Are all stressors bad? What are some examples of good stress? What is the feeling of being *stressed out*, and how does it relate to distress?

2. Explain the two coping mechanisms that can be implemented to minimize the impact of stress. Where does exercise fit?

3. Discuss the consequences of stress on the development and progression of disease and evidence that exercise may buffer this relationship.

4. Before encountering a stressful event, how can a person prepare to manage the event and avoid becoming stressed?

5. What are examples of healthy stress management? Discuss three techniques or approaches for handling and decreasing perceived stress, the potential benefits of each, and how they might be integrated into a fitness program.

REFERENCES

1. American Psychological Association. *Stress in America*. Washington (DC): American Psychological Association; 2019. 9 p.

2. Cohen S, Janicki-Deverts D, Miller GE. Psychological stress and disease. *J Am Med Assoc*. 2007;298(14):1685–7.

3. McEwen BS, Eiland L, Hunter RG, Miller MM. Stress and anxiety: structural plasticity and epigenetic regulation as a consequence of stress. *Neuropharmacology*. 2012;62(1):3–12.

4. Berger BG, Tobar DA. Physical activity and quality of life: key considerations. In: Tenenbaum G, Eklund RC, editors. *Handbook of Sport Psychology*. 3rd ed. Hoboken (NJ): Wiley; 2007. 960 p.

5. Rout UR, Rout JK. *Stress Management for Primary Health Care Professionals*. New York (NY): Kluwer Academic; 2002. 218 p.

6. Lazarus RS, Folkman S. *Stress, Appraisal and Coping*. New York (NY): Springer; 1984. 445 p.

7. Selye H. *The Stress of Life*. Revised ed. New York (NY): McGraw-Hill; 1976. 515 p.

8. McEwen BS. Protective and damaging effects of stress mediators. *N Engl J Med*. 1998;338(3):171–9.

9. Taylor SE. *Health Psychology.* 8th ed. New York (NY): McGraw-Hill; 2012. 576 p.

10. Stults-Kolehmainen MA, Tuit K, Sinha R. Lower cumulative stress is associated with better health for physically active adults in the community. *Stress.* 2014;17(2):157–68. doi:10.3109/10253890.2013.878329.

11. McFarlane AH, Norman GR, Streiner DL, Roy RG. The process of social stress — stable, reciprocal, and mediating relationships. *J Health Soc Behav.* 1983;24(2):160–73. doi:10.2307/2136642.

12. Cohen F, Lazarus RS. Coping and adaptation in health and illness. In: Mechanic D, editor. *Handbook of Health, Health Care, and the Health Professions.* New York (NY): Free Press; 1983. 806 p.

13. Lazarus RS. *Stress and Emotion: A New Synthesis.* New York (NY): Springer; 1999. 360 p.

14. Sarafino EP. *Health Psychology: Biopsychosocial Interactions.* 4th ed. New York (NY): Wiley; 2002. 599 p.

15. Glanz K SM. Stress, coping, and health behavior. In: Glanz K, Rimer B, Viswanath K, editors. *Health Behavior and Health Education: Theory, Research, and Practice.* 4th ed. San Francisco (CA): Jossey-Bass; 2008. p. 209–36.

16. Taylor SE, Kemeny ME, Aspinwall LG, Schneider SG, Rodriguez R, Herbert M. Optimism, coping, psychological distress, and high-risk sexual-behavior among men at risk for Acquired-Immunodeficiency-Syndrome (AIDS). *J Pers Soc Psychol.* 1992;63(3):460–73. doi:10.1037//0022-3514.63.3.460.

17. Baider L, Perry S, Sison A, Holland J, Uziely B, DeNour AK. The role of psychological variables in a group of melanoma patients — an Israeli sample. *Psychosomatics.* 1997;38(1):45–53.

18. Trask PC, Paterson AG, Hayasaka S, Dunn RL, Riba M, Johnson T. Psychosocial characteristics of individuals with non-stage IV melanoma. *J Clin Oncol.* 2001;19(11):2844–50.

19. Webb TL, Miles E, Sheeran P. Dealing with feeling: a meta-analysis of the effectiveness of strategies derived from the process model of emotion regulation. *Psychol Bull.* 2012;138(4):775–808. doi:10.1037/a0027600.

20. Folkman S, Lazarus RS. Coping as a mediator of emotion. *J Pers Soc Psychol.* 1988;54(3):466–75. doi:10.1037/0022-3514.54.3.466.

21. Folkman S, Lazarus RS, Dunkelschetter C, Delongis A, Gruen RJ. Dynamics of a stressful encounter — cognitive appraisal, coping and encounter outcomes. *J Pers Soc Psychol.* 1986;50(5):992–1003. doi:10.1037//0022-3514.50.5.992.

22. Faries MD, Boroff CS, Stults-Kolehmainen M, Bartholomew JB. Does a visual representation impact the affective response to body composition testing? *Pers Individ Dif.* 2011;50(4):502–5.

23. Faries MD, Kephart W, Jones EJ. Approach, avoidance and weight-related testing: an investigation of frontal EEG asymmetry. *Psychol Health Med.* 2015. doi:10.1080/13548506.2014.959530.

24. Selye H. *The Stress of Life.* New York (NY): McGraw-Hill; 1956. 324 p.

25. McEwen BS, Wingfield JC. The concept of allostasis in biology and biomedicine. *Horm Behav.* 2003;43(1):2–15. doi:10.1016/s0018-506x(02)00024-7.

26. Lundberg U. Coping with stress: neuroendocrine reactions and implications for health. *Noise Health.* 1999;1(4):67–74.

27. McEwen BS, Stellar E. Stress and the individual — mechanisms leading to disease. *Arch Intern Med.* 1993;153(18):2093–101. doi:10.1001/archinte.153.18.2093.

28. Pike JL, Smith TL, Hauger RL, et al. Chronic stress alters sympathetic, neuroendocrine, and immune responsivity to an acute psychological stressor in humans. *Psychosom Med.* 1997;59(4):447–57.

29. Stults-Kolehmainen MA, Bartholomew JB. Psychological stress impairs short-term muscular recovery from resistance exercise. *Med Sci Sports Exer.* 2012;44(11):2220–7. doi:10.1249/MSS.0b013e31825f67a0.

30. Stults-Kolehmainen MA, Bartholomew JB, Sinha R. Chronic psychological stress impairs recovery of muscular function and somatic sensations over a 96 hour period. *J Strength Cond Res.* 2014;28(7):2007–17. doi:10.1519/JSC.0000000000000335.

31. Mann TN, Lamberts RP, Lambert MI. High responders and low responders: factors associated with individual variation in response to standardized training. *Sports Med.* 2014;44(8):1113–24. doi:10.1007/s40279-014-0197-3.

32. Bartholomew JB, Stults-Kolehmainen MA, Elrod CC, Todd JS. Strength gains after resistance training: the effect of stressful, negative life events. *J Strength Cond Res.* 2008;22(4):1215–21. doi:10.1519/JSC.0b013e318173d0bf.

33. American Institute of Stress. 50 Common signs and symptoms of stress. Fort Worth (TX): American Institute of Stress; [cited 2015 Sep 29]. Available from: http://www.stress.org/stress-effects/.

34. Mayer EA. The neurobiology of stress and gastrointestinal disease. *Gut.* 2000;47(6):861–9. doi:10.1136/gut.47.6.861.

35. Lipton RB, Silberstein SD, Stewart WF. An update on the epidemiology of migraine. *Headache.* 1994;34(6):319–28. doi:10.1111/j.1526-4610.1994.hed3406319.x.

36. Pothmann R, Frankenberg SV, Müller B, Sartory G, Hellmeier W. Epidemiology of headache in children and adolescents: evidence of high prevalence of migraine among girls under 10. *Int J Behav Med.* 1994;1(1):76–89. doi:10.1207/s15327558ijbm0101_5.

37. Sauro KM, Becker WJ. The stress and migraine interaction. *Headache.* 2009;49(9):1378–86.

38. Lake AE. Headache as a stressor: dysfunctional versus adaptive coping styles. *Headache.* 2009;49(9):1369–77.

39. Stults-Kolehmainen MA. The interplay between stress and physical activity in the prevention and treatment of cardiovascular disease. *Front Physiol.* 2013;(4):346. doi:10.3389/fphys.2013.00346.

40. Schnall PL, Pieper C, Schwartz JE, et al. The relationship between job strain, workplace diastolic blood-pressure, and left ventricular mass index: results of a case-control study. *JAMA.* 1990;263(14):1929–35. doi:10.1001/jama.263.14.1929.

41. Manuck SB. Cardiovascular reactivity in cardiovascular disease: "once more unto the breach". *Int J Behav Med.* 1994;1(1):4–31. doi:10.1207/s15327558ijbm0101_2.

42. Sherwood A, Turner JR. Hemodynamic responses during psychological stress: implications for studying disease

processes. *Int J Behav Med.* 1995;2(3):193–218. doi:10.1207/s15327558ijbm0203_1.

43. Malkoff SB, Muldoon MF, Zeigler ZR, Manuck SB. Blood-platelet responsivity to acute mental stress. *Psychosom Med.* 1993;55(6):477–82.

44. Patterson SM, Zakowski SG, Hall MH, Cohen L, Wollman K, Baum A. Psychological stress and platelet activation: differences in platelet reactivity in healthy mean during active and passive stressors. *Health Psychol.* 1994;13(1):34–8. doi:10.1037/0278-6133.13.1.34.

45. Lundberg U. Stress hormones in health and illness: the roles of work and gender. *Psychoneuroendocrinology.* 2005;30(10):1017–21.doi:10.1016/j.psyneuen.2005.03.014.

46. Patterson SM, Matthews KA, Allen MT, Owens JF. Stress-inducted hemoconcentration of blood-cells and lipids in healthy women during acute psychological stress. *Health Psychol.* 1995;14(4):319–24. doi:10.1037/0278-6133.14.4.319.

47. Vitaliano PP, Russo J, Niaura R. Plasma lipids and their relationships with psychological factors in older adults. *J Gerontol Ser B-Psychol Sci Soc Sci.* 1995;50(1):P18–24.

48. Cohen S, Frank E, Doyle WJ, Skoner DP, Rabin BS, Gwaltney JM. Types of stressors that increase susceptibility to the common cold in healthy adults. *Health Psychol.* 1998;17(3):214–23.

49. Lovallo WR. *Stress & Health: Biological and Psychological Interactions.* 2nd ed. Thousand Oaks (CA): Sage; 2005. 296 p.

50. Cohen S, Tyrrell DAJ, Smith AP. Psychological stress and susceptibility to the common cold. *N Engl J Med.* 1991;325:606–12.

51. Glaser R, Rice J, Stout JC, Speicher CE, Kiecoltglaser JK. Stress depresses interferon production by leukocytes concomitant with a decrease in natural-killer cell-activity. *Behav Neurosci.* 1986;100(5):675–8. doi:10.1037/0735-7044.100.5.675.

52. Hernandez-Reif M, Ironson G, Field T, et al. Breast cancer patients have improved immune and neuroendocrine functions following massage therapy. *J Psychosom Res.* 2004;57(1):45–52. doi:10.1016/s0022-3999(03)00500-2.

53. Locke SE, Kraus L, Leserman J, Hurst MW, Heisel JS, Williams RM. Life change stress, psychiatric symptoms and natural killer cell activity. *Psychosom Med.* 1984;46(5):441–53.

54. Leserman J. Role of depression, stress, and trauma in HIV disease progression. *Psychosom Med.* 2008;70(5):539–45. doi:10.1097/PSY.0b013e3181777a5f.

55. Segerstrom SC, Taylor SE, Kemeny ME, Reed GM, Visscher BR. Causal attributions predict rate of immune decline in HIV-seropositive gay men. *Health Psychol.* 1996;15(6):485–93. doi:10.1037//0278-6133.15.6.485.

56. Mohr DC, Hart SL, Julian L, Cox D, Pelletier D. Association between stressful life events and exacerbation in multiple sclerosis: a meta-analysis. *Br Med J.* 2004;328(7442):731–3. doi:10.1136/bmj.38041.724421.55.

57. Ackerman KD, Heyman R, Rabin BS, et al. Stressful life events precede exacerbations of multiple sclerosis. *Psychosom Med.* 2002;64(6):916–20. doi:10.1097/01.psy.0000038941.33335.40.

58. Stults-Kolehmainen MA, Sinha R. The effects of stress on physical activity and exercise: a systematic review. *Sports Medicine.* 2014;44(1):81–121. doi:10.1007/s40279-013-0090-5.

59. Lupien SJ, de Leon M, de Santi S, et al. Cortisol levels during human aging predict hippocampal atrophy and memory deficits. *Nat Neurosci.* 1998;1(1):69–73. doi:10.1038/271.

60. Pearlin LI, Schooler C. Structure of coping. *J Health Soc Behav.* 1978;19(1):2–21. doi:10.2307/2136319.

61. McGonagle KA, Kessler RC. Chronic stress, acute stress, and depressive symptoms. *Am J Community Psychol.* 1990;18(5):681–706. doi:10.1007/bf00931237.

62. Brown GW, Harris T. *Social Origins of Depression: A Study of Psychiatric Disorder in Women.* New York (NY): Free Press; 1978.

63. Bandura A, Reese L, Adams NE. Microanalysis of action and fear arousal as a function of differential levels of perceived self-efficacy. *J Pers Soc Psychol.* 1982;43(1):5–21. doi:10.1037/0022-3514.43.1.5.

64. Borcela E, Perez-Alvarez L, Herreroa AI, et al. Chronic stress in adulthood followed by intermittent stress impairs spatial memory and the survival of newborn hippocampal cells in aging animals: prevention by FGL, a peptide mimetic of neural cell adhesion molecule. *Behav Pharmacol.* 2008;19(1):41–9.

65. Sandi C, Davies HA, Cordero MI, Rodriguez JJ, Popov VI, Stewart MG. Rapid reversal of stress induced loss of synapses in CA3 of rat hippocampus following water maze training. *Eur J Neurosci.* 2003;17(11):2447–56. doi:10.1046/j.1460-9568.2003.02675.x.

66. Lupien SJ, Evans A, Lord C, et al. Hippocampal volume is as variable in young as in older adults: implications for the notion of hippocampal atrophy in humans. *Neuroimage.* 2007;34(2):479–85. doi:10.1016/j.neuroimage.2006.09.041.

67. Lupien S, Lecours AR, Lussier I, Schwartz G, Nair NPV, Meaney MJ. Basal cortisol levels and cognitive deficits in human aging. *J Neurosci.* 1994;14(5):2893–903.

68. Marin MF, Lord C, Andrews J, et al. Chronic stress, cognitive functioning and mental health. *Neurobiol Learn Mem.* 2011;96(4):583–95. doi:10.1016/j.nlm.2011.02.016.

69. Sapolsky RM, Krey LC, McEwen BS. The neuroendocrinology of stress and aging: the glucocorticoid cascade hypothesis. *Endocr Rev.* 1986;7(3):284–301.

70. Van der Linden D, Keijsers GPJ, Eling P, Van Schaijk R. Work stress and attentional difficulties: an initial study on burnout and cognitive failures. *Work Stress.* 2005;19(1):23–36. doi:10.1080/0267837050065275.

71. de Sousa AFM, Medeiros A, Del Rosso S, Stults-Kolehmainen M, Boullosa D. The influence of exercise and physical fitness status on attention: a systematic review. *Int Rev Sport Exerc Psychol.* 2018;12(1):202–34. doi:10.1080/1750984x.2018.1455889.

72. Hillman CH, Erickson KI, Kramer AF. Be smart, exercise your heart: exercise effects on brain and cognition. *Nat Rev Neurosci.* 2008;9(1):58–65. doi:10.1038/nrn2298.

73. Thayer RE, Newman JR, McClain TM. Self-regulation of mood: strategies for changing a bad mood, raising energy, and reducing tension. *J Pers Soc Psychol.* 1994;67(5):910–25. doi:10.1037//0022-3514.67.5.910.

74. Ensari I, Greenlee TA, Motl RW, Petruzzello SJ. Meta-analysis of acute exercise effects on state anxiety: an update of randomized controlled trials over the past

25 years. *Depress Anxiety.* 2015;32(8):624–34. doi:10.1002 /da.22370.

75. Petruzzello SJ, Landers DM, Hatfield BD, Kubitz KA, Salazar W. A meta-analysis on the anxiety-reducing effects of acute and chronic exercise — outcomes and mechanisms. *Sports Med.* 1991;11(3):143–82.

76. Bartholomew JB, Moore J, Todd J, Todd T, Elrod CC. Psychological states following resistance exercise of different workloads. *J Appl Sport Psychol.* 2001;13(4):399–410. doi:10.1080/104132001753226265.

77. Ekkekakis P, Parfitt G, Petruzzello SJ. The pleasure and displeasure people feel when they exercise at different intensities decennial update and progress towards a tripartite rationale for exercise intensity prescription. *Sports Med.* 2011;41(8):641–71.

78. Bixby WR, Hatfield BD. A dimensional investigation of the State Anxiety Inventory in an exercise setting: cognitive vs. somatic. *J Sport Behav.* 2011;34(4):307–24.

79. Bartholomew JB, Morrison D, Ciccolo JT. Effects of acute exercise on mood and well-being in patients with major depressive disorder. *Med Sci Sports Exerc.* 2005;37(12): 2032–7. doi:10.1249/01.mss.0000178101.78322.dd.

80. Mata J, Hogan CL, Joormann J, Waugh CE, Gotlib IH. Acute exercise attenuates negative affect following repeated sad mood inductions in persons who have recovered from depression. *J Abnorm Psychol.* 2013;122(1):45–50. doi:10.1037/a0029881.

81. Asmundson GJG, Fetzner MG, DeBoer LB, Powers MB, Otto MW, Smits JAJ. Let's get physical: a contemporary review of the anxiolytic effects of exercise for anxiety and its disorders. *Depress Anxiety.* 2013;30(4):362–73. doi:10.1002/da.22043.

82. Broocks A, Bandelow B, Pekrun G, et al. Comparison of aerobic exercise, clomipramine, and placebo in the treatment of panic disorder. *Am J Psychiatry.* 1998;155(5):603–9.

83. Diaz AB, Motta R. The effects of an aerobic exercise program on posttraumatic stress disorder symptom severity in adolescents. *Int J Emerg Ment Health.* 2008;10(1):49–59.

84. Cutter CJ, Schottenfeld RS, Moore BA, et al. A pilot trial of a videogame-based exercise program for methadone maintained patients. *J Subst Abuse Treat.* 2014;47(4): 299–305. doi:10.1016/j.jsat.2014.05.007.

85. Gerber M, Pühse U. Do exercise and fitness protect against stress-induced health complaints? A review of the literature. *Scand J Public Health.* 2009;37(8):801–19. doi:10.1177/1403494809350522.

86. Norris R, Carroll D, Cochrane R. The effects of physical activity and exercise training on psychological stress and well-being in an adolescent population. *J Psychosom Res.* 1992;36(1):55–65. doi:10.1016/0022-3999(92)90114-h.

87. Hamer M, Taylor A, Steptoe A. The effect of acute aerobic exercise on stress related blood pressure responses: a systematic review and meta-analysis. *Biol Psychol.* 2006;71(2):183–90. doi:10.1016/j.biopsycho.2005.04.004.

88. Lutz RS, Stults-Kolehmainen MA, Bartholomew JB. Exercise caution when stressed: stages of change and the stress-exercise participation relationship. *Psychol Sport Exerc.* 2010;11(6):560–7. doi:10.1016/j.psychsport.2010 .06.005.

89. Stults-Kolehmainen MA, Lu T, Ciccolo JT, Bartholomew JB, Brotnow L, Sinha R. Higher chronic psychological stress is associated with blunted affective responses to strenuous resistance exercise: RPE, pleasure, pain. *Psychol Sport Exerc.* 2016;22:27–36.

90. Stults-Kolehmainen MA, Ciccolo JT, Bartholomew JB, Seifert J, Portman RS. Age and gender-related changes in exercise motivation among highly active individuals. *Athl Insight.* 2013;5(1):45–63.

91. Segar ML, Eccles JS, Richardson CR. Rebranding exercise: closing the gap between values and behavior. *Int J Behav Nutr Phys Act.* 2011;8:14. doi:10.1186/1479-5868-8-94.

92. Cohen S, Janicki-Deverts D. Who's stressed? Distributions of psychological stress in the United States in probability samples from 1983, 2006, and 2009. *J Appl Soc Psychol.* 2012;42(6):1320–34. doi:10.1111/j .1559-1816.2012.00900.x.

93. Cohen S, Kamarck T, Mermelstein R. A global measure of perceived stress. *J Health Soc Behav.* 1983;24(4):385–96.

94. Cohen S, Williamson G. Perceived stress in a probability sample of the United States. In: Spacapam S, Oskamp S, editors. *The Social Psychology of Health: Claremont Symposium on Applied Social Psychology.* Newbury Park (CA): Sage; 1988. p. 31–67.

95. Thoits PA. Mechanisms linking social ties and support to physical and mental health. *J Health Soc Behav.* 2011;52(2):145–61. doi:10.1177/0022146510395592.

96. Berkman LF, Glass T. Social integration, social networks, social support, and health. In: Berkman LF, Kawachi I, editors. *Social Epidemiology.* New York (NY): Oxford University Press; 2000. p. 158–62.

97. House JS. *Work Stress and Social Support.* Reading (MA): Addison-Wesley; 1981. 156 p.

98. Cohen S, Wills TA. Stress, social support, and the buffering hypothesis. *Psychol Bull.* 1985;98:310–57.

99. Heaney CA, Israel BA. Social networks and social support. In: Glanz K, Rimer B, Viswanath K, editors. *Health Behavior and Health Education: Theory, Research, and Practice.* 4th ed. San Francisco (CA): Jossey-Bass; 2008. p. 189–210.

100. Taylor RL, Lam DJ, Roppel CE, Barter JT. Friends can be good medicine: an excursion into mental-health promotion. *Community Ment Health J.* 1984;20(4):294–303. doi:10.1007/bf00757078.

101. MacFarlane A, Norman G, Streiner D, Roy R. The process of social stress: stable, reciprocal, and mediating relationships. *J Health Soc Behav.* 1983;24:160–73. doi:10.2307/2136642.

102. Suls J, Mullen B. Life change and psychological distress: the role of perceived control and desirability. *J App Soc Psychol.* 1981;11(5):379–89. doi:10.1111/j.1559-1816 .1981.tb00830.x.

103. Pruessner JC, Hellhammer DH, Kirschbaum C. Burnout, perceived stress, and cortisol responses to awakening. *Psychosom Med.* 1999;61(2):197–204.

104. Sandler IN, Lakey B. Locus of control as a stress mediator: the role of control perceptions and social support. *Am J Community Psychol.* 1982;10(1):65–80. doi:10.1007 /bf00903305.

105. Marshall GN. A multidimensional-analysis of internal health locus of control beliefs: separating the wheat from the chaff. *J Pers Soc Psychol.* 1991;61(3):483–91.

106. Bandura A. Self-efficacy — toward a unifying theory of behavioral change. *Psychol Rev.* 1977;84(2):191–215. doi:10.1037//0033-295x.84.2.191.

107. Rodgers WM, Sullivan MJL. Task, coping, and scheduling self-efficacy in relation to frequency of physical activity. *J Appl Soc Psychol.* 2001;31(4):741–53. doi:10.1111/j.1559-1816.2001.tb01411.x.

108. Bandura A, Taylor CB, Williams SL, Mefford IN, Barchas JD. Catecholamine secretion as a function of perceived coping self-efficacy. *J Consult Clin Psychol.* 1985;53(3):406–14. doi:10.1037//0022-006x.53.3.406.

109. Holahan CK, Holahan CJ, Belk SS. Adjustment in aging: the roles of life stress, hassles and self-efficacy. *Health Psychol.* 1984;3(4):315–28. doi:10.1037/0278-6133.3.4.315.

110. Gilson TA, Heller EA, Stults-Kolehmainen MA. The relationship between an effort goal and self-regulatory efficacy beliefs for Division I football players. *J Strength Cond Res.* 2013;27(10):2806–15. doi:10.1519 /JSC.0b013e31828151ca.

111. Peveler RC, Johnston DW. Subjective and cognitive effects of relaxation. *Behav Res Ther.* 1986;24(4):413–9. doi:10.1016/0005-7967(86)90006-9.

112. Jain S, Shapiro SL, Swanick S, et al. A randomized controlled trial of mindfulness meditation versus relaxation training: effects on distress, positive states of mind, rumination, and distraction. *Ann Behav Med.* 2007;33(1): 11–21. doi:10.1207/s15324796abm3301_2.

113. Martarelli D, Cocchioni M, Scuri S, Pompei P. Diaphragmatic breathing reduces postprandial oxidative stress. *J Altern Complement Med.* 2011;17(7):623–8. doi:10.1089/acm.2010.0666.

114. Davis M, Eshelman ER, McKay M. *The Relaxation and Stress Reduction Workbook.* 6th ed. Oakland (CA): New Harbinger Publications; 2008. 392 p.

115. Jacobson EJ. *Progressive Relaxation.* Chicago (IL): University of Chicago Press; 1938.

116. Critchley HD, Melmed RN, Featherstone E, Mathias CJ, Dolan RJ. Brain activity during biofeedback relaxation — a functional neuroimaging investigation. *Brain.* 2001;124:1003–12. doi:10.1093/brain/124.5.1003.

117. Budzynsk T, Stoyva JM, Adler CS, Mullaney DJ. EMG biofeedback and tension headache: controlled outcome study. *Psychosom Med.* 1973;35(6):484–96.

118. Field TM. Massage therapy effects. *Am Psychol.* 1998; 53(12):1270–81.

119. Moyer CA, Rounds J, Hannum JW. A meta-analysis of massage therapy research. *Psychol Bull.* 2004;130(1): 3–18. doi:10.1037/0033-2909.130.1.3.

120. Hilbert JE, Sforzo GA, Swensen T. The effects of massage on delayed onset muscle soreness. *Br J Sports Med.* 2003;37(1):72–5. doi:10.1136/bjsm.37.1.72.

121. Benson H, Rosner BA, Marzetta BR, Klemchuk HP. Decreased blood-pressure in borderline hypertensive subjects who practiced meditation. *J Chronic Dis.* 1974;27(3):163–9. doi:10.1016/0021-9681(74)90083-6.

122. MacLean CRK, Walton KG, Wenneberg SR, et al. Effects of the transcendental meditation program on adaptive mechanisms: changes in hormone levels and responses to stress after 4 months of practice. *Psychoneuroendocrinology.* 1997;22(4):277–95. doi:10.1016/s0306-4530(97)00003-6.

123. Solberg EE, Ingjer F, Holen A, Sundgot-Borgen J, Nilsson S, Holme I. Stress reactivity to and recovery from a standardised exercise bout: a study of 31 runners practising relaxation techniques. *Br J Sports Med.* 2000;34(4):268–72.

124. Ai AL, Dunkle RE, Peterson C, Bolling SF. The role of private prayer in psychological recovery among midlife and aged patients following cardiac surgery. *Gerontologist.* 1998;38(5):591–601.

125. Kabat-Zinn J. Mindfulness-based interventions in context: past, present, and future. *Clin Psychol-Sci Pract.* 2003;10(2):144–56. doi:10.1093/clipsy/bpg016.

126. Brown KW, Ryan RA, Creswell JD. Mindfulness: theoretical foundations and evidence for its salutary effects. *Psychol Inq.* 2007;18(4):211–37.

127. Astin JA. Stress reduction through mindfulness meditation — effects on psychological symptomatology, sense of control, and spiritual experiences. *Psychother Psychosom.* 1997;66(2):97–106.

128. Prakhinkit S, Suppapitiporn S, Tanaka H, Suksom D. Effects of Buddhism walking meditation on depression, functional fitness, and endothelium-dependent vasodilation in depressed elderly. *J Altern Complement Med.* 2014;20(5):411–6.

129. Chong CSM, Tsunaka M, Tsang HWH, Chan EP, Cheung WM. Effects of yoga on stress management in healthy adults: a systematic review. *Altern Ther Health Med.* 2011;17(1):32–8.

130. Jin PT. Efficacy of tai chi, brisk walking, meditation and reading in reducing mental and emotional stress. *J Psychosom Res.* 1992;36(4):361–70. doi:10.1016/0022-3999(92)90072-a.

131. Li AW, Goldsmith CAW. The effects of yoga on anxiety and stress. *Altern Med Rev.* 2012;17(1):21–35.

132. Naves-Bittencourt W, Mendonça-de-Sousa A, Stults-Kolehmainen M, et al. Martial arts: mindful exercise to combat stress. *Eur J Hum Mov.* 2015;34:34–51.

133. Ekkekakis P, Hall EE, VanLanduyt LM, Petruzzello SJ. Walking in (affective) circles: can short walks enhance affect? *J Behav Med.* 2000;23(3):245–75. doi:10 .1023/a:1005558025163.

Business

14 Legal Structure and Terminology

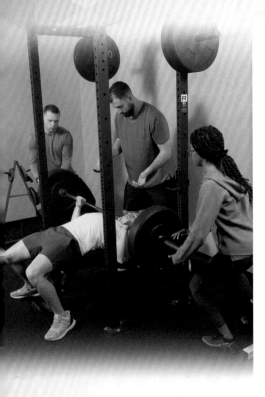

OBJECTIVES

- To understand basic concepts of the law and legal system.
- To understand the potential for legal liability and areas of primary concern.
- To appreciate the significance of industry standards and guidelines.
- To become acquainted with risk management strategies.
- To become acquainted with administrative responsibilities.

INTRODUCTION

What is the relevance of understanding the law and legal system by the certified exercise physiologist (EP)? With the recognition that the EP is a more qualified instructor than those typically found within the fitness industry, it is understandable that he or she will be held to a higher "standard of care." Therefore, it is incumbent on the EP to be knowledgeable of the basic structure and function of our legal system. Being aware of how this system may be used either as an asset or as a liability to the client–instructor relationship enables the EP to take advantage of protective mechanisms afforded by the system and to avoid pitfalls that can threaten not only the safety of his or her clients but also the livelihood of the EP.

The EP who trains within a fitness facility will most likely find that an injured party will pursue a claim against the facility rather than the EP because the facility is viewed as having more extensive financial resources. Nevertheless, claims have been filed jointly against facilities and instructors wherein multiple judgments have been rendered.

In this chapter, the EP is exposed to those tenets of the standard of care that are promulgated by industry leaders and available to protect the instructor. The focus is on essential client services and, more importantly, protective actions that help insulate the EP against litigation while simultaneously promoting professionalism.

The Law and Legal System

The EP must be knowledgeable about the basic concepts of the law and the legal system. Along with this is the accompanying terminology that will provide the EP with insight into issues affecting his or her business and potential exposure to liability. The EP needs to understand the various divisions of the law, and especially the division of civil law, where tortuous and contract claims are areas within which the EP is most likely to become legally embroiled. The anatomy of a lawsuit should be understood such that the EP can navigate the sequence of legal proceedings and requirements to successfully support or defend a negligence claim or contract violation.

The EP must understand that negligence is defined as one's failure to act, or as more likely will be the case, one's substandard performance. There are four elements of a negligence claim that must be documented to bring a successful suit against the EP. If in fact these elements are substantiated, then the court can assess monetary damages against the EP. Each element is discussed in more detail later in this chapter.

The EP needs to be aware of those varied situations wherein an instructor may create a risk of insult, injury, or possibly death because these all present a potential case of negligence. There exists a myriad of settings to be considered when determining one's susceptibility to a negligence lawsuit, and these areas of vulnerability can primarily be found within the five stages of the instructor–client relationship. In short, if the EP can remember the acronym STEPS (Fig. 14.1), this will be helpful in avoiding the distressing experience of litigation. By being attentive and applying the standard of care to the details of each one of these five steps, the EP can successfully navigate through potentially litigious waters (1).

Primary Sources of Law

The primary sources of law can be divided into four categories: (a) constitutional law, (b) statutory law, (c) case law, and (d) administrative law. The federal government and all states have constitutions that not only provide the authority for government but also define how it will function and

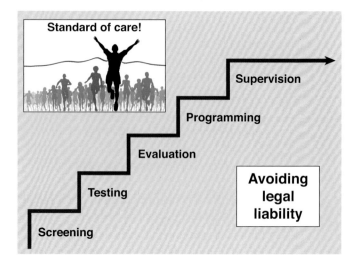

FIGURE 14.1. STEPS to success: avoiding legal liability.

what its responsibilities are. Statutory laws or legislative laws are enacted by mandates from federal, state, and municipal governments, and this codification of law imposes duties or restrictions on individuals. However, in the case of the Good Samaritan law, immunity is granted to those persons who in good faith try to protect, serve, and tend to others who are injured or ill. It should be noted, though, that the Good Samaritan law does not apply to the EP while on the job. Case law, sometimes referred to as common law, is based on decisions of courts and administrative tribunals. Common law is founded on unwritten law (not codified) and is based on customs and general usages, whereas case law is based on reported judicial decisions of selected lower and appellate courts. Administrative law is found within specialized bodies or agencies that have been granted lawmaking power to regulate specific activities. Federal agencies such as the Occupational Safety and Health Administration (OSHA), along with numerous state agencies, draft and enforce regulations that impact a wide range of individuals and entities, including fitness instructors and health facilities (2). Primary sources of law then are official bodies with the authority to make laws that can affect the legal rights of citizens.

In addition, our system of jurisprudence is subdivided into the two domains of criminal law and civil law, both of which dispose the citizenry to act in a way that benefits society. Whereas criminal law governs the conduct of both individuals and groups toward society as a whole, civil law pertains to personal responsibilities that an individual or a group must observe when dealing with other individuals or groups. This division of law addresses expressed grievances and judicial remedies between individuals, between an individual and a group, or between groups.

When individuals or groups violate criminal laws, they are subject to the penalties for misdemeanors and felonies, including fines, imprisonment, or both. Although the EP is less likely to violate criminal law, there is the possibility that he or she could be charged with the unauthorized practice of medicine or unauthorized practice of an allied health field such as physical therapy or dietetics. For example, after screening a client for resting blood pressure, the EP cannot diagnose him or her as hypertensive, as such a diagnosis remains only within the purview of a licensed physician. It could also be considering encroaching upon the realm of physical therapy by conducting postural analyses and providing corrective exercises, or encroaching upon the field of dietetics by providing clients with specific meal plans to correct nutritional deficiencies. The EP could be found guilty of committing a first-degree misdemeanor that not only is punishable by a severe fine but also could be punishable by imprisonment. Therefore, it is especially wise for the EP, and any other unlicensed provider, to remain well within his or her scope of practice.

When individuals or groups violate civil law, they are subject to the jurisprudence of civil courts that adjudicate noncriminal cases. Civil lawsuits handle disputes between individuals, organizations, businesses, and governmental agencies wherein two parties, the plaintiff (*e.g.*, the injured party or representative of an injured or deceased individual) and the defendant (*e.g.*, the EP and/or the facility that he or she represents), present their cases for litigation (2). Whereas criminal law requires that a prosecutor provide proof beyond a reasonable doubt to find the defendant guilty, civil law only requires that the plaintiff demonstrate that the preponderance of the evidence supports his or her claim to find the defendant liable. This again emphasizes that the EP should stay within the stated scope or practice, as to avoid any potential issues of negligence that may lead to litigation.

When considering lawsuits against instructor personnel and fitness facilities, the plurality of such cases falls within the domain of civil law. The typical civil law violation falls under the categories of either tort law or contract law.

Tort Law

A tort is a breach of legal duty amounting to a civil wrong or injury for which a court of law will provide compensation/damages. Therefore, tort law governs the legal rights and obligations between individuals as well as between collective bodies in relationship to injuries, deaths, or civil wrongdoings (3). A tort by definition is a wrongful act, whether intentional or accidental, from which an insult, injury, or death occurs to another person or perhaps an organization that sustains pecuniary damage. The individual or group that is injured or sustains pecuniary damage is known as the plaintiff, whereas the individual or group responsible for the tortuous act is known as the defendant or tortfeasor. When an injury, death, or wrong is documented and attributed to the defendant, a remedy, usually in the form of a financial judgment, is then levied against the defendant. This levy, applied by the civil court, provides relief to the plaintiff. A tort does not include a breach of contract that also can lead to adjudication and compensation in the form of monetary damages.

Torts do include all negligence cases as well as intentional wrongdoings that result in injury or death. There also exists a tort due to "no fault" conduct. Therefore, tortuous acts are divided into the following three categories: (a) intentional misconduct, (b) negligent conduct, and (c) "no fault" conduct. "No fault" conduct falls under the category of strict liability and relates to ultrahazardous activities and product liability that will not be addressed in this chapter (2). An intentional tort is indicative of an act that willfully caused an injury, a death, a financial distress, or a damaged reputation. Because it is extremely difficult to document an intentional tort, courts typically give the benefit of doubt to the defendant and presume that the tort is one of negligence.

Negligence

When considering the lawsuits filed against fitness facilities and/or fitness instructors, the overwhelming majority are suits alleging negligence. The definitions of "negligence" and "standard of care" are similar in that they both are concerned with prudence and caution in dealing with clients. Standard of care refers to the application of a degree of prudence and caution required by an individual or organization that owes a duty of care. As it relates to the fitness industry, the standard of care is the degree of care that a reasonably prudent fitness instructor or reasonably prudent facility management would use under similar circumstances. A failure to exercise that degree of care used by prudent instructors or management represents negligence. The failure to do, or the failure to avoid, that which the prudent instructor would have done or not done may lead an individual to becoming liable for negligence. As a certified practitioner, the EP will be held to a higher standard than most other instructors. Figure 14.2 provides an image of the components of negligence.

For the plaintiff to prosecute a successful tort claim, four basic elements of negligence must be well documented (4). First, a legal duty must be established from the relationship between the client and the EP, a duty in which the EP is required to provide safe and effective instruction without

FIGURE 14.2. Minimizing negligence through risk management.

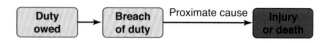

exposure to risks that could be the cause of injury and, perhaps, even death. Second, a breach of that legal duty, which is either substandard performance or a failure to act, is determined to have taken place. Third, the breach of duty owed was the factual or proximate cause of the injury or death. Fourth, the negligent act or failure to act resulted in well-documented damages or losses to the plaintiff, both economic damages (*e.g.*, medical costs and lost wages) and noneconomic damages (*e.g.*, pain and suffering).

In *Corrigan v. Musclemakers, Inc.* (1999) (5), the plaintiff (Corrigan) was a 49-year-old woman who had joined Gold's Gym and signed up for three 1-hour sessions with a personal trainer. She had never patronized a health facility or gym and claimed to never have been on a treadmill. During the first session, the personal trainer set her to walk on a treadmill at 3.5 mph for 20 minutes. The trainer then left the plaintiff alone, without instructions on how to adjust the treadmill's speed, stop the belt, or operate the control panel. Early in the exercise, the plaintiff was unable to keep up with the speed of the treadmill and drifted back on the belt. As Corrigan attempted to walk faster, she was thrown off the machine and suffered a broken ankle. She filed a lawsuit against the health facility for negligence in an effort to recover damages for the injuries she sustained. Corrigan's negligence claims included (a) the trainer did not properly instruct her on how to use the treadmill and its control panel and (b) failed to supervise her while using the machine. The defendant claimed that they only needed to ensure facility conditions were safe and that the plaintiff's voluntary participation meant she assumed the inherent risk of the "sporting" activity. The court disagreed, citing that the plaintiff specifically informed the personal trainer that she was sedentary and a newcomer to the gym. It was also undisputed that the personal trainer failed to inform the plaintiff of the treadmill's operation before using it, and the court pointed to the operator's manual that states informing users of how to properly operate the machine was a guideline for safe operation. The court found the personal trainer was negligent in his or her conduct, thus breaching the duty of care owed to the plaintiff. The negligent actions were specifically attributed to the injury sustained by the plaintiff, resulting in a ruling in favor of Corrigan (5).

EPs can use three major risk management strategies to lessen the chances of becoming embroiled in legal liability with a negligence tort. First, the EP must adhere to the standard of care in the screening process, fitness profiling, evaluation, programming, and supervision of clients. Second, the EP must use waivers and assumption of risk forms in varied venues of the client–instructor relationship. Third, the EP must ensure that he or she has purchased appropriate liability insurance for the activities in which his or her client is engaged.

Regarding adherence to the standard of care, the grasp of safe and effective fitness practices is dealt with in other chapters within this resource manual. However, the prudent and cautious EP is unlikely to be faced with litigation because of his or her commitment to providing such safe and effective practices. This is the first line of defense in risk management. Waivers and assumption of risk forms provide a second line of defense and must be understood in light of their implementation and limitations.

Protective legal documents exist in different forms, of which the three most common are informed consent, agreement to participate, and prospective waivers or releases. However, before discussing the legal protection each of the aforementioned documents provides, it is necessary to review the three major causes of injury or death associated with physical activity:

- *Inherent*: injuries due to accidents that are not preventable and are no one's fault
- *Negligence*: injuries due to the fault of the defendant (sometimes the plaintiff)
- *Extreme forms of negligence*: injuries due to the gross negligence, willful and wanton, or reckless conduct of the defendant (3)

When lawsuits are filed due to an inherent injury such as a sprained ankle on a fitness facility's basketball court, an informed consent or agreement to participate provides the best legal protection by strengthening what is termed an *assumption of risk defense*. For this reason, informed consents are used prior to fitness testing or exercise programming and participation. Therefore, despite the fact that the client has been advised and warned of the risks, he or she declares that the risks are understood, appreciated, and voluntarily assumed. Although this defense is generally upheld in court for injuries due to inherent causes, it is sometimes used unsuccessfully by defendants for various reasons; for example, the injury was due to negligence of the defendant or the plaintiff did not fully understand and appreciate the inherent risks prior to participation. Chapter 2 of this textbook covers preparticipation screening in greater detail.

When lawsuits are filed due to negligence on the part of the instructor, a prospective waiver or release provides the best legal protection to thwart potential liability. Within the waiver, there exists an "exculpatory" clause explicitly stating that the instructor is released from liability due to any negligence. This clause is designed to document that the client has relinquished his or her right to pursue litigation. The validity of waivers to provide protection from negligent torts is determined by state law, which can vary greatly from state to state. In some states, waivers provide no protection from liability due to negligence, whereas in other states, lenient, moderate, or rigorous requirements (6) must be upheld to protect the instructor from negligence.

Gregory Pederson, a personal trainer, was the defendant in a lawsuit after one of his clients of 17 sessions, Victor Berisaj, filed a complaint alleging negligence, gross negligence, and willful and wanton misconduct (*Berisaj v. LTF Club Operations Company, Inc.*, 2019) (7). The plaintiff suffered a back injury in an auto crash in 2014, completed physical therapy for lower back pain, and then began personal training sessions with Pederson. Berisaj trained with Pederson for 17 sessions before he stopped attending due to back pain. He then sued Pederson and Life Time Fitness (LTF), with the defendants responding that the plaintiff signed two waivers when he joined LTF and when he purchased the personal training package. The trial court ruled the waivers protected LTF and Pederson from liability of ordinary negligence, and there was no genuine issue of material fact regarding gross negligence and willful and wanton misconduct. The court found that Pederson had kept plaintiff's limitations in mind and never forced Berisaj to perform any unsafe or dangerous exercises, the plaintiff failed to demonstrate that Pederson intended to harm him, and Pederson submitted text messages that showed he was invested in the plaintiff's well-being. Multiple waivers and other documentation protected LTF and Pederson from this negligent tort claim (7).

To ensure that waivers and releases are legally binding, EPs should engage legal counsel to draft their exculpatory forms, recognizing that state laws not only vary but also change periodically. Therefore, if the EP has been using waivers or releases for an extended period, it is wise to have legal counsel review the forms to ensure that they remain compliant with current law. Frequently, the EP can obtain samples of waivers and releases from seminars or copies in texts such as American College of Sports Medicine (*ACSM*) *Health/Fitness Facility Standards and Guidelines* (8). Although this may save the cost of hiring a lawyer, the EP should be aware that these documents might not be applicable and legally enforceable in his or her state.

When lawsuits are filed due to extreme or gross negligence, there are generally no protective legal documents. A few states may permit the use of a waiver or release to provide such protection, but this is rarely the case (6). Extreme forms of negligence exist when the defendant is aware of the potential danger and risk of an activity or exercise but fails to warn the client and instead allows the performance of that activity or exercise. In such cases, punitive damages may be awarded, and normally, liability insurance policies will not cover the instructor who is liable of extreme negligence.

As discussed, protective legal documents are an important line of defense for the EP in that they can provide evidence in a court of law that the client was made aware of risks but decided to assume such risks as outlined. In addition, an exculpatory clause may provide a defense in case of an inadvertent lapse in the EP's performance related to either an act of commission or an act of omission.

Frequently, protective legal documents in the form of prospectively signed waivers or exculpatory agreements may prevent a claim from going forward because a judge can dismiss a case through a pretrial motion termed a *summary judgment*. Summary judgment is a judgment entered by a court where a decision is based on statements and admissible evidence without going to trial.

Joey Herren joined Nonstop Fitness Incorporated gym and began working with a personal trainer. A few weeks into his training, he obtained a non–U.S. Food and Drug Administration (FDA)-approved dietary supplement from a former coworker called R.A.G.E. and began taking the supplement. During one exercise session, Herren suffered a stroke. Herren filed a lawsuit against the fitness facility, the owner, his personal trainer, a management company, and the original seller of the dietary supplement. He argued he suffered the stroke as a result of overexercising and taking the dietary supplement and claimed negligence and gross negligence of all defendants. The defendants filed for summary judgment, contending that Herren had signed three separate agreements containing exculpatory clauses, which waived and released them from liability prior to an exercise program with a trainer. The defendants claimed Herren assumed the risk of his injuries by signing the documents and then participating, but Herren asserted that the agreements were not a defense for gross negligence. Although the trial court agreed that the plaintiffs' exculpatory clauses did not bar claims against the defendants based on gross negligence allegations, the exculpatory clauses were binding and enforceable regarding ordinary negligence claims. The court granted summary judgment for the defendants, and Herren unsuccessfully appealed his case (9).

Insurance Coverage

As previously stated, liability insurance is an important component of an EP's risk management strategy. There are multiple types of insurance coverage available to the EP; however, those of interest should be "general" and "professional" liability insurance that affords protection from negligence claims. The EP can obtain a general liability insurance policy, which protects from "ordinary" negligence, from a commercial general liability firm, or CGL (10).

Professional liability insurance (PLI), also called professional indemnity insurance (PII) but more commonly known as errors and omissions (E&O), protects individuals who provide professional advice and service as part of their job responsibility. This insurance is similar to malpractice insurance purchased by physicians. When the EP is employed in a health care provider setting, he or she is more likely to be regarded as conducting professional services and, therefore, should have PII. However, because CGL firms may attempt to avoid a payoff by claiming their policy excludes coverage for "professional services," the EP should hold both general liability insurance and PLI (2).

The last line of defense in risk management is the possession of both general liability insurance and PLI. With this coverage, the EP can be assured that an untoward event at work resulting in a negligence claim will not dampen his or her future but that he or she can continue to enjoy a personally rewarding and financially secure career as a fitness professional.

EPs should be sure to understand what the extent of their insurance policy covers before there is an issue. In *York Insurance Company v. Houston Wellness Center, Inc* (2003) (11), the insurance company argued they had no duty to indemnify and defend Houston Wellness Center in a bodily injury suit filed against the center. A fitness center member (Vandalinda) filed a negligence lawsuit against the wellness center after she was injured using one of their exercise machines. Vandalinda was using an exercise machine that develops triceps when she tried to release the machine using her arms, as instructed by one of Houston's employees. Allegedly, the machine improperly released, causing an injury to Vandalinda's left arm, requiring surgery. The plaintiff claimed the employee gave her improper instructions, thus causing the error in the machine release. The wellness center filed the claim with their insurance carrier, York Insurance Company, so they would defend their suit. The CGL insurer denied the request, filing a lawsuit contending it had no duty to defend the facility, based on explicit language of the insurance policy issued. The policy specifically excluded "bodily injury," "property damage," or "personal and advertising injury" that arose out of the rendering or failure to render service, treatment, advice, or instruction relating to physical fitness. Although the trial court initially ruled in favor of the facility, the insurance company appealed the ruling and won. This case serves as a reminder to review policies before issues arise, and to consider purchasing additional insurance, continue to use exculpatory agreements for client participation, and always have strong risk management practices.

Federal Laws

Key laws, in which both employers and EPs should be well versed, include those pertaining to sexual harassment, workplace safety, and maintaining privacy of clients and employees. Each of these is critical to promoting a safe and inviting environment and conducting business in the most professional manner possible. Ideally, legal counseling will be retained to make sure the place of business is in compliance with the various aspects of each law.

Sexual Harassment

The definition of sexual harassment is any kind of intimidation, browbeating, bullying, or coercion of a sexual nature; the inappropriate promise of promotions in exchange for sexual favors; or the threat of loss of job security for failure to provide such favors (12). Both sexes may be guilty of sexual harassment, although, more often, complaints are lodged against men. The EP could be the victim of sexual harassment by peers as well as superiors; of course, the EP could also be accused of sexual harassment in relation to clients. Sexual harassment is a form of sex discrimination and as such can lead to litigation.

Title VII of the Civil Rights Act of 1964 prohibits sex discrimination in the workplace, and since that time, the courts have extended this prohibition to include sexual harassment. In 1980, the U.S. Equal Employment Opportunity Commission (EEOC) amended its "Guidelines on Discrimination Because of Sex" to include sexual harassment and helped solidify judicial acceptance of this cause of action (12).

Sexual harassment could include a range of behaviors from seemingly mild transgressions and annoyances to actual sexual abuse or sexual assault. In some circumstances, sexual harassment may be not only unethical but also illegal and, therefore, a violation of criminal law. In the workplace, sexual harassment is a form of illegal employment discrimination. For many fitness facilities, preventing sexual harassment among personnel and defending employees from sexual harassment charges have become key goals of managers.

In *Sheppard v. River Valley Fitness One* (2002) (13), the plaintiffs (Mary and Robert Sheppard) brought a sexual harassment suit against their employer and supervisors, River Valley Fitness One. Mary alleged that over half a year, her supervisor had continuously given her unwanted kisses on her cheek, made sexually charged comments and jokes, and would "leer" at women while making inappropriate gestures. Sheppard claimed she was afraid of retaliation after she reported the harassment. The allegation also included charges that the owners refused to properly investigate or remedy the harassment and attempted to intimidate employees who complained about harassment. The club's manager, Robert Aubin, filed a separate lawsuit alleging that he was fired in retaliation for reporting Mary's complaints about harassment. This case became messier after there was misrepresentation of documents in a settlement negotiation, but the overall theme of this case is not necessarily uncommon in workplaces, so EPs must be mindful of their and others behavior.

The EP must also be aware that charges of sexual harassment by clients can be made against him or her, and therefore, the EP needs to choose his or her words carefully, to be cautious with touching as in assisting and spotting clients, and to avoid any suggestion of impropriety. For example, when the male EP is conducting body fat testing with skinfold calipers within the confines of a testing center, it would be wise to have a female employee assisting, thereby ensuring that no unjust accusations may be directed against the examiner.

Occupational Safety and Health Administration Guidelines

Under the U.S. Department of Labor, the OSHA is the principal federal agency charged with the enforcement of safety and health legislation in the workplace. In an effort to improve worker safety, OSHA has established regulations that have some specific implications for the fitness industry. The health code relating to blood-borne pathogens presents a formidable challenge to facility managers and often their EPs who, as a result of their higher level of certification, are assigned the task of implementing a safety policy to prevent the possibility of employees contracting HIV and hepatitis B and C viruses.

EPs frequently become responsible for understanding, recognizing, and dealing with the blood-borne pathogen threat inherent within fitness center operations, especially during an emergency response. There are potential dangers for pathogen exposure to both staff and members, and therefore, the EP may have to educate employees how to protect not only themselves but also their members through necessary preventive techniques.

EPs should become familiar with OSHA's published guidelines that provide directives on the training and record-keeping procedures of how to avoid and handle blood-borne pathogens. To adequately protect both staff and members, the EP may need to educate facility employees on the following:

- What is a blood-borne pathogen?
- What is meant by *occupational exposure* to blood-borne pathogens?
- What are potential infectious materials, and how to prevent exposure to them?
- What are the possible methods of disease transmission, and how can they be controlled?
- What protective equipment is required to safeguard the first responder in an emergency situation? (1)

An explanation of the stated concerns along with additional information of interest is available from OSHA, with regional offices located throughout the country that can provide fitness facility personnel with written materials and advice on how to meet OSHA requirements and how to improve workplace safety. Furthermore, the International Health, Racquet & Sportsclub Association (IHRSA), the professional trade association of the fitness industry, has published a briefing paper for its member facilities regarding the OSHA blood-borne pathogens requirements (14). Failure to meet OSHA's legally enforceable standards may result in facility citations and penalties.

Besides blood-borne pathogens, employees and perhaps even facility members may be exposed to potentially hazardous substances such as swimming pool chemicals and cleaning agents. Therefore, the EP may be assigned the task of advising facility employees, including independent contractors, of potentially harmful materials other than blood-borne pathogens. This may be accomplished through the posting of placards, notices, and memoranda. To this end, the *ACSM's Health/Fitness Facility Standards and Guidelines* indicates under Appendix B, Supplement 3, that "The OSHA Hazard Communication Standard requires you to develop a written hazard communication program" (8).

Health Insurance Portability and Accountability Act Guidelines and Recommendations

Under the U.S. Department of Health and Human Services, the Health Insurance Portability and Accountability Act of 1996 (HIPAA) was established to protect the privacy of health information. The Office for Civil Rights is provided the legal authority to enforce the HIPAA Privacy Rule, a rule that protects the privacy of an individual's identifiable health information. The HIPAA Security Rule sets national standards for the security of electronically protected health information and also for the confidentiality of such information (15).

HIPAA requires that all information gathered about a client's health status must be kept confidential in the fitness facility. The EP will frequently oversee the health screening process and therefore needs to guarantee that all information from medical histories, physical exam reports, and lifestyle questionnaires are only available to the appropriate individuals and that this information will be properly maintained and secured.

The HIPAA Privacy Rule provides federal protections for personal health information held by covered entities such as health care providers, health plans, and health care clearinghouses. The Privacy Rule gives patients an array of rights regarding the privacy of their information. Concurrently, the Privacy Rule is balanced by permitting the disclosure of personal health information that is required by legitimate health care professionals for patient care. Although fitness facilities are not technically listed as covered entities because they have access to members' health information, they have an obligation to guarantee the confidentiality, integrity, and security of that information, or they could be found in violation of the Privacy Rule.

 ## Client Rights and Responsibilities

The EP is expected to have a mature grasp of instructor–client relations and what it means to provide professional service to his or her clientele. The EP should know what is included in the rights of the client, such as making informed choices and knowing how to voice grievances. Likewise, it is often the duty of the EP to ensure that clients in turn know their responsibilities to the facility and instructor, which could mean being truthful about their health history and assisting in keeping the workout environment safe.

Client Rights

Clients have the right to receive quality service that is provided in a respectful manner without offensive or defamatory remarks or any form of discrimination. Clients should be provided with an overview of services provided and what would be typical health and fitness requirements to safely participate in these physical activities. This information allows clients to make informed choices about services and programs that would be suitable to their needs and capabilities.

Clients have the right to know the qualifications of staff members and the educational requirements met to achieve different certifications. Client should be well informed about any activities in which they will be exposed and any inherent risks as well as risks created through the inability to carry out activities as directed by instructors.

Clients not only have the right to an appropriate health screening but also have the necessity to be screened prior to physical activity. In addition, they have the right for a thorough orientation to the facility, operation of equipment to be used, and physical activity programs available while also being advised of how to respond to potential emergencies within the facility.

Clients have a right to timely responses to their requests and inquiries along with reasonable continuity and coordination of any services provided. Any charges for services should be openly disclosed and discussed, and if there are any complaints, clients have a right to know how to voice their grievances about services provided or omitted.

In line with the HIPAA Privacy Rule as well as described in ethical statements published by ACSM and other professional organizations, clients have the right to expect confidentiality regarding health information that is disclosed to facility staff. In addition, if there is other personal and financial information shared with a facility, it must be handled discreetly and securely.

Client Responsibilities

Clients have the responsibility to give accurate information about their physical and mental health, any substance abuse, or any other conditions or circumstances that could adversely impact their physical activity programming. If during activities clients experience pain or any injuries, it is their responsibility to report such concerns to instructor personnel in a timely and forthright manner.

Clients are to assist instructor personnel in maintaining a neat and safe environment, such as in putting weights back in their racks or not leaving clothing or bottles on the floor where they could become a hazard to others. This means respecting not only the workout areas but also other areas such as lounges or locker rooms.

Personal training clients are responsible for notifying their trainers well in advance if they cannot make appointments or if appointments need to be rescheduled. Likewise, clients should also notify facilities well in advance if they have to suspend a membership. If clients' addresses or phone numbers have changed, facilities must be advised. Clients are responsible for working with their instructors or trainers in reviewing, planning, or changing programs to ensure that programs meet their needs, capabilities, and schedules. In this respect, clients should also be quick to inform instructors or trainers if they are having any concerns or problems with the service being provided.

Both IHRSA and the ACSM have addressed a facility's responsibilities to its membership and therefore the rights to be anticipated by clients (8,14). Both *IHRSA's Standards Facilitation Guide* (14) and *ACSM's Health/Fitness Facility Standards and Guidelines* (8) publications outline important responsibilities addressing preactivity screening, orientations, education, and supervision of membership; risk management; and emergency policies. These responsibilities, and more, are owed to the client; in addition, there are responsibilities outlined that the member/client has to the facility and its staff.

Contract Law

The law of contracts governs agreements that are enforceable in court. Contracts are agreements pertaining to the legal rights and obligations between individuals as well as between collective bodies. The contract is a stipulation to which both parties consent and recognize as legally enforceable. This agreement or promise gives rise to a legal obligation that one will perform or not perform some activity or venture. An offer is proposed by one party and then accepted by the other. In effect, there exists a promised exchange between the parties, and this promised exchange may be written, oral, and even implied. This agreement or promised exchange within the health/fitness industry usually amounts to a service (availability of a facility and exercise instruction) for money (financial remuneration). Examples of contracts used in the health/fitness field are (a) employment contracts for employees and independent contractors, (b) informed consents, (c) waivers, and (d) membership contracts.

Personal trainers enter into agreements, or contracts, with clients that could promise to provide specialized workout routines tailored to the client. The contract may include that they, the personal trainers, are responsible for providing the client with the proper knowledge on how to use gym equipment and how to do the exercises. Should the client injure himself or herself due to the negligence of the trainer, he or she may have grounds for a personal injury lawsuit along with a breach of contract claim.

Employer and Employee Rights and Responsibilities

When individuals are hired by a facility to work as an EP, there is in effect a contract regarding the rights and responsibilities of the employee. The employee has agreed to perform certain services for which he or she will be remunerated. And the employee has the recognizable expectation that he or she will be treated with a degree of propriety and decorum while in the conduct of his or her service, whether it be from fellow workers, management, or even clientele.

Employers and employees have responsibilities to each other, and they should expect their rights to be upheld while their responsibilities are met. Regarding employee rights, one expects that he or she will be presented with a well-defined job description and that there will be periodic reviews of work performance with accompanying critiques and recommendations for improvement or, hopefully, recognition for exemplary performance.

Employees can expect that the provision of their terms and conditions of employment will be explicitly spelled out. They can expect that the terms and conditions will set forth what their primary and secondary duties are, to whom they are accountable, their rates of pay, and other entitlements such as vacation time, health benefits, sick leave, and the like.

Employees can expect that there will be no discrimination of any kind (to include sexual harassment) and that there will be equal opportunities for advancement with appropriate pay adjustments. Equal opportunity legislation mandates that all employees must receive the same pay and same work conditions for carrying out the same or similar work. There are also specific laws relating to gender, racial, and disability discrimination (16).

Employees are expected to conduct their services in a manner that has regard to the safety of others, both staff and clientele. In this vein, employees have a serious obligation to educate clients about the safe operation of exercise equipment, in addition to the safety practices involved with all physical activities that clients perform not only in the facility but also outside of the facility.

Regarding OSHA requirements, employees must be advised and have every right to expect that management will caution them about any potential hazards, whether of a physical or chemical nature. This caution may be delivered through verbal warnings or written and posted notices that are readily observable. As previously stated, there exist specific regulations about the manner in which potentially harmful substances should be used, stored, and recognized by both staff and clientele, and this information should be clearly posted for all to see.

In light of the stated requirements, employers are expected to abide by numerous regulations such as providing safe equipment, carrying out regular maintenance and safety checks, ensuring the training of employees in health and safety issues, and carrying out a risk assessment to assess the dangers of the unique work environment within fitness facilities. In short, during their employment, workers can anticipate that management will place a priority on their health and safety.

Employers and employees are expected to meet minimum legal requirements in the area of health and safety at work as well as minimum standards and conditions related to hours, pay scales, and the treatment of people in the workplace. Along with rights for employees, there are corresponding responsibilities such as the expectation that employees will work in a safe manner and will have regard for the safety of their colleagues and clientele. In addition, employees are responsible for conducting all their relations with management, fellow workers, and clientele with the respect and decorum, reflecting ethical and collegial behavior.

Federal Employment Laws

When in a position to hire personnel, the EP must understand the myriad laws that govern hiring. These laws cover issues related to civil rights, disabilities, and more; such laws are continually changing. It is not legally defensible to simply claim that a hiring law changed and you were unaware. Instead, similar to what was mentioned regarding earlier federal laws, legal counsel should be retained to ensure complete compliance with all local, state, and federal hiring laws.

Hiring and Prehiring Statutes

There are federal employment regulations or statutes regarding the hiring and prehiring of individuals and related regulations that apply to the fitness industry and other industries. The two important federal laws that prohibit employment discrimination related to preemployment inquiries include the Civil Rights Act of 1964 and the Americans with Disabilities Act of 1990 (ADA).

The Civil Rights Act of 1964 prohibits discrimination on the basis of race, color, gender, religion, and national origin (17). Therefore, unfair inquiries related to the stated characteristics or preferences within job application forms, preemployment interviews, or any type of inquiry made of job applicants are unlawful. Questions that appear to take a candidate's race; creed; color; national origin; age; gender; marital status; or any physical, mental, or sensory handicap into consideration for discriminatory purposes must be avoided. However, these rules do not prevent employers from asking questions to determine which candidates are most qualified to perform the specific functions or tasks of a given job. These rules were developed to prevent characteristics or conditions that have nothing to do with an individual's ability to perform the job from influencing the process of candidate selection. Understandably, certain physical and mental conditions in addition to personality traits would prevent some individuals from successfully performing various staff duties within a fitness facility, including exercise instruction.

The ADA prohibits employment discrimination on the basis of disabilities or perceived disabilities (18). The ADA addresses the "Dos and Don'ts" regarding preemployment inquiries, specifically those questions to be avoided at the preoffer stage. This means that employers cannot directly ask whether an applicant has a particular disability or ask questions that are closely related to disability issues at any time during the hiring process. The reason for this prohibition is that this information has been used in the past to exclude applicants with disabilities prior to an evaluation of their ability to perform the job.

Both the Civil Rights Act and the ADA make it clear that anyone involved in the interviewing process must avoid asking unfair preemployment questions. Interview questions are considered fair only when they specifically relate to an individual's ability to perform the actual duties of the job. Within the fitness industry, there are many staff positions that can be handled by individuals with disability. In addition, there are individuals with disability who can carry out many of the functions of an EP and, in some cases, may be the ideal candidate to offer classes for individuals with disability.

In light of the ADA, it is unfortunate that many barriers still exist that prevent individuals with disability from participating in mainstream society. Sadly, too many fitness facilities cannot accommodate individuals with disability, even though federal requirements mandate such accommodation. In addition to limited accessibility to the fitness facility as a whole, which in itself is an impediment to hiring, it is not uncommon to find rooms within the facility so overcrowded with exercise equipment that individuals who use a wheelchair cannot maneuver between machines nor have proper access to them, which is a clear violation of the ADA.

There are two other federal employment regulations related to hiring, which bear mentioning, background checks, and drug testing. A background investigation is normally the process of researching criminal records, commercial records, and, in some cases, financial records of an individual. Background checks are frequently requested by employers interviewing job applicants, especially applicants pursuing positions that require high security or substantial trust, such as in schools, hospitals, financial institutions, airports, and government. As background checks are normally conducted by government agencies or private enterprises for a fee, most fitness facilities conduct their own checks and are principally interested in criminal history and past employment verification. Such checks allow management to also evaluate qualifications such as education and certifications, along with character.

However, although a fitness facility may want more information on an applicant than that stated earlier, management does not have unlimited rights to investigate an applicant's background and personal life. As employees have a right to privacy in certain areas of their life, they can take legal action if they feel these rights have been violated. Consequently, it is essential that management understands what is permitted when doing further investigation on a potential employee's background and work history.

Under the Federal Trade Commission's Fair Credit Reporting Act (FCRA), applicants must give written permission to prospective employers if employers wish to obtain applicants' credit reports (19). If an employer decides not to hire an applicant or to promote an existing employee based on his or her credit report, then that applicant or employee must be provided a copy of the report, so he or she may challenge the veracity of the report. Statutes regulating the use of investigations of credit reports vary from state to state, and some states have very serious restrictions on obtaining credit reports.

As stated earlier, although fitness facilities have a vested interest in an applicant's potential criminal past, the extent to which a facility's management may consider one's criminal history in making a hiring decision varies from state to state. Owing to this wide variation, management should consult a lawyer or do further legal research on state laws before probing into whether or not an applicant does in fact have a criminal past.

The Drug-Free Workplace Act of 1988 and the mandatory guidelines for federal drug testing programs were specifically designed for federal employees with certain sensitive occupations relating to safety and security (18). Although the Drug-Free Workplace Act only applied to federal employees, many state and local governments followed suit and adopted similar programs under state laws and drug-free workplace programs. However, challenges to drug testing arose based on contested violations of the fourth and fifth amendments to the constitution. Generally, applicants are deemed to have a lesser expectation of privacy than current employees, and therefore, employers do enjoy greater freedom to test applicants without the same concerns of constitutional violations being invoked.

Drug testing may be of interest to the fitness facility not only because nondrug users make better employees but also because some facilities may insist that staff, particularly instructors, not engage in the use of steroids or other quasi-illegal performance-enhancing drugs. Although employers rightfully argue that the safety of clientele and coworkers may depend on the alertness of fellow employees and that employers will be liable if an employee under the influence of narcotics or alcohol injures a staff member or client, there are understandable concerns about the invasion of one's privacy. This idea of invasion of one's privacy is not only of concern to the American Civil Liberties Union (ACLU) but also deeply upsetting to many Americans who value their rights and privacy of person and property.

Owing to the stated concerns, there has been the tendency to limit the type and extent of drug testing in the workplace. Specifically, some states have found their courts more restrictive than the federal legislature in regard to preemployment drug testing as well as ongoing drug testing in the workplace. Consequently, it is essential that before designing a drug-free workplace with a testing program, management not only familiarizes itself with both state and federal regulations but also secures legal counsel specializing in labor relations and law.

An additional federal regulation and requirement related to prehiring and hiring is the Equal Pay Act of 1963, which prohibits different pay rates on the basis of gender (17). This act was necessitated because over the years, women have received lower wages for the exact same duties performed by men. Another employment regulation is the Age Discrimination in Employment Act (ADEA), which prohibits discrimination on the basis of age for people older than 40 years (17). Yet, another necessary regulation is the Immigration Reform and Control Act of 1986 (IRCA), which requires all employers to complete an employment eligibility verification form on individuals hired after November 6, 1986 (17).

The EEOC enforces federal laws that make it illegal to discriminate against a job applicant or employee based on a myriad of factors (16). In one such case, the EEOC filed suit against LTF (*EEOC v. Life Time Fitness, Inc.*, Civil Action No. 8:16-cv-02936-DKC) (20) on behalf of Emily Carpenter in 2016. Emily had applied to the location in Rockville, Maryland, and was told to come in and complete new hire paperwork so that she could be placed on the schedule. After she e-mailed her work availability and included that she was 35 weeks pregnant, the gym refused communication with her and did not schedule her for work. Two weeks later, a manager let Emily know that her position was put on hold and two other people were subsequently hired. She was informed she could apply for a different position at another facility after she gave birth. The EEOC attempted to reach a prelitigation settlement but ended up moving forward filing suit against the fitness facility alleging discrimination on the basis of pregnancy. LTF agreed to pay $86,000 in monetary relief to Carpenter, along with a 3-year consent decree that enjoined the company from failing to hire based on sex, including pregnancy. The company also agreed to revise its nondiscrimination policy to be distributed to all current and newly hired employees, along with annual antidiscrimination training to all managers and hiring personnel at its Montgomery County, Maryland, facilities. LTF also had to report to the EEOC on compliance with the consent decree, including how it handles complaints of alleged pregnancy discrimination, and had to post a notice regarding the settlement.

These are but a few of the important requirements that employers need to address when hiring staff for their fitness facilities. In order to be thoroughly versed with prehiring and hiring requirements, employers should visit the U.S. Department of Labor Web site and search under the "Hiring" section for information related to these and numerous other concerns such as affirmative action, the hiring of veterans and foreign workers, and the employment of workers younger than 18 years (17).

Facility Policies and Procedures

A fitness facility's policies and procedures represent a type of contract with employees as the applicant is agreeing to abide by such policies and procedures as a term of his or her employment. The development and implementation of policies and procedures provides businesses, such as fitness facilities, with operational uniformity and consistency. The adherence to policies and procedures is recognized to be one of the most important keys to profitability within a business. Policies and procedures are guidelines as well as mandates to the daily operation of a facility, and observing these assists employees in becoming more proficient because of the implied consistency of practice. This consistency, and proficiency, is noted by members and engenders greater confidence in the staff as a whole.

There are numerous policies and procedures related to the efficient conduct of business and financial operations within a facility. Unfortunately, many facilities fail to develop a comprehensive policy and procedure manual, and instead, it is the responsibility of the EP to work with management to develop and implement such a manual. Once developed, the number one priority of any facility should be the health and safety of its membership. Within this context of health and safety, there are certain policies and procedures that should take precedence: membership screening, fitness testing, orientations, instructor qualifications, supervision, equipment maintenance, facility cleanliness, and emergency procedures.

Regarding the development and implementation of proper policies and procedures, in *Beglin v. Hartwick College* (2009) (21), Michael Beglin was a student at Hartwick College, and while working out at the school's fitness center, the weight machine his friend was using became jammed. While Michael was examining why the plates were stuck, the weights (approximately 140 lb total) dislodged and fell on his hand. Beglin sued, as a result of his injury, saying that the college should have had, or already had, actual notice of the dangerous condition of the weight machine. The college claimed they had no knowledge of the danger and had met its duty to Beglin. Beglin, however, argued that the college failed in their duty by not having a plan in place to address any potential issues with machines or other risks in the center.

The college provided two employee testimonies that no one had knowledge of the danger, but Beglin was able to present testimony from the fitness center custodian. The custodian said when he would clean the machine, the metal plates on the weight machine could become easily jammed if an accessory weight was improperly placed on the machine. The custodian (Cook) claimed this was a recurring problem, and he had actually notified employees of the fitness center of this issue. Another issue at hand was whether Beglin saw and ignored warning signs to not put his hand under a certain spot in the machine. However, the court eventually ruled in his favor.

A way to mitigate this kind of risk in the future is to have a proper policy and procedural manual. Had a plan been in place, the fitness center supervisor would have known quickly of the danger presented by the allegedly defective machine. The fitness center custodian would have known exactly who to report to and how to report something, and then the supervisor would have had a plan in place to correct the issue. By failing to develop, implement, and manage a risk management plan, the college allowed itself to be open to liability and a big financial loss.

Screening members through health risk appraisals is essential to determine whether they are ready for the stress of exercise or whether medical clearance is needed. The health risk appraisal is the procedure by which a facility can identify those members who are at an increased risk for experiencing exercise-related cardiovascular incidents as well as musculoskeletal problems and the consequent need for physician referral before exercise programming can commence. Therefore, this appraisal should be completed and a review for potential risk concluded prior to finalizing a membership agreement and paying for services (1). The current standard of care dictates that screening procedures be practiced without exception. Additionally, it should be noted that too frequently abbreviated screening devices such as the Physical Activity Readiness Questionnaire (PAR-Q) are used when more comprehensive health risk appraisals are warranted.

Although it is possible for facilities to require that all members undergo a fitness assessment in conjunction with their health appraisal, it is typical that most facilities only offer and, hopefully, encourage members to avail themselves of this valuable service. There are numerous advantages for the member who participates in such an assessment or fitness profile. The real advantage to the facility, however, is the ability to design safer and more effective programs for clientele, thereby minimizing the chances of injuring a client or creating an untoward incident and consequently lessening the potential for litigation, an obvious priority for any facility.

Managers have a primary responsibility to ensure that facility members receive a formal and comprehensive orientation related to the effectiveness and safety in exercise programming. During the orientation, members should be apprised of the advantages of personal training, to include fitness profiling, which will enhance their chances of program success. Other program services and benefits can be outlined with appropriate cautionary notes regarding one's preparedness for some of the more demanding activities. A walk-through of the facility highlighting both aerobic and resistance equipment should be available, with an emphasis on equipment operation and safety concerns. There are numerous topics to be covered during the orientation, and these should be explicitly detailed in the procedure manual.

Of paramount importance are policies relating to instructor qualifications, particularly regarding education, certifications, and prior work experience. However, it is important to remember that although instructors may possess appropriate education, certification, and experience requirements and, therefore, appear qualified, this does not guarantee effective and safe training on their part. Too often, apparently qualified instructors demonstrate poor judgment and a lack of common sense, thereby endangering their clients. In effect, they may be certified and qualified but not justified in their actions (22).

In addition to the required knowledge, skills, and ability, instructors must be evaluated and advised on their interpersonal relations with fellow workers and members. Hiring policies must be clear as to which qualifications are most desirable and which qualifications meet minimal requirements. Performance reviews, along with continuing education expectations, should also be clearly detailed in the policy and procedure manual.

Policies regarding supervisory responsibilities ensure that personnel are always available to assist members having difficulty with equipment operation or the technique of specific exercises. Floor supervisors must be aware of potentially unsafe activities and alert to their anticipated implementation. Safe floor monitoring also requires that equipment is arranged in a manner that allows for all areas to be readily visible by personnel on duty and that there are no blind spots in which a member could become endangered without being observed.

Policies regarding equipment maintenance should be in writing and regularly observed. There are general, everyday maintenance requirements and inspections that can be carried out by staff members such as checking cables, pull pin security, loose belts, gated snap hooks, and so on, along with the routine cleaning and wiping down of equipment. Policies regarding equipment should also include timely and proper reporting of any defects to be listed in maintenance and repair logs. Posted warnings or out-of-order signage is to be visibly secured on inoperable equipment if the equipment cannot be removed from the floor. Besides in-house inspection and cleaning, management should have service contracts with outside vendors who are certified in the inspection and repair of equipment. In addition to regularly scheduled appointments for servicing aerobic and resistive equipment, vendors should also be available for short notice or emergency calls.

Policies regarding facility cleanliness not only lead to member satisfaction and retention but also, more important, lead to hygienic safety that can lessen the potential for litigation. An undercover investigation of fitness facilities indicated that "gyms" are some of the most likely environments for the transmission of germs (10). Accordingly, management needs to establish policy and procedures for daily equipment cleaning and hiring a professional cleaning service for nightly or early morning operations. Increased awareness of germ transmission has led many fitness facilities to provide members with clean towels and, more recently, with antiseptic spray bottles, germicidal wipes, paper towel dispensers, and antibacterial hand gel throughout the exercise floor. However, this cannot take the place of policies requiring regular and thorough cleaning provided by staff and professional services.

Of all facility policies, the emergency policy, and particularly the emergency medical policy, is the most consequential. It is incumbent on management to develop a written, venue-specific emergency response plan to deal with any reasonably foreseeable untoward event within the facility. The emergency plan's primary purpose is to ensure that minor problems do not escalate into major incidents and that major incidents do not intensify to fatal events. Possible emergencies could be fires, floods, tornadoes, earthquakes, hurricanes, severe storms, bomb threats, and even terrorist activities.

However, the most likely emergency is a "Code Blue" or "member down," indicating that a client is having a heart attack, stroke, or some other potentially fatal event. This emphasizes the need for an emergency response plan to include an explicit medical emergency policy in which all staff must be well versed. Such a policy dictates that sufficient staff members are certified in first aid and cardiopulmonary resuscitation (CPR) with automated external defibrillator (AED). Another important consideration, too often overlooked, is the availability of supplemental oxygen that is probably one of the most important steps that can be taken in treating the suspected heart attack. Additionally, in the case of a sudden cardiac arrest, an oxygen source attached to a resuscitation mask dramatically increases the chance of survival (1).

A well-rehearsed emergency response plan guarantees a timely response in carrying out the multiple duties expected of staff, such as who coordinates the scene, who are first and assistant responders, who takes charge of crowd control, who meets and directs paramedics to the scene, and who is responsible for securing the member's file along with notifying the nearest relative. If these policies and procedures are lax, or staff rehearsal is not frequent, the potential for litigation increases exponentially. Therefore, anticipative management is considered not only imperative but also "good insurance" (2).

SUMMARY

The key to the health and safety of facility members is the availability of knowledgeable, skilled, and conscientious fitness instructors capable of establishing a safe exercise environment. This requires that staff members at all levels must not only be appropriately qualified to carry out their respective duties but also be sufficiently motivated to do the job to the best of their abilities.

Today, however, the public is beginning to hold health facilities and fitness instructors more accountable than in the past. As a result, there has been an upsurge in the number of personal injury lawsuits against facilities and instructors along with a concurrent rise in the costs of relevant liability insurance. Even with the obvious deterrent of prospectively executed waivers and releases, the public appears more willing to take their grievances to court.

The current escalation of litigation is a reflection of a serious industry problem regarding client expectations and service delivery. Too frequently, individuals are injured as a result of certified instructors not being truly qualified professionals, and too often, individuals die while pursuing a healthier lifestyle because of insufficient screening, ineffective instruction, improper supervision, and/or an inadequate emergency response.

To lessen the possibility of litigation, facility personnel must be capable of thoroughly screening potential members, providing suitable fitness tests, evaluating health assessments and fitness profiles, designing appropriate exercise programs, and attentively supervising member activities. In addition, staff should constantly be aware of potentially dangerous situations and be empowered with the responsibility as well as the accountability to immediately correct hazardous conditions and respond effectively to emergency situations. This can only occur if management is knowledgeable about the field of exercise science and if instructors are properly qualified.

EPs are typically placed in positions of not only conducting fitness programming but also managing facility operations. Therefore, their knowledge of exercise science must be complemented with a well-rounded knowledge of the many different areas within which management and personnel can become legally embroiled. Too often, the many administrative and legal concerns of a health/fitness facility have gone unrecognized or have been misunderstood. The truly knowledgeable EP recognizes the numerous responsibilities in managing and operating a facility that is totally committed to the health, fitness, and safety of its membership as well as the professionalism of the health and fitness industry.

STUDY QUESTIONS

1. What are those incidents in which an EP would most likely become legally embroiled?
2. Identify major risk management strategies to lessen the chances of litigation.
3. What is the last line of defense in risk management?
4. List some of the municipal, state, and federal administrative requirements in the hiring of personnel and the operation of a fitness facility.
5. List various roles of responsibility in handling a medical emergency such as a sudden cardiac arrest.

REFERENCES

1. Bates M, editor. *Health Fitness Management: A Comprehensive Resource for Managing and Operating Programs and Facilities.* 2nd ed. Champaign (IL): Human Kinetics; 2008. 400 p.

2. Eickhoff-Shemek J, Herbert D, Connaughton D. *Risk Management for Health/Fitness Professionals: Legal Issues and Strategies.* Philadelphia (PA): Lippincott Williams & Wilkins; 2009. 407 p.

3. Earle R, Baechle T, editors. *NSCA's Essentials of Personal Training.* Champaign (IL): Human Kinetics; 2004. 676 p.

4. American College of Sports Medicine. *ACSM's Guidelines for Exercise Testing and Prescription.* 6th ed. Philadelphia (PA): Lippincott Williams & Wilkins; 2000. 368 p.

5. Corrigan v. Musclemakers, Inc., N.Y. App. Div. LEXIS 1954. (1999).

6. Cotten D, Cotten M. *Legal Aspects of Waivers in Sport, Recreation and Fitness Activities.* Canton (OH): PRC Publishing; 1997. 206 p.

7. Berisaj v. LTF Club Operations Company, Inc., Mich. Ct. App. (2019).

8. American College of Sports Medicine. *ACSM's Health/ Fitness Facility Standards and Guidelines.* 5th ed. Champaign (IL): Human Kinetics; 2019. 232 p.

9. Herren et al., v. Sucher, Ga. Ct. App. (2003).

10. ABC News. Is your health club unhealthy? [Internet]. New York (NY): ABC News; [cited 2005 Jan 13]. Available from: http://abcnews.go.com/Primetime/Fitness/story?id=410907.

11. York Insurance Company v. Houston Wellness Center, Inc., Ga. Ct. App. (2003).

12. Paul E. Sexual harassment as sex discrimination: a defective paradigm. *Yale Law Policy Rev.* 1990;8(2):333–65.

13. Sheppard v. River Valley Fitness One, LP, 218 F. Supp. 2d 38. (D.N.H. 2002).

14. International Health, Racquet & Sportsclub Association. *IHRSA's Standards Facilitation Guide.* 2nd ed. Boston (MA): International Health, Racquet & Sportsclub Association; 1998.

15. U.S. Department of Health and Human Services Web site [Internet]. Washington (DC): U.S. Department of Health and Human Services; [cited 2017 Feb 7]. Available from: https://www.hhs.gov.

16. U.S. Equal Employment Opportunity Commission Web site [Internet]. Washington (DC): U.S. Equal Employment Opportunity Commission; [cited 2017 Feb 7]. Available from: https://www.eeoc.gov.

17. U.S. Department of Labor. Hiring issues [Internet]. Washington (DC): U.S. Department of Labor; [cited 2017 Feb 7]. Available from: https://www.dol.gov/general/topic/hiring.

18. U.S. Department of Labor Web site [Internet]. Washington (DC): U.S. Department of Labor; [cited 2017 Feb 7]. Available from: https://www.dol.gov.

19. Federal Trade Commission Web site [Internet]. Washington (DC): Federal Trade Commission; [cited 2021 April 13]. Available from: https://www.ftc.gov.

20. EEOC v. Life Time Fitness, Inc., Civil Action No. 8: 16-cv-02936-DKC. (2016).

21. Beglin v. Hartwick College, 67 A.D. 3d 1172. (2009).

22. Abbott A. Fitness professionals: certified, qualified and justified. *Exerc Stand Malpract Rep.* 2009;23(2):17, 20–2.

15 Leadership and Management

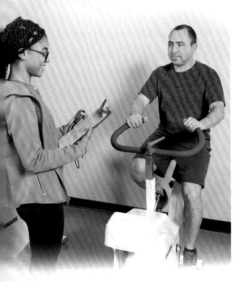

INTRODUCTION

The context of the health/fitness industry is complex and volatile and, like most other industries, is constantly changing. There is a steady stream of changing regulations, evolving accreditation standards, emerging or reorganized regulatory agencies, new research, and an onslaught of fitness fads. In addition to satisfying many stakeholders (*e.g.*, clients and fitness club owners and peers), there is now the need to have and develop sufficient leadership and management skills for sustained success.

Leadership has become a fundamental expectation of all American College of Sports Medicine Certified Exercise Physiologists® (ACSM-EPs®) regardless of their work context. Although not every ACSM-EP is a leader with a formal organizational role, every ACSM-EP should practice leadership. As the practice of exercise physiology becomes more closely associated with the mainstream health care industry, leadership practices within the profession and during the socialization process become critical. In 1998, the Pew Health Professions Commission recommended that all health professionals in the 21st century, whether they seek management positions or not, should practice leadership (1). In other words, leadership behaviors have not only become an industry standard but also a professional standard that transcends the work place. Leadership, apart from management, should be practiced consistently and intentionally. The aim of this chapter is to instill a sense of responsibility in the ACSM-EP to introduce and cultivate a working leadership philosophy into their professional practice.

 ## Defining Leadership and Management

The construct of leadership has hundreds of nuances, anecdotes, gradations, and theories. So much literature exists on leadership and its development, which can make sorting through and implementing leadership strategies a difficult process. In the past, many of the concepts and ideas concerning organizational effectiveness and motivation focused solely on management techniques. Recently, however, there has been a clear swing toward leadership competencies as a means of achieving organizational effectiveness and employee motivation. Management and leadership, whether independent of each other or in combination, are necessary within the health/fitness industry (2). There are clear differences between leadership and management (3). Generally, *people* require leadership and *resources* require management. The ACSM-EP should try to avoid falling into the trap of managing people. Although management is a necessary skill, it should not be substituted for leadership. The temptation to manage people usually results from the perception that managing is easier than leading. For example, managing might lead to "punishing" by enforcing established policies and procedures, whereas leading may involve discussion, negotiation, and established new ways of operating.

Operational Definitions

Operationally, leadership is the ability to facilitate and influence others (*i.e.*, superiors, peers, and subordinates) to make recognizable strides toward shared and unshared objectives (2). Management is the ability to use organizational resources to accomplish predetermined objectives (2). Leadership transcends the workplace, whereas management is often confined to the workplace. For example, in a health/fitness setting, leadership is demonstrated when the ACSM-EP motivates and inspires clients or patients to make needed lifestyle changes. However, management in this situation may require the ACSM-EP to add additional or longer training days, make a referral to other health professionals, or schedule additional consultations. This would require having a well-organized, managed schedule and referral system in place.

Management and leadership are not always different. In fact, both usually have similar outcome objectives, project power, and use influence. However, the differences between leadership and management may best be delineated in the examination of intended outcomes and processes (4). The intended outcome of leadership is typically change, vision casting, and innovation; the intended outcome of management is predictability, vision implementation, and maintaining the efficient status quo. These two constructs often require different techniques and operate from fundamentally different frameworks. Dye and Garman (5) describe management as the "science" of mitigating risk, whereas "leadership is the art of taking risks." Therefore, leadership tends to use vision casting, alignment, meaningful communication, self-reflection, and self-assessment to develop willing followers, whereas management uses "planning, organizing, controlling, and coordinating," regardless of the subordinates' willingness (6). Stated another way, management is a function or role within an organization, and leadership is a relationship between the follower and the leader, regardless of the organizational context (7). Any time something occurs despite the context, complexity is involved. This further helps us to distinguish between management and leadership. Leadership takes place in a complex environment where boundaries and borders are not clearly delineated. With both leadership and management, there are many variables to consider in the decision-making process. In the complex leadership environment, those variables are usually interdependent and not easily separated. On the other hand, management is often understood as complicated (as opposed to complex), and typically, those variables can be separated and operate independently.

Another distinguishing factor is that management is required when problems arise of a technical nature, which requires preestablished policies and procedures to be enacted. On the other hand, leadership is required when problems do not have preestablished solutions and instead require adaptability, critical thinking, creativity, and innovation (8).

Although management and leadership are generally accepted as distinct, they are not necessarily exclusive because both need to exist to efficiently operate a health/fitness facility. Therefore, the ACSM-EP should be able to manage a facility (budget, mitigate risk, use policy and procedures, etc.) while also leading people (inspire, communicate, motivate, exhibit empathy and ethical behavior, etc.). Figure 15.1 is an adaptation of a relationship matrix for the integration of leadership and management — the higher the value, the greater the competency. Table 15.1 outlines the central tendencies that differentiate leadership and management.

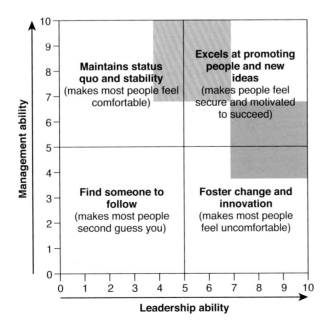

FIGURE 15.1. Integrating leadership and management. (From Kutz MR. *Leadership and Management in Athletic Training: An Integrated Approach.* Baltimore [MD]: Lippincott Williams & Wilkins; 2010. 331 p.)

Table 15.1	Differences between Leadership and Management
Leadership's Tendencies	**Management's Tendencies**
■ Change oriented	■ Predictable
■ Vision caster	■ Vision implementer
■ Innovates	■ Maintains status quo
■ Motivated to take risk	■ Motivated to analyze risk
■ Influence/authority transcends the organization	■ Influence/authority confined to within the organization
■ Solves unexpected and novel problems with creativity	■ Solves known and technical problems with established policy and procedure
■ Proactive	■ Reactive
■ Focus on long term	■ Focus on short term
■ Identifies opportunities	■ Identifies obstacles
■ Idea and person centered	■ System and plan centered
■ Shares information freely	■ Shares "need-to-know" information
■ Uses interpersonal skills to handle conflict	■ Uses precedent, policy, procedure to handle conflict
■ Places emphasis on team accomplishments	■ Places emphasis on individual performance
■ Works to prevent conflict or problems	■ Works to solve existing conflicts or problems

Evidence-Based Management

One way to make the process of management more effective is a relatively new concept of evidence-based management. As ACSM-EPs, we are familiar with the concept of evidence-based practice, but the rapid growth and complexity of the health care system has required the introduction of evidence-based management. Evidence-based management helps the ACSM-EP to use the best available management research combined with the practitioner's experience and stakeholder expectations. The ultimate outcome of evidence-based management is to make efficient and reliable decisions. Evidence-based management is a decision-making process that considers equally three inputs. The first input is the best available research. Of course, the key is "best available," which implies that the ACSM-EP knows how to evaluate and consume the *best* research, not just *any* research. Because leadership and management tend to be social sciences, ACSM-EPs may need to familiarize themselves with nonexperimental or social scientific study design techniques in order to evaluate this research accurately. The second input is the personal experience of the ACSM-EP. Of course, this does not mean clinical experience, but decision-making and management experience. When this is lacking, say in the instance of a novice, the ACSM-EP may have the tendency to overrely on research for input. To mitigate that risk, seek opportunities to lead and manage even if that means volunteering outside of your employer, professional organization, or even health care. Valuable leadership and management experience can be gained from involvement in civic and social organizations. The third input for effective evidence-based management is understanding and knowing stakeholder expectations. This means the ACSM-EP must be familiar with the values and desires of several stakeholders. Stakeholders can be patients or clients, but they can also be physicians, coworkers, other allied health care professionals, and administrators. Importantly, these three inputs should be considered when learning to manage (and lead). When one strives to integrate all three inputs equally, decision making improves.

⬢ Leadership: Past, Present, and Future

Although leadership theory is dynamic and continually evolving, four major models of leadership theory are consistently referenced in the literature: classical, transactional, visionary, and organic (9,10). Collectively, these four leadership models serve as a philosophical foundation from which leadership is practiced.

Through the early 1970s, the classical model dominated leadership theory. Under this model, a leader's power or influence was considered innate, and having a vision was not considered necessary to ensure follower support. Often, a leader's influence was based on fear or respect. A leader's position or placement was rarely challenged. Of course, as workers became more skilled and knowledgeable, this model became less popular and was less able to motivate subordinates.

Transactional Model

The transactional model also began to gain popularity in the 1970s and signaled the era of the manager. Under this model, vision was neither necessary nor articulated. Instead, influence was based on contractual negotiations of rewards and punishments between the leader and subordinates. Considerable effort was taken by transactional leaders to create "environments" conducive to management intervention. In other words, the focus was on the manager's ability to generate policies and procedures that capitalized on productivity and efficiency. This model rewarded management for generating systems where a manager could intervene. Productivity was considered an outcome of "good" management, and any role employees had in productivity was minimized.

The transactional model is still in full use in many health/fitness enterprises today. For example, most health care clinics, hospitals, and related facilities are bureaucratic and require transactional behaviors to operate. Transactional behaviors include the use of job descriptions, core competencies, and annual performance evaluations, which are based on those job descriptions and competencies. Furthermore, the typical transactional practices include the use of contracts or incentives. Formal agreements, such as an agreed-on salary in exchange for 40 hours of work per week, is a transactional leadership technique. The ACSM-EP may incentivize a patient to pursue a certain goal or reach a certain objective (*e.g.*, lose 10 lb, decrease body fat percentage, or increase healthy eating habits). The drawback to using transactional techniques is the absence of internal or intrinsic motivation. Patients might revert back to former (poor) habits when incentives or contracts are removed or satisfied. Nonetheless, transactional techniques are efficient and productive (albeit shortsighted), which is why they remain.

Visionary Model

The visionary model emerged shortly thereafter (mid-1980s) and still has many proponents today, although it has lost some popularity. Visionary leadership (also called charismatic or transformational leadership) involves the leader using emotion to inspire and create buy-in of the followers. Interestingly, with the entrance of the visionary model, the language changed from "subordinates" to "followers." Within this model, vision became fundamental and followers were encouraged to contribute to the leader's vision.

The visionary model is a frequently used technique. However, these visionary techniques require a different type of skill and intentionality. Transactional practices depend on technical competency and expert power. Visionary techniques require the skillful application of soft skills. Soft skills fall outside the domain of technical competencies and include abilities such as empathy, creativity, work ethic, critical thinking, adaptability, and resiliency. As noted earlier, the visionary model is closely related to charismatic or transformational leadership. Importantly, the ACSM-EP should focus on developing visionary leadership habits, paying particular attention to the intrinsic motivation of the client. Intrinsic motivation occurs when the client desires to improve because improvement itself is the best thing and its own reward. The ACSM-EP can use visionary tactics by getting clients to envision living a healthy lifestyle or accomplishing a certain goal (*e.g.*, losing weight, finishing a 10K run). In this instance, the ACSM-EP uses interpersonal techniques to inspire and motivate the client to want to accomplish these goals for his or her own sake and well-being.

Organic Model

The most recent model, organic, tends to overlap with visionary. The organic leadership model centers on a collective vision of the group as a team. A vision is important but is not "owned" only by the leader; instead, the vision is created collectively, and the leader helps implement the will of the team. Influence is based on the relationship and mutuality of the team and the endorsement of a leader. Organizational charts from an organic model tend to look like an amoeba instead of the pyramid shape of the other models. The organic model is most unique from a leadership development standpoint. In the previous three models, leadership development occurs by traditional means. In traditional leadership development, the external institutions (*e.g.*, a university) have the responsibilities of socializing members and providing formal leadership instruction. However, within the organic model, leadership development is grass roots. That means, leadership development takes place within the organization, and socialization occurs as one is practicing his or her profession and not *before* he or she enters the profession. This, of course, has huge implications for hiring leaders. In the other models, leaders would be searched for from outside and imported, whereas in an organic model, leaders are looked to and developed from within.

The organic leadership model is growing in popularity. The ACSM-EP is traditionally educated and certified from an outside agency, such as the national accrediting agency (*e.g.*, ACSM) or university. Therefore, this traditional process is not strictly organic. However, there are several very popular organic-based systems growing in popularity. The most obvious examples are structured and membership-based high-intensity interval training programs (HIIT; *e.g.*, CrossFit). These types of programs are highly dependent on a local community working together to motivate and inspire each other toward collaborative goals. This is the epitome of the organic model of leadership. These programs often offer their own training and certifications that are often pursued by members within the local HIIT community. The ACSM-EP can use organic leadership techniques by aligning clients to peers with similar goals and creating a social support system between other clients, ACSM-EPs, and the client's peers. For the ACSM-EP to be successful in using organic leadership techniques, interprofessional practice (*i.e.*, working closely with professionals from other disciplines) is a prerequisite. Competition between health care facilities and other health/fitness professionals takes a "backseat" to client's outcomes.

Leadership Theory and Model

As new and more research emerges, leadership models and theories will continue to evolve. As this evolution occurs, there will always be the temptation for leaders to operate out of multiple models, some of which are in conflict with each other. For example, having a personal belief that leadership is something people are born with and is innate (classical model) is very different from the open leadership development programs to anyone interested (organic model) or soliciting feedback on strategic plans from nonleaders (visionary model). Applying different leadership *models* during the practice of management or leadership is contradictory. However, mixing leadership *behaviors* or *styles* is encouraged. Transitioning between or mixing leadership styles is appropriate when confronted with new problems or situations. For example, in a particular situation or with certain personnel, a leader may have to demonstrate servant leadership and then use a path–goal approach or apply situational style in a different situation.

The seminal work of Ralph Stogdill (11) in the 1950s identified 1,800 separate leadership behaviors. Stogdill was eventually able to identify two key behaviors rated by the vast majority of subordinates as critical to leadership: "initiating structure" and "consideration" (12). Initiating structure means organizing and defining relationships in a group (12). Consideration is defined as the degree to which the leader creates an environment of emotional support, warmth, friendliness, and trust (12). These two constructs have served as the foundation for much of how leadership is practiced and understood.

Leadership Behaviors and Theories

Many of the following leadership behaviors and theories have developed and emerged over time. In one way or another, all are still applicable today. There are many different situations where each behavior or theory may be appropriate as well as situations where they may not be appropriate. The important thing to realize is that each one — depending on the context — may or may not be relevant. For instance, trait theories (defined in the following text) are less prominent today than ever before; however, many agencies still hire individuals based on certain expected traits. The perfect example of this is the expectation that health/fitness professionals (*e.g.*, personal trainers, strength and conditioning specialists, and ACSM-EPs) be physically active and "look the part." Despite having the requisite knowledge or expertise, failing to be physically active or "look the part" may disqualify certain candidates to some employers.

Trait Theory

The "great man" (or woman) theory promoted the idea that being a "superior leader" is an issue of genetics, in which one is born to lead and has an innate set of leadership qualities and abilities (11). The "great man" ideology still has proponents today. For example, a popular leadership book states, "Leadership cannot be manufactured. It cannot be mustered up. It's an innate gifting" (13).

Trait theory postulates two forms — (a) leadership traits are innate or a divine endowment (*i.e.*, great man theory) or (b) an individual can awaken dormant traits over time (14). Regardless of whether leadership is innate, divine endowment, or learned, those who might have innate leadership ability still must improve their leadership skills through years of practice and experience (5).

Situational Leadership Theory

Situational leadership was originally developed by Blanchard and Hersey in the 1960s. Situational leadership's purpose is to open up communication and to increase the quality and frequency of conversations about performance and development (15). Situational leadership suggests that leadership style is adapted by the leader on the basis of the leader's "diagnosis" of the "development level" of the subordinate (15). The development level or "situation" of a subordinate is based on a relationship between two factors: competence and commitment (15). For example, subordinates with high competence and high commitment (*i.e.*, experts) warrant delegation with little supervision (*i.e.*, a "leader who empowers them to act independently, affirming and confirming their decisions") (16). On the other hand, subordinates who demonstrate low competence but high commitment warrant direction aimed at "developing competence" (Fig. 15.2) (15).

Situational leadership is used almost every day by ACSM-EPs and allows the ACSM-EP to address the different levels of a patient's motivation and willingness to perform certain activities. In particular situations, a client may be more motivated (*e.g.*, has high competence and

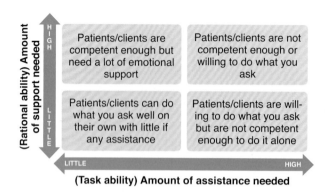

FIGURE 15.2. Situational leadership.

high commitment) or less motivated to perform. Depending on the level of motivation and the experience of the ACSM-EP, different types of engagement with the client or patient are needed. For example, a patient who is very knowledgeable and enthusiastic about cardiovascular training but fears or has little experience with resistance training warrants different types of engagement from the ACSM-EP. Using the situational leadership mindset, the ACSM-EP should use different techniques to motivate and inspire the client during resistance training. For instance, using a more hands-on and direct supervision approach when the patient is performing resistance training may be more appropriate compared to when the patient performs cardiovascular training.

Path–Goal Leadership Theory

Path–goal theory was popularized by House in the 1970s and is a modification of contingency or situational leadership. This theory involves the leader setting a path to a specific goal for a specific member or team on the basis of that member's personality or team's dynamics (12). Path–goal theory is about how leaders motivate employees to accomplish their designated goals (16). This theory draws heavily on motivational theory and emphasizes how the leader's style is influenced by both the work setting and subordinates (16).

Path–goal leadership techniques are similar to situational techniques; however, in this case, the ACSM-EP collaborates with the client or patient to predetermine specific goals and then uses different techniques to motivate that client to accomplish those goals. The difference is that the ACSM-EP does not use the same technique(s) for every patient or client. The techniques that the ACSM-EP uses to motivate and inspire one patient toward his or her goals will be determined by the personality and needs of the individual client or patient. In other words, the ACSM-EP refuses to motivate and inspire all of the patients and clients the same way and is intentional about learning the specific techniques that individual patients respond to the best.

Transformational and Transactional Leadership

Burns (17) identified two types of leadership: transformational and transactional. Transformational leadership can be summarized as that which inspires and motivates others. Followers are influenced by the leader's creativity, admiration, and respect (17). Transformational leaders give respect and admiration to their followers and are likewise typically admired and respected by their followers. Transformational leadership is considered similar to charismatic or visionary leadership (12).

Transformational leaders give "individual attention, inspire others to excel and stimulate people to think in new ways" (18). Stated another way, transformational leadership fosters innovation in coworkers and followers. There are five "practices" associated with transformational leadership: "challenging the process, inspiring a shared vision, enabling others to act, modeling the way, and encouraging the heart" (18).

Transactional leaders view leadership as the process of "exchanging one thing for another" (17). Often, transactional leadership comes down to exchanging rewards (salary and benefits) for performance or work (17). Transactional leaders operate under different circumstances and from a different motivation than transforming leaders. Burns (17) pointed out the divergent nature of the two leadership types. Transactional leadership is about the "individual interest" of the leader and is not concerned with the "collective interest of followers"; on the other hand, transformational leadership concerns itself with the follower's interests (17). "The transactional leader's behavior closely resembles that of a manager" (18). Although followers prefer transformational leadership, this leadership style is not necessarily the most efficient.

Lewin's Leadership Styles

In 1939, Kurt Lewin identified three styles of leadership that were commonly used in the decision-making process of managers: autocratic, democratic, and laissez-faire (19). In the autocratic style, the leader makes decisions on his or her own and typically does not consult with others. Autocratic style often results in the highest level of discontentment among subordinates and followers. An autocratic style typically only works well in an "emergency" situation.

In the democratic style, the leader involves his or her peers and subordinates in the decision-making process. One often misunderstood aspect of democratic leadership is that consensus or the will of the followers should override the leaders. However, true democratic leadership may still make the unpopular decision; in this style, the leader always reserves the authority to make the ultimate decision. The democratic style is often highly valued by followers. However, a democratic style can be challenging when there are wide ranges of opinions.

The third style is laissez-faire, which virtually eliminates any leadership involvement in decision making. In other words, followers usually make their own decisions. This is problematic because the "leader" is still ultimately responsible for the group's decisions. This style can work when followers take ownership of the process and are competent and willing to make decisions. However, this style was found to be the least rewarding and often showed low morale of followers.

Servant Leadership

Servant leadership theory was introduced by Greenleaf in the early 1970s and shares many traits with transformational leadership (20). The one major difference is that in the decision-making process of servant leadership, the individual's interest is considered. Although transformational leadership implies that the organization is considered first, servant leadership establishes that organizational performance is secondary to the relationship between the leader and the follower (20). The servant leader is said to be a servant first and leader second. Leading and directing are part of their roles and functions, but that role and function is secondary to the desire or need to promote others.

Servant leadership is incredibly relevant today. The ACSM-EP should always strive to serve the best interest of the clients and patients as well as the other stakeholders (*e.g.*, employer, ACSM) by intentionally serving. The hallmark of servant leaders is placing the interests of patients and stakeholders before their own. Obviously, every ACSM-EP should put the interest of the patient's well-being and health before personal ambition. Being a servant leader sometimes requires you to alter your schedule and adjust break periods or lunch times and maybe even vacation time to accommodate patients' needs. A reasonable effort should be made for these accommodations; however, a servant leader should not feel guilty when he or she cannot accommodate certain needs and should never let employers or patients take advantage of him or her.

Leader–Member Exchange Theory

Leader–member exchange (LMX) theory centers on the "interactions" between the leader and the follower (16) and was intended to help establish a more mature leadership relationship (21). LMX theory is based on vertical dyad research, which establishes *in-groups* and *out-groups* (16). In-groups are those leader–follower relationships that allow for subordinate's roles to be expanded and negotiated; out-groups are those leader–follower relationships based purely on formal contract and predefined roles (16). Followers falling into the in-group category tend to achieve more and receive more of the leader's time and attention (16). Out-group members do what they are told and stick to formal procedures. Typically, out-group members are treated fairly by leaders but do not get "special attention." Current LMX research is based on how the leader can make relationships with every subordinate so that each one feels he or she is part of the in-group (16).

Emotional Intelligence

Although more of a concept than a theory, emotional intelligence (EI) is recognized as a set of skills (*i.e.*, street smarts) that include awareness of self and others and the ability to handle emotions and relationships (21–23). EI is the capacity to reason about emotions and use emotions to enhance thinking (24). EI includes the ability to accurately perceive emotions, to access and generate emotions to assist thought, to understand emotions and emotional knowledge, and to effectively regulate emotions (23,24).

Theoretically, EI involves the relationship between cognition and emotion and works closely with other intelligences such as social, practical, and personal (24). Practicing EI involves four critical skills. Those skills are as follows: (a) being able to recognize and perceive emotions of others; (b) using emotions to assist (not hinder) thoughts and thinking; (c) ability to analyze and understand emotions; and (d) managing personal emotions based on personal goals, self-knowledge, and social awareness (24).

Goleman (25) has written extensively on the topic of EI and has popularized its concept. Successful leaders have a high EQ, which appears to be directly related to EI. In fact, leaders with very high expertise and technical knowledge (*i.e.*, high IQ) fail in certain leadership initiatives because of low EQ (10). The "How to Identify Emotional Intelligence" box shows key elements that must be present to identify a leader with EI.

HOW TO — **Identify Emotional Intelligence**

EI is a trait that works closely with social, practical, and personal intelligence and allows leaders to accurately perceive others feelings and emotions. To recognize someone with high levels of EI, you should note the following four factors.

Internal Factors

1. *Self-awareness*: someone who is aware of his or her own emotions and feelings
2. *Self-management*: someone who can regulate his or her own emotions and feelings

External Factors

1. *Social awareness*: someone who displays empathy or is aware of others' emotions and feelings
2. *Relationship management*: someone who can successfully regulate emotional aspects of work-related relationships

Contextual Intelligence and Three-Dimensional Thinking

Contextual intelligence (CI) is also a concept that has great implications for leadership and management. CI has been described by researchers in psychology, education, and athletic training as well as by intelligence theorists as the ability to adapt or respond appropriately to any number of different contexts, where the context is determined by environmental factors and stakeholder values (26–29). CI is a cluster of individual leadership skills that are integrated and demonstrated simultaneously (Table 15.2). Sternberg (28) is recognized as introducing the term *contextual intelligence* as a subtheme of practical intelligence. CI is typically associated with tacit knowledge (30,31) and is closely associated with wisdom gained from experience; however, recently strategies for teaching and learning CI have also emerged (26,32). As opposed to academic intelligence, often

Table 15.2	Leadership Skills Associated with Contextual Intelligence
Future minded	Has a forward-looking mentality and sense of direction and concern for where the organization should be in the future
Influencer	Uses interpersonal skills to ethically and noncoercively affect the actions and decisions of others
Mission minded	Understands and communicates how the individual performance of others influences subordinate's, peer's, and supervisor's perception of how the mission is being accomplished
Socially responsible	Expresses concern about social trends and issues (encourages legislation and policy when appropriate) and volunteers in social and community activities
Embraces new ideas	Promotes diversity in multiple contexts, aligns diverse individuals by creating and facilitating diversity, and provides opportunities for diverse members to interact in nondiscriminatory manner
Multicultural leadership	Can influence and affect the behaviors and attitudes of peers and subordinates in an ethnically diverse context
Diagnoses context	Knows how to appropriately interpret and react to changing and volatile surroundings
Change agent	Has the courage to raise difficult and challenging questions that others may perceive as a threat to the status quo
	Proactive rather than reactive in rising to challenges, leading, participating in, or making change (*i.e.,* assessing, initiating, researching, planning, constructing, and advocating)
Constructive use of influence	Demonstrates the effective use of different types of power in developing and demonstrating influence
Intentional leadership	Assesses and evaluates own leadership performance and is aware of strengths and weaknesses
	Takes intentional action toward continuous improvement of leadership ability
	Has an action guide and delineated goals for achieving personal best
Critical thinker	Cognitive ability to make connections, integrate, and make practical application of different actions, opinions, and information
Consensus builder	Exhibits interpersonal skill and convinces other people to see the common good or a different point of view for the sake of the organizational mission or values by using listening skills, managing conflict, and creating win-win situations

measured by IQ, CI has been shown to be the best predictor of success in real-life performance situations (33,34).

CI requires the integration of knowledge gained from a person's total experiences. In other words, problems are solved or solutions are generated on the basis of knowledge built from all experiences (direct and indirect), and this does not exclude experiences that might seem to be unrelated or irrelevant. For the contextually intelligent leader, solutions are based on the use of knowledge acquired in the past and the present, combined with what is currently anticipated about the future. This phenomenon has been described as thinking in three dimensions or 3D (32).

The 3D-thinking model of CI is the simultaneous integration of three distinct time orientations: hindsight, insight, and foresight (32). Lessons learned from the past are referred to as hindsight. Hindsight requires accurately reflecting on the past and ensuring that the lessons learned from the past are always being reevaluated for new lessons. Therefore, hindsight requires intentionally applying lessons learned from the past in every new context the ACSM-EP may find himself or herself. Accurately understanding the present is referred to as insight. Insight is knowing what to do in the moment you are in right now, the present. Insight occurs after the convergence of hindsight and foresight. Foresight is being able to accurately articulate the future—not any future, but your future. Simply, foresight is the ability to answer the questions what sort of future are you hoping for and how specifically are you going to accomplish your vision. Once hindsight and foresight begin working together, insight is a natural consequence (32). The CI model has a lot of promise for helping leaders learn to manage complex and ambiguous environments while still bringing the most value to stakeholders. However, practicing CI and its related 3D-thinking framework is not without obstacles. Specifically, there are four obstacles to CI that need to be addressed. Those four obstacles (32) are presented in Table 15.3.

Table 15.3   Obstacles and Solutions for Contextual Intelligence

Obstacle to Contextual Intelligence	Description	Recommended Solution
The pace of change	Change often happens so quickly that there is no time to respond without some element of guesswork or reflexive reaction.	Intentionally "extract" lessons from any and all experiences and be prepared to apply those lessons in seemingly unrelated situations or events.
Complexity	The ever-increasing number of external and internal variables that have an impact on people and organizations	Realize that as complexity increases, the amount of information/data required for accurate decision making decreases.
Learned behavior	Past success often creates incredible obstacles to adapting or responding to changing contexts. People are often strongly biased by their existing knowledge and rarely can interpret what they see without that bias.	Adopt a new commitment to learn what informs the behaviors and attitudes of self, others, society, and the organization. Do not rely as heavily on precedent or actions that lead to previous success.
Inappropriate orientation to time	Most people when faced with a decision will disproportionately pull and apply information from one of three time orientations (past, present, and future), rarely are all three time orientations consulted proportionately.	One solution is to think in 3D. Thinking in 3D requires a proportionate awareness of how the past, present, and future are influencing the current context.

Management Techniques

Management techniques are viewed as distinct from leadership styles, skills, or behaviors. The term *technique* was chosen because this word implies that something can be implemented by anyone in a position to do so and does not necessarily require any prerequisite skill for the technique to be used. Therefore, management techniques can be applied even if one does not possess leadership skills or demonstrate leadership behaviors. Obviously, the management techniques can be improved, or applied with greater success, if combined with appropriate leadership skills in the management application or implementation.

Management Grid (Blake and Mouton)

The management grid is intended to measure the relationship between one's concern for people and production. The grid allows the ACSM-EP to identify which of five major styles he or she exhibits in order to better use his or her leadership and management skills. For the concern of people, the ACSM-EP considers the needs of team members and their interests when deciding how best to accomplish goals. For the concern of production, the ACSM-EP emphasizes efficiency and productivity when deciding how best to accomplish goals. The five major styles identified by Blake and Mouton are as follows:

1. *Improvised management*: a low concern for people and production. The manager's main motivation is to stay out of trouble and maintain the status quo. Effort is at a minimum, and they are satisfied to simply pass orders from superiors.
2. *Country-club management*: high concern for employees but low concern for production. The goal of the manager is to satisfy needs of employees and provide a friendly atmosphere.
3. *Authoritarian management*: high concern for production and efficiency but low concern for employees. Managers often perceive personal needs as irrelevant or perhaps even harmful to goals. Often, authority is used to coerce subordinates to meet goals.
4. *Middle-of-the-road management*: moderate concern for production and employee satisfaction.
5. *Team or democratic management*: high concern for both production and morale. Team or democratic managers often try to develop committed work groups and focus.

Scientific Management (Frederick W. Taylor)

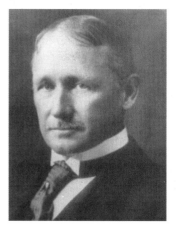

Scientific management is the organization and supervision of jobs and duties based on the manager's direct observation of the job. The manager's job was to create rules and procedures on how to do a given job that replaced "rule of thumb," and these were based strictly on the manager's direct and "scientific" observation of that job. Any deviation from the manager's scientifically prescribed procedures is punished. Scientific management's basic tenet was that monetary payment was the only motivation employees needed. In fact, when Taylor published *The Principles of Scientific Management* in 1911, he suggested that sole responsibility of the organization rests with the manager and that only the manager needed to be concerned with working conditions and outcomes. According to Taylor, a manager's responsibility was to provide detailed and specific instructions on how to do the assigned task and that the organization was more important than the individual (35,36). Scientific management is no longer a popular model; however, remnants of this model can be seen in bureaucratic and transactional behaviors. Eventually, the presuppositions that framed scientific management were rejected, but Taylor's contribution to management practice has served as a foundational framework for much of what is practiced today.

Although scientific management is out of vogue, there are still those within health care who use scientific management techniques. The most common scientific management technique is autocratic leadership or requiring subordinates to obey purely because they have the formal organizational authority or expertise to require such obedience. For instance, the ACSM-EP who requires patient compliance and adherence and then punishes or retaliates against a patient when they fail to comply or adhere is a scientific management strategy. However, individuals rarely use scientific management strategies unless the organization's operational policies reinforce them. For example, the organization may be arranged in such a way where managers and staff are encouraged to compete with each other to reach sales goals, a specific revenue, or other measurable outcome. Competing with peers to achieve a revenue goal may encourage the ACSM-EP to retaliate against patients who fail to reach goals or comply with their exercise prescription. When teams who, by definition, should be collaborating and helping each other accomplish goals are encouraged to compete, team morale is destroyed and unethical behavior is fostered.

Bureaucratic Model of Management (Max Weber)

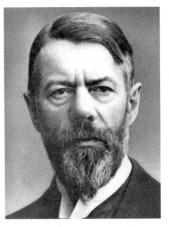

Unless individually or privately owned and operated, almost every health care system, because of the plethora of accrediting agencies and governmental oversight, is forced to be a bureaucratic organization. Thus, the ACSM-EP needs to be familiar with bureaucratic models of management. Bureaucratic structures are typically formalized and centralized, have a firm hierarchy, and divide labor between specialists (12). Bureaucracy requires standardized rules in the forms of policy and procedure. By creating a reference point for action and reducing variability, bureaucracy provides benefit for an unskilled labor force. However, critics of bureaucratic management point out that minimized variability is not as effective with today's knowledgeable workers (12). Weber believed bureaucracy to be a set of official functions bounded by rules with a clear division of labor, and qualification replaced favoritism as the basis of selection for certain jobs. Bureaucracy, as Weber showed, leveled the playing field for many workers and increased their social equality. Although today, elements of bureaucratic management remain, even Weber was able to foresee the risk of bureaucracy and warned of the potential for the organization to dominate policy and individuals.

Total Quality Management (W. Edwards Deming)

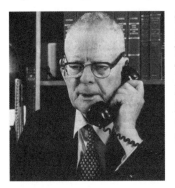

Originally adopted and practiced in Japan, total quality management (TQM) was not favored in the United States until the United States began to fall behind in global competition (14). Deming described TQM as 14 separate aspects of quality management, including such points as "create consistency of purpose for the improvement of product and service," "cease dependence on inspection to achieve quality," and "put everyone in the company to work to accomplish the transformation" (32).

One additional point that is consistently used by ACSM-EPs as they work with clients and customers toward reaching their goals is to "remove barriers that rob people of pride and workmanship."

Management by Objective (Peter Drucker)

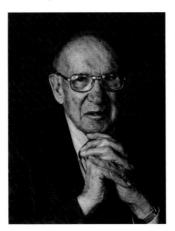

Management by objective (MBO) was the idea that preestablished objectives should be used in the appraisal of every aspect of an organization and that performance relies on defining and assessing those objectives and requires collaboration, strategic planning, and goal setting (37). MBO seeks employee buy-in and participative decision making for departmental or organizational objectives. MBO managers commonly allow, and even require, employees to develop their own career or job development action plan.

For MBO objectives to work, they must be SMART (specific, measurable, achievement oriented, realistic, and time oriented). Drucker believed that every goal or objective must have each of these five elements of SMART in order to be actionable. Finally, MBO requires appraisal, which is routine clarification and assessment of progress toward previously agreed on goals and objectives. Participating in MBO appraisals is an involved process that includes identifying obstacles that have been hindrances to employees accomplishing their objectives and creating new ones once original objectives have been met.

Motivator-Hygiene Theory (Fredrick Herzberg)

The motivator-hygiene theory was first popularized in business management and states that there are factors that contribute separately to both job satisfaction and dissatisfaction (2). Job satisfaction elements are also known as motivators, which when present add to employee satisfaction. These might include work that is intellectually challenging, recognition of superior performance, and increasingly greater levels of responsibility. Hygiene factors are those that when not present increase worker dissatisfaction. They may include status, job security, salary, and fringe benefits. Hygiene factors do not give satisfaction, but if they are absent, they result in dissatisfaction.

A career as an ACSM-EP can serve as a highly satisfying one; there is often a high degree of responsibility and intellectually challenging work. However, there may be hygiene factors, salary and job security, that in spite of the motivators, may lead the ACSM-EP to become dissatisfied.

The motivator-hygiene theory is not only practical for ACSM-EPs in their own career but also for understanding their clients and patients. For example, certain patients will be motivated to comply or adhere to the exercise prescription due to hygiene factors and others for motivator factors. For example, a motivator factor for a patient losing weight might be the recognition from coworkers or even the jealousy that coworkers would feel when they see the patient's success. A hygiene factor for a patient losing weight would be the ability to perform a certain job or task with less effort or more ease. The fact is, most everyone is driven by both hygiene and motivator factors. Although determining these factors for their clients is not the ACSM-EP's responsibility per se, the ACSM-EP should recognize that there are a multitude of motivations, some of which are *motivator* and some of which are *hygiene* factors.

Theory X and Y (Douglas McGregor)

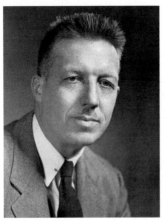

McGregor was a management professor who proposed that human motivation is based on one of two tendencies, which he called X and Y as part of his Theory X and Theory Y of human motivation and management. Theory X is the assumption that most people (followers) are inherently lazy and if given the chance will try to avoid work (2). Belief in Theory X has a profound effect on how a leader would choose to motivate his or her employees. For example, managers who subscribe to Theory X would need to closely monitor and supervise their employees, likely employing a high degree of micromanagement.

Theory Y is the assumption that employees are self-motivated, desire responsibility, and exercise self-direction (2). Managers who hold to Theory Y tend to believe that if given the chance, employees will be creative and productive. Therefore, managers who subscribe to Theory Y often delegate and share responsibility and can be more transformational leaders.

The ACSM-EP uses Theory X and Theory Y unknowingly almost daily. These two theories, X and Y, are rooted in the ACSM-EP's assumptions about why people do what they do. This is specifically a management ideology but crosses over into the assumptions the ACSM-EP holds about patient motivation. For example, if the ACSM-EP believes that *most people generally* fit into Theory X, they will lead their teams and staff a certain way (*e.g.*, transactionally or micromanage them) and assume that their clients or patients will inherently try to get out of or "cheat" on their exercise prescription when no one is looking. On the other hand, if they believe that most people fit into Theory Y, they are more likely to give their staff and their patients the benefit of the doubt. Under Theory Y, the ACSM-EP is more likely to assume all interested parties will be intrinsically motivated to perform even when no one is looking. Obviously, holding a Theory X or Theory Y assumption influences how one leads and interacts with others. ACSM-EPs should take time to ask themselves if they believe most people fit into either a Theory X or Theory Y category, so they are aware of their own implicit biases.

Behavioral Approach (Mary Parker Follet)

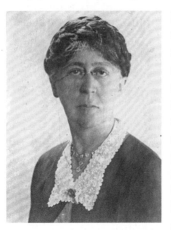

Mary Parker Follett introduced the behavioral model of management and is perhaps the single greatest contributor to how management practice is understood today. Follett was a political scientist and is credited with advancing the democratic style of management. Follett was a "management philosopher" and believed that an organization was a microcosm of society (35,36). The behavioral model of management placed a large emphasis on the individual's ability to define and shape his or her own roles and life and was the precursor to what eventually became known as human resource management (35,36). Within this model, communication flowed both up and down (vertically), as opposed to the more traditional horizontal communication pathways of the time. Follett was a pioneer who suggested that leadership could be learned, and anyone who did not learn leadership would always remain in a subordinate position. Follet also emphasized how important it was for followers to realize the necessity of the instructions for a job rather than follow instructions blindly or mindlessly. Leaders need to understand the jobs themselves and need to be able to communicate the short- and long-term aspects of the job from the worker's perspective.

Organizational Behavior

Understanding the fundamental management techniques and certain theories of leadership provides a foundation for understanding or effectively navigating organizations. Organizational behavior, similar to human resource management, is the capacity to understand, explain, and improve the attitudes and behaviors of individuals and groups within organizations (38). This brings clarity to why the ACSM-EP must be equipped to practice both leadership and management. Many organizational interactions require dealing with human resources, which ultimately require mastery of leadership skills, abilities, and behaviors. Dealing with nonhuman resources (budgets, facilities, information and knowledge, etc.) requires correct application of different management techniques, with the understanding that there may be overlap or integration of leadership and management.

Colquitt (38) presents an integrated model of organizational behavior that includes five major elements:

1. *Individual outcomes*: These are what happens as a result of the other four elements and include job performance and commitment to the organization. For the ACSM-EPs, this would represent competency (*i.e.*, proficiency toward ACSM-EPs exam content outline) and commitment (to his or her customers and employer).
2. *Individual mechanisms*: These consist of five areas that directly impact individual outcomes: (a) job satisfaction — how ACSM-EPs feel about their job when not at the job as well as how well they feel in their day-to-day operations, (b) stress — dealing with the psychological responses to the demands of the job, (c) motivation — the energy ACSM-EPs put into their work, (d) trust and ethics — how ACSM-EPs believe their employer handles business in terms of honesty and integrity, and (e) learning and decision making — how ACSM-EPs acquire and apply new knowledge and continuing education for their job.
3. *Individual characteristics*: These include ACSM-EPs' abilities or skills (*i.e.*, how well they could do their job respective to the expectations and complexity of the job) and personality.
4. *Group mechanisms*: These include how leadership uses power and implements different leadership styles within the ACSM-EP's organization.
5. *Organizational mechanisms*: These include the larger concepts of organizational culture and structure.

ACSM-EPs should consider all five of these elements when diagnosing how well they fit into an organization while also realizing that these elements play a critical role in their own individual and organizational success.

Strategic Planning

Strategic planning is another major component of good leadership and management. Strategic planning is the process of diagnosing the organization's external and internal environments and includes deciding on a vision and mission, developing overall goals, creating and selecting general strategies to be pursued, and allocating resources to achieve the organization's goals (39). Strategic thinking requires conceptualizing the past, present, and future from the organization's and stakeholder's vantage point. This requires understanding the relevant history of the decision at hand, including the factors that helped or hindered the process up until the present day. Also important is to account for relevant present-day activities that occur locally, professionally, or globally (*i.e.*, perceptions, new research, and changing regulations or reforms). Only after historical information and present-day environment have been evaluated can the process of planning for the future begin. Planning for the future must include innovation and a willingness to navigate change.

The overall strategic process is multifaceted and includes delineating organizational, stakeholder, and individual values; creating vision and mission statements; setting goals and objectives; doing program analysis; and establishing a decision-making process. Therefore, planning is a fundamental aspect of leadership and management, including in the health/fitness context, and should include the following steps:

- *Determining stakeholders*: All enterprises in every industry across the globe have stakeholders. Stakeholders are anyone affected by the actions or plans of an organization, department, or individual. For example, the stakeholders for the ACSM-EP in a private health club might include the manager, members, clients, other employees, vendors, sales department, and the neighborhood or community where the club is located. A fundamental component to proper planning is to realize that all decisions and actions are likely to affect most if not all stakeholders.

- *Delineating values*: Values are those practices or attitudes that are predetermined to be celebrated (18). Values are a list of ideals that the organization focuses its time, attention, and resources on; later, these same values will guide the vision and mission statements. Delineating values, therefore, serve a critical role in any organization.

- *Creating a vision*: "Without a vision people perish" (40). A clear and articulate vision is essential for the successful operation of any enterprise and is an ideal image of the future one seeks to create (18,40). Vision is the goal or direction an organization, individual, or team strives toward. This concept of vision suggests an orientation toward the future, and a key leadership practice is to visualize an ideal future (41). The ACSM-EP can facilitate the advancement of his or her industry and profession by maintaining a clear and articulate vision.

- *Drafting a mission*: Mission statements expand on the vision by adding "how" the vision will be accomplished. There is a fundamental difference between vision and mission: The vision statement is future oriented, and the mission statement is oriented toward current services and conditions — visions challenge; missions anchor (42). The mission statement keeps the ACSM-EP focused on who is being served and how to best serve them. A clearly defined mission can help drive leadership decisions and actions (43,44).

- *Establishing goals and objectives*: Goals and objectives are critical to tie together all the planning. Objectives are dynamic endpoints that can be stated quantitatively (we want to sell 25% more memberships) or qualitatively (we want to be the best fitness center in the city). The ACSM-EP should strive to create SMART goals, each with a realistic objective. Once goals and objectives are identified, actions can be taken toward implementing the devised strategy. Figure 15.3 is an overall schematic of the strategic planning process.

After the strategy is implemented, it is necessary to evaluate the progress. Evaluation is most commonly done with a SWOT analysis (strengths, weaknesses, opportunities, and threats). Strengths and weaknesses are internal factors that identify the good and the bad of what is happening and can be controlled and changed within the organization by leaders and managers. The opportunities and threats are external factors that cannot be controlled. Strengths and opportunities are considered positive, whereas weaknesses and threats are typically negative. All strategic plans must be evaluated regularly, and the ACSM-EP should be familiar with the stages of strategic planning and how to perform a SWOT analysis.

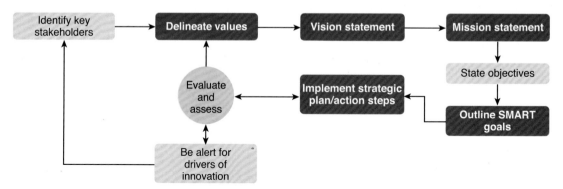

FIGURE 15.3. Strategic planning process. (Reproduced with permission from Kutz MR. Contextual intelligence: overcoming hindrances to performing well in times of change. *Develop Learn Organ*. 2011;25[3]:8–10.)

The Case of Jeanie

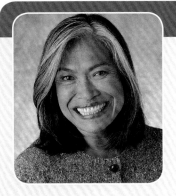

Submitted by **Carol Jean Dale, ACSM-EP, North Mississippi Medical Center — Pontotoc Wellness Center, Pontotoc, MS**

Jeanie Dale, an ACSM-EP manager and a 25-year veteran of hospital-based wellness operations, has used varying styles of management during the constantly changing outcomes-based expectations for the industry. For Jeanie, management is not just about efficiency but also about empowering people to care about their work and the work of others.

Narrative

I work at the Pontotoc Wellness Center, a medical fitness center located in Pontotoc, Mississippi, and at a satellite facility of North Mississippi Medical Center (NMMC), located in Tupelo, Mississippi. NMMC was the 2006 recipient of the Malcolm Baldrige Quality Award, the nation's highest presidential honor for organizational performance excellence. As a manager, I walk a fine line to ensure safety and a rigorous standard of care while introducing commercially relevant current trends and meeting the needs of our stakeholders. We want to serve diverse populations while being able to provide the more resource-demanding special populations that are referred by our Exercise is Medicine® (EIM®) program.

Initially, we had a medical board of physicians who helped our team set up our EIM program so that we could all be clear about the expectations the physicians had for us serving their patients. We looked at ease of entry into the program, safety, and reducing physician time. We also considered the educational, nutritional, and exercise components of our services to make our program affordable to the clients referred. The referral system has now broadened from physicians to other health care practitioners such as physical therapists, behavioral psychologists, nurse practitioners, and professionals from specialty programs including our cancer clinics, cardiac, gastric bypass, and pulmonary rehabilitation. The EIM program is a successful venture and continuing to thrive and develop.

I encourage my team to submit ideas for excellence for our department. Although our mission and vision are rooted in the mission of the institution, the organizational plans for wellness services are in continual development. We implemented a dynamic evaluation involving a 90-day action plan process to assess our progress toward achieving our annual goals and outcomes. This organic style of leadership is practiced system-wide and is encouraged by our director of wellness services. The collection of good ideas from everyone helps find the best idea for a particular circumstance and improves morale of the team at our wellness center.

We also use tools that evaluate our team by having coworkers give feedback to each employee on what we do well and what improvements we need. Because our field is emerging, we need to empower dynamic, independent thinkers who play an important role in preventing disease and reducing risk factors. These frontline professionals will directly impact future health care costs and serve to bridge the gap from rehabilitation into improved functional capacity and healthier lifestyles. The transformational leadership style I try to demonstrate is primarily to encourage individuals to work with autonomy, commitment, and care to improve the quality of life of both clients and coworkers. The EIM program provides a framework for us to work as a team to challenge mediocrity and implement evidence-based practices within the context of a medical fitness facility.

QUESTIONS

- Provide an example of management and an example of leadership in the implementation of the EIM program.
- How does Jeanie exemplify transformational leadership style?
- Which of the approaches to management and leadership align most closely with the way Jeanie manages the team at Pontotoc Wellness Center?

SUMMARY

Leadership and management are separate constructs that have overlapping outcomes. The two are equally valuable aspects of performance for ACSM-EPs, particularly as they seek to advance their career. Leadership is a relationship with people based on the ethical use of influence, whereas management accomplishes goals and objectives by controlling and organizing resources. Leadership research and theory have evolved from a classical approach, which is based on giftedness of the leader, to an organic model, which is a grassroots approach in which everyone can demonstrate leadership. Once ACSM-EPs have a grasp on the differences between leadership and management and on the framework for developing their own philosophical underpinnings, they will be well on their way to making a lasting and meaningful difference in their organization and the lives of their customers.

STUDY QUESTIONS

1. Explain why leadership research and theory are important in developing sound leadership practices across different contexts.
2. What are some key applications of the different leadership concepts and theories discussed in this chapter that an ACSM-EP can use?
3. How can CI be used to increase leadership effectiveness in the health/fitness industry?
4. What are the primary differences between leadership and management? How might these differences be seen in the day-to-day operation of a health/fitness facility?
5. Describe which management techniques might be easiest and most difficult to implement in a health/fitness facility.

REFERENCES

1. O'Neil EH. *Recreating Health Professional Practice for a New Century*. San Francisco (CA): Pew Health Professions Commission; 1998. 142 p.
2. Kutz MR. *Leadership and Management in Athletic Training: An Integrated Approach*. 2nd ed. Burlington (MA): Jones & Bartlett Learning; 2019. 336 p.
3. Nellis SM. Leadership and management: techniques and principles for athletic training. *J Athl Train*. 1994;19(4):328–35.
4. Yukl GA. *Leadership in Organizations*. Upper Saddle River (NJ): Prentice Hall; 2002. 508 p.
5. Dye CF, Garman AN. *Exceptional Leadership: 16 Critical Competencies for Healthcare Executives*. Chicago (IL): Health Administration Press; 2006. 227 p.
6. Kent T. Leading and managing: it takes two to tango. *Manag Decis*. 2005;43(7/8):1010–7.
7. Maccoby M. Understanding the difference between management and leadership. *Res Technol Manag*. 2000;43:57–9.
8. Heifetz R. Anchoring leadership in the work of adaptive progress. In: Hesselbein F, Goldsmith M, editors. *The Leader of the Future 2: Visions, Strategies, and Practices for the New Era*. San Francisco (CA): Jossey-Bass; 2006. p. 73–84.
9. Antonakis J, Cianciolo A, Sternberg R. *The Nature of Leadership*. Thousand Oaks (CA): Sage; 2004. 448 p.
10. Avery G. *Understanding Leadership*. London (United Kingdom): Sage; 2004. 328 p.
11. Stogdill RM. *Handbook of Leadership*. New York (NY): Free Press; 1974. 613 p.
12. DuBrin AJ. *Leadership: Research Findings, Practice, and Skills*. New York (NY): Houghton Mifflin; 2004. 538 p.
13. Maxwell JC. Foreword. In: Kouzes J, Posner B, editors. *Christian Reflections on the Leadership Challenge*. San Francisco (CA): Jossey-Bass; 2004. p. x.
14. Yoder-Wise P. *Leading and Managing in Nursing*. St. Louis (MO): Mosby; 2003. 612 p.
15. Hersey P, Blanchard KH, Johnson DE. *Management of Organizational Behavior: Leading Human Resources*. Upper Saddle River (NJ): Prentice Hall; 2001. 516 p.
16. Northouse PG. *Leadership: Theory and Practice*. Thousand Oaks (CA): Sage; 2004. 360 p.
17. Burns JM. *Leadership*. New York (NY): Harper & Row; 1978. 530 p.
18. Kouzes JM, Posner BZ. *The Leadership Challenge*. San Francisco (CA): Jossey-Bass; 1995. 416 p.

19. Lewin K, Lippitt R, White RK. Patterns of aggressive behavior in experimentally created "social climates." *J Soc Psychol*. 1939;10:271–99.

20. Winston B, Patterson K. An integrated definition of leadership. *Int J Leadersh Stud*. 2005;1(2):6–66.

21. Graen GB, Uhl-Bien M. Relationship-based approach to leadership: development of leader–member exchange (LMX) theory of leadership over 25 years: applying a multi-level multi-domain perspective. *Leadersh Q*. 1995;6:219–47.

22. Bolman LG, Deal TE. *Reframing Organizations*. San Francisco (CA): Jossey-Bass; 2003. 483 p.

23. Salovey P, Mayer JD. Emotional intelligence. *Imagin Cogn Pers*. 1990;9(3):185–211.

24. Mayer J, Salovey P, Caruso D. Emotional intelligence: theory, findings, and implications. *Psychol Inq*. 2004;15(3):197–215.

25. Goleman D. Leadership that gets results. *Harv Bus Rev*. 2000;78(2):78–90.

26. Hays KF, Brown CH. *You're On! Consulting for Peak Performance*. Washington (DC): American Psychological Association; 2004. 328 p.

27. Kutz MR. Toward a conceptual model of contextual intelligence: a transferable leadership construct. *Leadersh Rev*. 2008;8:18–31.

28. Sternberg RJ. *Beyond IQ: A Triarchic Theory of Human Intelligence*. New York (NY): Cambridge University Press; 1985. 411 p.

29. Teremzini PT. On the nature of institutional research and the knowledge and skills it requires. *Res High Educ*. 1993;34(1):1–9.

30. Wagner R. Practical intelligence. In: Sternberg RJ, editor. *Handbook of Intelligence*. New York (NY): Cambridge University Press; 2000. p. 380–95.

31. Wagner RK. Tacit knowledge in everyday intelligent behavior. *J Pers Soc Psychol*. 1987;52(6):1236–47.

32. Kutz MR. *Contextual Intelligence: How Thinking in 3D Can Help Resolve Complexity, Uncertainty and Ambiguity*. London (United Kingdom): Palgrave MacMillan; 2017. 164 p.

33. Knight W, Moore M, Coperthwaite C. Institutional research: knowledge, skills, and perceptions of effectiveness. *Res High Educ*. 1997;38(4):419–33.

34. Sternberg RJ. Intelligence and wisdom. In: Sternberg RJ, editor. *Handbook of Intelligence*. New York (NY): Cambridge University Press; 2000. p. 631–50.

35. Miller T, Vaughan B. Messages from the management past: classic writers and contemporary problems. *SAM Adv Manag J*. 2001;66(1):4–20.

36. Robinson D. Management theorists: thinkers for the 21st century? *Train J*. 2005:30–1.

37. Muczyk J, Reimann B. MBO as a complement to effective leadership. *Acad Manag Exec*. 1989;3(2):131–8.

38. Colquitt JA, Lepine JA, Wesson MJ. *Organizational Behavior: Improving Performance and Commitment in the Workplace*. New York (NY): McGraw-Hill; 2010. 630 p.

39. Hellriegel D, Jackson SE, Slocum JW. *Management: A Competency-Based Approach*. Cincinnati (OH): South-Western Thomson Learning; 2002. 561 p.

40. Senge P. Leadership in living organizations. In: Hesselbein F, Goldsmith M, Somerville I, editors. *Leading Beyond the Walls*. San Francisco (CA): Jossey-Bass; 1996. p. 73–90.

41. Brown MG. Improving your organization's vision. *J Qual Particip*. 1998;21(5):18–21.

42. Pointer D, Orlikoff J. *The High Performance Board: Principles of Nonprofit Organization Governance*. San Francisco (CA): Jossey-Bass; 2002. 208 p.

43. Bart C, Hupfer M. Mission statements in Canadian hospitals. *J Health Organ Manag*. 2004;18(2–3):92–110.

44. Umbdenstock R, Hageman W, Amundson B. The five critical areas for effective governance of not-for-profit hospitals. *Hosp Health Serv Adm*. 1990;35(4):481–92.

General Health Fitness Management

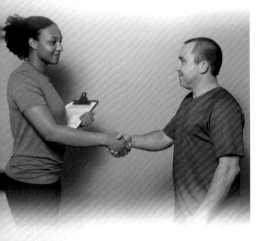

- To know the basics of human resource management, including the procedures necessary to recruit and staff a fitness facility.
- To recognize the relationship between employee training and development and employee performance and retention.
- To recognize the importance of organizational culture in fostering a cohesive team of employees.
- To understand the basic financial instruments used in managing a fitness business and how to use these financial instruments to manage the business.
- To recognize the primary sources of revenue and the key expense categories impacting the financial performance of a fitness facility.
- To understand how to create a budget for a fitness facility.
- To understand the standards and guidelines relating to facility operations and management and how to apply them.
- To understand the basic principles of marketing and sales as they relate to the operation of a fitness facility.
- To understand the basic principles of programming as it relates to the success of a fitness facility.
- To understand the inherent differences between a clinical and a nonclinical health/fitness facility setting.
- To understand the basic principles and practices of risk management in the fitness business.

INTRODUCTION

This chapter provides an overview of the core responsibilities involved in managing and leading a fitness-based facility in either a clinical or nonclinical setting. Although a manager should have knowledge and experience in the fitness industry, management positions also require competency in areas such as human resources, financial planning, facility operations, marketing, programming, risk management, and sales. The role of the manager in fostering organizational culture and providing the leadership necessary to recruit, develop, retain, and empower a team of employees is also covered. Basic financial principles relating to the operation of a fitness center and an overview of facility management and operations are also presented. Finally, the basic principles of marketing and sales and their role in building a successful fitness business are addressed.

 ## Human Resource Management

One of, if not the most important, contributors to the success of any fitness-based business is the team of individuals tasked with delivering the customer experience. To ensure customers are satisfied with their experience and, consequently, make the conscious decision to remain a customer, it is critical to build a team of highly qualified individuals who can establish strong relationships with customers while providing a friendly and inspirational fitness environment.

Organizational Culture and Teamwork

In his book entitled *The Five Dysfunctions of a Team*, Patrick Lencioni exclaimed, "It is teamwork that remains the ultimate competitive advantage. Both because it is so powerful and so rare." Teamwork begins with the institutionalization of a compelling and relevant organizational culture. Culture provides the framework, purpose, and inspiration to bring people together to work toward a common goal and outcome. Furthermore, culture defines the priorities of your business in respect to the employee and customer experience. Howard Schulz, the former chief executive officer (CEO) of Starbucks Coffee Company, said of culture, "Culture defines priority . . . it is your road map."

A relevant organizational culture is composed of several important building blocks, and without them in place, it is nearly impossible for management to provide a roadmap for how employees in the organization should behave when dealing with each other and the customers. So, what are the key cultural building blocks?

- Purpose. An organization's purpose provides a relevant and compelling reason for why a company does what it does. The purpose is the underlying reason for the work being done. Purpose provides meaning to the objectives of the business and to the roles and responsibilities of each employee. Howard Schulz, founder and former CEO of Starbucks Coffee Company, said of an organization's purpose, "When you're surrounded by people who share passionate commitment around a common purpose, anything is possible."
- Vision. An organization's vision speaks to its dream, or the destination of its work efforts. Vision provides employees with a sense of ownership in a common and aspirational pursuit.
- Values. Values represent the beliefs of the organization. Values are the principles that underlie each and every decision and action management and staff take during the course of business. Values are the foundation of a firm's ethical compass. In addition, values are critical for attracting and retaining talent. Employees sharing a common set of values lay the foundation for a cohesive team.

Beyond these three primary building blocks, an empowering organizational culture also includes traditions, which celebrate the underlying tenets of the culture; stories that translate the information about the culture into an emotional spark; and finally, storytellers who are able to share these stories with everyone in the organization. Steve Jobs, the founder of Apple, said that storytellers are the most powerful people in the world.

Staffing

How you staff your fitness facility is dependent on a host of variables, the most influential being the facility's business model (*e.g.*, budget club, premium club, medical fitness center, recreational facility, Young Men's Christian Association [YMCA], and boutique fitness studio) and organizational culture. Having clarity around the business model and accompanying culture will then dictate the types and number of positions needed at different levels throughout the organization. This process should consider the following questions:

- How many people will it take to fulfill the business model's value proposition?
- What staff-to-member ratio will provide sufficient support of the value proposition?
- What job roles will be needed to deliver on the fitness facility's value proposition?
- What responsibilities will be held by each type of position?
- How many hours will the facility be in operation during the week?
- How many members and clients will the fitness facility serve?
- What member or client demographics will the facility be serving (*e.g.*, adults older than the age of 55 yr, adults 25–34 yr, youth younger than the age of 18 yr, individuals with disabilities, apparently healthy adults)?

These are just a few of the key questions that will help a manager determine the staffing needs for their particular fitness facility. As a point of reference, the International Health Racquet & Sportsclub Association (IHRSA) shared the staffing parameters for different club business models in its *2018 Profiles of Success* (1).

As reflected in Table 16.1, employee counts can vary significantly, even when the only screening criteria used is the square footage of the fitness facility.

Types of Positions

Regardless if a fitness facility is corporate, for-profit commercial, hospital-based, nonprofit community-based, or fitness studio, similar positions appear in each facility type. One of the best resources for identifying the types of positions typically found in the fitness facility industry can be found in IHRSA's *Employee Compensation and Benefits Report* (the most recent edition published in 2017 [2]) or *Fitness Management*, fourth edition (published in 2018 by Healthy Learning and authored by Stephen Tharrett [3]). Table 16.2 lists some of the most common positions in a fitness facility along with a general description of their core responsibilities.

Table 16.1	Average Number of Employees per Square Feet of Facility		
	Average No. of Employees	Average No. of Full-time Employees	Average No. of Part-time Employees
Less than 20,000 ft^2	17	4	13
35,000–60,000 ft^2	83	15	68
Greater than 60,000 ft^2	168	37	131

Table 16.2	Common Positions in the Fitness Industry
Job Position	**Job Roles**
General manager	Responsible for the overall operations of the facility, including fiduciary responsibility; develops core values, creates and implements strategic plan, develops relationship with complementary business services, oversees annual budget and marketing development and distribution, and manages all on-site supervisors
Sales manager	Oversees the sales activities of the fitness facility, including creating the sales plan, hiring and training sales staff, monitoring sales activity, and managing all sales-related activities
Fitness director	Oversees the activities and functions of the fitness department, which typically includes the fitness floor and group exercise areas creates and implements member fitness programs; markets fitness services; encourages members to achieve fitness goals through offered programs and services; and oversees on-site fitness employees, including personal trainers, fitness instructors, and group exercise instructors
Group exercise director	Responsible for creation and implementation of group exercise programs; oversees all on-site group exercise instructors
Personal training director	In facilities with large personal training and small group training programs, oversees the personal training activities, including recruiting, hiring, and coaching personal trainers; establishing the standards and systems for personal training; leading the personal training staff
Personal trainer	Markets and sells personal training packages, leads one-on-one or small-group personal training sessions, may perform initial fitness evaluations and reassessments, conducts fitness orientations for all new and returning members, and supervises members while circulating fitness floor
Group exercise instructor	Teaches group-based exercises classes and programs for members
Fitness instructor	Supervises the general activities of the fitness floor, may perform fitness evaluations, conducts new and returning member fitness orientations, and assists members with their workouts while on the fitness floor

Employee versus Independent Contractor

Many positions in the health/fitness industry are filled by hiring employees or retaining independent contractors. According to Internal Revenue Service (IRS) (4) release FS-2017-09 from July 20, 2017, an independent contractor is an individual for whom the business has the right to control or direct only the result of the work, not what will be done and how it will be done. For example, if a business retains a personal trainer as an independent contractor, then the business can't set the rates the personal trainer charges, set the hours the personal trainer works, and cannot dictate the uniform the personal trainer wears. If, instead, the business hires the personal trainer as an employee, the business is allowed to direct and control the work of the employee. For example, if a personal trainer were hired as an employee, the business can dictate the hours the personal trainer works, specify the rates to be charged for the services the employee renders, dictate the policies the personal trainer must follow while on duty, and the type of attire the personal trainer can wear. A manager must review the tasks and responsibilities of each job, along with the level of control the business wants to have of the individual's work to determine whether hiring an individual as an employee or retaining them as an independent contractor is more appropriate. Table 16.3 provides an overview of the key differences between an employee and independent contractor.

Table 16.3	Factors Defining Employees and Independent Contractors	
Factors	**Employees**	**Independent Contractors**
Behavior control	Subject to the business's instructions about when and where to do work, is provided a job description, instructed how to perform job duties, shown what equipment or tools to use, told what standards are to be followed, have their hours set for them, etc.	Typically make their own business decisions about how and when to do work, maintain their own office or workspace off-site, use personal tools and equipment, set their own hours, etc.
	Must complete a job application, may have a job description, receives regular performance evaluations, etc.	Have a legally binding contract with the employer that stipulates the expectations and obligations of each party to the contract
	May be trained to perform services in a particular manner or required to obtain company-mandated certifications or continuing education	Not eligible for employer-offered education and training unless stipulated in contract or paid for by the independent contractor
Financial control	Most expenses incurred while working for the business are reimbursed.	Typically responsible for all expenses associated with performing their duties as an independent contractor
	Use facility and tools owned and maintained by business	Have a significant investment in the facilities/tools used in performing services for someone else
	Work for the business, typically do not market their services/skills to other businesses	Are free to seek out business opportunities, advertise, and maintain public business location and are available to work in the relevant market
	Generally guaranteed a regular wage by hour per week or other period of time. If paid by the hour, eligible for overtime pay. Eligible for employer-sponsored benefits such as paid health insurance, vacation time, paid time off, participation in employer-sponsored retirement program, covered by business insurance, etc. Employer pays portion of social taxes.	Often paid a flat fee or on a time and materials basis for the job; not eligible for any employer-sponsored benefits and must pay their own federal and state taxes, including social taxes; must provide own insurance
	Fees charged for employees' services are established by the business.	Establish fees for their services
Type of relationship	Receive employee benefits, such as insurance, pension plan, vacation pay, sick time, etc.	Do not receive employee benefits from employer and must provide their own insurance coverage
	Indefinite relationship	Relationship lasting for a specific project or period of time specified by a contract

Table 16.4	Criteria for Exempt and Nonexempt Positions
Exempt	**Nonexempt**
Must supervise a department or subdepartment of the business (*e.g.*, fitness, group exercise, pools)	Does not have supervisory responsibilities as primary part of their job
Falls into one of the following six FLSA categories: executive, professional, administrative, computer employee, outside sales, and highly compensated	Does not meet the FLSA exempt status criteria
Must be paid a salary of at least $684 a week ($35,568 annually)	Paid an hourly wage and eligible for overtime pay
Must supervise at least two full-time employees or the equivalent of	
Must have the authority to hire and dismiss an employee	

Exempt versus Nonexempt

Another consideration for managers when recruiting is whether an employee should be classified as exempt or nonexempt. An exempt employee, according to the Fair Labor Standards Act (FLSA), is a professional who falls into one of seven categories as well as meeting certain other tests established by FSLA. A nonexempt employee is an employee who does not meet the FSLA criteria for exemption. Table 16.4 provides an overview of the differences between an exempt and nonexempt employee based on the criteria established under FLSA.

Full-time versus Part-time

An additional consideration that managers must make in respect to an employee's status is determining whether they can be classified as full-time or part-time. The regulations that determine an employee's status as either full-time or part-time are established by the same department of the federal government that puts forth the rules around exempt and nonexempt status. The current rules stipulate that a part-time employee cannot work more than 1,000 hours annually; the equivalent of 17.5 hours a week if they were to work 52 weeks a year. The "test" applied to part-time status is based on annual hours, not weekly hours, and consequently, assuming an employee did seasonal work, they could work up to 29 hours a week or 130 hours a month as long as they didn't exceed 1,000 hours annually. Table 16.5 provides a general overview of the criteria associated with

Table 16.5	Criteria for Full-time and Part-time Status
Employment Status	**Criteria Established by Labor Department**
Part-time	Cannot work over 1,000 h in a calendar year
	Must work less than 30 h in any given week and less than 130 h in any given month
Full-time	Employee who works more than 1,000 h in a calendar year
	Must work more than 30 h over the course of any week and more than 130 h a month over the course of any given month

full-time and part-time employment status. In the previously mentioned *2018 Profiles of Success* published by IHRSA (1), the data shows that on average, clubs have anywhere from 2 to 4 times as many part-time employees as they do full-time employees.

Job Descriptions

Detailed job descriptions, or job models as many human resource professionals refer to them, are important to the recruiting process and, once an individual is hired, to guiding the performance of the employee. During the recruiting process, job descriptions help define for candidates the overall accountabilities of the role they are seeking along with the competencies and skills necessary to perform the job. The job description also provides a framework for the types of interview questions a candidate may be asked. Ultimately, this contributes to the selection of the best candidate for the position. Once a position has been filled, the job description becomes a framework for employees around which they can base their performance. A detailed job description (see "How to Create a Job Description" box) should include the job title, main purpose of the job, accountabilities of the job, required skills, required education and/or certifications, reporting structure, conditions of employment, and performance measures.

Recruiting and Selection

Recruiting refers to the process of finding and attracting new employees. Selection refers to the process of screening candidates to find the one most suitable to fill the open position. Collectively, these two processes, recruitment and selection, are vital to the formation of a purpose-driven team of employees.

Recruiting Strategies

The most effective recruiting strategies allow management to fill positions quickly, effectively, and efficiently. So what are the most effective strategies for recruiting the best candidates to fill positions in a fitness facility?

- Employee referral. Employee referral is considered one of the most effective ways of attracting talent that fits with your organization. Existing employees are familiar with the culture and the expectations of management and consequently are in the best position to know if individuals are a good fit for the team. Although most employee referrals are organic in nature, many fitness facility operators have formal employee referral programs in place that reward employees for referring individuals who are later retained as employees.
- Internship programs. Internship programs serve a dual purpose. First, they provide students with an opportunity to gain hands-on experience in their chosen field. Second, they provide management with a chance to assess a candidate's potential under real-time conditions. IHRSA has developed an internship manual that fitness facilities can leverage to help implement an internship program.
- Recruit members. Within the fitness facility industry, management commonly find talent within its membership ranks. Active members are often the best candidates for positions such as group exercise instructor, personal trainer, front desk, etc.
- Have a career center on your Web site. Candidates spend considerable time online exploring their options. Offering a career page on your Web site will encourage potential candidates to go online and apply. Fitness companies such as 24 Hour Fitness, Equinox, and Life Time Fitness have career sites.

HOW TO — Create a Job Description

Creating a job description requires a clear understanding of what the organization expects out of an individual serving in this role. There are plenty of variables to consider if you want to craft a job description that will attract an outstanding pool of applicants and furthermore provide the framework for how each employee performs once they are hired. Following is the description of key items to consider when drafting a job description.

Position Overview

This is the section that gives candidates and employees a general sense of the primary responsibilities and accountabilities of their job. A typical position overview for a fitness director could look like this:

Responsible for supervising the performance of all employees and contractors in the fitness department, responsible for creating an annual business plan and budget for the department and monitoring that performance on a regular basis to make sure desired key performance indicators are met, delivering programs and services that foster member delight, and championing the company culture during interactions with employees and members.

Job Accountabilities

Describing job accountabilities is one of the keys to a quality job description. Laying out these key accountabilities of the job is critical so that applicants and, more importantly, employees know what is expected of them and so the employer has an objective basis for future performance evaluations. Listing each and every area of accountability may not be necessary, but clearly delineating accountabilities management will hold an employee responsible for is critical (*e.g.*, meet financial targets, achieve specific levels of member satisfaction, achieve certain levels of employee satisfaction). Many human resource professionals will separate accountabilities into two categories: essential and secondary. Essential accountabilities are absolutes, whereas secondary accountabilities are less important to the performance of the job. Below are examples of two broad categories of accountabilities that might be found in a facility manager's job accountabilities.

Supervisory: Oversee all facility employees including personal trainers, group exercise instructors, front desk staff, spa services staff, and maintenance staff; recruit, hire, and train all staff in facility; and conduct performance reviews and create development plans for each employee.

Facility Operations: Manage all facility services (group exercise, personal training, day care program); track operating expenses and revenues while monitoring budget guidelines; oversee maintenance and purchase of equipment; coordinate group exercise and personal training programs and schedules; manage employee payroll and benefits; participate and manage daily operations including floor supervision, class instruction, and fitness appointments when appropriate; develop marketing strategies; determine individual and team goals; and review goals on a monthly, quarterly, and annual basis.

Reporting Lines

It is important that employees, including prospective employees, understand how their role aligns with other jobs in the organization. This section of the job description needs to clarify who they report to (directly and indirectly), whom they supervise, and whom they may need to collaborate with. For example, a fitness director in a multichain facility operation may report directly to the club manager but indirectly to the corporate head of fitness. Likewise, they may have to collaborate with the sales manager and have supervisory responsibility for personal trainers, group exercise instructors, activity coaches, and massage therapists.

Continued

Position Credentials

This category can also be called "qualifications," "skills required," or any number of other words or phrases that clearly state the background expected of all serious applicants and future employees. This section must list everything you feel is critical to performing the job. A typical Credentials section could look like this:

High school diploma required, Bachelor's degree preferred; 5+ years of relevant work experience; experience in working in a team environment with the ability to delegate workload and responsibilities; competence in management skills including quality management, risk management, and achievement of goals; strong verbal and written communications; time management and organizational skills; ability to design, deliver, and evaluate programs and services; provide exceptional customer service; knowledge of fitness management software; experience in the performance of fitness assessments; basic computer literacy; budget tracking and management experience; current cardiopulmonary resuscitation (CPR)/automated external defibrillator (AED) and first aid certification; current fitness certification from an accredited organization (*e.g.*, American College of Sports Medicine [ACSM], American Council on Exercise [ACE], National Academy of Sports Medicine [NASM], or National Strength and Conditioning Association [NSCA]).

Employee Status

This section is relatively straightforward and indicates the working hours, including if the position is exempt or nonexempt and full-time or part-time.

- Place job postings on industry-based career sites, in particular when seeking individuals for positions such as group exercise instructor, personal trainer, group exercise coordinator, or fitness director. The ACSM, ACE, and IHRSA all maintain career sites designed to help link candidates with employers.
- Place job postings on the leading online recruiting sites such as Indeed.com, Glassdoor.com, and ZipRecruiter.com. These sites are among the most popular for posting jobs and finding potential candidates.
- Consider working with local universities and/or colleges to establish an internship program.

Selection Process

Once a number of applications have been compiled from recruiting efforts, the selection process can begin. Selection is the process of sorting through the applicants to find qualified individuals who will be taken through the interview process. Depending on the size and scope of a facility, a manager might create a search committee to screen and interview potential candidates. The search committee should be composed of employees from key areas within the facility; for example, the group exercise director may have a unique role in the hiring of individuals who may be needed to teach group exercise. Forming a committee also allows for greater collaboration among employees. The first step a manager or committee must take is to create a checklist or matrix of the qualifications and responsibilities needed for the position. Each resume and cover letter should be reviewed within the framework of the matrix, looking for past experiences and knowledge that match the crucial items outlined on the matrix. Checking professional references also provides insight into the work habits and skills of the applicant. Applicants whose resumes, cover letters, and references pass the matrix test should be contacted to start the interview process. Sometimes, in larger organizations, the human resources department conducts this initial screening and works with the appropriate department head to select the most suitable candidates to interview.

Interview Process

A multiple-stage interview process should be applied to each candidate who passes the initial selection process. The first interview, typically referred to as a "cultural fit" interview, is designed to uncover whether the candidate's character and values are aligned with the fit organization's culture. The goal is to ascertain upfront whether the individual is someone whose values and work style are in alignment with the firm's culture. Absent a fit, there is no need to interview further. A cultural fit interview may be done in person, over the phone, or possibly via a video conference platform such as Google Hangouts, Skype, or Zoom. In large organizations, this interview is typically conducted by a member of the human resources department, whereas in smaller businesses such as an independent fitness facility, the cultural fit interview might be conducted by the department supervisor.

If a candidate successfully gets through the cultural fit interview, the next step is to conduct a structured interview. The structured interview can involve one individual, typically the department supervisor, or can involve several individuals within the organization. During the structured interview, the candidate is asked questions from a prepared list of questions structured around the accountabilities of the job. Very often, these structured interview questions involve role-play situations. If a candidate is deemed worthy after the structured interview, many organizations will schedule a third interview called a team interview where the candidate is interviewed by a team of employees, often employees whose jobs will have them interacting with this individual if they are hired. The primary focus of the team interview should be on personality and team dynamics to ensure that the applicant is an appropriate fit to the current team.

Once candidates have completed the interview process, they should be ranked by both the position's immediate supervisor, employees involved in the team interview, and possibly by the employees in the department in which the open position exists. In the case when there is a search committee, the chair of the committee makes a recommendation to the hiring manager based on the discussion and vote of the committee. In some cases, more than one name can be submitted, and the hiring manager makes the final decision. Once the candidates are ranked, an offer should be extended to the applicant with the highest rank first.

Compensation

Compensation is not limited to wages. When offering a position to a candidate, it is important to outline the additional benefits that may be included with employment. Organizations vary greatly on what types of supplemental benefits can be offered to augment wages. Some organizations provide professional development funds for employees to support conference attendance or the cost of obtaining additional specialty certifications. Other organizations provide partial or whole health care, dental, vision, or mental health benefits. In addition, childcare or adult care opportunities, flexible schedules, vacation time, or incentives to earn additional income all provide an attractive package for candidates. For some employees, job security and work–life balance are equally as important as salary. Providing opportunities for advancement and professional development aids in recruiting and maintaining a satisfied and productive workforce. Table 16.6 outlines the average wages paid to various positions in the fitness facility industry, along with some of the more common benefits offered by operators based on information found in IHRSA's *2017 Employee Compensation and Benefits Report* (2). Another source of information on compensation levels for various positions in the fitness facility industry can be found on Glassdoor.com.

Table 16.6	Wages and Benefits in the Fitness Facility Industry		
Position	**Exempt or Nonexempt**	**Median Wage**	**Benefits**
General manager	Exempt	$90,000	Medical insurance for employee
Fitness director		$65,000	91% pay in full or partially
Sales manager		$55,000	Dental insurance
Accountant		$61,600	73.6% pay in full or partially
			Educational assistance program
			53% pay in full or partially
			Section 125 plan
			49% pay in full or partially
Personal trainer	Nonexempt	$30 an hour	Medical insurance for employee
Specialty personal trainer		$35 an hour	79.1% pay in full or partially
Pilates instructor		$33.38 an hour	Dental insurance
Yoga instructor		$30 an hour	57% pay in full or partially
Group cycling instructor		$27.50 an hour	Educational assistance program
Front desk staff		$11.15 an hour	41% pay in full or partially
			Section 125 plan
			38% pay in full or partially

Employee Orientation, Development, and Training

New employee orientations are important to any facility because a well-planned orientation will make onboarding easier for the new individual as well as for current staff and members. According to the SHRM Foundation, a nonprofit affiliate of the Society for Human Resources Management, approximately 93% of companies offer a new employee orientation. These programs are used to introduce the new employee to the organizational culture, to reduce an employee's uneasiness and anxiety that comes with starting a new position, to prepare the employee to start his or her new position, and to create a strong and positive relationship between the new employee and the organization. According to an article entitled "The Purpose of New Employee Orientations" appearing in the April 29, 2019, online edition of Bizfluent.com (5), the author states that if a new employee orientation is conducted properly, work performance can be enhanced by 11% and improve employee retention by 25%.

The approach and extent of a new employee orientation is often dependent on both the organization's culture and the position in question. Regardless of the approach taken, new employee orientations should include an overview of the company culture and facility policies and, finally, teach the new employee job-related skills.

A properly conceived and structured new employee orientation process should include the following:

■ *The structural and cultural organization of the company, facility, and department*: A discussion should be held regarding the organization's mission statement and its importance to the new employee's position and the organizational culture and the expectation it creates. Any employee in a fitness facility must understand the hierarchy and chain of command that exists within the organization, from CEO to general manager, fitness director to personal trainers, maintainers, and desk staff.

■ *Human resource policies and procedures applicable to all employees*: Although information about benefits and compensation is often provided when a position is offered, new employees must be equipped with all company/facility policies and procedures that apply to them and their position. A human resources associate or department supervisor should discuss pay, absenteeism and tardiness, benefits, and the processes the employee needs to follow to access him or her as well as highlight key areas in the employee handbook, such as job performance and reviews.

Job-specific orientation, typically conducted by an immediate supervisor or department mentor, should include the following:

■ *Informing the employee of specific job responsibilities and expectations*: A written job description should be given to the new employee, outlining job tasks and accountabilities. At this point, a time frame should be decided on by the new employee and immediate supervisor regarding when the individual will be able to perform the job independently, signifying the completion of the orientation sessions. A probationary period may be used to ensure employee performance in a timely manner. The typical probationary period is 90 days.

■ *Laying out the workspace to be used by the new employee*: An aquatic exercise class instructor would need an in-depth tour of the pool area and changing rooms, whereas a certified exercise physiologist (EP) would need to be shown where equipment is kept, places to find paperwork for members, and a tour of the entire facility before working independently.

■ *Including an introduction to immediate coworkers*: Meeting coworkers will allow a new employee to settle in to his or her position quickly and will provide the employee with potential mentors as he or she gains more experience. For example, group exercise instructors often gain valuable information from other instructors, including member preferences, equipment issues, and class structure.

■ *Shadowing an existing employee*: Many fitness facility operations will have a new employee shadow an existing employee for a period of time. For example, a new personal trainer may be asked to shadow one of the facility's best trainers for a period of time as a means of helping them assimilate the expectations of the facility.

Performance Management and Employee Retention

During the onboarding process, new employees should be equipped with the knowledge of what is expected of someone in their position. Expectations must be clearly defined by an organization and the position's immediate supervisor in order for an employee to be successful. For example, if employees on the membership sales team do not know that they are expected to sell 50 memberships each month, they will be frustrated when they are disciplined or penalized for selling only 30 memberships. Unknown expectations create a sense of uneasiness among employees, and this can lead to poor performance and increased turnover. Instead, make each employee's specific expectations clear and revise the expectations when needed.

Setting Goals

Expectations should be set with employees on an annual basis, emphasizing the commitment a company has to its employees' development over time. Annual goals give employees insight into where the company plans to be in a year as well as provide them guidance as to how they can help the company succeed. It is the responsibility of a manager to meet with each employee, explain the goals of the company, and help the employee determine how his or her position can contribute to the accomplishment of those goals.

Table 16.7	SMART Goal-Setting Principle
Specific	A specific goal answers the questions "Who?" "What?" "Where?" "When?" and "Why?" and has a much greater chance of being accomplished because the goal has definition. An example of a specific goal for a personal trainer might be to average 20 sessions a week or generate $1,000 a week in sales.
Measurable	Goals must be stated with either a quantitative or qualitative assessment. To determine if a goal is measurable, ask "How much? How many? What determines success?" An example for a group exercise instructor might be to have an average attendance of 12 clients per class.
Attainable/achievable	The goal must be attainable given the employee/employer resources. To establish stretch targets knowing they are unachievable will generate negative outcomes.
Relevant	Goals need to relate to an employee and his or her position and hold some significance or meaning. For example, a fitness director's targets should involve areas he or she directly influences such as personal training revenues, class participation, fitness payroll, member satisfaction, etc.
Time-based	A goal needs a time frame in which to be accomplished. For example, you might have a goal that states average attendance for yoga classes will reach 120 by November 1.

Goal setting should be a collaborative effort between the employee and the immediate supervisor. It is important to maintain a distinction between ongoing tasks or responsibilities, goals related to a company's overall performance, and goals connected to living the company culture. Goals should be specific, measurable, achievable, relevant, and time-based — five qualities known as the SMART criteria for goal setting (Table 16.7).

Performance Appraisals

Many companies conduct formal performance appraisals, typically on an annual basis but sometimes on a semiannual basis. Some managers, fearing conflict or confrontation, prefer this method to be an informal process. In reality, regularly scheduled evaluations give the manager an opportunity to gather both positive and constructive feedback about employees over the course of the year and make an informed decision about employees' progress. However, this technique of analyzing and critiquing an employee's performance does not replace day-to-day performance management and can sometimes lead to negative experiences for both the employee and the immediate supervisor. For example, a manager observes a front desk employee ignoring members as he or she enters the facility. If the manager waits months before telling the employee that he or she needs to be acknowledging members while signing in, the employee will continue to perform incorrectly, and the manager will become increasingly frustrated. Instead, feedback, both positive and constructive, should be delivered to employees on both a regular and as-needed basis.

Formal performance appraisals should be held annually, giving the employee and the immediate supervisor a chance to assess the goals set at the beginning of the review year as well as provide the opportunity for discussion of future goals. Performance evaluation forms should be completed by the employee first and then by the immediate supervisor. Once the forms have been completed by the respective parties, a session should be held where the two parties discuss their respective assessments. This meeting allows the two parties to discuss their respective perspectives and allows for a fair and equitable appraisal of performance to be reached. Using this method allows a supervisor to understand how the employee thinks he or she has been performing. Performance evaluation forms should include sections for the following:

1. Employee strengths
2. Employee weaknesses and opportunities
3. Goals from the review period, with explanations of achievements or challenges that were met in the process of achieving success
4. Company-defined skills and competencies

All reviews, whether informal or formal, should be documented by the immediate supervisor, acknowledged by the employee, and kept in the employee's folder.

Employee Retention

An effective performance appraisal process can positively affect employee performance and retention. More frequent performance checks can help maintain favorable relations between an immediate supervisor and his or her employees, improving employee loyalty and retention. Additionally, other more informal employee morale activities are beneficial for employee retention.

Section Summary

The EP in management positions will typically find themselves involved in staffing or restaffing their facility. It is imperative for the EP to understand the recruiting, selection, and hiring processes and to collaborate with the appropriate departments (*i.e.*, human resources and talent acquisition). Good team dynamics and hardworking and dedicated employees are important to running a successful fitness facility.

 Risk Management

As the fitness industry continues to grow, the EP has a great opportunity to work in a variety of settings and make a powerful difference in people's lives. More professional opportunities, however, increase expectations of responsible professional conduct, which means greater potential for liability for failing to act responsibly. Today's EP must understand these areas of risk exposure and the legal issues and industry standards and guidelines that surround them and be able to deliver services confidently and proactively.

Risk management is both an initial and ongoing process to identify relevant risks associated with the delivery of a service and, thus, is a critical area of concern to any EP manager. This process occurs through the application of various approaches intended to recognize, eliminate, reduce, or transfer risk through the implementation of operational strategies to the program activities of the facility.

The role of the EP manager in creating and maintaining a safe work environment is critical to the success of any fitness facility. A comprehensive and effective risk management plan should be developed, which minimizes unsafe conditions and practices while maximizing safety by establishing policies and procedures that address safe practices and protect the assets of the company.

Standards and Guidelines for Risk Management and Emergency Procedures

The ACSM has identified 35 fundamental standards relating to risk management and emergency procedures as documented in the fifth edition of *ACSM's Health/Fitness Facility Standards and Guidelines* (6) (Table 16.8). Because the EP may offer services in a variety of locations, including a

Table 16.8	ACSM Health/Fitness Facility Standards as of Fifth Edition

1. Facility operators shall offer a self-guided or professionally guided exercise preparticipation health screening tool (*e.g.*, Pre-activity Screening Questionnaire [PASQ], the Physical Activity Readiness Questionnaire for Everyone [PAR-Q+], and/or Health History Questionnaire [HHQ]) to all new members and prospective users.

2. Exercise preparticipation health screening tools shall provide an authenticated means for new members and/or users to identify whether a level of risk exists that indicates that they should seek consultation from a qualified health care professional prior to engaging in a program of physical activity.

3. Exercise preparticipation health screening tools shall be reviewed by qualified staff (*e.g.*, a qualified health/fitness professional or health care professional), and the results of the review shall be retained on file by the facility for a period of at least 1 yr from the time the tool was reviewed. All health data and related communications shall be kept in such a manner that it is private, confidential, and secure.

4. If a facility operator is told that a member, user, or prospective user has known cardiovascular, metabolic, or renal disease or any other self-disclosed medical concern that may affect the individual's ability to exercise safely, medical clearance is recommended before beginning a physical activity program.

5. Facilities shall provide a means for communicating to existing members the value of completing an exercise preparticipation health screening tool on a regular basis (*e.g.*, preferably once annually) during the course of their membership, or if they experience a significant change in health status. Such communication can be done through a variety of mechanisms, including, but not limited to, the facility membership agreement, online communications, personal correspondence, and/or signage.

6. Once a new member or prospective user has completed a preparticipation health screening process, facility operators shall then offer the new member or prospective user a general orientation to the facility.

7. Facilities shall provide a means by which members and users who are engaged in a physical activity program within the facility can obtain assistance and/or guidance with their efforts.

8. Facility operators must have written emergency response policies and procedures, which shall be reviewed regularly and physically rehearsed a minimum of twice annually. These policies shall enable staff to respond to basic first-aid situations and other emergency events in an appropriate and timely manner.

9. Facility operators shall ensure that a safety audit is conducted that routinely inspects all areas of the facility to reduce or eliminate unsafe hazards that may cause injury to employees and health/fitness facility members or users.

10. Facility operators shall have a written system for sharing information with members and users, employees, and independent contractors regarding the handling of potentially hazardous materials, including the handling of bodily fluids by the facility staff in accordance with the guidelines of the U.S. Occupational Safety and Health Administration (OSHA).

11. In addition to complying with all applicable federal, state, and local requirements relating to AEDs, all facilities (staffed or unstaffed) shall have as part of their written emergency response policies and procedures a public access defibrillation (PAD) program in accordance with generally accepted practice.

12. AEDs in a facility shall be located to allow a time from collapse, caused by cardiac arrest, to defibrillation of 3–5 min or less. A 3-min response time can be used to help determine how many AEDs are needed and where to place them.

13. A skills review, practice sessions, and a practice drill with the AED shall be conducted a minimum of every 6 mo, covering a variety of potential emergency situations (*e.g.*, water, presence of a pacemaker, children).

14. A staffed facility shall assign at least one staff member to be on duty, during all facility operating hours, who is currently trained and certified in the delivery of CPR and in the administration of an AED.

Table 16.8	ACSM Health/Fitness Facility Standards as of Fifth Edition (continued)

15. Unstaffed facilities must comply with all applicable federal, state, and local requirements relating to AEDs. Unstaffed facilities shall have as part of their written emergency response policies and procedures a PAD program as a means by which either members and users or an external emergency responder can respond from time of collapse to defibrillation in 5 min or less.

16. Health/fitness professionals who have supervisory responsibility and oversight responsibility for the physical activity and exercise training programs as well as the staff who administer them shall have appropriate levels of professional education, work experience, and/or certification. Examples of health/fitness professionals who serve in a supervisory role include the fitness director, group exercise director, aquatics director, and program director.

17. Health/fitness professionals who serve in counseling, instruction, and physical activity supervision roles for the facility shall have appropriate levels of professional education, work experience, and/or certification. The primary professional staff and independent contractors who serve in these roles are fitness instructors, group exercise instructors, personal trainers, and health and wellness coaches.

18. Health/fitness professionals engaged in preactivity screening or prescribing, instructing, monitoring, or supervising of physical activity programs for facility members and users shall have current AED and CPR certification from an organization qualified to provide such certification. A CPR or AED certification should include a hands-on practical skills assessment.

19. Facilities shall have an operational system in place that monitors, either manually or technologically, the presence and identity of all individuals (*e.g.*, members and users) who enter into and participate in the activities, programs, and services of the facility.

20. Facilities that offer a sauna, steam room, or whirlpool shall ensure that the temperature settings are appropriate and the equipment is well maintained. There should also be appropriate warning signage in place to notify members and guests of the risks associated with these amenities, including unsafe changes in temperature and humidity.

21. Facilities that offer members and guests access to a pool or whirlpool shall provide evidence that they comply with all water-chemistry safety requirements mandated by state and local codes and regulations.

22. A facility that offers youth services or programs shall provide evidence that it complies with all applicable state and local laws and regulations pertaining to their supervision.

23. The registration policy of a facility that provides childcare shall require that parents or guardians of all children left in the facility's care complete a waiver (when permitted by law), an authorization for emergency medical care, and a release for the children whom they leave under the temporary care of the facility.

24. The facility shall require that parents and guardians provide the facility with names of persons who are authorized by the parent or legal guardian to pick up each child. The facility shall not release children to any unauthorized person, and furthermore, the facility shall maintain records of the date and time each child checked out and was dropped off and the name of the person to whom the child was released. Facility personnel should verify the identity of the adult picking up the child (*e.g.*, using a numbered photo identification, or a photo in the member management system or computer system).

25. Facilities shall have written policies regarding children's issues, such as requirements for staff providing supervision of children, age limits for children, restroom practices, food, and parental presence on site. Facilities shall inform parents and guardians of these policies and require that parents and guardians sign a form that acknowledges they have received the policies, understand the policies, and will abide by the policies.

26. Facilities shall properly secure physical and electronic data concerning its employees and potential, present, and future members to protect against a data breach and the release of their personal information.

Continued

Table 16.8	ACSM Health/Fitness Facility Standards as of Fifth Edition (continued)

27. Facilities, to the extent required by law, must adhere to the standards of building design that relate to the designing, building, expanding, or renovating of space, as detailed in the Americans with Disabilities Act (ADA).

28. Facilities must be in compliance with all federal, state, and local building codes.

29. Facilities must provide adequate clearance to the side and at the rear of all types of continuous-motion exercise equipment.

30. The aquatic and pool facilities must provide the proper safety equipment according to state and local codes and regulations.

31. Facility operators shall post proper caution, danger, and warning signage in conspicuous locations where facility staff know, or should know, that existing conditions and situations warrant such signage.

32. Facility operators shall post the appropriate emergency and safety signage pertaining to fire and related emergency situations, as required by federal, state, and local codes.

33. Facility operators shall post signage indicating the location of any AED and first aid kits, including directions on how to access those locations.

34. Facilities shall post all ADA and OSHA signage required by federal, state, and local laws and regulations.

35. All cautionary, danger, and warning signage shall have the required signal icon, signal word, signal color, and layout as specified in ASTM International F1749.

health/fitness facility, the outdoors, or a client's home, basic precautions should be taken to ensure that every exercise setting is safe.

Developing an emergency response policy should involve the establishment of a risk management or safety team. This team might consist of a health care professional (*e.g.*, licensed physician or registered nurse), a local emergency medical service professional (*e.g.*, paramedic), and key staff members. The emergency response policy should include the procedures for responding to critical incidents such as sudden cardiac arrest or heat illness as well as less life-threatening incidents requiring first aid. Emergency response policies also need to include evacuation procedures in case of fire, natural disaster, or active shooter situation. The risk management team is charged with the responsibility of training and practicing the emergency response plan so that every employee is prepared in the event of an emergency. For additional suggestions on preparing a comprehensive emergency response plan, the author refers to you to Chapter 3 of the fifth edition of *ACSM's Health/Fitness Facility Standards and Guidelines* (6). The EPs who are sole proprietors of a fitness business or provide in-home training should also have written emergency policies and procedures.

Types of Business Liability Insurance

An important element of risk management involves acquiring the proper types of insurance to protect your business, its customers, and its employees. The five main categories of business insurance include the following:

- General liability insurance. This insurance protects your business if someone pursues a legal claim as a result of experiencing bodily injury or property damage incurred as a result of an interaction with your business. A typical commercial general liability plan will provide 1 million dollars in coverage per incident with a cumulative total of at least 2 million dollars.

- Professional liability insurance. This insurance protects not only your business but also your employees in the event someone pursues a legal claim for the professional misconduct of an employee. Misconduct refers to an error or omission in what would be considered standard practice.
- Workers compensation insurance. This insurance protects your employees and business from claims resulting from employment-related accidents, injuries, and even death. Most states require an employer to retain this type of insurance coverage.
- Property insurance. This insurance protects the physical assets of your business by covering the cost to fix or replace physical assets damaged or destroyed due to an incident.
- Business interruption insurance. This insurance coverage replaces income lost by a business due to direct physical damage from a natural disaster (*e.g.*, hurricane) or, in some instances, forced closure due to government actions or policies (*e.g.*, coronavirus disease 2019 [COVID-19] mandated gym closures).

Risk Management Summary

Risk management is an initial and ongoing process to identify relevant risks associated with the delivery of a service. This occurs through the application of various approaches to identify, eliminate, reduce, or transfer those risks through the implementation of operational strategies. The EP is critical in the development of a team of individuals working together to establish and maintain a safe environment for both employees and clients. Although a clearly defined written emergency plan is essential, cultivating meaningful relationships with members and developing a vigilant attitude around safety will create an atmosphere of security and well-being for all. The EP may also be responsible for facility operations that extend beyond acute emergency situations.

Facility Management and Operations

Fitness facilities vary greatly in respect to their operating model, programming focus, square footage, usage, equipment, layout, and member access. However, there are several key principles of facility management that pertain to every facility regardless of capacity. *ACSM's Health/Fitness Facility Standards and Guidelines*, fifth edition (6), provides critical information required to meet industry benchmarks. The EP may be involved in different aspects of facility management. Therefore, a brief description of the role of the EP from the perspective of operations and equipment usage will be presented.

Clinical and Nonclinical Health/Fitness Facility Settings

In 2019, there were over 39,000 fitness facilities in the United States and more than 200,000 fitness facilities operating around the globe. The growth and evolution of the fitness industry has led to a host of different business models, including for-profit and not-for-profit. According to the IHRSA, the core business models in the fitness industry are the following:

- Fitness only. These are for-profit facilities that have fitness centers, group exercise spaces, locker rooms, social areas, and occasionally a pool or gymnasium (sport court).
- Multipurpose. These are for-profit facilities that not only include all the elements of a fitness-only facility but also offer racquet sports and are more likely to have pools and gymnasiums.
- Not for profit. These are facilities (fitness or multipurpose) operated by local communities (park and recreation), colleges and universities, the military, and government.
- YMCA/Young Women's Christian Association [YWCA]/Jewish Community Center [JCC]. These facilities are not-for-profit facilities (fitness or multipurpose) operated by nongovernmental institutions, which are focused on serving a specific community.

- Corporate fitness. These are fitness facilities operated by corporations for the sole purpose of providing a fitness and wellness benefit for the employees of a company. Corporate facilities are typically operated on a not-for-profit basis.
- Boutique fitness studios. These are for-profit specialized fitness facilities that are typically less than 10,000 ft^2 (1,000 m^2) in size and focus on delivering a specific type of fitness format to its clients.

In addition to the aforementioned business models, a fitness operation can choose to operate in either a clinical or nonclinical environment.

Clinical Fitness Setting

A clinical fitness setting is associated with a health care or medical-based facility. In a clinical setting, the vast majority of clients will have an underlying health condition that requires additional consideration in respect to prescribing and monitoring the patients or clients exercise routines. Examples of these underlying health conditions best served in a clinical fitness setting include diabetes, cardiovascular disease, orthopedic conditions, and disorders of the neuromuscular and respiratory systems. In most instances, a clinical fitness setting will retain a diverse staff of health care and fitness professionals, including athletic trainers, physical therapists, registered nurses, certified fitness professionals (EP), and physicians.

Clinical settings exist in many of the aforementioned fitness industry business models. Among the most common clinical fitness settings are the following:

- Hospital-based medical fitness centers. These are fitness facilities incorporated into a hospital setting. These fitness centers will often have cardiac rehabilitation services, physical therapy services, and related medical elements integrated within the fitness offerings of the facility. These fitness settings have health care and fitness professionals working together on the delivering of fitness. Hospital-based medical fitness facilities typically have a Medical Fitness Facility Certification from the Medical Fitness Association (MFA). Examples of hospital systems that operate medical fitness centers include the Baylor Health Care System in Dallas, Texas, and John Hopkins Health System based in Baltimore, Maryland.
- For-profit medical fitness facilities. These are for-profit commercial clubs (fitness-only and multipurpose) that have chosen to build their value proposition around offering a medically based service similar to what a hospital-based facility would offer. In most instances, these medical fitness facilities have obtained Medical Fitness Facility Certification from MFA. For-profit commercial clubs such as The Atlantic Club, New Jersey; Atlantic Coast Athletic Clubs, Virginia; and Cedardale Health & Fitness, Massachusetts, are all certified by MFA as medical fitness centers.
- Boutique sports medicine studios. These are boutique fitness studios that have chosen to deliver a sports medicine–based offering. In the majority of instances, these clinical settings focus on programming to assist those in various stages of recuperation from an orthopedic or neuromuscular injury. An example is D1 Sports Training, a chain of sports medicine–oriented fitness studios in the United States. Their model involves physicians, physical therapists, athletic trainers, and certified fitness professionals.
- Hospital-based cardiac rehabilitation facilities. These are fitness centers dedicated solely to providing medically supervised cardiac rehabilitation.

Nonclinical Fitness Settings

A nonclinical fitness setting primarily serves an apparently healthy population and individuals with no known underlying medical condition or serious health risk factors. Nonclinical fitness settings are not positioned to serve individuals with underlying health and medical conditions; instead, they are designed to serve the general public. These nonclinical settings don't retain the health care staff a clinical setting would employ, and the fitness professionals that serve in these settings tend not to have the appropriate certifications for serving an unhealthy or medically compromised population.

Operations

In addition to human resource functions relating to scheduling and supervision, facility operations may involve a great variety of tasks relating to the supervision and coaching of members, availability of equipment for members and guests, temperature control, music and sound functions, information technology, and overall facility maintenance. The EP must always take into consideration the well-being of all members and staff when it comes to developing and implementing operational practices. Although facility dependent, there are certain operating practices common to all facilities including greeting members and guests within the facility; monitoring access to and usage of the facility; maintaining proper water temperature and chemical balance for saunas, steam rooms, and/or whirlpools; providing the proper oversight of member and guest activities; and employing appropriate supervision for youth programing (6).

From an operational perspective, the ACSM Health/Fitness Facility Standards were written to ensure expectations regarding supervision, responsibility, and duty are clearly defined. Facilities that are nontraditional in respect to hours of operation, such as facilities that offer 24-hour 365-day access, also have an obligation to provide clear policies and procedures around the supervision and access of members and guests. In addition, creating a safe physical environment for users and employees involves relevant and thoughtfully placed signage that communicates the expectations, responsibilities, risks, and actions required to maintain a successful fitness operation. Considering the policies and procedures around equipment and supplies is also important.

Equipment

Although it is the responsibility of every member, guest, and employee to respect equipment, the EP may be charged with the task of monitoring, inspecting, and maintaining equipment. There are several key questions to ask when considering the care and use of equipment. Table 16.9 offers an example of the most common preventive maintenance practices for resistance equipment, free weight equipment, and the leading pieces of cardiovascular training equipment.

1. Is the equipment being used for the purpose it was designed?
2. Is the preventive maintenance schedule adequate given the equipment usage?
3. Is the preventive maintenance schedule for the equipment in adherence with the recommendations of the manufacturer?
4. Is the manufacturer's warranty reasonable given the equipment usage?
5. Is the equipment thoughtfully and safely positioned within the facility?
6. Is the equipment stored properly?
7. Is the equipment being replaced on a reasonable usage cycle?
8. Is the equipment reflective of the facility's value proposition?
9. Is the equipment intuitive and user-friendly?

In addition to the responsibility to provide clean and well-functioning equipment to clients, members, and guests, the EP has a responsibility to provide clear instructions about the use and misuse of equipment. Empowering members with the knowledge to safely and properly use all the equipment is paramount.

Table 16.9	Sample Equipment Care Checklist			
Equipment	**Daily**	**Weekly**	**Monthly**	**As Needed**
Variable-resistance equipment	Clean frames with mild soap and water. Clean upholstery with mild antibacterial soap and water.	Check all cables and bolts and tighten as needed. Check moving parts and adjust as needed.	Lubricate guide rods with lightweight oil.	Repair or replace pads. Replace cables if needed.
Free weight benches	Clean frames with mild soap and water. Clean upholstery with mild antibacterial soap and water.	Check all cables and bolts and tighten as needed. Check moving parts and adjust as needed.		Repair or replace pads. Replace cables if needed.
Dumbbells and bars	Clean off bars with dry cloth.	Check all screws and bolts and tighten as needed.	Use lightweight oil on cloth to remove any rust.	Repair or replace broken bars and dumbbells.
Bikes	Clean off control panel with dry cloth. Clean off handles with mild antibacterial soap and damp cloth. Clean off seats with mild antibacterial soap and damp cloth.	Check equipment diagnostics through control panel for any potential troubles. Check all screws and bolts and tighten as needed. Vacuum underneath.	Remove bike housing and clean out dust and lint that may have collected.	Refer to manufacturer's guidelines.
Elliptical trainers	Clean off control panel with dry cloth. Clean off handles with mild antibacterial soap and damp cloth. Clean off foot pedals with damp cloth.	Check equipment diagnostics through control panel for any potential troubles. Check all screws and bolts and tighten as needed. Vacuum underneath.	Remove elliptical housing and clean out dust and lint that may have collected.	Refer to manufacturer's guidelines.
Treadmills	Clean off control panels with dry cloth. Clean off housing with mild antibacterial soap and damp cloth.	Check equipment diagnostics through control panel for any potential troubles. Check all screws and bolts and tighten as needed. Vacuum underneath.	Clean belt using a damp cloth. Check belt and deck surface and lubricate as needed and per manufacturer's specifications.	Replace belt if needed. Refer to manufacturer's guidelines.

The EP must understand potential areas of risk exposure surrounding facility operations to deliver services confidently and to proactively manage risk. The professionalism that such vigilance requires increases the personal and professional rewards of life as a fitness professional while also ensuring lasting business success. The most successful EP will always keep in mind that his or her top priority is to protect the best interests of the participant at all times and in all ways. Protecting the client also means acting with ethics and integrity.

Financial Management

For any fitness facility, accurate financial planning and management are crucial to succeeding in the industry. Fitness managers need a basic understanding of accounting and financial processes to create facility budgets, provide financial forecasts, and monitor overall financial performance. Following are some of the key accounting terms every EP should be familiar with.

Accounts payable: money the business owes to another individual or business. Examples include outstanding invoices, property taxes, etc.

Accounts receivable: money owed to the business by individuals or businesses. Examples include dues balances from annual contracts, balances from personal training packages, etc.

Asset: any property owned by a business that has monetary value. Assets can be either short term, meaning they can be converted to cash within the next year (cash in bank, short-term Certificate of Deposit [CD], or small equipment that can be sold), or long term, meaning the assets are likely to take more than 1 year to convert to cash (*e.g.*, property, equipment, leasehold improvement, and deducted depreciation).

Balance sheet: a financial statement that presents the assets, liability, and equity of a business at a specific point in time. This is the primary tool used to assess a business's overall financial health.

Budget: a plan forecasting expected income, expenses, and profit for a given period

Capital: money, goods, land, or equipment used to produce other goods and services

Cash flow: movement of money in and out of a business through the collection of revenue and payments of expenses, especially as it impacts the liquidity of the business

Depreciation: a decline in the value of any given asset over a period of time due to wear and tear or age. Depreciation schedules are used to determine the amount and period of depreciation for the assets of a business.

Earnings Before Interest, Taxes, Depreciation, and Amortization (EBITDA): This is a management metric and not an accounting metric as defined by U.S. Generally Accepted Accounting Principles (GAAP). EBITDA is equal to gross revenues minus operating expenses but before accounting for interest payments, federal/state business income taxes, depreciation allowances, and amortization.

Equity: the monetary value of all shareholder interests in a business after subtracting business liabilities from business assets. Equity is typically in cash or stock.

Income statement: a financial statement that includes the revenue, expenses, and net income/loss of a business for a specified period, very often referred to as a profit and loss statement

Liability: a debt owed to an individual or business. Liabilities can be short term, meaning they will become due and payable in the next year (*e.g.*, accounts payable items, income taxes due, and deferred revenue), and long term, meaning they will come due and payable beyond the next year (*e.g.*, future interest and principal payments, deferred revenue from long-term contracts, and deferred rent).

Liquidity: a term for cash on hand

Net income: gross income less all expenses including amortization, interest, and tax expenses. This represents the taxable profit of a business for a specific period.

Variance: the difference between an expected and an actual result

Accounting is the process of recording and summarizing business and financial transactions and analyzing, verifying, and reporting the results. These financial records provide information needed to make decisions about the future state of the business.

Accrual and Cash Accounting

A standard method of recording business transactions is necessary to maintain accurate financial records. The most common methods used in the fitness industry are cash accounting, sometimes called checkbook accounting, and accrual accounting. In cash accounting, transactions are recorded when money is actually received or paid out. Using this method, membership dues would be recorded on the day the payment was received from the member. Another example of how cash accounting works is to consider rent payments. In cash accounting, the expense of rent is accounted for the day rent is paid. In contrast, accrual accounting requires transactions to be recorded when they occur. Therefore, membership dues would be recorded on the day a membership payment is considered due regardless of whether or not the payment has been received. If we take the previous example of rent for cash accounting, in accrual accounting, the total rent for the year would be spread out across each month regardless of when it is actually paid. Cash accounting is typically used by smaller fitness businesses such as fitness studios, whereas accrual accounting is the preferred method for larger fitness businesses, especially multiple unit operations.

Financial Statements

Financial statements are a financial report card informing management and shareholders about a summary of the business's financial performance. These statements are also important for institutions invested in the business, such as a bank that has loaned money or private investor who has given the business money. Balance sheets and profit and loss statements are two of the most important financial statements a manager needs to understand.

Balance Sheet

A balance sheet (Fig. 16.1) indicates the financial status of a business at any given time and is separated into assets, liabilities, and owner's equity. In order for a balance sheet to be accurate, the total assets must always be equal to the total liabilities plus total equity.

1. Assets are anything a company owns that has monetary value (*i.e.*, cash, buildings, land, and equipment). Assets are typically divided into two categories: current (short term) and fixed (long term).

    Current assets are those that can and are expected to be turned into cash within the next 12 months. Examples of current assets include the following:

    - Cash and cash equivalents
    - Inventory
    - Accounts receivable
    - Prepaid expenses

    Fixed assets are those that have been acquired for long-term use by the business. These assets include the following:

    - Property (land and buildings)
    - Equipment
    - Office furniture

Balance Sheet for ABC Fitness Center June 30, 20XX **Assets**		
Current assets		
Cash	200,000	
Cash equivalents	90,000	
Inventory	25,000	
Accounts receivable	130,000	
Total current assets	$445,000	
Fixed assets		
Equipment	845,000	
Building	1,500,000	
Land/property	675,000	
Accumulated depreciation		200,000
Total fixed assets	$2,820,000	
Total assets	$3,265,000	
Liabilities		
Current liabilities		
Accounts payable		115,000
Accrued expenses		65,000
Deferred taxes		9,500
Total current liabilities		$189,500
Non–current liabilities		
Notes payable (bank)		1,650,000
Others		120,000
Total non–current liabilities		$1,770,000
Total liabilities		$1,959,500
Owner's equity		
Capital stock		985,000
Retained earnings		215,500
Paid in capital		105,000
Total owner's equity		$1,305,500
Total liabilities and owner's equity		$3,265,000

FIGURE 16.1. Sample balance sheet.

2. Liabilities are financial obligations or credits owed by the business. Liabilities are defined as current (short term) or noncurrent (long term).

   Current liabilities are debts the business is obligated to pay within the next 12 months. Examples include the following:

   ■ Accounts payable
   ■ Income taxes
   ■ Accruals
   ■ Deferred revenue, rent, or taxes

   Noncurrent liabilities are debts and expenses that are not due in the next 12 months. Examples include the following:

   ■ Future payments on loans
   ■ Deferred revenue, rent, or taxes

3. Owner's equity is the owner's investment in the business plus any profits or minus any losses. How equity appears on a balance sheet is determined by how the business was established — either as a corporation, limited liability corporation, partnership, or sole proprietorship.

Profit and Loss Statement

A profit and loss statement, also referred to as an income statement (Fig. 16.2), summarizes the financial performance over a specific time (month, quarter, or year). This financial tool includes actual expenses and revenues in the stated time frame as well as a look at how those numbers compare with a year-to-date plan and, in the case of many institutions, comparison to prior year performance. Revenues are primarily generated by membership sales, fitness programs, and

ABC Fitness Center Income Statement for the quarter ending March 31, 20XX

	Actual Year to Date	**Forecast YTP**	**Variance**
Revenue			
Membership dues	$397,500	$357,750	$39,750
Enrollment fees	$21,000	$26,250	($5,250)
Personal training	$315,965	$280,860	$35,105
Pilates instruction	$1,527	$2,290	($763)
Pro shop	$2,384	$1,500	$884
Miscellaneous	$11,934	$10,000	$1,934
Total revenue	**$750,310**	**$678,650**	**$71,660**
Expenses			
Payroll and benefits			
Wages	$124,876	$130,000	($5,124)
Commission	$32,000	$30,000	$2,000
Payroll costs	$22,478	$23,400	($922)
Benefits	$18,433	$20,000	($1,567)
Total payroll and benefits expenses	*$197,787*	*$203,400*	*($5,613)*
Fitness			
Locker room supplies	$4,765	$4,500	$265
Equipment maintenance	$5,500	$7,000	($1,500)
Entertainment fees	$1,254	$1,200	$54
Total fitness expenses	*$11,519*	*$12,700*	*($1,181)*
Utilities			
Electricity	$95,988	$100,000	($4,012)
Gas	$17,934	$16,000	$1,934
Water	$16,223	$15,000	$1,223
Total utilities expenses	*$130,145*	*$131,000*	*($855)*
Other			
Advertising	$9,241	$11,500	($2,259)
Office supplies	$1,329	$2,000	($671)
Landscaping	$23,925	$33,320	($9,395)
Total other expenses	*$34,495*	*$46,820*	*($12,325)*
Fixed			
Depreciation	$73,453	$75,680	($2,227)
Insurance	$126,177	$123,725	$2,452
Total fixed expenses	*$199,630*	*$199,405*	*$225*
Total expenses	*$573,576*	*$593,325*	*($19,749)*
Pretax operating income	**$176,734**	**$85,325**	**$91,409**

FIGURE 16.2. Sample income statement.

miscellaneous profit centers, whereas expenses reflect the costs incurred to collect revenue and operate the facility.

Budgeting

Effective financial management relies on a well-thought-out budget, created to lay out the allotment of funds spent or brought in by a business and its various operating units. Budgeting, the process of coordinating resources and expenditures required for business functions, is essential for any business to survive. Budgets span a minimum of one fiscal year (typically January 1 to December 31 or July 1 to June 30). Being conservative when estimating revenues and liberal when predicting expenses is often beneficial for a business. Underestimating expenses or overestimating revenue streams can put a business in a challenging position, where expenses cannot be paid and profits will not be made.

Types of Budgets

Two of the most common budget processes in the health/fitness industry are zero based and trend line. Zero-based budgeting is the process often used when opening a new facility or when making significant changes in the operation of an existing facility. This process uses assumptions regarding business expenses and revenues to develop a budget rather than relying on prior years' actual numbers. Trend-line budgeting is the most common process used and involves using previous years' financial data and applying some general assumptions to develop the budget for the current and upcoming years. This process makes the assumption that facility expenses and revenues will continue on the trend seen over the past years.

Creating a Budget

Once the method of creating the budget has been determined, there are four main steps to follow to develop a complete and accurate budget:

1. *Establish budget expectations*: Any limitations must be determined before starting the development of a budget. Limitations may include restrictions to keep overall expenses close to the previous year's budget or even possibly to cut the expenses to a percentage less than the previous year. For example, when the author worked for ClubCorp, one of the budget assumptions was building in a 2-point spread where revenues were budgeted to grow 2 percentage points more than expenses.
2. *Forecast revenues*: Using previous years' data and assumptions regarding future conditions, a manager can estimate the revenue coming into the facility for the next fiscal year. It is important to include any new sources of revenue that may not have existed in the previous year (*e.g.*, usage fees from a new childcare facility opening in the next fiscal year).
3. *Forecast expenses*: Determine operating costs for the upcoming year, making sure to include percentage increases for salaries, increases in maintenance and repairs, escalations in rent, etc.
4. *Project profits and losses*: Comparing revenue and expense streams will determine the overall profits or losses for the projected budget. Revisit the first step to ensure that the profits/losses fall within the limitations set for the budget. Most for-profit fitness facilities establish an EBITDA target, which is the most common business metric for assessing profitability in the fitness facility industry.

Remember that a budget is only a tool; a budget is a map to follow throughout the fiscal year to ensure the facility can continue to operate profitably. A manager must revisit the budget on a monthly or quarterly basis, reviewing the year-to-date revenue and expenses and how they measure up to budget projections. On the basis of the direction the finances are headed, adjustments may need to be made for the rest of the fiscal year to stay on track financially.

Income Management

All revenue, which is reported on the income statement, must be diligently tracked throughout the year. Areas of revenue include the following:

- *Membership dues*: Membership and entrance fees are generally a facility's main sources of revenue. According to IHRSA's *2018 Profiles of Success* (1), the average U.S. fitness facility in 2017 generated 68% of total revenues from membership.
- *Fitness center*: This category would include fees for fitness programs, personal training, specialty group exercise sessions, and locker/towel rentals. IHRSA typically divides fitness-related income into subdepartments such as personal training, small group training, and group exercise. According to the aforementioned IHRSA report, in 2017, the median percentage of revenue generated by personal training represented 10% of a fitness facility's total revenue.
- *Food and beverage*: Often a small-profit center, facilities have started to include a snack/smoothie bar as an incentive to members. According to the aforementioned IHRSA report, in 2017, the median percentage of total revenues generated from food and beverage was 3.1% of total revenues.
- *Other services*: Depending on the type and size of the facility, a spa department offering services such as massage, youth center, on-site childcare, racquet sports, or a pro shop selling clothing or fitness equipment can provide other sources of revenue. According to the aforementioned report from IHRSA, in 2017, the median percentage of total revenue that fitness facilities generated from spas was 4.6%.

Controlling and tracking accounts receivable is critical to the survival of a fitness facility. Decisions must be made on how to collect and manage revenue streams. Otherwise, a fitness business may find itself in a weak cash position. Managing accounts receivables can be a time-intensive task, and most fitness organizations use software programs or third-party systems to facilitate the collection of revenue.

The collection of revenue will be fairly straightforward in most instances; however, all businesses must have procedures in place for delinquent accounts. Aged trial balance reports, listing all outstanding balances by category (1–30 d, 31–60 d, 61–90 d, and 901 d), should be run on a scheduled basis to facilitate the collection of funds.

Expense Management

Expenses are as important to a company's financial stability as revenue and in many instances are easier to manage than revenues. If spending is out of control, revenue streams may not be enough to keep a business functioning while still producing a profit. Expenses can be broken down into two broad categories: variable or fixed. Variable costs are those that fluctuate on the basis of usage of resources or participation in a program. Possible variable expenses include payroll, benefits, employee education and training, supplies, marketing, equipment maintenance and repairs, and inventory. Fixed expenses are those that are relatively consistent year after year and include insurance, rent, property tax, management fees, and principal and interest owed on any debts or loans. Another way fitness businesses look at expenses is to define them as distributed operating expenses, undistributed operating expenses, and capital expenses. Specifically,

- Distributed expenses are expenses that can be allocated to a specific department such as childcare, fitness, racquet sports, and spa. These expense areas include payroll, payroll costs, supplies, and education.

- Undistributed expenses are expenses that can't be definitively assigned to any single department such as rent, utilities, marketing, and insurance.
- Capital expenses represent the cost associated with the purchase of equipment or property that can be depreciated.

The goals of any manager should include eliminating excess spending in any areas within his or her control. Fixed expenses typically cannot be negotiated but in certain instances can. Most variable expenses can be effectively reduced by following a few guidelines:

1. When purchasing equipment, outsourcing services, and acquiring supplies, obtain at least three quotes from different suppliers to find the right price for the best product. Be sure to repeat this process on a regular basis for any items that may be purchased repeatedly to ensure the cost reflects industry norms. Negotiate with vendors to get the best deal on goods and services.
2. Eliminate unnecessary expenses. Examine every cost center and determine its expendability. Fill empty spaces or cost centers with profit centers (*i.e.*, make an office or storage closet into a massage room).
3. Contract out services (*i.e.*, landscaping, food and beverage, spa) to limit staff costs, equipment and training expenses, and liability concerns.
4. Use internal resources when possible. A business may prefer to hire a few part-time employees to create and publish all marketing efforts instead of signing a contract with a marketing firm.

Regardless of the methods used, managers must constantly review the budget to keep expenses in control while also making sure revenue streams meet their targets.

Section Summary

Using budgeting and financial planning skills, an EP can successfully manage a facility's profits and losses. Exposure to different types of facilities will allow managers to develop a variety of financial skills, enhance their ability to accurately forecast a facility's budget, and provide their investors with an annual profit.

Marketing and Sales

Marketing, and its close companion sales, is an often-neglected consideration in the toolkit of fitness facility managers. P.T. Barnum, the founder of the Barnum and Bailey Circus, said, "Without promotion, something terrible happens . . . nothing." In the business of fitness, whether your objective is to increase membership sales, drive personal training revenues, increase group exercise participation, or introduce a new program, your objective can't happen unless effective promotion takes place. EPs who wish to ascend to a leadership or management role need to have an understanding of and appreciation for marketing and sales and furthermore should pursue every opportunity to master the basics of marketing and sales.

Marketing

Marketing is a modern-day form of storytelling whose purpose is twofold. First is to generate attention and awareness of a particular facility, program, or service. Before consumers or clients can engage with a fitness facility, whether it's to purchase a membership or sign up for a program, they have to be aware of the offering. Second, marketing is about creating purchase intent, getting individuals to make the thoughtful decision to purchase a product or service. Absent customer awareness and purchase intent, no facility, program, or service can be sold or used.

There are three broad categories of marketing: image or brand marketing, content marketing, and call-to-action marketing.

- Image or brand marketing. Image marketing involves communicating to your audience who and what your brand is. This type of marketing relays to consumers your value proposition and your brand promise and defines what you stand for. The overarching goal of image marketing is to generate awareness of your brand and to establish in the consumer's mind a particular image of what your brand stands for (*i.e.*, family oriented, trendy, medical based). Two brands in the fitness industry that do an excellent job conveying who they are and what their value proposition is through image marketing are Equinox and SoulCycle.

- Content marketing. Content marketing is designed to educate and inform consumers about your brand. The goal is to help consumers make an informed decision about the relevance and value of a particular brand in respect to the individual's interests and underlying lifestyle preferences. Content marketing can drive both brand awareness and purchase intent. Content marketing has emerged as a powerful promotional approach in the past decade with the advent of blogs and podcasts. The emergence of industry influencers can be directly tied to content marketing and the followers that can be generated with outstanding content.

- Call-to-action marketing. This approach to marketing has one and only one purpose: to get consumers to take action. This may include getting consumers to sign up for a free class, visit a particular Web site, or participate in a free trial. In order to achieve this objective, call-to-action marketing strategies involve introducing scarcity, promoting discounts, offering free trials, and promoting reduced or cheap prices. One fitness firm that is highly effective at call-to-action marketing is Planet Fitness.

Broadly speaking, a fitness facility needs to use all three marketing approaches if it wants to enhance awareness of its brand and concurrently generate purchase desire among its targeted audience.

Marketing Tools

To effectively market your fitness facility or its programs, there are some basic marketing tools an EP should be familiar with, including direct mail, print advertisements, word-of-mouth (WOM)/referral promotions, Internet advertisements, e-mail blasts/SMS blasts, and social media posts.

- Direct mail involves sending a promotional offer to a targeted audience that encourages the recipients to take action (call, visit, or write). Most direct mail promotions involve the use of a postcard, flyer, coupon, or similar print item. The typical response rate for direct mail falls in the 0.5%–3% range, meaning for every 100 pieces sent out, 1–3 people respond.

- Print advertisements can either be image driven or call to action. Large fitness groups such as 24 Hour Fitness, Equinox, Life Time Fitness, and Planet Fitness will place print advertisements in local newspapers and magazines with the intent of creating enhanced awareness of their brand and in other instances to drive traffic to their doorstep.

- WOM speaks to marketing efforts that informally leverage the voice of existing clients and customers. In the instances where a fitness facility takes a more formal approach to WOM, the method is called a client referral program. Client referral programs typically offer existing customers a reward for bringing forward the names of friends and associates or inviting them in as a guest.

- Internet advertising has overtaken print advertising as a leading tool for conducting image and call-to-action advertising for many fitness facilities. Google Ads and Facebook Business are the two most prevalent means of conducting Internet or digital advertising. According to the *2018 International Fitness Industry Trend Report — What's All the Rage* conducted by ClubIntel (7), 41% of U.S. fitness operators reported using Internet advertising. Equinox and Planet Fitness rely heavily on Internet advertising for promoting their brands and driving client traffic.

■ E-mail blasts and SMS blasts are digital versions of traditional direct mail. Like direct mail, e-mail and SMS blasts are used primarily for call-to-action promotions with the intent of driving foot traffic. In the case of an e-mail blast, open rates (the percentage of recipients that open the e-mail) can range from 20% to 50% and the click through rate (percentage that actually open an attachment or click on an offer) typically ranges from 3% to 5%.

■ Social media posts are a digital extension of WOM in which a fitness business posts compelling content and images on its social media sites in an effort to generate awareness and, in some instances, drive call to action. The most popular social media platforms for posting marketing related content are Facebook, Instagram, and Twitter.

In addition to the aforementioned marketing tools, Web sites that are search engine optimized and mobile applications are powerful platforms for marketing a fitness business.

Sales

Sales occur once marketing has performed its job: brought attention to your offer and fostered purchase intent in the consumer's mind. For most fitness professionals, the word *sales* conjures up negative impressions, most often associated with high-pressure sales techniques such as those experienced by visiting a new or used car dealership or possibly a low-price commercial fitness facility. Sales represent a process of discovery, a means of identifying a solution to address a particular individual's needs. Sales involve taking an individual who has expressed an interest in your offer, such as a fitness assessment or personal training session, and guiding them in making the purchase decision. As an EP, you will likely find yourself in a situation where possibly you have to manage the sales of a fitness facility, or more likely have to sell a particular program or service. Consequently, as an EP, you should be familiar with the basic steps of selling at the personal level, a process that takes an individual from a place of interest to making a purchase decision. Following are the key steps in the selling process:

■ Build a relationship with the prospect. People are more inclined to make a purchase when they know someone.

■ Foster trust. Beyond establishing a relationship with the prospect, you want to build trust. Individuals are more inclined to purchase from people they trust than those they don't.

■ Listen. B.C. Holwick is quoted as saying, "Good listeners generally make more sales than good talkers." By actively listening to people, it is easier to discover what their needs and interests are. Once you identify what is important to an individual, you can then guide them to make the correct purchasing decision.

■ Confirm what you've heard before introducing the product you wish the individual to purchase. People will make a purchase when they believe the offer you have meets their need. Confirming what you've heard reinforces for the individual that you understand their need, which in turn makes introducing them to your offer easier.

■ Once they have confirmed their need and the value of what you are offering, then it's time to ask for the sale.

To learn more about the process of relationship selling, consider reading the book written by Jim Cathcart entitled *Relationship Selling*.

Section Summary

Marketing and sales are as important to business success as building a great team, preparing a budget, and having quality operating systems. Marketing is the process of making the market aware of what your fitness facility offers, what your facility stands for, and, finally, generating purchase intent among those in your targeted audience. Sales are a very personal process allowing a professional to connect with an individual who has expressed purchase intent and then guide them to make the purchase decision.

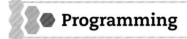

Programming

Programming encourages clients and members of a fitness facility to become engaged. Other than individuals who visit a fitness facility and jump on a piece of equipment, most individuals who use a fitness facility do so because of interest in a particular type of program activity. Programming helps foster connections between a fitness facility, its staff, and its clients/members. Through effective programming, a fitness facility can inspire people, help clients overcome boredom, address individual interests and needs, and finally make fitness fun.

Programs in Demand

One important element of great programming is offering activities and events that appeal to your target audience. Table 16.10 provides a list of some leading program activities that are popular among health club consumers as brought forth in IHRSA's *2019 Health Club Consumer Report* (8), whereas Table 16.11 identifies several leading program trends among U.S. fitness facility operators based on the *2018 International Fitness Industry Trend Report — What's All the Rage* conducted by ClubIntel (7).

Steps to Successful Programming

Programming that engages and empowers individuals in the pursuit of a healthier lifestyle requires EPs to be versed in the key elements of great programing, as brought forward in the following text.

1. Understand your market. To deliver programs that are appealing, empowering, and inspiring, management needs to be clear about who their audience is and what their interests and needs are. This can be accomplished in several ways, including gathering information on client interest and behaviors at the time they join the fitness facility, conducting focus group sessions among various client groups, and conducting surveys.

Table 16.10	Leading Consumer Program Activity Preferences in the United States for 2018
Program Activity	**Percentage of Consumers Who Participate in Activity**
Yoga	21%
HIIT	20%
Calisthenics	19%
Dance, step, and other choreography	15%
Cross-training–style activities	11%
Aquatic exercise	10%
Group cycling	9%

HIIT, high-intensity interval training.

Table 16.11	Top 10 Program Trends in United States Fitness Facilities in 2018
Program	**Facility Adoption Percentage**
Personal training	90%
Free weight training	83%
Functional resistance training	83%
Smal-group fee-based personal training	77%
Boot camp–style conditioning classes	74%
Senior fitness/active aging programs	72%
Traditional yoga	67%
HIIT small group training	65%
Group cycling classes	63%
Suspension training classes	63%

HIIT, high-intensity interval training.

2. Have an overarching purpose and vision for programming. When you have a unifying purpose and vision for programming, defining the parameters of the facility's programming is easier. For example, is programming at the facility there to drive revenues, create greater member engagement, or both? Understanding and codifying the purpose and vision of your programming will help introduce a program calendar that aligns with both the facility's overall purpose and the interests of its clients.

3. Get everyone involved. This speaks to the importance of getting your clients and employees involved in programming. When people are involved, they take ownership, and when they take ownership, they will serve as advocates for the facility's programs. Involvement can include having a member committee that works with management on program ideas, having a team of employees responsible for overseeing different aspects of the facility's programs, and engaging a select group of clients and employees to brainstorm program ideas to establishing an incentive program that encourages employees and clients to bring in participants.

4. Build a program plan. Developing an annual program plan is critical for a facility manager. This program plan should address specific targets, establish a calendar with milestones, frame the promotional efforts that will be implemented to inform clients about the programs, and, finally, identify individual employees who will be accountable for the success of each program.

5. Promote, promote, and promote. Make it everyone's job to get the word out about each and every program using all available resources. The best marketing approaches for communicating the facility's programs include facility newsletter, facility's Web site, facility's social media sites, e-mail blasts, and WOM.

6. Gather feedback after each program. Soliciting client feedback, and even employee feedback, around each program provides a framework for ensuring future programming efforts are successful.

Section Summary

Programming, like talent management, operations, finance and accounting, and marketing, is a competency that EPs should become comfortable with. By mastering the essentials of programming, a facility manager can foster a fitness environment that is compelling, inspirational, and relevant to its customers.

SUMMARY

Managing a fitness-based facility requires experience across many specialties. As discussed in this chapter, managers need knowledge and experience in the fitness industry; management positions also require competency in areas such as human resources, financial planning, facility operations, marketing, programming, risk management, and sales.

Customer service is such an important draw for potential customers in the fitness industry, such that a manager must make it a top priority to foster organizational culture and provide the leadership necessary to recruit, develop, retain, and empower a team of employees. Using budgeting and financial planning skills, an EP can successfully manage a facility's profits and losses. Marketing and sales are as important to business success as building a great team, preparing a budget, and having quality operating systems. Finally, by mastering the essentials of programming, a facility manger can foster a fitness environment that is compelling, inspirational, and relevant to its customers.

STUDY QUESTIONS

1. Provide an example of how employee recruitment strategies used by a corporate fitness center may differ from a local commercial fitness center.
2. How can the professional development of employees impact budget decisions? What are some strategies to empower employees to gain additional experience without putting a strain on financial resources?
3. Describe the difference between a trend-line budget and a zero-based budget. When is one budget process more appropriate to use?
4. If your fitness facility's primary client audience is young adults between the ages of 20 and 35 years, describe what marketing strategies would you leverage to gain the greatest traction.
5. How might your programming strategy be different for serving clients ages 55 years and older versus a programming strategy for 25- to 34-year-old millennials?

REFERENCES

1. International Health Racquet & Sportsclub Association. *2018 Profiles of Success*. Boston (MA): International Health Racquet & Sportsclub Association; 2018.
2. International Health Racquet & Sportsclub Association. *2017 IHRSA Employee Compensation and Benefits Report*. Boston (MA): International Health Racquet & Sportsclub Association; 2018.
3. Tharrett S. *Fitness Management*. 4th ed. Monterey (CA): Healthy Learning; 2018. 678 p.
4. Internal Revenue Service, U.S. Department of the Treasury. Understanding employee vs. contractor designation [Internet]. Washington [DC]: Internal Revenue Service; [cited 2019 Aug 20]. Available from: https://www.irs.gov/newsroom/understanding-employee-vs-contractor-designation.
5. Picincu A. The purpose of new employee orientations [Internet]. San Francisco (CA): Bizfluent.com; [cited 2019 Aug 20]. Available from: https://bizfluent.com/facts-5128586-purpose-new-employee-orientation.html.
6. Sanders M. *ACSM's Health/Fitness Facility Standards and Guidelines*. 5th ed. Champaign (IL): Human Kinetics; 2019. 232 p.
7. ClubIntel. *2018 International Fitness Industry Trend Report — What's All the Rage. A Comprehensive Study of Global Fitness Industry Behavior*. Dallas (TX): ClubIntel; 2018. 106 p.
8. International Health Racquet & Sportsclub Association. *2019 Health Club Consumer Report*. Boston (MA): International Health Racquet & Sportsclub Association; 2019.

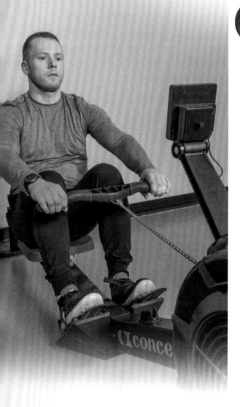

17 Marketing

OBJECTIVES

- To identify the different aspects of the marketing mix, including the five Ps.
- To recognize the concepts behind the acquisition of new clients and/or participants.
- To apply marketing strategies to business development and growth.

INTRODUCTION

This chapter is designed to provide the American College of Sports Medicine Certified Exercise Physiologist® (ACSM-EP®) with a basic understanding of the marketing mix relating to the ACSM-EP's specific job profile. An overview of the marketing mix and the application of the strategies that may be used to promote health and fitness services and products is presented.

Marketing Basics

The marketing mix represents a basic building block of marketing for the ACSM-EP. At its core, marketing is a function of the aspects that make up product, place, price, and promotion, also known as the four Ps. However, the fitness industry lends itself to one additional "P," representing "people." Knowing and understanding the customers, stakeholders, and target markets enables the ACSM-EP to apply a tailored marketing strategy to increase revenues and promote fitness efficiently and effectively. The following is a breakdown of the five Ps:

1. People (not formerly considered part of the marketing mix)
2. Place
3. Product
4. Price
5. Promotion

People

The first function relating to people involves learning more about the individuals and groups who will be served by fitness-related businesses and services. Understanding the demographic, psychographic (attitudes, values, and opinions), and physical activity attributes of potential customers enables the ACSM-EP to employ deliberate marketing strategies and build sustainable relationships. For example, once the ACSM-EP decides to establish a fitness business, a demographic analysis needs to be performed to better understand the people most likely to frequent the facility. Demographic analyses can provide public information about people residing in any specific geographic area. Researchers have found that individuals who reside within 1- to 5-mi radius of a fitness or recreational facility tend to be more physically active and thus become a target audience (1,2). Alternatively, a demographic analysis can be performed for an entire trade area or city in an attempt to learn more about a broader client base. Either way, the goal is to evaluate data that can provide information necessary to make good decisions with regard to successful marketing practices. A demographic search can be performed with a variety of online resources, including the United States Census Bureau, which is updated every 10 years, providing easily accessed, reliable data at no cost (http://2010.census.gov/2010census/).

Because of the vast amount of information available, finding a trade area and requesting demographic data can be overwhelming. Therefore, distinguishing which data are relevant to both the industry and the product is important. In the health/fitness industry, the major factors to examine in a demographic profile are number of people, number of households, household income, and gender breakdown.

The Centers for Disease Control and Prevention (CDC) also provides important information about the exercise and leisure-time habits of individuals. Accessing and synthesizing CDC information enables the ACSM-EP to consider both demographic profiles of a particular area and epidemiological data relating to a particular population. For example, almost regardless of the region of the country, approximately 25% of all adults in the United States perform no leisure-time

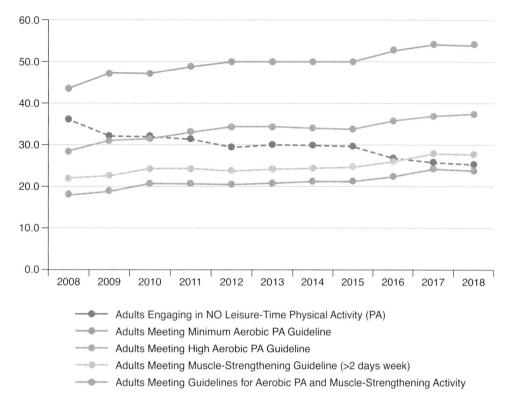

FIGURE 17.1. Trends in meeting the 2008 Physical Activity Guidelines, 2008–2018. (Reproduced from Centers for Disease Control and Prevention. 2008 Physical activity guidelines for Americans. Trends in meeting the 2008 Physical Activity Guidelines, 2008—2018 [Internet]. Atlanta [GA]. Available from: https://www.cdc .gov/physicalactivity/downloads/trends-in-the-prevalence-of-physical-activity-508.pdf.)

physical activity (Fig. 17.1) (3). This segment of the population may be a very difficult target for a new ACSM-EP.

However, the remaining 75% of adults are active and therefore more likely to respond to physical activity marketing. In addition, given that the target population should specifically include those living within 1–5 mi of a potential location (4), the ACSM-EP can quickly assess the number of potential customers willing to purchase some type of health and fitness services. Having demographic and epidemiological data enables the ACSM-EP to make informed decisions about possible services and programs to develop and promote these programs effectively.

Successful program development requires an ability to distinguish between trends and fads. Several organizations provide reliable survey data to help make informed decisions about program development. The annual ACSM Survey of Worldwide Survey of Fitness Trends provides information about the top 20 fitness trends within a historical perspective (5). Listed in the following text are the top 20 fitness trends for 2019 (5).

1. Wearable technology
2. Group training
3. High-intensity interval training (HIIT)
4. Fitness programs for older adults
5. Body weight training
6. Employing certified fitness professionals
7. Yoga
8. Personal training
9. Functional fitness training

10. Exercise is Medicine® (EIM®)
11. Health/wellness coaching
12. Exercise for weight loss
13. Mobile exercise apps
14. Mobility/myofascial devices
15. Worksite health promotion and workplace well-being programs
16. Outcome measurements
17. Outdoor activities
18. Licensure for fitness professionals
19. Small group personal training
20. Postrehabilitation classes

The International Health, Racquet, & Sportsclub Association (IHRSA) also provides research reports on industry data and fitness club trends (http://www.ihrsa.org).

Although these data may seem plentiful, more information is usually needed to determine whether a program can be successful, including issues related to possible competitors and market demand in a particular area. Data about people alone are not enough to develop a comprehensive marketing plan. Therefore, product development and implementation is the next critical component of the marketing mix.

Product

Product can be both tangible (selling a membership) and nontangible (helping someone achieve a fitness goal). Possibly, the most common product of ACSM-EPs is personal training services, which can include something to sell (*i.e.*, training sessions) or something to achieve (*i.e.*, increase strength), or both. The ACSM-EP might work in a clinical, community, corporate, or private setting, and each of these will determine the type of product available. The product may be an incentive program, educational series, or community-based boot camp class. Regardless of product type, it is important for ACSM-EPs to recognize themselves and their services as an integral part of the product, so they can appropriately market the product in the best possible way. The skills and knowledge required to become an ACSM-EP must not be undervalued by the individual who has attained them. As a matter of principle, marketing success begins with believing in the value of the product. Every ACSM-EP must first believe in himself or herself.

Practically, one approach might include viewing the product in a different way than originally thought. What is the intention of a client purchasing a fitness-related product, and what does the consumer want or expect from the product? The top reasons cited for joining a fitness center are consistently reported as improving health and fitness and improving appearance (6). The job of the ACSM-EP is to market himself or herself as a professional with the skills and knowledge to help the client achieve these exact results. Although the ACSM-EP is continually educating clients about evidence-based practices, it is important not to sell a product purely for the sake of the sale without regard for client interest. Where the product is located can play a pivotal role in the sales and marketing process.

Place

Place refers to where the product can be purchased and/or delivered. For most ACSM-EPs, the service will be delivered out of a particular physical location such as a commercial, corporate, or private fitness facility or clinic. However, others may elect to conduct in-home or online personal training services with their clients. In addition, current market practices dictate the need for creating a virtual environment to deliver personal training services over and above the brick-and-mortar setting. The ACSM-EP will need to identify how to properly market his or her services, within a specific environment, whether that be cyberspace, a fitness center, or a client's home.

| HOW TO | **Develop an Incentive Program Incorporating Exercise Is Medicine** |

As a grassroots effort, EIM is a scientifically sound tool that can be used to promote fitness and wellness. As an educational initiative endorsed by many major health, medical, and fitness organizations, EIM initiatives can reach a broad base of consumers across several levels of expertise and engagement. Although the objectives of this program may go beyond a single incentive program, ACSM-EPs can focus on one aspect of health, for example, blood pressure, or choose to create a broader connection between fitness and disease prevention. Below are examples of ways to incorporate EIM into programmatic incentives. Creating a team to develop the EIM strategy is the first place to start.

Step 1: Develop Objectives

The vision of EIM to make physical activity and exercise a standard part of a global disease prevention and treatment medical paradigm that can be adopted as the vision of any fitness facility.
Objective 1: Increase awareness among members, staff, and the local medical community about EIM initiatives.
Objective 2: Increase member usage of fitness testing programs by 25%.
Objective 3: Increase membership of health care professionals by 10%.

Step 2: Develop Strategies to Address Objectives

Objective 1: Increase awareness of EIM.
  Strategy 1: Create an EIM team composed of facility members, human resources representatives, local medical professionals, and local educators.
  Strategy 2: Offer free blood pressure screening to provide initial information about the connection between exercise and the prevention of hypertension.
  Strategy 3: Provide members with a blood pressure form they can bring to their primary care physician.
Objective 2: Increase membership of health care professionals by 10%.
  Strategy 1: Provide trial or discounted memberships to health care professionals.
  Strategy 2: Invite health care professionals to "lunch-and-learn" sessions.
  Strategy 3: Develop a strategic partnership with Institute of Lifestyle Medicine (http://www.institute oflifestylemedicine.org) to provide educational incentives to health care professionals.

Step 3: Develop an EIM Incentive Program Action Plan

On the basis of the objectives and strategies listed above, develop an action plan to implement the strategies. The resources available for the implementation of an EIM initiative are numerous and are listed at https://www.exerciseismedicine.org.
Action item: Using the theme of May is EIM month, prepare news releases and other media information relating to exercise and disease prevention to send to local newspapers.
Action item: Develop a reward system for members who access fitness assessment programming.
Action item: Host "lunch-and-learn" series for local medical professionals to network and share ideas about exercise as a disease prevention tool.
Action item: Connect with local college or university to enlist kinesiology students as ambassadors of EIM message.
Action item: Use social media to create opportunities to provide information about EIM.
Action item: Organize fitness-related event as culminating EIM month activity.

Step 4: Evaluation

Schedule a meeting of the EIM team as soon as possible after event to discuss ways in which the objectives were met.
Develop simple questionnaire for members about effectiveness of EIM campaign.
Follow up with medical professionals about effectiveness of EIM campaign.

By clearly defining "place," the ACSM-EP can better understand his or her market. For instance, if the place is a private fitness center, considerations must be made for the physical environment of the club in terms of how the product is perceived. Considering the impact a place, including physical location or Web site, can have on the perceived value of the product is important (7). An easily navigated Web site and/or impeccably clean training studio set forth an image of professionalism, organization, and quality. Consideration should be given to any sensory perception of the place where the product will be delivered. Sensitivity to scents, appropriate music, and comfortable temperatures are just a few of the many factors that relate to a customer's perception of the product as related to the place of delivery. Facility attractiveness and operation has been identified as a key component for customer satisfaction (8). Interconnected with place is the function of price, which involves not only the actual costs of operation but also the perceptions of quality and value.

Price

Determining the appropriate price of the product is multifaceted and critical to the success of any business (1). Basic issues affecting price include cost of developing and/or delivering, profit margin, and market value (real and perceived).

Cost of delivery — The most important factor is the cost of delivering the service. Cost includes marketing, materials (*e.g.*, paper or online), equipment, facility, and the time value of the ACSM-EP. Unless subsidized, the price must at least cover the costs of delivery. It is important to be comprehensive in calculating these costs so as not to under- or overprice the product.

Acceptable profit margin — The cost as noted earlier includes everything except a profit, which is one of the ultimate goals of delivering the product. Therefore, the price above the cost of delivery becomes the actual profit margin. The higher the margin, the more profitable the business. However, set the margin too high, and the product becomes unaffordable to many and overall profit may suffer. An acceptable profit margin varies depending on the type and goals of the business (not for profit vs. for profit) and what the current market will bear. If there are similar products being offered locally, the profit margin should be set with due consideration to competitors pricing. If the price is set too high, many potential customers will be tempted to patronize a lower priced competitor. If the price is too low, people may be skeptical of the product's quality. Therefore, thoroughly assessing what the local market will bear in terms of overall price becomes critical to the success of the product.

Market value — Another important pricing factor is the balance between perceived value and actual demand for a product. A product with high demand, yet low perceived value ("yes we want it, but we are not willing to pay much for it"), may have to be priced very differently than a product with low demand but great perceived value (a select few want it and are willing to pay handsomely for it). Ideally, develop a product that falls somewhere in the middle such that reasonable demand exists and the product is perceived as valuable. Researchers have found that the consumer behaviors of fitness center members have shifted in the perceptions of the costs associated with fitness club memberships (9), which further emphasize value and perception. In the past, members paid only for programs they would consume. Today, members are more likely than ever to try a new program (10). This may be in part due to the variety of membership options available and the increased popularity of nontraditional programming.

Like many other industries, the pricing of fitness-related services also varies according to region. Facilities located on the West Coast may be able to set pricing at a much higher rate than their Midwest counterparts, which may largely be a function of cost-of-living differences. Another issue influencing pricing is the demand for access to fitness facilities, and given the West Coast has higher rates of physical activity participation, the demand is also naturally higher. Of course, demand and price are linearly related, which is then reflected in the average income of the ACSM-EP (Fig. 17.2).

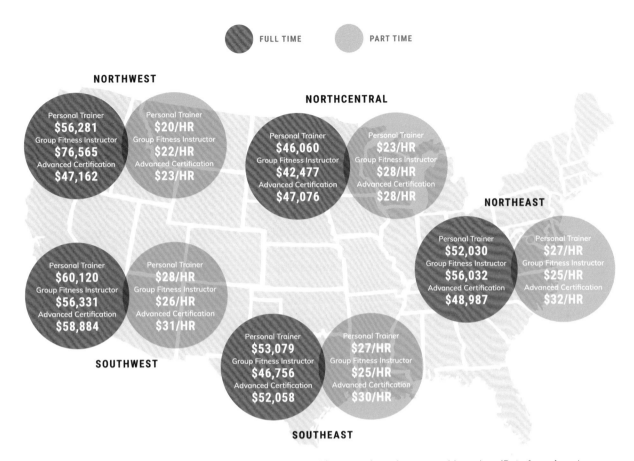

FIGURE 17.2. Average income of personal trainers and general fitness trainers by geographic region. (Data from American Council on Exercise. Salary report for health and fitness professionals [Internet]. San Diego [CA]: American Council on Exercise. Available from: https://acewebcontent.azureedge.net/assetportfoliodownloads/ACE_SalarySurvey.pdf.)

ACSM-EPs who develop marketing plans that incorporate an appreciation of the customer (people) with an understanding of the product and recognition of the perceptions related to price and value are able to apply myriad promotional strategies to achieve and sustain successful business practices.

Promotion

As the fifth "P" in the marketing mix, promotion is an ever-expanding and complex process of educating, presenting, and engaging stakeholders so that consumer loyalty and sustained relationships develop, grow, and are maintained. Following a brief explanation of branding, this section provides a limited overview of promotional strategies related to the following areas:

1. Advertising
2. Referrals
3. Direct mail/e-mail
4. Internet
5. Business to business
6. Sponsorship
7. Personal sales
8. Public relations

Branding

While considering the five Ps, the ACSM-EP can also evaluate strategies for reaching the appropriate target market with a suitable message. Deciding how to package the message helps determine the best marketing strategies to implement. Branding is an important consideration for the ACSM-EP to convey. What about the product or services makes them special, unique, or different from other products in the same industry? Why should a potential customer want to purchase fitness services or memberships from you or your facility as opposed to someone else? The ACSM-EP working privately has to be able to answer questions about his or her education, experience, and ability in a way that can be successfully branded. If the ACSM-EP is employed in a corporate or clinical setting, what is the mission and vision of the organization? What distinctive qualities does the organization have that enables the fitness services to serve a special niche, fulfill a unique need, or carry a particular association? Once these questions are answered, the ACSM-EP will have a clearer picture of how to brand the product. As an intangible, brand development is often accomplished by focusing on the health and wellness outcomes associated with fitness. Incorporating vicarious achievement and nostalgia have been found to build brand loyalty (11). In addition, the concept of building a "brand community" has been proposed as an effective mechanism to engage stakeholders both physically and virtually (12). A second consideration in marketing is the image being portrayed. Many fitness professionals create a logo, trade character, or image that relates in some way to health, wellness, and exercise. The logo is another tool to create brand awareness that can be used on business cards and other marketing materials. Increasing brand recognition builds brand loyalty within the target market of potential customers. Creating a professional and unique brand enables the ACSM-EP to employ marketing strategies across multiple mediums with a comprehensive design that is easily recognized and identified by stakeholders and potential customers.

Advertising

Advertising can be both a general and a targeted approach to spreading the word about a product. Commonly used advertising mediums in the health/fitness industry include print media such as newspapers, trade magazines, television, radio, and billboard. Social media and directed use of the Internet is fast becoming an effective advertising medium (13). The ACSM-EP may consider using one or more of these resources to advertise, although cost needs to be considered. Each advertising medium has unique pros and cons that will vary depending on the goals of the promotion, available resources, and breadth of the marketing plan (14). In addition, word of mouth recommendations have long been considered a highly successful means of promoting products and services, especially in the fitness industry.

Referral

The business of fitness has traditionally been a face-to-face process, although online options are becoming increasingly popular. A rapport built with faithful clientele is deep and long-lasting. Consequently, one of the most effective ways to market services to new clients is to ask for referrals from existing clients. Existing clients are the best sales team because they have experienced the impact of incorporating fitness into their lifestyle and the role a particular ACSM-EP can play in bringing about positive change over a period. When clients do refer a new prospect who then becomes a client, recognizing the referring member with some type of reward is important. A free personal training session or group exercise goes a long way toward future referrals.

Direct Mail/E-mail

Direct mail is an expensive but effective method of reaching a target market because of the ability to select the specific households to pursue. Traditionally, direct mail efforts produce a return rate between 1% and 3%. E-mail marketing has been found to be effective in reaching specific customers with similar interests (15). The key for creating effective e-mail blasts is to compile a list of potential customers. The ACSM-EP can build an e-mail list through referrals, existing clients, and, if permissible, club e-mail listings. A good e-mail blast can be a powerful message and include images, videos, and coupons that are tailored to a specific type of customer. Typical response rates from e-mail blasts run between 5% and 15%. E-mail marketing has also been found to be an effective strategy for health promotion and behavior change (16). Therefore, carefully crafting the e-mail message is critical to the success of any program or promotion (8). Virtual exchanges provide another opportunity for an ACSM-EP to connect with a client or potential client. Facebook, Twitter, and other social network sites provide outstanding mediums to promote the ACSM-EP's services.

Internet

Integrated marketing strategies that include e-mail communications and a Web site presence have been found to be more effective than print messages alone (17,18). Web site development, however, can be complex or simple. Trade magazines relating to health/fitness management and Internet businesses offer excellent advice on the choices and process of launching a health/fitness Web site (19). A simple Web site would include basic information about the product, place, price, and promotions. More dynamic Web sites can provide a virtual tour and engage a client at a personal level. Interactive Web opportunities can also be developed using social media tools.

Social media can be an excellent marketing tool when used correctly. Facebook, Instagram, Twitter, and other Internet sites have proven useful in referral-based businesses such as fitness because potential clients can make contact quickly and ask questions with relative anonymity. Social media sites can provide an opportunity for exchanges about topics that may be uncomfortable to discuss in face-to-face settings (13,20).

Business to Business

Like client referrals, business-to-business (B2B) referrals can be a very inexpensive and powerful way to reach a target audience. Taking the extra time to meet business owners in the area can pay huge dividends in terms of reaching new prospects. The key to developing strategic relationships in the community is to seek out businesses and individuals whose client bases overlap. Some ways to connect with other business professionals may be to attend a chamber of commerce event, host an open house, serve on a city or town committee, or volunteer and/or sponsor a local road race or event. Bartering for services is also an excellent way to build relationships with other professionals. B2B associations provide opportunities for collaboration and growth that can increase profitability with minimal use of resources.

Sponsorship

Sponsorship is also an effective means of promoting fitness-related products and growing B2B connections. Many small business owners seek ways to encourage physical activity for employees (21). Sponsorship enables the ACSM-EP to allocate resources toward a specific event and particular target market. Sponsorship also provides an opportunity for the ACSM-EP to practice good citizenship by being actively involved in a local community. Sponsorship builds brand recognition

Table 17.1	Cost-Benefit Breakdown of Common Marketing Tools		
Method	**Type**	**Cost**	**Impact**
Advertising	Internet	Low	Moderate/high
	Television	High	High
	Radio	High	Moderate
	Newspaper/magazine	Moderate	Low
Personal contact	Referrals	Free	High
B2B	Chamber of commerce	Low	High
Sponsorship	Event/cause marketing	Moderate	High

with vendors, participants, and spectators; provides a means of distributing print and media communications; and actively engages current fitness club members in the prospect of participating in a cause-related activity. Research has found that corporations primarily use sponsorship as a means of seeking exclusivity and raising public awareness and a positive image (22). Effective sponsorships include an evaluation on the return on investment that enables the sponsor to negotiate tailored packages that best meet the needs of those involved (23). Table 17.1 provides an illustration of the cost-benefit breakdown of common marketing tools.

Personal Sales

When evaluating the performance of fitness center employees, sales revenues are often included in the employee evaluation process (24). Most academic programs do not provide extensive sales training for students majoring in exercise science or kinesiology. However, fitness-related majors tend to be more physically active and appreciate the relationship of physical activity to greater quality of life (25). Translating that personal experience to the sale of health and fitness is the key to success for the ACSM-EP. Having confidence in the value of the fitness product is important to conveying a genuine attitude. Research cites empathy, ego drive, high energy level, integrity, an ability to learn, positive self-image, and an ability to forge relationships as critical characteristics of successful salespeople (26). To be a maven about a product (27) has also been cited as a significant quality to possess. A maven salesperson is described as someone who has an expertise in a given area or subject, is passionate about the subject, and wants to share that knowledge with others. Confidence in the product coupled with an ability to find and follow leads can lead to a successful career for an ACSM-EP.

Finding Leads

In sales, a lead is defined as someone who fits the profile of a target market and has shown an interest in the product or service. The marketing and advertising process is designed almost entirely to help identify leads through e-mail, phone calls, or Web site inquiries. Ideally, leads are individuals who have been exposed to one of the marketing mediums described earlier and have indicated a desire for more information about the product or service for sale. Each lead is a potential client. For this reason, having a system of managing leads is imperative, as each phone call, e-mail, or Web site inquiry that comes in is a potential customer. To be successful, the ACSM-EP will develop an organizational plan to include the lead on a spreadsheet and contact the person as soon as possible. The spreadsheet should include all relevant information about the lead, including home address, e-mail address, phone number, and any other personal details the lead provided when he or she responded to the marketing campaign. The more information gathered about the lead, the more personalized response can be provided. The lead spreadsheet should also include the date of each attempted contact and the eventual status of the lead.

Qualifying Prospects

Once a solid lead list is in place, the goal is to turn those leads into prospects. A lead becomes a prospect when he or she has expressed a need for the fitness product or service after an initial contact has been made. Qualifying prospects is a process that involves talking to the prospect and learning as much about the potential client as possible. The key to qualifying the prospect is (a) asking open-ended questions that will allow the ACSM-EP to learn the maximum amount possible about the individual ("What do you see as the next action steps?" "What is your timeline for implementing/purchasing this type of service/product?" "What concerns do you have?"), (b) listening to the potential client's responses and remembering relevant information, and (c) helping the prospect realize that what you offer can meet the needs he or she has expressed. Essentially, the goal is to become familiar with the individual and learn why he or she is interested in the services and products being promoted.

The Art of the Deal

Many ACSM-EPs will be able to positively impact their own compensation by attracting and closing new clients. Learning and adhering to specific sales guidelines should improve closing percentages and overall success.

Closing the deal is an extension of the "qualifying prospects" strategies. At this stage, the ACSM-EP will have adequate knowledge of the demographic, psychographic, exercise motivations, and activity goals of the potential client. The key to an effective close is to connect the fitness product or service with a need the prospect mentioned during the qualifying process. For example, a prospect may have identified a need to engage a personal trainer because he or she has little knowledge in the area of strength training. An appropriate closing strategy would be to reiterate this need verbally to the prospect and then highlight how personal training with you will enhance the prospect's strength training knowledge base. Once the prospect confirms that this benefit serves his or her personal need, the sale is likely to occur. Typically, many needs are uncovered during the prospect qualification process. If possible, try to highlight a second benefit that can be met with the fitness services being promoted and ask the prospect to confirm that the benefit exists. Complimenting a potential customer and engaging in active listening have been found to increase sales of add-on features of fitness equipment (28).

After the prospect has acknowledged at least two needs that can be met with the services being promoted, the groundwork is in place to ask for the sale. At this point, having some options for the prospect to consider is important. When asking for the sale, highlight two or three options that fit the prospect's needs that were previously identified. The final step is to actually ask the question: "Which of these packages would be the best fit for you?" The framing of this question allows for a positive "either/or" response rather than a "yes or no" response. With proper preparation by really trying to understand where the client is coming from (empathy) and engaging in active listening, the sales process is often more an educational opportunity for both the ACSM-EP and the client to learn and understand in greater depth about the challenges and opportunities available for individuals choosing active lifestyles.

Public Relations

Unlike costly advertising, public relations strategies provide an opportunity to promote fitness products and services using minimal financial resources. Although advertising is effective in communicating information about a product or service, public relations give potential customers an opportunity to consider the product or service at a more emotional level (29). Public relations can be used in several ways from writing a news release to announce a new program or service to writing a weekly column or blog in a local paper or Web site about exercise and physical activity. Both examples provide an opportunity to gain exposure, build brand community, and increase consumer confidence. Although public relations has traditionally been part of a print communication process, online media outlets often use expert bloggers to support different content areas. The ACSM-EP is qualified and capable of serving as a valuable resource for disseminating evidence-based information about fitness and exercise. Writing is therefore a prerequisite proficiency for preparing quality promotional materials. Seven suggestions for writing simple and effective news releases are provided (16):

1. Identify and address the target audience.
2. Keep it simple and short (never longer than a page).
3. The basics of who, what, when, where, why, and how belong in the first short paragraph.
4. Use short paragraphs and emphasize one major point in each paragraph.
5. Avoid acronyms and technical jargon.
6. With permission, quote authority.
7. Be careful and deliberate.

Careful and deliberate use of public relations can support other promotional efforts by providing positive exposure that may create opportunities for future ventures and collaborations.

The Case of the Continuum Performance Center

Submitted by **Chris Worrell, ACSM-EP, NSCA-CSCS; and Geoff Sullivan, ACSM-EP, NSCA-CPT, Continuum Performance Center, East Longmeadow, MA**

A team of certified professionals reinvented themselves to develop a unique brand identity and create a fitness business that defines success by individual client achievement.

Narrative

The Continuum Performance Center (CPC) was created by industry professionals who worked within the confines of an outdated commercial system and witnessed countless active individuals become turned off by the membership structure of "gyms." All of CPC's programming is centered around the active individual or those who truly desire to become recreationally involved in activity and movement on a deeper level.

CPC opened its doors with one employee-owner and has grown to support three full-time and one part-time nationally certified employees who are referred to as "coaches." Within one calendar year, CPC has grown its "subscriber" (title for members) base from 9 unique subscribers to over 160 subscribers who actively train at the facility at least one time every 14 days.

CPC's floor plan has a unique design. Although constant functional movements are promoted to all subscribers in all training areas at all times, CPC has separate training spaces, totaling 50 ft^2. The north end of CPC is dedicated for group programming in a more functional training environment with a large tie into TRX Suspension Training. The south end of CPC offers a more traditional strength environment, but CPC coaches still place a large emphasis on movement.

Branding: Don't Talk About It. Be About It.

CPC established itself as the alternative to traditional fitness facilities through its tag line: Don't talk about it. Be about it. By using challenge-oriented Facebook posts, dynamic uploaded video on Vimeo and YouTube, and an information stream from Constant Contact to relay tips, advice, and reminders, CPC has grown 200% within its first year of business. On a daily basis, CPC gets more than 50 hits on Facebook and Twitter and has an 88% open rate on their Constant Contact campaigns. CPC relies solely on social media and e-mail communication with its subscribers to deliver inspiration, motivation, and information. Subscribers have come primarily through word-of-mouth sales and Facebook "shares."

To keep subscribers involved, CPC rotates programming on a consistent basis to keep interest and motivation high. By having subscribers take ownership of the space and the offerings, it allows CPC to grow at a consistent and positive rate.

Collaboration

Through the CPC 1,500 (a muscular endurance challenge involving 1,500 repetitions of five exercises), TRX Suspension Training, and partnerships with other like-minded area small business such as Fit to Ride and Heartsong Yoga Center, members are able to connect to others and take on a physical and mental challenge in a safe, supervised, and challenging environment.

CPC is a neighborhood place for regular people trying to incorporate exercise that is fun, challenging, and variable into their busy lives. Subscribers are from every walk of life, but they have one thing in common — they *want* to be healthy and they've made a commitment to be well. CPC's commitment to the community doesn't stop with its subscribers or other businesses. Giving back to the community is essential to the organization's growth and the core of the mission. Partnering with organizations such as The Food Bank of Western Massachusetts, Toys for Tots, and the American Red Cross, CPC sets a standard of community involvement that resonates with CPC subscribers.

Using social media has enabled CPC to not only reach a broader base of subscribers but also gain critical feedback about what are the "likes" and "dislikes" of any given demographic. As CPC grows, we hope to continue to be about it and not just talk about it!

QUESTIONS

- How does CPC develop the tangible and intangible aspects of their product?
- How has CPC branded itself?
- How does CPC sell its brand?

SUMMARY

This chapter focused on the marketing mix and strategies the ACSM-EP can use when initiating and developing a marketing plan for health/fitness-related products, services, and programs. An overview of the five Ps of people, place, product, price, and promotion was provided. Examples of how the ACSM-EP could apply strategies to different promotional programs were also presented. Several aspects of the promotions function of marketing were discussed in the context of the experience of the ACSM-EP. In addition to personal selling, B2B promotions, sponsorship, and social media promotions, a brief overview of the benefits and uses of public relations as a marketing tool was provided. As a health/fitness professional, the ACSM-EP is uniquely qualified to act both as an advanced personal trainer and as a manager. As the fields relating to health/fitness expand, knowledge and skills relating to management, marketing, and business also expand. The ACSM-EP is well positioned to serve in a managerial role, seeking additional training when necessary and building on the competencies and skills inherent in the professional nature of the field.

STUDY QUESTIONS

1. How does advertising differ from public relations? What are the similarities and differences?
2. Explain the five Ps of marketing.
3. What role does the mission and vision of an organization have on the development and implementation of fitness services and products?

REFERENCES

1. Bates M. *Health Fitness Management: A Comprehensive Resource for Managing and Operating Programs and Facilities*. 2nd ed. Champaign (IL): Human Kinetics; 2008. 381 p.
2. Kaczynski A, Henderson K. Environmental correlates of physical activity: a review of evidence about parks and recreation. *Leisure Sci*. 2007;29(4):315–54.
3. Centers for Disease Control and Prevention. Data and statistics [Internet]. Atlanta [GA]: Centers for Disease Control and Prevention; [cited 2020 Jan 15]. Available from: https://www.cdc.gov/physicalactivity/data/index.html.
4. Roux A, Moore L, Evenson KR, et al. Availability of recreational resources and physical activity in adults. *Am J Public Health*. 2007;97(3):493–9.
5. Thompson W. Worldwide survey of fitness trends for 2019. *ACSMs Health Fit J*. 2018;22(6):10–7.
6. Mullen S, Whaley D. Age, gender and fitness club membership: factors related to initial involvement

and sustained participation. *Int J Sport Exerc Psychol.* 2010;8(1):24–35.

7. Ferrand A, Robinson L, Valette-Florence P. The intention-to-repurchase paradox: a case of the health and fitness industry. *J Sport Manag.* 2010;24(1):83–105.

8. Papadimitriou D, Karteroliotis K. The service quality expectations in private sport and fitness centers: a reexamination of the factor structure. *Sport Mark Q.* 2000;9(3):157–64.

9. Wang B, Wu C, Quan W. Changes in consumers behavior at fitness clubs among Chinese urban residents — Dalian as an example. *Asian Soc Sci.* 2008;4(10):106–10.

10. Wang H, Lin H. An investigation into exercisers at fitness clubs in Dalian. *J Phys Educ Issue.* 2000;14(4):22–4.

11. Filo K, Funk D, Alexandris K. Exploring the role of brand trust in the relationship between brand associations and brand loyalty in sport and fitness. *Int J Sport Manag Mark.* 2008;3(1/2):39–57.

12. Devasagayam P, Buff C. A multidimensional conceptualization of brand community: an empirical investigation. *Sport Mark Q.* 2008;17(1):20–9.

13. Frimming RE, Polsgrove MJ, Bower GG. Evaluation of a health and fitness social media experience. *Am J Health Educ.* 2011;42(4):2–7.

14. Tharrett SJ, Peterson JA. *Fitness Management.* 2nd ed. Monterey (CA): Healthy Learning; 2008. 579 p.

15. Reed J. Examining the impact of an email campaign to promote physical activity and walking in adult women six-weeks and one-year post-intervention. *ICHPER-SD J Res.* 2009;4(1):64–9.

16. Perry DJ. Writing for the media. *Tech Commun.* 1992;39(4):638–42.

17. Marshall A, Owen N, Bauman A. Mediated approaches for influencing physical activity: update of the evidence on mass media, print, telephone and website delivery of interventions. *J Sci Med Sport.* 2004;7(1 Suppl):74–80.

18. Parrott M, Tennant L, Olejnik S, Poudevigne M. Theory of planned behavior: implications for an email-based physical activity intervention. *Psychol Sport Exerc.* 2008;9(4):511–26.

19. Alsac B. Maximizing your social media investments. *IDEA Fitness J.* 2010(July–August):42–7.

20. Gold J, Lim M, Hocking J, Keogh L, Spelman T, Hellard M. Determining the impact of text messaging for sexual health promotion to young people. *Sex Transm Dis.* 2011;38(4):247–52.

21. Suminski R, Poston W, Hyder M. Small business policies toward employee and community promotion of physical activity. *J Phys Act Health.* 2006;3(4):405–14.

22. Copeland R, Frisby W, McCarville R. Understanding the sport sponsorship process from a corporate perspective. *J Sport Manag.* 1996;10(1):32–48.

23. Zinger J, O'Reilly N. An examination of sports sponsorship from a small business perspective. *Int J Sport Mark Sponsorship.* 2010;11(4):283–301.

24. Wen-Yu C, Yuan-Duen L, Tsai-Yuan L. Performance evaluation criteria for personal trainers: an analytical hierarchy process approach. *Soc Behav Pers Int J.* 2010;38(7):895–905.

25. Huddleston S, Mertesdorf J, Araki K. Physical activity behavior and attitudes toward involvement among physical education, health and leisure services pre-professionals. *Coll Stud J.* 2002;36(4):555–73.

26. Mayer D, Greenberg H. What makes a good salesman? *Harv Bus Rev.* 2006;84(7/8):164–71.

27. Adidam P. Mavenness: a non-explored trait of quality salespeople. *Paradigm.* 2009;13(1):6–7.

28. Dunyon J, Gossling V, Willden S, Seiter JS. Compliments and purchasing behavior in telephone sales interactions. *Psychol Rep.* 2010;106(1):27–30.

29. Hoyle LH. *Event Marketing: How to Successfully Promote Events, Festivals, Conventions and Expositions.* New York (NY): Wiley; 2002. 4 p.

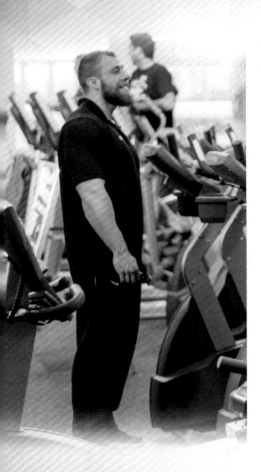

18 Professional Behaviors and Ethics

OBJECTIVES

- To briefly trace the historical development and identify the breadth of certified American College of Sports Medicine (ACSM) professionals.
- To identify the settings and skills defined in the scope of practice of the exercise physiologist (EP).
- To distinguish boundaries of professional practice between the EP and other allied health professionals.
- To encourage the use of referral tools for clients outside the scope of practice.
- To demonstrate behaviors that meet professional standards.

INTRODUCTION

Ethics, as a branch of philosophy, can be viewed as an abstract concept focusing on morals and values that inform decisions and behaviors. Ethics is also defined in terms of systematic rules or principles governing right conduct (1). Each practitioner, upon entering a profession, is invested with the responsibility to adhere to the standards of ethical practice and conduct set by the profession. Professional ethics, as presented in this chapter, is immensely practical. An initial examination of the historical context with which American College of Sports Medicine (ACSM) first offered certifications provides an opportunity to consider the development of the profession and the demand for standards of practice. As certified professionals, understanding the expectations articulated in our Code of Ethics is critical. This chapter applies the Code of Ethics to specific challenges facing the certified exercise physiologist (EP), operationalizing the concept of scope of practice through several research-based examples. In addition, a useful tool to assist the EP in ethical decision making relating to scope of practice is provided. Professional ethics includes identifying conflicts of interest as well as disseminating evidence-based information. Professional ethics also includes personal practices relating to responsibility and accountability, staying current and maintaining a certification, as well as demonstrating personal behaviors that exemplify the professional nature of the EP. The need for qualified, competent, and engaged fitness professionals is well documented (2,3). Professional ethics is the foundation for continuing the tradition of excellence initiated and sustained by the founders and fellows of ACSM.

Therefore, this chapter provides a basic overview of professional ethics as applied to the practice of the EP. A brief overview of the role ACSM has played in the development of fitness-related certifications is presented, along with a close examination of the ACSM's Code of Ethics, with particular focus on the scope of practice for the EP. Additional areas related to conflict of interest, developing evidence-based practices, maintaining certification, and defining professional behaviors are examined.

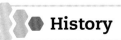 History

Eleven physicians, physiologists, and physical educators founded ACSM in 1954 to provide a professional society for individuals sharing a common interest in health and fitness. As part of ACSM's efforts to gain new interest, growth, and visibility, the College hosted an "Invitational Conference on Implementation of ACSM's Exercise Testing and Exercise Prescription Guidelines" in Aspen, Colorado, in December 1974. Here, a small group of ACSM members finalized plans for a proposed certification process for Exercise Program Directors and Exercise Leaders. In May 1975, *ACSM's Guidelines for Graded Exercise Testing and Exercise Prescription* were first published. The following month at Pennsylvania State University, ACSM held its first Exercise Program Director's Certification Conference, with 35 professionals earning the first-ever ACSM certification. Later, in September of 1975, 20 individuals were certified by ACSM as exercise specialists. The Exercise Test Technician certification began the following year, 1976, with 92 individuals earning certification. ACSM Certified Exercise Physiologist® (ACSM-EP®) certification (originally the Health Fitness Instructor) started in 1982, followed by the Health Fitness Director and Exercise Leader certifications in 1986 (4). In the 20 years since, ACSM certifications have evolved, and as part of this evolution, some certifications are no longer offered, some are new, and some have been dramatically redefined. All of these changes, however, are a tribute to ACSM's commitment to reflect the current state of the fitness and wellness industry. Figure 18.1 provides a basic timeline in relation to the development of ACSM certifications, particularly the EP.

Accreditation

In 2004, ACSM collaborated with six other leading fitness organizations to establish the Committee on the Accreditation for the Exercise Sciences, or CoAES (5). CoAES is responsible for establishing

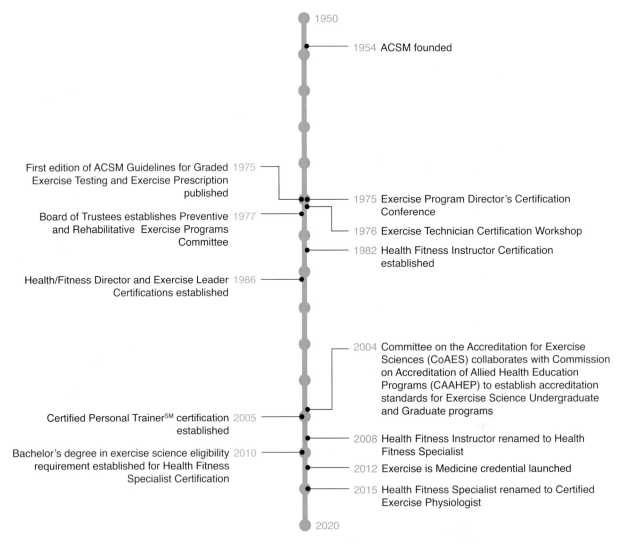

1950

1954 ACSM founded

First edition of ACSM Guidelines for Graded 1975
Exercise Testing and Exercise Prescription
published

1975 Exercise Program Director's Certification
Conference

Board of Trustees establishes Preventive 1977
and Rehabilitative Exercise Programs
Committee

1976 Exercise Technician Certification Workshop

1982 Health Fitness Instructor Certification
established

Health/Fitness Director and Exercise Leader 1986
Certifications established

2004 Committee on the Accreditation for Exercise
Sciences (CoAES) collaborates with Commission
on Accreditation of Allied Health Education
Programs (CAAHEP) to establish accreditation
standards for Exercise Science Undergraduate
and Graduate programs

Certified Personal Trainer^SM certification 2005
established

2008 Health Fitness Instructor renamed to Health
Fitness Specialist

Bachelor's degree in exercise science eligibility 2010
requirement established for Health Fitness
Specialist Certification

2012 Exercise is Medicine credential launched

2015 Health Fitness Specialist renamed to Certified
Exercise Physiologist

2020

FIGURE 18.1. ACSM historical timeline for certifications and accreditation. (Adapted with permission from Berryman JW. *Out of Many, One: A History of the American College of Sports Medicine.* Champaign [IL]: Human Kinetics; 1995. 283 p.)

standards and guidelines for academic programs that prepare students seeking employment in the health, fitness, and exercise industry. In addition, CoAES establishes and implements a process of self-study, review, and recommendation for all exercise science–related academic programs seeking accreditation through the Commission on Accreditation of Allied Health Education Programs (CAAHEP). Today, there are four postsecondary program accreditations through CAAHEP: Associate or Certificate in Personal Fitness Training, Bachelor of Science in Exercise Science, Master of Science in Applied Physiology, and Master of Science in Clinical Exercise Physiology. Accreditation, like certification, is a critical component for ensuring a consistent and standardized set of knowledge and skills, which is essential for industry professionals and is conveyed to students through their academic experience.

The need for certified professionals who are competent and proficient in a subject area and who are evaluated through the successful completion of a psychometrically sound, objective examination has grown exponentially. ACSM currently offers four primary certifications and four specialty credentials (6), with more than 35,000 ACSM-certified professionals practicing worldwide. The clinical certification (Table 18.1) is the ACSM Certified Clinical Exercise Physiologist® (ACSM-CEP®). Also listed in Table 18.1 are the fitness certifications, which include the ACSM-EP, the ACSM Certified

Table 18.1	Current Levels of ACSM Certifications
ACSM-CEP	Health care professional with a Master's degree[a] in clinical exercise physiology who uses scientific rationale to design, implement, and supervise exercise programming for those with chronic diseases, conditions, and/or physical shortcomings. Services provided by an ACSM-CEP include, but are not limited to, individuals with cardiovascular, pulmonary, metabolic, orthopedic, musculoskeletal, neuromuscular, neoplastic, immunological, and hematological disease.
ACSM-EP	Health/fitness professional with a Bachelor's degree in exercise science who performs preparticipation health screenings, conducts physical fitness assessments, interprets results, develops exercise prescriptions, and applies behavioral and motivational strategies to apparently healthy individuals and individuals with medically controlled diseases and health conditions
ACSM-CPT	Fitness professional with a high school diploma who plans and implements exercise programs for healthy individuals or those who have medical clearance to exercise. The ACSM-CPT facilitates motivation and adherence as well as develops and administers programs designed to enhance muscular strength, endurance, flexibility, cardiorespiratory fitness, body composition, and/or any of the motor skills related components of physical fitness.
ACSM-GEI	Fitness professional with a high school diploma who works in a group exercise setting with apparently healthy individuals and those with health challenges, who have been cleared by their physicians for independent exercise to enhance quality of life, improve physical fitness, manage health risk, and promote lasting health behavior change

[a]A Bachelor's degree in exercise science with 1,200 h of clinical experience is also acceptable.

Personal Trainer® (ACSM-CPT®), and the ACSM Certified Group Exercise Instructor® (ACSM-GEI®). In addition, four specialty credentials focus on serving individuals with unique needs: ACSM/American Cancer Society Certified Cancer Exercise Trainer (ACSM/ACS-CET), ACSM/National Center on Health, Physical Activity and Disability Certified Inclusive Fitness Trainer (ACSM/NCHPAD-CIFT), ACSM/Exercise Connection (EC) Autism Exercise Specialist, and ACSM/National Physical Activity Society Physical Activity in Public Health Specialist (ACSM/NPAS-PAPHS).

What was for many years known as the Health Fitness Instructor certification was renamed the Health Fitness Specialist, or HFS, in 2008. The eligibility requirements of the HFS were changed in 2010 to limit the certification to those holding a Bachelor of Science degree in Kinesiology, Exercise Physiology, or Exercise Science. In 2015, the name was changed again to Certified Exercise Physiologist or ACSM-EP. The change in the education prerequisite evolved to better support the job tasks associated with this profession. The change in the name of the certification resulted from a commitment on the part of ACSM to adopt a uniform professional title, that of Exercise Physiologist, for degreed exercise professionals in both fitness and clinical tracks. The title aligns with positive perceptions and name recognition by both internal and external constituencies (7). Attainment of the ACSM-EP certification implies specialized training and competencies for degreed individuals to pursue careers in university, corporate, commercial, hospital, and community settings, serving healthy individuals and individuals with controlled conditions released for independent physical activity. The Exercise is Medicine® (EIM®) credential provides further support for the unique characteristics of the ACSM-EP.

The EIM credential was developed and launched in 2012 to support the EIM initiative and provide health care providers with an identifiable exercise professional qualified to work with different clients (8). A description of the three-tiered EIM credential is presented in "Exercise is Medicine Connection" box.

EXERCISE IS MEDICINE CONNECTION

Exe**R**cise is Medicine®

The EIM credential contains three levels based on the health status of the patient referrals (8). All three levels require exercise professionals to be certified by an NCCA- or American National Standards Institute (ANSI)-International Organization for Standardization (ISO)–accredited certification. ANSI is the American representative to the ISO (9), a worldwide federation of accrediting organizations, each of which performs a similar function to NCCA. Those with formal education in exercise science (Bachelor of Science or Master of Science degree) are able to qualify for the higher levels of certification.

Level 1: Individuals at Low or Moderate Risk Who Have Been Cleared for Independent Exercise

NCCA- or ANSI-ISO–accredited fitness professional certification

Successful completion of the EIM credential course and EIM credential examination

EIM course and examination exempt for those with an NCCA- or ANSI-ISO–accredited fitness certification and a Bachelor's degree in exercise science/exercise physiology/kinesiology

Level 2: Individuals at Low, Moderate, or High Risk Who Have Been Cleared for Independent Exercise

Bachelor's degree in exercise science/exercise physiology/kinesiology

NCCA- or ANSI-ISO–accredited fitness professional certification

Successful completion of the EIM credential training course and EIM credential examination

EIM course and examination exempt for those with certifications with an emphasis on special populations (ACSM-EP, ACSM-CEP, American Council on Exercise [ACE] Medical Exercise Specialist)

Level 3: Individuals at Low, Moderate, or High Risk, Including Those Requiring Clinical Monitoring

Approved Master of Science/Master of Arts Exercise Science/Exercise Physiology/Kinesiology *or* approved Bachelor of Science/Bachelor of Arts in Exercise Science/Exercise Physiology/Kinesiology plus 4,000 hours of experience in a clinical exercise setting

NCCA-accredited clinical exercise certification (ACSM-CEP)

No EIM credential course or EIM credential examination necessary, just a completed application/exemption form

Organizations with NCCA-Accredited Health/Fitness and/or Clinical Exercise Certifications

- ACTION certification (ACTION)
- ACSM
- ACE
- Athletics and Fitness Association of America (AFAA)
- Collegiate Strength and Conditioning Coaches Association (CSCCa)
- International Fitness Professionals Association (IFPA)
- National Academy of Sports Medicine (NASM)
- National Council for Certified Personal Trainers (NCCPT)
- National Council on Strength and Fitness (NCSF)
- National Exercise and Sports Trainers Association (NESTA)
- National Exercise Trainers Association (NETA)
- National Federation of Professional Trainers (NFPT)
- National Strength and Conditioning Association (NSCA)
- Personal Training Academy Global (PTAG)
- Pilates Method Alliance
- World Instructor Training Schools

Committee on the Certification and Registry Board

The Committee on Certification and Registry Boards (CCRB), a volunteer committee composed of ACSM members, oversees the process of regularly reviewing and revising the job definition, eligibility requirements, and scope of practice for each certification. In addition, each certification undergoes a rigorous external review through the National Commission for Certifying Agencies (NCCA). The NCCA is a nonprofit, external certifying agency whose mission is to safeguard public safety and well-being through the assessment and evaluation of professional competencies and standards. The NCCA provides accreditation to a broad range of professions, including nursing, respiratory therapy, and counseling (10). The guiding principle of advancing health through science, education, and medicine that inspired the early community of ACSM members is kept alive today by the oversight provided internally by members of the CCRB and externally through ACSM's commitment to adhere to the standards set by the NCCA.

ACSM Code of Ethics

The ACSM Code of Ethics states, "The principal purpose of the College is the generation and dissemination of knowledge concerning all aspects of persons engaged in exercise with full respect for the dignity of people" (11). The Code of Ethics is further defined by four standards:

Section 1: Members should strive continuously to improve knowledge and skill and should make available to their colleagues and the public the benefits of their professional expertise.
Section 2: Members should maintain high professional and scientific standards and should not voluntarily collaborate professionally with anyone who violates this principle.
Section 3: The College, and its members, should safeguard the public and itself against members who are deficient in ethical conduct.
Section 4: The ideals of the College imply that the responsibilities of each fellow or member extend not only to the individual but also to society with the purpose of improving both the health and the well-being of the individual and the community (11).

Although each standard implies many personal and public practices that define the professional nature of an EP, the following five areas are of great importance:

1. Practicing within one's scope of practice
2. Acknowledging conflicts of interest
3. Providing evidence-based information
4. Maintaining certification
5. Personal characteristics of professional behavior

Scope of Practice

Scope of practice is the range of responsibility that determines the boundaries within which a profession operates (12). Each phrase in a scope of practice is critical in defining what tasks a professional can do, with whom the professional can work, what settings are appropriate, and what type of oversight is necessary. This book is devoted to the knowledge and skills that are needed to practice as an EP. As such, the text operationalizes the EP scope of practice. In other words, if a given practitioner in the field adheres to the job tasks and skills described in this text, then he or she is operating within the boundaries of the defined field of the EP, a requirement for practicing ethically sound behavior. The fundamentals of the scope of practice of the EP are outlined in the following job definition developed by the CCRB.

The ACSM-EP works with apparently healthy clients and those with medically controlled diseases to establish safe and effective exercise and health lifestyle behaviors to optimize both health and quality of life. The ACSM-EP conducts preparticipation health screenings; submaximal graded exercise tests; and assessments of strength, flexibility, and body composition. The ACSM-EP subsequently develops and administers programs designed to enhance cardiorespiratory fitness, muscular strength and endurance, balance, and range of motion. The ACSM-EP has a minimum of a Bachelor's degree in exercise science and is usually self-employed or employed in commercial, community, studio, worksite health promotion, university, and hospital-based fitness settings (13).

The scope of practice is a living document that is regularly reviewed by ACSM's EP subcommittee. Each of the ACSM certifications has a subcommittee that operates as part of the CCRB. The components of the scope of practice are verified in a systematic manner through a job task analysis (JTA) of practicing EPs (13). The JTA is a survey sent to EP practitioners to gather information about what tasks they are doing in their daily work. On the basis of the survey data, EP subcommittee members review the scope of practice, the knowledge and skill statements (KSs), and the content of publications related to EP work (such as this book) to make sure all are in line with the evolution of the profession.

Defining the scope of what an EP does (*e.g.*, risk classification, fitness assessment, exercise prescription, and lifestyle behavior change), the job definition and JTA also serve as a guide as to what may lie *outside* the boundary of the EP's scope. Figure 18.2 and Table 18.2 show that although there may be overlap between scopes of practice of various professionals working with similar clientele as the EP, there are distinct areas within which each profession functions. The challenge can be figuring out where the EP practice ends and the practice of another professional begins. The purpose of this section is to provide some examples and guidelines so that EP practitioners can make sound decisions to operate within their defined scope of practice. First, a decision tree is introduced. Practitioners can use the decision tree to check that the tasks they are performing are firmly within the EP scope of practice. Then, three scenarios are presented to delineate the boundaries between some of the professions depicted in Figure 18.2 and Table 18.2.

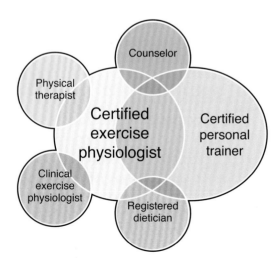

FIGURE 18.2. A visual representation of the overlapping scopes of varying health care, allied health, and health/fitness professionals.

Table 18.2	Areas of Overlapping Scope of Practice between the Certified Exercise Physiologist and Other Professions
Overlap: Certified Exercise Physiologist and	
Personal trainer	Health screening, exercise assessment, and exercise prescription for apparently healthy individuals and for those with health challenges who are capable of independent exercise
Dietitian	Promotion of healthy eating, hydration, and energy consumption to optimize; physical performance, recovery from and adaptation to exercise training and competition, and weight management
Clinical and/or counseling psychologist, health coach	Promotion of healthy living through behavior change, motivational interviewing, and cognitive restructuring strategies
Clinical exercise physiologist	Adjusting and adapting exercise training for special populations, including those living with chronic diseases and conditions
Physical therapist and/or athletic trainer	Adjusting and adapting exercise training for special populations, including those living with chronic musculoskeletal and neuromuscular conditions, or athletes or clients with acute injury

Consider the following scenarios to better understand the complex and delicate issues that arise when faced with scope of practice decisions.

Scenario 1

A client asks about recommending a piece of aerobic exercise equipment for his home. The client is a healthy 40-year-old man with hypertension controlled by diet and exercise.

If a practitioner is unsure whether the request in scenario 1 is permitted in his or her scope of practice, then the first place to look might be the most recent EP JTA. In the 2017 JTA, under Domain II Exercise Prescription and Implementation, Job Task B states, "Implement cardiorespiratory exercise prescriptions for apparently healthy clients based on current health status, fitness goals, and availability of time" (14).

Figure 18.3 shows a decision tree designed to help the EP assess whether they are practicing within the boundaries of the EP scope of practice (15). Because the client has asked for recommendations on a *type* of exercise equipment, this task is clearly permitted. If the client asked about a specific type of equipment that the practitioner was unfamiliar with, then the EP must progress further down the decision tree. The EP knows the task is permitted but should ask question 4 on the decision tree: "Do I personally have the education needed?" If the practitioner is not knowledgeable about that piece of equipment, then they need to gather enough information to advise the client *or* refer the client to someone else with specific knowledge about that particular piece of equipment.

Nutritional counseling is an area with potential overlap for the EP, as clients requesting dietary advice is not unusual (16). The EP does have training in basic nutrition, so it seems reasonable that an EP should be able to work with clients' diets to some extent. In fact, there are 30 KSs in the most recent JTA related to nutrition and weight management. Most of them are KSs under the Job Task IIE, "Implement a general weight management program as indicated by personal goals, as needed" (13). The EP should have knowledge of basic nutritional principles related to weight management, should be able to make referrals to scientifically based resources, and should be familiar

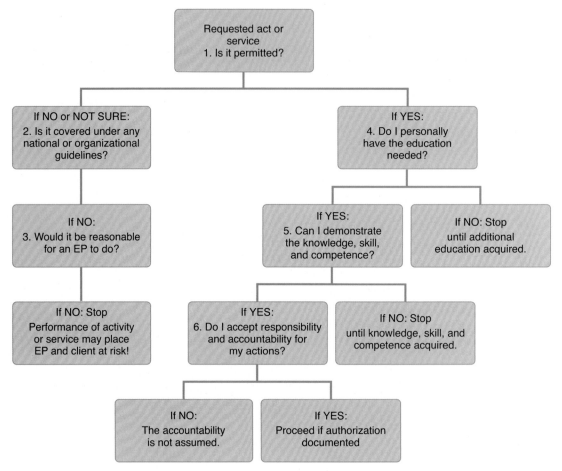

FIGURE 18.3. Scope of practice decision tree. (Adapted with permission from O'Sullivan-Maillet J, Skates J, Pritchett E. American Dietetic Association: scope of dietetics practice framework. *J Am Diet Assoc.* 2005;105[4]:634–40.)

with ergogenic aids and supplements and their risks and benefits. However, there is no KS indicating that an EP should be involved in individual nutritional counseling or therapeutic nutritional advice (17). Table 18.3 provides clear guidance on what nutritional information is acceptable for an EP to share with clients.

Scenario 2

The lawsuit *Capati v. Crunch Fitness* provides an instructive example of crossing this line. In 1997, a personal trainer at Crunch Fitness in New York City recommended dietary supplements to Anne Marie Capati. Capati had high blood pressure, and one of the supplements contained Ephedra, contraindicated for those with hypertension. Capati suffered a massive stroke that took her life, hours after a workout at the gym (18). This is an extreme example of what can occur when stepping outside the boundary of scope of practice. Even if the consequences are not life-threatening, exceeding one's scope of practice reflects poorly on one's professional practice and calls to question his or her ethics.

If the personal trainer working with Anne Marie Capati had applied the decision tree to his actions, would this tragedy have been avoided? That is difficult to know; however, following the decision tree provides timely and prudent guidance whenever the task at hand is in question. Question 1 asks, is it permitted, in this example, to recommend a particular supplement for a client

Table 18.3	The Practice of Dietetics versus General Nonmedical Nutritional Information
Activity	**Definitions**
Practice of dietetics; limited to licensees[a]	▪ Nutritional assessment to determine nutritional needs and to recommend appropriate nutritional intake, including enteral and parenteral nutrition ▪ Nutritional counseling or education as components of preventive, curative, and restorative health care ▪ Development, administration, evaluation, and consultation regarding nutritional care standards
General nonmedical nutrition information not restricted[b]	Providing information on the following: ▪ Principles of good nutrition and food preparation ▪ Food to be included in the normal daily diet ▪ The essential nutrients needed by the body ▪ Recommended amounts of the essential nutrients ▪ The actions of nutrients on the body ▪ The effects of deficiencies or excesses of nutrients or food and supplements that are good sources of essential nutrients

[a]Dietetics. Ohio Rev, Code Ann x 4759-2-01(A), 2006.

[b]Dietetics. Ohio Rev, Code Ann x 4759-2-01(M), 2006.

Adapted with permission from Sass C, Eickhoff-Shemek JM, Manore MM, Kruskall LJ. Crossing the line: understanding the scope of practice between registered dieticians and health fitness professionals. *ACSMs Health Fit J.* 2007;11(3):12–9.

who is trying to lose weight? An EP would refer to the most current EP JTA, whereas the personal trainer working with Capati would refer to the current CPT JTA. In either case, the practitioner would have to answer no to question 2; the service of recommending specific supplements is not covered under the guidelines for CPTs or EPs. If the practitioner was still unsure, then he or she could consult the Code of Ethics for ACSM-certified professionals and the licensure laws related to the practice of dietetics in his state (17). If the answer was still no, then question 3 asks whether it would be reasonable for the practitioner to perform this service. In this case, he or she might look to position stands, place a call or e-mail to the appropriate certification subcommittee chair, and ask whether the service is routinely performed by other practitioners. In the Capati case, the personal trainer would have found no supporting documentation or practice to support a recommendation of a nutritional supplement to a client.

Looking at this case from a different angle, how might this personal trainer have better handled the query about weight loss supplements? He could have shared evidence-based information about the supplement, including papers that had been published. He could have referred Capati to a registered dietitian, especially because one of the job tasks for the EP is to maintain relationships with other health professionals and to have skill in referral to those professionals.

Scenario 3

Another area that has the potential to be unclear is the differences in scopes of practice between the EP and the CEP.

A 58-year-old woman who is newly diagnosed with heart disease signs up to work with an EP at a local fitness facility. She had two stents inserted 6 weeks ago, and her doctor told her to exercise.

She has Type 2 diabetes and is taking an oral hypoglycemic drug. The client is obese (body mass index [BMI] = 35 kg · m^{-2}) with stage 1 Parkinson disease (PD) and is also taking medication for PD. The EP working with her is conscientious, so they have already asked the client to get a referral from a medical doctor (MD), which she has supplied. The referral states, "OK to exercise." The EP is unsure as to whether the client should be supervised during exercise and whether she should be scrutinized more closely by a clinical exercise professional. This puts the EP at question 2 in the decision tree: Is this situation covered under any national or organizational guidelines? The EP's scope of practice defines the population that EPs can work with as "apparently healthy and with controlled conditions released for independent exercise." This client is not apparently healthy as she has a metabolic disease, a cardiovascular disease, and a neuromuscular disease. Are all her diseases in a controlled condition? If the EP was unsure, then he or she must conservatively answer no to question 2 and ask question 3: Should an EP work with a patient who has postsurgical heart disease and two comorbidities? Even with the MD referral, the wiser option would probably be for this client to begin in a cardiac rehab program or other clinically supervised program and then eventually graduate to the services of the EP. In a best practice scenario, the EP would contact the referring MD and suggest this alternative.

In most day-to-day situations, the tasks of the EP will fall squarely within the defined framework for an EP. However, as Table 18.2 indicates, there are many areas of overlap, so the potential for stepping out of scope of practice is real. Recently, EPs have embraced functional movement screening and corrective exercise prescription. In fact, functional training was rated ninth of the top 10 fitness trends for 2019 (19). Is there potential for this trend to overlap with physical therapy, athletic training, or manual therapy? Table 18.4 outlines some guidelines differentiating preventive versus rehabilitative practices. As the professional practices of the EP evolve, practicing EPs need to be conscientious about using all available professional resources to guide them in scope of practice issues.

Table 18.4	The Practice of Preventive versus Rehabilitative Exercise Prescription
Activity	**Definitions**
Practice of preventive exercise prescription	■ Assessment leads to identification of balance, stability, range of motion, endurance, and/or strength deficits. ■ Exercises prescribed improve balance, stability, strength, alignment, and range of motion and reinforce optimal neuromuscular patterning within a pain-free range. ■ Modalities like foam rolling are applied by the client on himself or herself. ■ Referrals are made when the client experiences pain and/or motion is limited by injury.
Rehabilitative exercise prescription	■ Assessment leads to diagnosis, prognosis related to pain, injury, or movement malfunction. ■ Exercises prescribed and modalities used alleviate pain, correct a movement malfunction, and resolve an injury. ■ Modalities are applied by a trained physical therapist or other licensed practitioner.

American Physical Therapy Association. Physical therapist's scope of practice. [Internet]. Alexandria (VA): American Physical Therapy Association; [cited 2019 Aug 6]. Available from: https://www.apta.org/apta-and-you/leadership-and-governance/policies/position -scope-of-practice; Mikeska D. A SWOT analysis of the scope of practice of personal trainers [Internet]. *Personal Train Q.* 2014 [cited 2019 Aug 6];2(1). Available from: https://www.nsca.com/education/articles/ptq/a-swot-analysis-of-the-scope-of-practice -for-personal-trainers/; and U.S. Department of Labor. *OSHA Letter of Interpretation: Preventive vs Therapeutic Exercise* [Internet]. Omaha (NE): U.S. Department of Labor; 2016 [cited 2019 Aug 6]. Available from: https://www.osha.gov/laws-regs/standard interpretations/2016-09-09-0.

Conflict of Interest

The hallmarks of professional ethics include the acknowledgment and awareness of potential conflicts of interest coupled with acting within one's scope of practice. The ACSM Ethics and Professional Conduct Committee has defined conflict of interest as "a significant financial interest in a business or other direct or indirect personal gain or consideration provided by a business that may compromise, or have the appearance of compromising, an ACSM member's professional judgment" (20). Conflict of interest has also been defined in terms of a situation in which financial or other personal considerations have the potential to compromise or bias professional judgment and objectivity (21). An example may be an EP who purchases equipment or services from a friend who in return provides a kickback or "refund." The EP has not provided fair access for other equipment vendors to bid or offer quotes. In the same way, conflict of interest is apparent in the fitness specialist who will only sell a particular type of nutritional product or clothing without acknowledging the commission base of the sale.

Collaborative models of rehabilitation treatment and fitness training have become more common modes of delivering services to clients. If a company has two divisions in which one provides a referral to the other division for services, this is generally not considered a conflict of interest unless personal gains (commissions) are provided to individual service providers without full disclosure to the customers they serve. In general, the concept of conflict of interest underscores the need to maintain social trust by clearly acknowledging any relationship that may provide personal gain to the professionals involved (22). Disclosure of significant relationships builds client trust and ensures that the professional standards developed to maintain the integrity of the profession are upheld. How information is obtained, discerned, and disseminated is another important aspect of professional ethics.

Providing Evidence-Based Information

The National Academy of Sciences identified evidence-based practice as a critical competency of all heath care practitioners (23,24). Evidence-based practice is defined as the integration of current and valid research with clinical judgment and patient preference to make decisions about care of a patient (25,26). Providing evidence-based information is a critical characteristic for the EP to cultivate and develop. Evidence-based information empowers both the client and the EP to ask important questions and seek fundamental answers. As a health/fitness professional working with individuals and groups with medically controlled disease, the EP should be fully immersed in evidence-based practices. There are multiple sources of information regarding the explanation and applications of evidence-based practice among allied health and health care providers. Two models of incorporating evidence-based practices are presented.

Amonette et al. (27) present a practical and systematic approach to incorporating evidence-based investigations into the regular practice of the EP. The four-step process can be used to disseminate scientifically sound information to clients without reliance on anecdotal myths and falsehoods that are so prevalent in fitness and nutrition.

Step 1: Develop a Question

The EP or the client can inspire questions. Client-driven questions provide important information to the EP about the level of understanding the client has about his or her physical, emotional, and psychological well-being. Client questions also require the EP to engage in active listening.

Step 2: Search for Evidence

Evidence can be found in three ways: personal experience, academic preparation, and research knowledge.

Personal Experience

Although personal experience can provide powerful evidence, this type of information is often anecdotal. An EP may have experience with one client that may not be applicable to another client.

Academic Preparation

Supporting personal and professional experience with academic preparation and research knowledge is helpful in the search for evidence. Every EP is required to hold a Bachelor's degree in exercise science or kinesiology. The discipline and knowledge gained through the process of obtaining that degree provide the EP with the tools to seek evidence from appropriate academic sources. However, academic preparation may not always provide the most recent information.

Research Knowledge

Research knowledge is the form of evidence that holds the least amount of bias. With the accessibility of the Internet, peer-reviewed journals can provide ample sources of evidence-based practices that can address a client question. When searching for information, the professional needs to be able to distinguish between quantitative and qualitative research in addition to other types of research studies, for example, a clinical case study or a meta-analysis. In addition, research disseminated at regional and national conferences is cutting edge and relevant.

Step 3: Evaluate the Evidence

The magnitude of information available can make the process of discerning appropriate information from inappropriate information difficult. The EP needs to be able to discriminate the evidence gathered and make thoughtful decisions about the best way to disseminate information to the client.

Step 4: Incorporate Evidence into Practice

The EP can build on his or her knowledge of the scientific foundations of exercise to use the evidence that best answers the original question. Tailoring the information to the client's needs has also been found to be an effective strategy for long-term behavior change (28). A graphic representation of how the four-step process is applied to an exercise prescription is presented in Figure 18.4.

A real-life example of the application of the four-step process of evidence-based learning may be found in the "How to Incorporate Evidence-Based Practice" box. Scott et al. (29) also provide an example of an effective application of evidence-based clinical decision making (EBCD) that has been used with physical and occupational therapy students and practitioners. Knowing and understanding the process is not enough. Practicing the skill of integrating EBCD in the context of real clients is necessary. The process, which was divided into three phases, is another application of the method outlined earlier by Amonette et al. (27) with a similar development and progression.

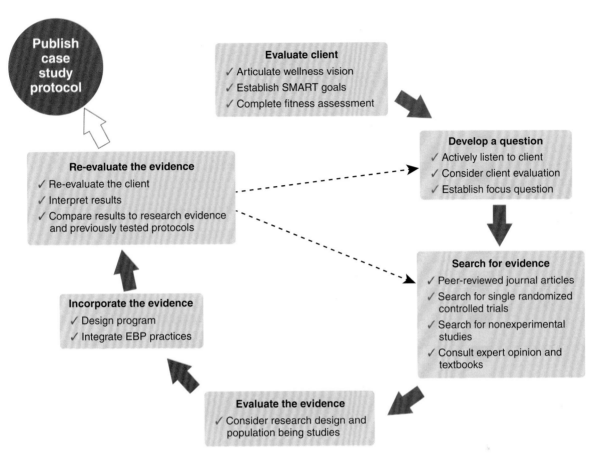

FIGURE 18.4. An example of the application of the evidence-based practice (EBP) model applied to an individualized exercise prescription. Dashed lines represent alternative or additional steps that may arise. (Used with permission from Amonette W, English K, Ottenbacher K. *Nullius in verba:* a call for the incorporation of evidence-based practice into the discipline of exercise science. *Sports Med.* 2010;40[6]:449–57.)

In phase 1, students were introduced to the different types of evidence available and given instruction on how to search for evidence and redesign questions using the PICO format (30): P = population; I = intervention; C = comparison; O = outcome. The therapists generated questions that pertained to real-life problems or practices in their clinics. The student teams selected one question to explore further and seek evidence-based solutions. In phase 2, the students collected evidence and then met with the therapists at the clinic to evaluate the evidence in the context of the question. In phase 3, the students learned about communicating the evidence to the different stakeholders as well as again meeting with the therapists to discuss their findings and get feedback on communication strategies (29).

Although the Scott et al.'s (29) article cited a collaborative arrangement from physical and occupational therapy settings, the application to the EP could be made as well. The EP who is working as part of a team of trainers can develop and pose questions to one other on the basis of the issues raised by current or past clients. Many fitness facilities also serve as internship sites for students seeking additional practical experience. The EBCD process can be incorporated into the internship experience through case studies, mentoring, and small group discussions.

Providing evidence-based information enables the EP to continually stay abreast of relevant and important information that impacts the health and well-being of clients. Maintaining the EP certification is another mechanism to stay current and involved with the growing fields of fitness and exercise.

HOW TO   Incorporate Evidence-Based Practice

You have a new client, a young woman who is apparently healthy and whose primary form of exercise is hot yoga four times a week. She tells you that she heard an interview on the evening news debating whether yoga is an adequate means of gaining aerobic health. She is perplexed because her yoga instructor has assured her that her yoga classes are all she needs for complete fitness (aerobic conditioning, flexibility, and whole body strengthening). Using evidence-based practice, you would follow the following steps.

Formulate a Question

Is yoga an effective means of improving cardiorespiratory endurance in young healthy populations?

Search for Evidence

You are able to find a video of the interview online, so you understand the source of the interview and the statements made.

Personal Experience

You have lots of experience with yoga, although you are not a certified yoga instructor. In some yoga classes, you have experienced physical exertion that seems strong enough to elevate your heart rate. The next time you take a yoga class, you take your heart rate twice during the class.

Academic Knowledge

Because you have a degree in exercise science, you know the Frequency, Intensity, Time, and Type (FITT) Guidelines for minimum physical activity levels required for cardiorespiratory adaptation. You know the physiology of the heart, vessels, and respiratory system and understand the dynamics of how exercise at a defined heart rate maximum can produce cellular changes that manifest to improve aerobic capacity.

Research Knowledge

A search for research related to yoga and cardiorespiratory endurance will reveal the current status of the literature. You carefully assess the quality of the studies you find to formulate your conclusions. Are the studies published in peer-reviewed journals? Are there randomized controlled trials generating consistent data across populations?

Evaluate the Evidence

Even if you are able to get your heart rate in range during your yoga classes, this is not strong enough evidence with which to advise your client. Only by looking further into the current research can you reach a conclusion backed by clear evidence, which may either support or refute the claim. Whatever the outcome, your competence as a health/fitness professional and your high ethical standards depend on your ability to educate yourself on the basis of the best evidence available at the time.

Incorporate Evidence into Practice

With an understanding of the strengths and the limitations of the current research related to your question, you can answer your client's question with integrity and create an exercise program for her that is backed by science.

Maintaining Certification

A profession continuously enlarges its body of knowledge, functions autonomously in formulation of policy, and maintains by force of organization or concerted opinion high standards of achievement and conduct. Members of a profession are committed to continuing education, place service above personal gain, and are committed to providing practical services vital to human and social welfare (31). The purpose of ACSM recertification is to ensure that ACSM-certified professionals enhance skills and knowledge above and beyond minimum competence. Periodic recertification occurs through the documentation of required continuing educational activities within the 3-year period following successful passing of an ACSM certification exam.

On the basis of the results from the JTA, along with a comprehensive review of recertification policies and procedures of similar credentials from other organizations, the CCRB determined that a 3-year duration was an appropriate window for a certified professional's recertification (14). EP recertification requirements include the following:

1. Accumulate 60 continuing education credits (CECs).
2. Maintain current cardiorespiratory resuscitation (CPR) certification.
3. Pay the required recertification fee.

Ways to Earn Continuing Education Credits

There are many ways to earn CECs. Continuing education enables the EP to build on his or her field experiences and engage in additional networking and scientifically based opportunities that focus and build a professional practice. Table 18.5 provides an overview of ways to earn CECs.

The professional responsibilities of practicing within an appropriate scope of practice, using evidence-based practices, maintaining certification, and adhering to a standard relating to conflict of interest all represent professional ethical behaviors that are informed and nurtured by personal characteristics reflective of a true professional.

Personal Characteristics

Cultivating and developing professional practices that reflect the nature of the EP certification are critical to growing respect for and continued growth of the role of the EP in the health/fitness industry. Employers in fields aligned with exercise science have articulated specific personal characteristics desirable in potential employees.

Melton et al. (3) interviewed fitness managers from both profit and nonprofit fitness facilities. The managers identified several positive characteristics of personal trainers seeking employment. Trainers who were comfortable interacting and who communicated effectively with a variety of individuals, who had a teachable attitude and aptitude, who were fit or provide evidence of engaging in fit behaviors, and who had the discipline and competence to obtain a relevant degree were seen as valuable employees. Likewise, the fitness managers described personal trainers who were arrogant and overconfident or who acted outside their scope of practice, specifically around nutritional advice, as a liability for the facility. The managers cited the consequences of such negative behaviors in terms of legal liability as well as loss of members, reputation, and revenue (3).

The American Fitness Professionals & Associates lists a number of qualities in their code of ethics document (32). Among them are "treating all with respect and dignity regardless of country of origin, gender, age, sexual orientation or ability; maintaining confidentiality with regard to information obtained from clients; recognizing and addressing stereotyping and prejudice; establishing appropriate boundaries with clients so that working relationships are not confused with friendships or other relationships" (32).

Similarly, the professional characteristics of athletic trainers have also been examined (33). Some of the defining features of quality athletic trainers include being personable, self-confident, mature, assertive, and enthusiastic (33). Likewise, among recreational staff personnel, characteristics such as patience, fun, creative, passionate, and people-oriented define successful professional

Table 18.5	Ways to Earn Continuing Education Credits		
Obtain a specialty certification.	ACSM/ACS-CET webinar series	9 CECs	
	ACSM/NCHPAD-CIFT webinar series	5 CECs	
Attend an ACSM certification workshop.	ACSM-CPT 2-d workshop	20.75 CECs	
	ACSM-EP 2-d workshop	16.0 CECs	
	ACSM Certified Group Exercise Instructor 2-d workshop	17.0 CECs	
Complete webinars, distance education, or other Internet-based continuing education programs on specific clinical or health/fitness-related topics.		Varies	
Attend professional education meetings from ACSM or other nationally recognized organizations.		Varies	
Take continuing education self-tests that offer CECs, CMEs, or CEUs from ACSM or other nationally recognized organizations.	*ACSMceOnline* (https://www.acsm.org/learn-develop-professionally/ceonline2)	Varies	
	ACSM's Health & Fitness Journal®	52 CECs per year	
Take and receive a passing grade in a health/fitness- or exercise science–related course from an accredited college or university.		10 CECs per credit hour[a]	
Author or coauthor books, peer-reviewed journal articles, or accepted abstracts.		10 CECs	
Teach academic courses; conduct classroom instruction; or present health, fitness, or clinical lectures at an organized professional conference.		Varies	

CME, continuing medical education; CEU, continuing education units.

[a]For example, a 3-credit-hour course is worth 30 CECs. Course must be health/fitness- or clinically related and completed with a grade of "C" or better.

Adapted from American College of Sports Medicine. Candidate handbook [Internet]. Indianapolis (IN): American College of Sports Medicine; 2021 [cited 2021 Apr 13]. Available from: https://www.acsm.org/get-stay-certified/policies-procedures.

behaviors (34). Honest, intelligent, and responsible were the top-rated attributes among nurses (35), as were a positive attitude and overall job satisfaction (36). Health care professionals are further described as respectful, reflective, and socially responsible (23,37). In a white paper focusing on the professional characteristics of pharmacy students, accountability, openness to new ideas, and willingness to learn were cited as important to individual success (38). Perhaps one of the most cited characteristics of the helping professions is patience, especially in the role of educator and teacher (39). The EP as a helping health care professional can gain insight into the favorable characteristics cited by professionals from related fields.

Another important arena in which EPs should be mindful is their social media presence. Being active on a number of platforms is encouraged and accepted as a vital and effective marketing tool, particularly for those in business for themselves. Blogs, Instagram, Facebook, and Twitter are excellent vehicles for branding, networking, selling, and educating. On the flip side, these same tools can quickly spiral downward if used in an unprofessional manner. Fortunately, there is guidance for best practice use of social media. Ventola (40) cites six major risks of social media engagement by health care professionals: poor quality of information, damage to professional image, breaches of patient privacy, violation of the patient–health care professional boundary, licensing, and legal issues. In addition, Gavejian and Gerling (41) focus on improper use of social media during work time and cite common problems with posts that contain inaccurate, inappropriate, discriminatory, or harassing content toward clients, coworkers, or work institutions. Even comments that are unrelated to the workplace can reflect poorly on an institution if that workplace is identified with an employee's personal site (41). A good rule of thumb is not to post anything that you would not say or show to your manager. Finally, check with your institution for its social media responsible use policy. Many institutions, especially those in health care, are attending to this important aspect of our world. At the end of this chapter is a case study that highlights an issue related to social media use.

The acronym WISE (Wisdom, Integrity, Stewardship, and Enthusiasm) provides a helpful summary of personal characteristics and behaviors important to the success of an EP.

Wisdom represents the individual seeking answers to sound questions with scientifically based evidence. Integrity signifies the individual respectful of appropriate boundaries while assisting clients in the achievement of holistic and meaningful change. Stewardship represents the individual who values the historical progression of the exercise science professions and acts thoughtfully and professionally as a steward of the future. Enthusiasm denotes the individual whose contagious positive attitude inspires others.

The Case of Maria, an Undergraduate Intern

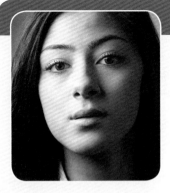

Submitted by **Randi Lite, MA, ACSM-CEP, NBC-HWC, FACSM, Simmons University, Boston, MA**

Maria is an intern at a corporate fitness center. She is asked by a member for advice and she responds directly to the client and then in a post. This case addresses issues of professional behavior on-site at a workplace and on social media.

Narrative

Maria Jones, a university senior, is an exercise science major who is interning at a corporate fitness site for ACME, a major company in her area. The fitness center is located on the ACME campus and is staffed with the fitness director, three group exercise instructors who also do personal training, and a physical therapist. Maria is at the center 3 d · wk^{-1} from 6:00 to 10:00 a.m. She has a certification as a group exercise instructor and runs a body sculpting class. She is responsible for designing and changing the bulletin board at the entry to the gym, writing a blog once per month for members, and orienting new members to the equipment, and she shadows the physical therapist and the personal trainers.

One day, she is on the floor by herself and a new member approaches her. The member has developed pain in their right shoulder, which is exacerbated when using the lat pull-down machine. Maria had recently been experimenting with an app to locate trigger points, and she has successfully reduced her own shoulder pain. She tells the member about the app, and together, they look up and identify a possible trigger point. Maria does manual massage for the member on that trigger point area and instructs the member how to do self-massage. Unbeknownst to the member, Maria takes a quick picture of the member with her own cell phone. After the client leaves, she posts the picture to her Facebook page and Instagram account with this description: "From intern to expert — helped my first client today! #triggerpointmassage #ACME"

QUESTIONS

- For each of Maria's actions below, discuss whether the action was permissible given her role as an intern, and if not, classify the action as a breach of confidentiality, overstepping scope of practice, unprofessional behavior, conflict of interest, or not evidence based.
  - Running a body sculpting class at her internship
  - Telling the member about the trigger point app
  - Identifying a possible trigger point from the app
  - Manual massage on the member by Maria
  - Instructing the member on self-massage
  - Taking a picture of the member with her cell phone
  - Posting the picture to her Facebook and Instagram accounts
  - Using her phone during her internship to make a personal post
  - Use of a hashtag connecting Maria to her workplace
- If Maria were an EP or a physical therapist, would any of your answers to the prior question be different?
- Brainstorm alternate responses for Maria in the situation described.

SUMMARY

The EP has a personal and professional responsibility to engage in behaviors that "do no harm" (22). After providing a brief history of ACSM certifications, this chapter has reviewed the ACSM Code of Ethics and provided a more in-depth examination of the professional responsibilities and personal characteristics of the EP. The professional responsibilities relating to scope of practice, conflict of interest, evidence-based practice, and maintaining certification have been reviewed. Personal characteristics represented by WISE have also been examined in the context of desirable personal characteristics of professionals in the helping professions.

STUDY QUESTIONS

1. The ACSM-EP is qualified to pursue a career in all EXCEPT
   a. local YMCA.
   b. hospital cardiac care unit.
   c. university fitness and wellness center.
   d. clinical research project related to childhood obesity.
2. The ACSM-EP scope of practice includes
   a. exercise testing of a healthy 76-year-old man with mild osteoarthritis.
   b. aerobic training of a 21-year-old woman with acute anorexia.
   c. therapeutic exercise to target a cancer survivor's chronic lymphedema of the left arm.
   d. interpreting a 12-lead electrocardiogram of a patient who has coronary artery bypass graft in a phase 2 cardiac rehabilitation program.
3. Henry's business card indicates that he is a certified EP working as a manager of an employee wellness center. In addition to his management responsibilities, he functions in the role as a personal trainer at the center for employees who want to pay an extra fee to the center for individualized services. Henry has a side business of selling essential oils and nutritional aids for health and longevity. Discuss whether each example is permissible for Henry to engage in.
   a. Henry has a side business of selling essential oils and nutritional aids for health and longevity.
   b. Henry pins his essential oils business card on a bulletin board in the wellness center where other business cards advertise massage services, nutritional counseling, physical therapy, and acupuncture.
   c. Henry gives his essential oils business card and a free sample to every client he works with at the wellness center.
   d. Henry makes essential oils recommendations within the context of a training session for a client at the wellness center.
   e. Henry makes essential oils recommendations within the context of a training session for a private client.
4. List some ways of maintaining one's EP certification.
5. Discuss personal characteristics that you deem important for professional conduct as an EP.
6. How do the personal behaviors of an EP impact the professional integrity of the field?

REFERENCES

1. The Free Dictionary. Ethics [Internet]. Huntingdon Valley (PA): Farlex; [cited 2019 Jul 15]. Available from: http://medical-dictionary.thefreedictionary.com/ethics.

2. U.S. Bureau of Labor Statistics. Occupational outlook handbook. Fitness trainers and instructors [Internet]. Washington (DC): U.S. Department of Labor; [cited 2019 Jul 26]. Available from: https://www.bls.gov/ooh/personal-care-and-service/fitness-trainers-and-instructors.htm.

3. Melton DI, Dail TK, Katula JA, Mustian KM. The current state of personal training: managers' perspectives. *J Strength Cond Res.* 2010;24(11):3173–9.

4. Berryman JW. *Out of Many, One: A History of the American College of Sports Medicine.* Champaign (IL): Human Kinetics; 1995. 283 p.

5. Committee on Accreditation of the Exercise Sciences. About us. [Internet]. Clearwater (FL): Committee on Accreditation of the Exercise Sciences; [cited 2019 Aug 6]. Available from: http://www.coaes.org.

6. American College of Sports Medicine. Get certified [Internet]. Indianapolis (IN): American College of Sports Medicine; [cited 2019 Jul 15]. Available from: https://www.acsm.org/get-stay-certified/get-certified.

7. Simpson WF. Progress for ACSM certifications: 2015 and beyond. 2015. *ACSMs Health Fit J.* 2015;19(2):30–1.

8. American College of Sports Medicine. ACSM Exercise is Medicine® credential [Internet]. Indianapolis (IN): American College of Sports Medicine; [cited 2019 Jul 15]. Available from: https://www.acsm.org/get-stay-certified/get-certified/specialization/eim-credential.

9. American National Standards Institute. U.S. representation in ISO [Internet]. New York (NY): American National Standards Institute; [cited 2019 Jul 15]. Available from: https://www.ansi.org/standards_activities/iso_programs/overview.

10. National Commission for Certifying Agencies. NCCA accreditation [Internet]. Washington (DC); [cited 2019 Aug 6]. Available from: https://www.credentialingexcellence.org/ncca.

11. American College of Sports Medicine. Code of ethics & membership refund policies [Internet]. Indianapolis (IN): American College of Sports Medicine; [cited 2019 Jul 15]. Available from: https://www.acsm.org/acsm-membership/membership/join/acsm-member-code-of-ethics.

12. The Free Dictionary. Scope of practice [Internet]. Huntingdon Valley (PA): Farlex; [cited 2019 Jul 15]. Available from: http://medical-dictionary.thefreedictionary.com/scope+of+practice.

13. American College of Sports Medicine. *ACSM Certified Exercise Physiologist^SM Exam Content Outline* [Internet]. Indianapolis (IN): American College of Sports Medicine; 2019 [cited 2019 Jul 15]. Available from: https://www.acsm.org/docs/default-source/default-document-library/acsm-ep-exam-content-outline-(2017).pdf?sfvrsn=15f8d9dc_0.

14. American College of Sports Medicine. Candidate handbook [Internet]. Indianapolis (IN): American College of Sports Medicine; 2017 [cited 2019 Aug 5]. Available from: https://www.acsm.org/docs/default-source/certification-documents/acsmcandidatehandbook_v12_2017.pdf?sfvrsn=49f62c5d_2.

15. O'Sullivan-Maillet J, Skates J, Pritchett E. American Dietetic Association: scope of dietetics practice framework. *J Am Diet Assoc.* 2005;105(4):634–40.

16. Muth ND. The elephant in the room: nutrition scope of practice. Where do fitness professionals draw the line when it comes to dishing out diet and nutrition advice? [Internet]. San Diego (CA): IDEA Health & Wellness Association; [cited 2019 Jul 8]. Available from: http://www.ideafit.com/fitness-library/the-elephant-in-the-room-nutrition-scope-of-practice.

17. Kruskall LJ, Manore MM, Eickhoff-Schemek MM, Ehrman JK. Drawing the line. Understanding the scope of practice among registered dietitian nutritionists and exercise professionals. *ACSMs Health Fit J.* 2017;21(1):23–32.

18. Sass C, Eickhoff-Shemek JM, Manore MM, Kruskall LJ. Crossing the line: understanding the scope of practice between registered dieticians and health fitness professionals. *ACSMs Health Fit J.* 2007;11(3):12–9.

19. Thompson WR. Worldwide survey of fitness trends for 2019. *ACSMs Health Fit J.* 2018;22(6):10–7.

20. American College of Sports Medicine. *Leadership Manual 2014-2015.* Indianapolis (IN): American College of Sports Medicine; 2014. 9 p.

21. Responsible Conducts of Research Courses Portal. Conflicts of interest [Internet]. New York (NY): Columbia University; [cited 2019 Aug 6]. Available from: http://ccnmtl.columbia.edu/projects/rcr/rcr_conflicts/foundation/index.html#1.

22. Brody H. Clarifying conflict of interest. *Am J Bioeth.* 2011;11(1):23–8.

23. de Cordova PB, Collins S, Peppard L, et al. Implementing evidence-based nursing with student nurses and clinicians: uniting the strengths. *Appl Nurs Res.* 2008;21(4):242–5.

24. Institute of Medicine. *Crossing the Quality Chasm: A New Health System for the 21st Century.* Washington (DC): National Academies Press; 2001. 360 p.

25. DukeHealth. Evidence-based practice series [Internet]. Durham (NC): DukeHealth; [cited 2019 Aug 5]. Available from: https://tutorials.mclibrary.duke.edu/ebpintro/.

26. The Free Dictionary. Evidence-based practice [Internet]. Huntingdon Valley (PA): Farlex; [cited 2019 Aug 6]. Available from: http://medical-dictionary.thefreedictionary.com/evidence-based+practice.

27. Amonette W, English K, Ottenbacher K. *Nullius in verba*: a call for the incorporation of evidence-based practice into the discipline of exercise science. *Sports Med.* 2010;40(6):449–57.

28. Eyles HC, Mhurchu CN. Does tailoring make a difference? A systematic review of the long-term effectiveness of tailored nutrition education for adults. *Nutr Rev.* 2009;67(8):464–80.

29. Scott PJ, Altenburger PA, Kean J. A collaborative teaching strategy for enhancing learning of evidence-based clinical decision-making. *J Allied Health.* 2011;40(3):120–7.

30. The Centre for Evidence-Based Medicine. Asking focused questions [Internet]. Oxford (United Kingdom): The Centre for Evidence-Based Medicine; [cited 2015 Oct 13]. Available from: http://www.cebm.net/index.aspx?o=1036.

31. The Free Dictionary. Profession [Internet]. Huntingdon Valley (PA): Farlex; [cited 2015 Oct 13]. Available from: http://medical-dictionary.thefreedictionary.com/profession.

32. American Fitness Professionals & Associates. Code ethics for personal trainers & fitness instructors [Internet]. Ocean City (NJ): American Fitness Professionals & Associates; [cited 2019 Aug 5]. Available from: https://store.afpafitness.com/code-of-ethics-for-personal-trainers-fitness-instructors/.

33. Kahanov L, Andrews L. A survey of athletic training employers' hiring criteria. *J Athl Train.* 2001;36(4):408–12.

34. Chase D, Masberg B. Partnering for skill development: park and recreation agencies and university programs. *Manag Leisure.* 2008;13(2):74–91.

35. Rassin M. Nurses' professional and personal values. *Nurs Ethics.* 2008;15(5):614–30.

36. Shields MA, Ward M. Improving nurse retention in the National Health Service in England: the impact of job satisfaction on intentions to quit. *J Health Econ.* 2001;20(5):677–701.

37. Beach M, Duggan P, Cassel C, Geller G. What does "respect" mean? Exploring the moral obligation of health professionals to respect patients. *J Gen Intern Med.* 2007;22(5):692–5.

38. American Pharmaceutical Association Academy of Students of Pharmacy/American Association of Colleges of Pharmacy Council of Deans Task Force on Professionalism. White paper on pharmacy student professionalism. *J Am Pharm Assoc.* 2000;40(1):96–102.

39. Tichenor MS, Tichenor JL. Understanding teachers' perspectives on professionalism. *Profession Educ.* 2004;27(1–2):89–95.

40. Ventola CL. Social media and health care professionals: benefits, risks, and best practices. *P T.* 2014;39(7):491–520.

41. Gavejian JC, Gerling ES. Fitness industry legal update — 2018. *Venulex Legal Summ.* 2018;30(7):1–3.

Appendix A

Editors from the Previous Two Editions of *ACSM's Resources for the Exercise Physiologist**

SECOND EDITION

Senior Editor

Peter Magyari, PhD, FACSM, ACSM EP-C
University of North Florida
Jacksonville, Florida

Associate Editors

Randi Lite, MA, ACSM-RCEP, ACSM-EIM3
Simmons College
Boston, Massachusetts

Marcus W. Kilpatrick, PhD, FACSM
University of South Florida
Tampa, Florida

James E. Schoffstall, EdD, FACSM, ACSM EP-C, ACSM-RCEP, ACSM/NCHPAD CIFT, ACSM/NPAS PAPHS
Liberty University
Lynchburg, Virginia

FIRST EDITION

Previously titled *ACSM's Resources for the Health Fitness Specialist*

Senior Editor

Gary Liguori, PhD, FACSM, ACSM-CES
Dean
College of Health Sciences
University of Rhode Island
Kingston, Rhode Island

Associate Editors

Gregory B. Dwyer, PhD, FACSM, ACSM-PD, ACSM-RCEP, ACSM-CEP, ACSM-ETT, EIM 3
Professor
Department of Exercise Science
East Stroudsburg University
East Stroudsburg, Pennsylvania

Teresa C. Fitts, DPE, FACSM, ACSM-HFS
Westfield State University
Westfield, Massachusetts

Beth A. Lewis, PhD
Associate Professor, Behavioral Aspects of Physical Activity
Director, Undergraduate Studies
University of Minnesota
School of Kinesiology
Minneapolis, Minnesota

*Degrees, certifications, and affiliations are current at the time of publication of the edition listed.

Contributors from the Previous Two Editions of *ACSM's Resources for the Exercise Physiologist**

SECOND EDITION

Anthony A. Abbott, EdD, FACSM, ACSM-CPT, ACSM EP-C, ACSM-CEP, ACSM/ACS CET, ACSM/NCHPAD CIFT
Fitness Institute International, Inc.
Lighthouse Point, Florida

John B. Bartholomew, PhD, FACSM
University of Texas at Austin
Austin, Texas

Keith Burns, PhD, ACSM EP-C
Walsh University
North Canton, Ohio

Katrina D. DuBose, PhD, FACSM
East Carolina University
Greenville, North Carolina

J. Larry Durstine, PhD, FACSM
University of South Carolina
Columbia, South Carolina

Gregory Dwyer, PhD, FACSM, ACSM-PD, ACSM-RCEP, ACSM-CEP, ACSM-ETT, EIM3
East Stroudsburg University
East Stroudsburg, Pennsylvania

Avery D. Faigenbaum, EdD, FACSM, ACSM EP-C
The College of New Jersey
Ewing, New Jersey

Mark D. Faries, PhD
Texas A&M University, AgriLife Extension Service
College Station, Texas

Diana Ferris Dimon, MS
Praxair, Inc.
Danbury, Connecticut

Charles J. Fountaine, PhD
University of Minnesota Duluth
Duluth, Minnesota

Benjamin Gordon, PhD
University of North Florida
Jacksonville, Florida

Sarah T. Henes, PhD, RD, LDN
Georgia State University
Atlanta, Georgia

Josh Johann, MS, EIM1
The University of Tennessee at Chattanooga
Chattanooga, Tennessee

Betsy Keller, PhD, FACSM, ACSM-ETT
Ithaca College
Ithaca, New York

Marcus W. Kilpatrick, PhD, FACSM
University of South Florida
Tampa, Florida

Matthew Kutz, PhD
Bowling Green State University
Bowling Green, Ohio

Beth Lewis, PhD
University of Minnesota
Minneapolis, Minnesota

Gary Liguori, PhD, FACSM, ACSM-CEP
The University of Rhode Island
Kingston, Rhode Island

Randi Lite, MA, ACSM-RCEP, EIM3
Simmons College
Boston, Massachusetts

Meir Magal, PhD, FACSM, ACSM-CEP
North Carolina Wesleyan College
Rocky Mount, North Carolina

*Degrees, certifications, and affiliations are current at the time of publication of the edition listed.

Peter Magyari, PhD, FACSM, ACSM EP-C
University of North Florida
Jacksonville, Florida

Linda May, PhD
Eastern Carolina University
Greenville, North Carolina

Jessica Meendering, PhD, ACSM EP-C
South Dakota State University
Brookings, South Dakota

Laurie Milliken, PhD, FACSM
University of Massachusetts Boston
Boston, Massachusetts

Nicole Nelson, MHS, LMT, ACSM EP-C
University of North Florida
Jacksonville, Florida

Neal Pire, MA, FACSM, ACSM EP-C, ACSM-EIM2
Castle Connolly Private Health Partners, LLC
New York, New York

Deborah Riebe, PhD, FACSM, ACSM EP-C
The University of Rhode Island
Kingston, Rhode Island

James E. Schoffstall, EdD, FACSM, ACSM EP-C, ACSM-RCEP, ACSM/NCHPAD CIFT, ACSM/NPAS PAPHS
Liberty University
Lynchburg, Virginia

John M. Schuna Jr., PhD
Oregon State University
Corvallis, Oregon

Katie J. Schuver, PhD
University of Minnesota
Minneapolis, Minnesota

John Sigg, PT, PhD
Ithaca College
Ithaca, New York

Matthew Stults-Kolehmainen, PhD, ACSM EP-C
Yale-New Haven Hospital
New Haven, Connecticut
Teachers College Columbia University
New York, New York

Kathleen S. Thomas, PhD, ACSM-CPT, ACSM EP-C
Norfolk State University
Norfolk, Virginia

FIRST EDITION
Previously titled *ACSM's Resources for the Health Fitness Specialist*

Anthony A. Abbott, EdD, FACSM
Fitness Institute International, Inc.
Lighthouse Point, Florida

Keith Burns, MS
Kent State University
Kent, Ohio

Dino Costanzo, MA, ACSM-RCEP, FACSM, ACSM-PD, ACSM-ETT
The Hospital of Central Connecticut
New Britain, Connecticut

Katrina DuBose, PhD, FACSM
East Carolina University
Greenville, North Carolina

J. Larry Durstine, PhD, FACSM
University of South Carolina
Columbia, South Carolina

Gregory B. Dwyer, PhD, FACSM ACSM-PD, ACSM-CES, ACSM-ETT, ACSM-RCEP
East Stroudsburg University
East Stroudsburg, Pennsylvania

Chris Eschbach, PhD, ACSM-HFS
Valencell, Inc.
Raleigh, North Carolina

Avery Faigenbaum, EdD, FACSM
The College of New Jersey
Ewing, New Jersey

Diana Ferris, MS, ACSM-HFS
ACSM/NPAS-PAPHS
Public Health Specialist
Stratford, Connecticut

Teresa C. Fitts, DPE, FACSM, ACSM-HFS
Westfield State University
Westfield, Massachusetts

Charles Fountaine, PhD
University of Minnesota Duluth
Duluth, Minnesota

Benjamin Gordon, MS, ACSM-CES
The University of South Carolina
Columbia, South Carolina

Sarah T. Henes, PhD, RD, LDN
East Carolina University
Greenville, North Carolina

Ernestine Jennings, PhD
Warren Alpert Medical School, Brown University
Providence, Rhode Island

Betsy Keller, PhD, FACSM
Ithaca College
Ithaca, New York

Riggs Klika, PhD, FACSM
Cancer Survivor Center
Aspen, Colorado

Matthew Kutz, PhD, ATC, ACSM-CES
Bowling Green State University
Bowling Green, Ohio

Beth Lewis, PhD
University of Minnesota
Minneapolis, Minnesota

Gary Liguori, PhD, FACSM, ACSM-CES
University of Tennessee Chattanooga
Chattanooga, Tennessee

Sarah Linke, PhD, MPH
University of California, San Diego
La Jolla, California

Randi Lite, MA, ACSM-RCEP
Simmons College
Boston, Massachusetts

Meir Magal, PhD, ACSM-CES
North Carolina Wesleyan College
Rocky Mount, North Carolina

Bess Marcus, PhD, FACSM
University of California, San Diego
La Jolla, California

Jessica Meendering, PhD, ACSM-HFS, ATC
South Dakota State University
Brookings, South Dakota

Laurie Milliken, PhD, FACSM
University of Massachusetts Boston
Boston, Massachusetts

Rob Motl, PhD
University of Illinois
Urbana, Illinois

Mark Nutting, ACSM-HFD, ACSM-HFS
Saco Sport & Fitness
Saco, Maine

Matthew W. Parrott, PhD, ACSM-HFS
H-P Fitness, LLC
Leawood, Kansas

Neal I. Pire, MA, FACSM
Inspire Training Systems
Ridgewood, New Jersey

Deborah Riebe, PhD, FACSM, ACSM-HFS
University of Rhode Island
Kingston, Rhode Island

John M. Schuna, Jr., PhD
Pennington Biomedical Research Center
Baton Rouge, Louisiana

Katie Schuver, MS
University of Minnesota
Minneapolis, Minnesota

John Sigg, PhD
Ithaca College
Ithaca, New York

Madeline Weikert, MS
Human Kinetics
Champaign, Illinois

Molly Winke, PhD
Hanover College
Hanover, Indiana

Index

Note: Page numbers followed by *b*, *f*, or *t* indicate boxes, figures, or tables, respectively.

A

Abdominal bracing, 185–186, 277
Abdominal (central) obesity, 204–205
ABI. *See* Ankle/brachial systolic pressure index
Abnormal responses, to exercise, 92
Absolute contraindications, 52
Absolute oxygen consumption, 77
Academic preparation, 496, 498
Accelerometers, 13, 351
Access
    ADA and, 407–408, 452*t*
    perceived, 356
Acclimation, 96
Acclimatization, 94, 96–97, 302
Accommodations, for functional movement, 176
Accounting, 457–461
Accounts payable, 457, 459
Accounts receivable, 457, 458, 462
Accreditation, ACSM, 485–489, 486*f*
Accrual accounting, 458
ACE inhibitors, 254*t*, 255
Acetaminophen, 270*t*
Acetaminophen + codeine, 270*t*
ACLS. *See* Aerobics Center Longitudinal Study
ACOG. *See* American College of Obstetricians and Gynecologists
ACSM. *See* American College of Sports Medicine
ACSM's Fitness Assessment Manual, 70
ACSM's Guidelines for Exercise Testing and Prescription, 30, 50–51, 110, 111, 300, 313
ACSM's Scientific Pronouncements: Physical Activity Guidelines for Americans, 10, 10*t*
Action, as stage of change, 328*t*, 330*b*, 357–358
Active Choices, 334
Active living, 3–4
Active Living Everyday, 334
Activities of daily living, 137, 282
Activity factors, in weight management, 215, 215*t*
Acute injuries, 271
Acute stress, 379
ADA (Americans with Disabilities Act), 407–408, 452*t*
Adaptations
    bone, 288
    functional movement and, 176
    periodization *versus*, 128
    principle of specificity and, 114–115
    stress and, 374–376, 379
Adenosine triphosphate (ATP), 61, 62–64, 63*f*, 64*f*
Administrative law, 397–398
Adolescents, 300–305
    behavior change and physical activity in, 336*b*
    body mass index of, 203

body size and composition of, 300–301
cardiorespiratory function in, 302
chronic exercise by, impact of, 302–303
exercise programming for, 303–305
motor skills and physical activity in, 302
muscular strength, flexibility, and motor performance in, 302
nutrition for, 221*t*
obesity in, 14–15, 14*f*, 201, 203, 302–305
physical activity and health in, 13–15
physical activity guidelines for, 11*t*, 12, 13–14
physical and physiological changes in, 300–302
recommended activity level for, 303
thermoregulation in, 302
weight management in, 304–305
Adoption, as stage of change, 327, 328*t*
ADP. *See* Air displacement plethysmography
Adults
    deconditioned, 310
    nutrition for, 221*t*
    older (*See* Older adults)
    physical activity and health in, 15–17, 17*t*
    physical activity guidelines for, 11*t*–12*t*, 12, 16, 16*f*
Adversity, cumulative, 373
Advertising, 464–465, 476, 478*t*
AED (automated external defibrillator), 412, 450*t*–452*t*
Aerobic activities, 3
Aerobic capacity. *See* Oxygen consumption
Aerobic dance, 88
Aerobic exercise
    for arthritis, 282–283, 284*f*
    for children and adolescents, 303
    for low back pain, 279*t*
    for older adults, 315
    for osteoporosis, 290*t*
    for persons with chronic diseases, 242*t*, 257
    in pregnancy, 306–309
    for stress management, 380
    for weight loss, 217
Aerobic glycolysis, 63–64
Aerobic machines, 88*t*
Aerobic respiration, 63–64, 63*f*, 64*f*
Aerobics Center Longitudinal Study (ACLS), 9
Affect (emotion)
    regulation of, 352–353, 373–374
    and self-efficacy, 330–333, 332*t*, 353, 354*t*
Affective expectations, 339–340
Age
    and body composition, 201
    and bone density, 286–287
    and CRF exercise prescription, 94
    and CRF/maximal aerobic power, 78*t*–79*t*
    and exercise across lifespan, 299–323
    and flexibility, 139
    and functional movement, 182
Age Discrimination in Employment Act (ADEA), 409
Agility training, for osteoporosis, 291
Agonist contraction, 142
Agonist muscles, 105, 181
Agreements (contract law), 406
AHA. *See* American Heart Association

Air displacement plethysmography (ADP), 211–213
Airex pad, 193
Alarm reaction, 375, 379
Alignment
    addressing issues in, 191–193
    common faults and corresponding muscles, 191*t*
    corrective exercises for, 191–193, 191*t*, 192*f*–193*f*
    fault checklist, 191*t*
    instability training for, 193, 194*t*, 195*f*
    stretching and self-myofascial release for, 194–196, 196*f*, 197*t*
Allostasis, 375–376
Allostatic load model, 375–376
Altitude, 94–97
Altitude acclimatization, 96–97
Ambivalence, about change, 361
American Academy of Pediatrics, on overweight and obesity, 304–305
American Association of Cardiovascular and Pulmonary Rehabilitation (AACVPR) risk stratification, 49, 50*t*
American Civil Liberties Union (ACLU), 409
American College of Cardiology/American Heart Association Task Force, 234–235
American College of Obstetricians and Gynecologists (ACOG), 305, 309
American College of Sports Medicine (ACSM)
    certification, 485–489, 486*f*
    Code of Ethics, 485, 489
    fitness trend survey, 471
    guidelines on exercise for weight loss, 218
    guidelines on exercise prescription, 485
    guidelines on exercise safety, 21
    guidelines on flexibility, 137
    guidelines on graded exercise testing, 485
    guidelines on physical activity, 9–10
    guidelines on preparticipation screening, 30, 450*t*
    guidelines on resistance training, 104, 124*t*
    guidelines on risk management and emergency procedures, 449–452
    Health/Fitness Facility Standards and Guidelines, 401, 404, 406, 449, 450*t*–452*t*, 453
    history of, 485, 486*f*
    metabolic formula, 82–84, 83*t*, 219
    Pollock and, 8
    risk factor assessment and defining criteria in atherosclerotic CVD, 52–53
    risk factor thresholds, 30, 31
    signs and symptoms of CMR disease, 46–48
American Fitness Professionals & Associates, 499
American Heart Association (AHA), 311
    certification in emergency care, 49
    contraindications to exercise testing, 51
    guidelines on physical activity, 9–10
    guidelines on preparticipation screening, 31–32
    on risk of sudden death, 55
    risk stratification, 49

American Institute of Stress, 376
American National Standards Institute (ANSI), 488
American Psychological Association
   mental health resources, 386
   Stress in America report, 372, 374
Americans with Disabilities Act (ADA) of 1990, 407–408, 452*t*
Amortization, 457
Amortization phase, 118
Amotivation, 338–339, 357
Anaerobic activities, 3
Anaerobic glycolysis, 62–64, 63*f*, 64*f*
Analgesics
   precautions in chronic diseases, 253, 255*t*
   for sprains and strains, 270*t*
Anasarca, 47
Anatomical planes, 114–115, 114*f*
Android (central) obesity, 204–205
Ankle, static stretches for, 166*f*, 166*t*–167*t*, 167*f*
Ankle/brachial systolic pressure index (ABI), 235, 239
Ankle edema, 47
Ankle sprain, 268
ANSI (American National Standards Institute), 488
Antagonist contraction, 142
Antagonist muscles, 105, 143, 181
Anterior cross-arm stretch, 140*f*
Anthropometric measures, 201–206. *See also specific measures*
Antibiotics, and musculoskeletal injuries, 154
Anxiety
   as barrier to physical activity, 355
   exercise to relieve, 380
   physique, 355
   referral to psychologist for, 386
   resistance training and, 104
   stress and, 378–379
Appraisal support, 382
Aquatic exercise
   advantages and disadvantages of swimming, 88*t*
   for arthritis, 282, 283
   for older adults, 314
   for pregnant women, 307
   program preferences/trends, 466*t*
   weight loss in swimming, 217
Arab Muslims, 367
Archimedes's principle, 211
Arm cycling, energy expenditure during, 83*t*
Arteries, 61–62
Arterioles, 61–62
Arthritis, 281–285. *See also* Osteoarthritis; Rheumatoid arthritis
   case study of, 292–294
   yoga for, 143
Art of the deal, 479
Aspirin, 253
Assessment. *See also specific assessment tools*
   body composition, 201–213
   cardiac events during exercise testing, 20, 55
   cardiorespiratory, 70–77
   contraindications to exercise testing, 51–53, 51*b*
   flexibility, 145–146, 146*f*, 147*t*–152*t*
   functional movement, 183–193
   muscular fitness, 108–111, 112
   preparticipation, 29–57, 411

stress (Perceived Stress Scale), 381–382
   stress associated with, 375
Assets, 457, 458
Associate or Certificate in Personal Fitness Training, 486
Assumption of risk defense, 401
Asthma, 237, 237*f*
   exercise concerns, precautions, and contraindications in, 251–252
   FITT considerations in, 245
   medications for, effects of, 256
Astrand-Rhyming Cycle Ergometer Test, 70*t*, 75, 76*f*
Astrand-Rhyming Step Test, 70*t*
Atherosclerosis
   in coronary artery disease, 233–234, 234*f*
   dyslipidemia and, 236
   exercise and, 238–239
   in peripheral artery disease, 235
   risk factor assessment and defining criteria in, 52–53
   stress and, 378
ATP. *See* Adenosine triphosphate
Atria, of heart, 61–62
Attainable goals, 349
Auscultation, 68
Authoritarian management, 427
Autism Exercise Specialist, ACSM/Exercise Connection, 487
Autocratic leadership, 423, 428
Automated external defibrillator (AED), 412, 450*t*–452*t*
Autonomy, 338–339, 356

B

Bachelor of Science in Exercise Science, 486
Background checks, 408–409
Back pain, low. *See* Low back pain
Balance sheet, 457, 458–459, 459*f*
Balance training
   in arthritis, 283, 284
   in osteoporosis, 290*t*
Ballistic flexibility, 139, 140
Balls, for SMR, 196, 196*f*
Balls and cords, for resistance training, 121
Band external rotation, 191*t*, 193*f*
Bands, for resistance training, 117, 119, 121
Band walks, lateral, 188*t*, 190*f*, 191*t*
Bariatric surgery, 223–224
Barometric pressure, 95–96
Barriers, to physical activity, 4–5, 7*t*, 336, 354–356
   actual, 354
   anxiety and, 355
   behavior change and (case study), 341–342
   body-related, 355
   for diverse populations, 366–367
   environmental, 354–356, 367
   health-related, 355
   IDEA method for solving, 355
   for older adults, 366–367
   perceived, 354
   perceived access and options, 356
   problem-solving, 354–356
   psychosocial, 355
   race/ethnicity and, 367
   relapse, 356, 357*b*
   stress as, 380
   working with diverse populations, 366–367

Barriers, to self-monitoring, 350
Beglin v. Hartwick College, 410–411
Behavior, client. *See* Behavior change
Behavior, leadership, 421
Behavior, organizational, 431–432
Behavior, professional, 484–505. *See also* Ethics
Behavior, transactional, 419
Behavioral control, 383
Behavioral factors, in social cognitive theory, 328–329, 331*f*
Behavioral model, of management, 430
Behavioral processes, of change, 331*t*
Behavioral Risk Factor Surveillance System, 13
Behavioral strategies, for weight loss, 224
Behavior change
   case studies of, 341–342, 362–366
   client's engagement scale for, 358–359
   communication and, 359–360
   emotional regulation in, 352–353
   evidence-based practice on, 348
   facilitating, 347–370
   goal setting for, 349
   health belief model of, 348
   hedonic theory of, 327, 339–340
   identifying benefits of, 348
   incorporation into practice, 357–359
   increasing options for physical activity in, 356
   motivational interviewing for, 339, 359, 360–366
   older adults and, 366–367
   practical resources for, 359*b*
   practical strategies for, 348–356
   problem-solving barriers to physical activity in, 354–356
   race/ethnicity and, 367
   relapse prevention in, 333, 356, 357*b*
   role of exercise physiologist in, 357–361
   self-determination theory of, 327, 338–339
   self-efficacy in, 329–333, 332*t*, 353, 354*t*
   self-monitoring for, 349–351
   skills and strategies for, 357*b*, 357*t*
   social cognitive theory of, 327, 328–333, 331*f*, 348
   social ecological model of, 327, 334–336, 335*f*, 336*b*
   social support for, 351–352
   theories of, 326–346
   theory-based interventions for, 348
   theory of planned behavior in, 327, 337–338, 338*f*
   theory translation to real world, 334
   transtheoretical model of, 327–328, 328*t*, 329, 330*b*, 357–358
   working with diverse populations, 366–367
Benefits, employee, 445, 446*t*
Berisaj, Victor, 401
Berisaj v. LTF Club Operations Company, Inc., 401
β₂-agonists, 256
β-blockers, 248–250, 254*t*, 255
BIA. *See* Bioelectrical impedance analysis
Biceps brachii, 105, 158*t*, 159*t*
Biceps curl exercise, 119
Bicycles, care of, 456*t*
Bicycling
   advantages and disadvantages of, 88*t*
   cardiorespiratory fitness in, 70*t*, 75, 76*f*
   energy expenditure during, 83–84, 83*t*
   weight loss in, 217

Bioelectrical impedance analysis (BIA), 209–210
Biofeedback, 384
Bird dog, 188*t*, 189*f*, 191*t*, 279–280, 280*f*
Bisphosphonates, 289*t*
Black Americans
    obesity in, 201
    participation in physical activity, 367
Blake-Mouton management grid, 427
Blood
    circulation of, 61–62, 62*f*
    deoxygenated, 61–62
    oxygenated, 61
Blood-borne pathogens, 404
Blood pressure
    assessment before, during, and after exercise, 68–69
    in children and adolescents, 301
    diastolic, 67–68, 234–235, 301
    elevated (*See* Hypertension)
    exercise and, 239–240
    in graded intensity exercise, 67–69, 67*f*
    medications affecting, 93, 253, 254*t*, 255–256
    muscular fitness and, 104
    in older adults, 311, 312
    in pregnant women, 305, 307
    regulation of, 68–69, 235
    resting, measurement of, 69*b*
    stress and, 378
    systolic, 67–68, 69, 234–235, 301
Blood vessels, 61–62
BMI. *See* Body mass index
Bodybuilding, resistance training *versus*, 105
Body composition, 200–230
    age and, 201
    bioelectrical impedance analysis of, 209–210
    body mass index of, 201, 202–204, 202*t*, 203*t*
    case study, 226
    children and adolescents, 300–301
    circumference measures of, 204–206, 204*t*, 205*f*, 206*t*
    as component of health-related fitness, 201
    importance of determining, 206
    laboratory measures of, 206, 211–213
    measurement of, 201–213
    older adults, 311
    percentage body fat in, 206–213, 207*t*, 208*t*
    skinfold measurements of, 207–210, 209*t*, 211*t*, 212*f*
    stress associated with testing, 375
    weight management and, 213–225
Body mass index (BMI), 201, 202–204, 236
    calculation of, 202, 203
    chart, 202*t*
    classifications of, 202–203
    disease risk based on, 202–203, 203*t*
    limitations of using, 203–204
    and osteoarthritis, 283
    in pregnancy, 306
    race and, 201, 205
Body-related barriers, to physical activity, 355
Body scan, for stress management, 384
Body size, of children and adolescents, 300–301
Body temperature
    children and adolescents, 302
    cold stress and, 94–95
    heat stress and, 94–95, 302
    obesity and, 302
    older adults, 312–313, 316
    pregnant women, 306, 309

Body weight exercises, 119–121, 120*f*
    for children and adolescents, 304–305
    for older adults, 315
Bone adaptation, 288
Bone growth/maturation, 286–287, 300–301
Bone health, 88, 105, 287–291, 288*t*, 290*t*.
    See also Osteoporosis
Bone mineral density, 266, 285–291
Bone-strengthening exercises, for children and adolescents, 304–305
Borg's Category Ratio Scale, 92
Borg's RPE scale, 92
Boutique fitness studios, 454
Brachial artery pressure, 235, 239
Brachialis, 105, 158*t*
Brachioradialis, 105, 158*t*
Bracing
    abdominal, 185–186, 277
    stabilization in, 179
    teaching, 185–186
    trunk, 185
Bradycardia, 47
Branding, 464, 476
Breach of duty, 400, 400*f*
Breast cancer, physical activity and reduced risk of, 16, 17*t*
Breathing, diaphragmatic, 186–187
    assessment and corrective methods, 186–187
    healthy *versus* altered, 186
    Hi-Lo assessment of, 186, 186*t*
    lifestyle recommendations, 197
    pattern progression for, 186–187, 187*t*
    for stress management, 384
Bridges/bridging
    for core strength, 125
    glute, 188*t*, 189*f*
    side (plank), 185, 188*t*, 190*f*, 191*t*, 278*f*, 279–280
Bronchitis, chronic, 237, 237*f*
Bronchodilators, 256
Brozek equation, 209
Budget(s)
    creating, 461–462
    definition of, 457
    types of, 461
Budgeting, 461–462
    expectations in, 461
    trend-line, 461
    zero-based, 461
Bureaucratic model of management, 428
Burnout, 379
Bursitis, 273
Business
    facility management, 453–457
    facility operations, 455
    financial management, 457–463
    general health fitness management, 436–468
    human resource, 437–449
    leadership and management, 415–435
    legal structure and terminology, 396–414
    marketing, 469–483
    professional behavior and ethics, 484–505
    programming, 466–467
    risk management, 400–403, 449–453
    sales, 466, 478–479
Business interruption insurance, 453
Business liability insurance, 452–453
Business models, 453–454
Business to business (B2B), 477, 478*t*

C

Cachexia, rheumatic, 281
Cadence, in resistance exercise, 127
Caffeine drinks, 224–225
Calcitonin, 289*t*
Calcium, 287, 288*t*, 289*t*
Calcium channel blockers (CCBs), 254*t*, 255
Calf pain (intermittent claudication), 47, 235, 239, 250
Call-to-action-marketing, 464
Calories
    calculating needs for, 216, 216*t*, 219, 220
    definition of, 219
    intake and expenditure of, 213–216
    restricted (dieting), 225
Calorimetry, indirect, 215
Cancer
    physical activity and, 16, 17*t*
    stress and, 376, 378
Cancer Exercise Trainer, ACSM/ACS Certified, 487
Capati v. Crunch Fitness, 492–493
Capillaries, 61–62
Capital, 457
Capital expenses, 462–463
Carbon dioxide, gas exchange of, 61–62
Cardiac events, during exercise testing, 20, 55
Cardiac output
    altitude and, 96
    blood pressure regulation in, 67–68, 235
    cold stress and, 95
    in Fick equation for $\dot{V}O_{2max}$, 66
    in graded intensity exercise, 66–67, 67*f*
    heat stress and, 95
    in older adults, 312
    in pregnant women, 305
Cardiac rehabilitation, 238–241, 244
    concerns, precautions, and contraindications, 247–250, 248*t*
    Pollock and, 8
    risk stratification, 49, 50*t*
Cardiopulmonary resuscitation (CPR), 412, 450*t*–451*t*, 499
Cardiorespiratory fitness (CRF), 60–102
    acclimatization and, 96–97
    altitude and, 94–97
    anatomy and physiology in, 61–64
    assessment of, 70–77
        benefits of, 70
        for healthy populations, 70–75
        interpreting results of, 76–77, 78*t*–79*t*
        selecting appropriate technique of, 71–72
        types of, 70–71, 70*t*
        $\dot{V}O_{2max}$ as gold standard in, 70–71
    case study, 98
    in children and adolescents, 301
    cold stress and, 94–95
    contraindications to training exercises, 93
    CVD and responses during exercise, 246–247
    definition of, 61
    exercises for enhancing, 87–88, 88*t*
    FITT framework for developing, 84–87, 85*t*
    frequency in, 84–85, 85*t*
    graded exercise responses in, 64–69
    guidelines on, 85
    heat stress and, 94–95
    high, benefits associated with, 61
    individual differences in, 87
    intensity in, 84–85, 85*t*, 89–92

Cardiopulmonary resuscitation (CPR)
(continued)
  interval training for, 89
  low, as predictor of disease, 77
  medications affecting, 93
  metabolic calculations for programming, 77–84, 82*f*, 83*t*
  musculoskeletal injuries in exercises, 93–94
  in older adults, 312
  overload in, 86
  oxygen uptake kinetics in
    during graded intensity exercise, 65–66, 66*f*
    sex/age and, 78*t*–79*t*
    during submaximal single-intensity exercise, 64–65, 65*f*
  in pregnant women, 305–306
  progression in, 86–87
  reversibility in, 86–87
  Rockport walking test of, 70*t*, 72
  specificity of training for, 87
  time in, 84–85, 85*t*
  type of activity in, 84–86, 85*t*
  as umbrella term, 70
  volume in, 86
Cardiovascular disease
  ACSM major signs or symptoms of, 46–48
  aerobic training guidelines in, 242*t*
  cardiac rehabilitation in, 238–241, 244
    concerns, precautions, and contraindications, 247–250, 248*t*
    Pollock and, 8
    risk stratification, 49, 50*t*
  cardiorespiratory fitness as predictor of, 77
  case study in, 258–259
  components of, 61–62
  contraindications to exercise testing, 51–53, 51*b*
  controlled, exercise for individuals with, 232–264
  economic costs of, 17
  epidemiology of, 233, 246
  events during exercise testing, 20, 55
  exercise concerns, precautions, and contraindications in, 93, 247–250, 248*t*
  exercise initiation in lieu of graded exercise test in, 249
  exercise prescription and programming in, 244
  exercise responses affected by, 246–247
  exercise role in mediating, 238–240
  FITT considerations in, 242*t*, 244, 243*t*, 257
  known, 46
  medication effects on exercise in, 253–256
  muscular fitness and, 104
  obesity and, 201, 202–203
  in older adults, 311
  PA epidemiology in, 8–9, 8*f*
  pathophysiology of, 233–235
  physical activity and reduced risk of, 15–17, 84
  preparticipation screening for, 29–47
    (*See also* Preparticipation physical activity screening)
  preventive *versus* rehabilitative exercise prescription in, 493–494, 494*t*
  resistance training guidelines in, 243*t*, 244
  rheumatic arthritis and, 281
  risk factors and defining criteria of, 52–53
  stress and, 376, 378
  sudden cardiac death in, 20, 55

  teaching and demonstrating exercises in, 256–257
  weight loss and, 217
Cardiovascular drift, 95
Cardiovascular endurance exercises, 87–88, 88*t*
Cardiovascular system. *See also* Cardiorespiratory fitness; Cardiovascular disease
  altitude and, 94–97
  anatomy and physiology of, 61–64
  in children and adolescents, 301
  cold stress and, 95
  goal/function of, 61, 62*f*
  graded exercise responses of, 64–69
  heat stress and, 95
  medications affecting, 93
  in older adults, 312
  in pregnant women, 305, 307
Career center, 442
Carotid pulse, 68
Case law, 397–398
Case studies
  behavior change, 341–342, 362–366
  cardiorespiratory fitness, 98
  chronic disease, 258–259
  Continuum Performance Center (CPC), 481–482
  flexibility, 170–171
  management, 433
  osteoarthritis, 292–294
  physical activity and health, 22–24
  pregnancy, 317–318
  preparticipation physical activity screening, 54–55
  professional behavior (intern), 502
  resistance training, 130–131
  stress management, 388–389
  weight management, 226
  wellness vision, 22–23
Cash accounting, 458
Cash flow, 457
Cathcart, Jim, 465
CCRB. *See* Committee on Certification and Registry Boards
CDC. *See* Centers for Disease Control and Prevention
CECs. *See* Continuing education credits
Center for Food Safety and Applied Nutrition, 225
Centers for Disease Control and Prevention (CDC)
  Behavioral Risk Factor Surveillance System, 13
  data on physical activity, 12–13, 470–471, 471*f*
  growth chart of, 203
  guidelines on physical activity, 9
Central (abdominal) obesity, 204–205
Certification, ACSM, 485–489, 486*f*
  continuing education credits for, 499, 500*t*
  maintaining, 498–499
Certified Autism Exercise Specialist, 487
Certified Cancer Exercise Trainer (CET), 487
Certified Clinical Exercise Physiologist (ACSM-CEP), 37, 486, 487*t*
Certified Exercise Physiologist (ACSM-EP)
  certification, 485–487, 487*t*
  conflict of interest, 495
  income of, 474
  job task analysis, 490–494
  nutritional role of, 491–492, 493*t*
  personal characteristics of, 499–501

  preventive *versus* rehabilitative practice, 493–494, 494*t*
  scope of practice, 489–494
Certified Group Exercise Instructor (GEI), 486–487, 487*t*
Certified Inclusive Fitness Trainer (CIFT), 487
Certified Personal Trainer (ACSM-CPT), 486–487, 487*t*
Change
  behavior (*See* Behavior change)
  processes of, 331*t*
  stages of, 327–328, 328*t*, 329, 330*b*, 357–358
Charismatic leadership, 419–420
Checkbook accounting, 458
Chest pain, 46, 52
Chest press, 110
Childhood obesity, 14–15, 14*f*, 201, 203, 302–305
Children, 300–305
  age classification of, 300
  body mass index of, 203
  body size and composition of, 300–301
  cardiorespiratory function in, 302
  chronic exercise by, impact of, 302–303
  exercise programming for, 303–304
  motor skills and physical activity in, 302
  muscular strength, flexibility, and motor performance in, 302
  nutrition for, 221*t*
  physical activity and health in, 13–15
  physical activity guidelines for, 11*t*, 12, 13–14
  physical and physiological changes in, 300–302
  recommended activity level for, 303
  thermoregulation in, 302
China, ancient, 7
Chin tucks, 191*t*, 192*f*
Chin-ups, 138
Cholecystokinin, 213
Cholesterol levels, 53, 236
  in coronary artery disease, 233–234
  exercise and, 240
  good *versus* bad, 236
  stress and, 378
Cholesterol-lowering medication, 254*t*, 255
Chronic bronchitis, 237, 237*f*
Chronic conditions, musculoskeletal, 266, 281–294. *See also specific conditions*
Chronic disease
  aerobic training guidelines in, 242*t*
  case study of, 258–259
  controlled, exercise for individuals with, 232–264
  exercise prescription and programming in, 241–246
  exercise responses affected by, 246–247
  exercise role in mediating, 238–241
  FITT considerations in, 241–246, 242*t*, 243*t*, 257
  medication effects on exercise in, 253–256
  pathophysiology of, 233–238
  resistance training guidelines in, 243*t*, 257
  teaching and demonstrating exercises in, 256–257
Chronic health conditions, adults with
  physical activity and health in, 17*t*, 18–19
  physical activity guidelines for, 12, 12*t*
Chronic kidney disease (CKD)
  aerobic training guidelines in, 242*t*
  controlled, exercise for individuals with, 232–264

exercise concerns, precautions, and contraindications in, 252–253
exercise role in mediating, 240–241
FITT considerations in, 242t, 243t, 246
medication effects on exercise in, 253–256
pathophysiology of, 238
resistance training guidelines in, 243t
teaching and demonstrating exercises in, 256–257
Chronic obstructive pulmonary disease (COPD), 237, 237f
exercise concerns, precautions, and contraindications in, 251–252
FITT considerations in, 245
Chronic restrictive pulmonary disease (CRPD), 238, 245, 252
Chronic stress, 372–373, 375–376, 379
Circulation, 61–62, 62f
Circumference measures, 204–206, 204t, 205f, 206t
Civil law, 398–399
Civil Rights Act of 1964, 403, 407–408
CKD. *See* Chronic kidney disease
Clam shell, 188t, 190f, 191t
Claudication, intermittent, 47, 235, 239, 250
Cleanliness, facility, 412
Clearance, medical, 39, 48–49, 108
Client engagement, 358–359
Client referral, 476
Client responsibilities, 406
Client rights, 405
Clinical Exercise Physiologist, certified, 37, 486, 487t
Clinical health/fitness facility settings, 454
Closed kinetic chain exercises, 124
ClubIntel, 464, 466, 467t
CoAES. *See* Committee on the Accreditation for the Exercise Sciences
Cobra stretch, modified, 188t, 189f
"Code Blue," 412
Code of Ethics, ACSM, 485, 489
Code of Ethics, American Fitness Professionals & Associates, 499
Cognition, stress and, 379
Cognitive control, 383
Cognitive processes, in behavioral change, 327–328
Cold acclimatization, 96
Cold and flu medication, 253, 254t
Cold stress, 94–95
Collins, Audrey M., 362–366
Colon cancer, physical activity and reduced risk of, 16, 17t
Commercial general liability, 402
Commission on Accreditation of Allied Health Education Programs (CAAHEP), 486
Committee on Certification and Registry Boards (CCRB), 489, 490
Committee on the Accreditation for the Exercise Sciences (CoAES), 485–486
Common law, 397–398
Communication
and behavior change, 359–360
leadership and, 417
and professional behavior, 499
Community factors, in social ecological model, 334–336, 335f
Companionship, 351
Compensation, 445, 446t
Competence, as psychological need, 338–339
Competencies, in leadership and management, 416

Concentric muscle contraction, 106–107, 118, 124
Confidentiality, 404–405
Conflict of interest, 495
Consciousness raising, 331t
Consent, informed, 37, 38f, 401
Consideration, in leadership, 421
Constitutional law, 397–398
ConsumerLab.com, 225
Contemplation, as stage of change, 327, 328t, 330b, 357
Content marketing, 464
Contextual intelligence, 425–426
definition of, 425
leadership skills associated with, 425, 425t
obstacles and solutions in, 426, 426t
3D-thinking model of, 426
Continuing education credits (CECs), 499, 500t
Continuous-Scale Physical Performance Test, 314
Continuum Performance Center (CPC), 481–482
Contract law, 406
Contractor, independent, 439, 440t
Contraindications
absolute *versus* relative, 52
in cardiovascular disease, 247–250
to cardiovascular training exercises, 93
in chronic diseases, 247–253
definition of, 52
to exercise in pregnancy, 309
to exercise testing, 51–53, 51b
in kidney disease, 252–253
in metabolic disease, 250–251
in pulmonary disease, 251–252
Controlled disease
aerobic training guidelines in, 242t
case study of, 258–259
exercise for individuals with, 232–264
exercise prescription and programming in, 241–246
exercise responses affected by, 246–247
exercise role in mediating, 238–241
FITT considerations in, 241–246, 242t, 243t, 257
medication effects on exercise in, 253–256
pathophysiology of, 233–238
resistance training guidelines in, 243t, 257
teaching and demonstrating exercises in, 256–257
Contusion, 268–269
Conversion factors, 77, 82f
Cooper Institute for Aerobics Research, 8
COPD. *See* Chronic obstructive pulmonary disease
Coping, 373–374. *See also* Stress management
definition of, 373
emotion-focused, 373–374
mind–body techniques for, 383–386
problem-focused, 373–374
transactional model of, 373
Cords, for resistance training, 121
Core exercises, 124–125, 276–281, 278f, 280f
for pregnant women, 306, 308
Core musculature, 124–125, 180, 276, 277t
Coronal (frontal) plane, 114–115, 114f
Coronary artery disease (CAD)
dyslipidemia and, 233–234, 236
exercise concerns, precautions, and contraindications in, 247–250, 248t
exercise initiation in lieu of graded exercise test in, 249
exercise's effect on, 238–239

Morris's study of, 84
obesity and, 202–203
pathophysiology of, 233–234, 234f
stress and, 378
Coronavirus (COVID-19) pandemic
business interruption in, 453
stress response to, 376
Corporate fitness, 454
Corrigan v. Musclemakers, Inc., 400
Corticosteroids
inhaled, 256
injection, exercise after, 273
oral, for arthritis, 284
Cortisol, 375–376, 378–379
Cost of delivery, 474
Cough suppressants, 253
Counterconditioning, 331t
Country-club management, 427
COVID-19 pandemic
business interruption in, 453
stress response to, 376
CPR (cardiopulmonary resuscitation), 412, 450t–451t, 499
C-reactive protein (CRP), 239
Creatine phosphate (CP), 62–64, 64f
Creativity, principle of, 113
Credit reports, 408–409
CRF. *See* Cardiorespiratory fitness
Criminal law, 398
Criterion-referenced standards, 76–77, 78t–79t
Cross-arm stretch, anterior, 140f
CRP. *See* C-reactive protein
CRPD. *See* Chronic restrictive pulmonary disease
Culture, organizational, 437–438, 446
Cumulative adversity, 373
Cureton, T.K., 7–8
Curl-ups, 119, 191t
Current (short-term) assets, 458
Current (short-term) liabilities, 459
Cycle ergometer tests, 70t, 75, 76f, 83–84

D

Dale, Carol Jean, 433
Dancing, 88, 316, 466t
DBP. *See* Diastolic blood pressure
DCER. *See* Dynamic constant external resistance training
Death, sudden cardiac, 20
Decisional control, 383
Decision making
clinical, evidence-based, 496–497
in evidence-based management, 418
in strategic planning, 431–432
Decision tree
preparticipation screening, 42f, 48
scope of practice, 490, 492f
Defendant, 399
Dehydration
heat stress and, 95
in older adults, 312, 316
Delayed-onset muscle soreness (DOMS), 218
Dementia, physical activity and reduced risk of, 17, 17t
Deming, W. Edwards, 428–429
Democratic leadership, 423
Democratic management, 427
Demographics, 470–472
Denosumab, 289t
Deoxygenated blood, 61–62
Depreciation, 457

Depression
    exercise and, 380
    referral to psychologist for, 386
    resistance training and, 104
    stress and, 378–379
Depth jumps, 118–119, 118f
Development, employee, 446–447
DEXA. See Dual-energy x-ray absorptiometry
Diabetes mellitus
    aerobic training guidelines in, 242t
    behavior change in, 328–328
    definition of, 53
    exercise concerns, precautions, and
        contraindications in, 250–251
    exercise prescription and programming in,
        244–245
    exercise role in mediating, 240
    FITT considerations in, 242t, 243t,
        244–245
    foot care in, 245, 250
    lifestyle modifications for, 252
    medical identification for persons with, 245
    medication effects on exercise in, 253,
        255t, 256
    muscular fitness and, 104
    obesity and, 201
    oral medications for, 255t, 256
    pathophysiology of, 236
    physical activity and reduced risk of,
        15–16, 17t, 19
    pregnancy and, 310, 317–318
    resistance training guidelines in, 243t
    risk factor assessment in, 53
    stress and, 378
    Type 1, 236
    Type 2, 236, 244–245, 252, 378
Diagnostic exercise testing, 48, 55
Diagonal PNF stretching, 141, 141f
Diaphragmatic breathing, 186–187
    assessment and corrective methods, 186–187
    healthy versus altered, 186
    Hi-Lo assessment of, 186, 186t
    lifestyle recommendations, 197
    pattern progression for, 186–187, 187t
    for stress management, 384
Diastasis recti abdominis, 306
Diastolic blood pressure (DBP), 67–68,
        234–235
    in children and adolescents, 301
Dietary Guidelines for Americans, 221–222
Dietary supplements, 223t, 224–225, 253, 402,
        492–493
Dietary Supplement Verified U.S.
        Pharmacopeia, 225
Dieting, 225
Digestive disorders, stress and, 376–377
Digitalis, 254t, 255, 256
Dill, D.B., 7
Direct mail, 464, 477
Disabilities, persons with
    legal rights of, 407–408, 452t
    physical activity and health in, 18–19
    physical activity guidelines for, 12, 12t
    trainers certified for working with, 487
Discrepancies, in motivational interviewing,
        361
Discrimination, 403, 407–410, 409
Distributed expenses, 462–463
Diuretics, 254t, 255, 256
Diverse populations, working with, 366–367
Dizziness, 47
Documents, for legal protection, 400–402
Domains of physical activity, 3–4, 3f
DOMS. See Delayed-onset muscle soreness

Double inclinometer, 146, 146f
Double product (rate pressure product), 69
Dowager's hump, 291
Dramatic relief, 331t
Drucker, Peter, 429
Drug-Free Workplace Act of 1988, 409
Drug testing, 408–409
Dual-energy x-ray absorptiometry (DEXA),
        206, 213, 285, 287, 375
Dues, membership, 462
Duty, and negligence, 399–400, 400f
Dynamic constant external resistance training
        (DCER), 116–117, 117f
Dynamic flexibility, 137, 142–143
Dynamic flexibility testing, 145
Dynamic muscle contractions, 3
Dynamic stretching, 108, 139, 142–143
    muscle performance affected by, 137, 169
    recommendations, 154–169
    sports performance affected by, 142–143
Dynamometers, 109, 117
Dyslipidemia, 53, 201, 202–203
    case study of, 258–259
    in coronary artery disease, 233–234, 236
    exercise and, 240
    exercise concerns, precautions, and
        contraindications in, 251
    medications for, exercise effects of, 254t,
        255
    in metabolic syndrome, 237
    pathophysiology of, 236
    stress and, 378
Dyspnea, 47, 245, 251–252

E

Earnings Before Interest, Taxes, Depreciation,
        and Amortization (EBITDA), 457,
        461
Eating pattern, healthy, 221–222
Ebbeling single-stage submaximal treadmill
        walking test, 74
EBITDA (Earnings Before Interest, Taxes,
        Depreciation, and Amortization),
        457, 461
Eccentric loading, for overuse injuries, 274,
        274f
Eccentric muscle action, 106–107, 118, 124,
        267
Ecological model of health behavior, 335
Edema, 269
    ankle, 47
    generalized, 47
Education
    academic preparation, 496, 498
    continuing, 499, 500t
EEOC. See Equal Employment Opportunity
        Commission
EEOC v. Life Time Fitness, Inc., 409–410
Effective listening, 359
EIM (Exercise is Medicine) credential, 487–488
EIMD (exercise-induced muscle damage),
        267, 269
EIM (Exercise is Medicine) promotional
        strategy, 473
Elastic tubing/bands, 117, 119, 121
Elbow, static stretches for, 158f, 158t–159t,
        159f
Elderly. See Older adults
Electronic Physical Activity Readiness
        Medical Examination
        (ePARmed-X+), 32, 48
Electron transport chain, 63–64
Elliptical trainers, 456t

E-mail blasts, 465
E-mail marketing, 477
Emergency policy and procedures, 412,
        449–452
Emotion, and self-efficacy, 330–333, 332t,
        353, 354t
Emotional expectations, 339–340
Emotional intelligence, 424
Emotional regulation, 352–353, 373–374
Emotional support, 351, 380–382
Emotion-focused coping, 373–374
Empathy, 361, 383, 479
Emphysema, 237, 237f
Employee Compensation and Benefits Report
        (IHRSA), 438, 445
Employee referral, 442
Employees
    average number per square feet of facility,
        438t
    background checks for, 408–409
    compensation for, 445, 446t
    drug testing of, 408–409
    exempt versus nonexempt, 441, 441t
    full-time versus part-time, 441–442, 441t
    goals for, 447–448, 448t
    hiring and prehiring inquiries, 407–410
    human resource management, 437–449
    versus independent contractor, 439, 440t
    interview process for, 408
    job descriptions for, 407, 442, 443–444
    orientation, development, and training,
        446–447
    performance appraisals of, 411, 448–449
    performance management of, 411
    positions in fitness facility, 438, 439t
    recruiting, 442–444
    retention of, 449
    rights and responsibilities of, 406–407
    safety for (OSHA), 398, 404, 407, 450t
    selection process for, 442, 444–445
    staffing, 438–442
    workplace safety, 404
Employers. See also Leadership; Management
    rights and responsibilities of, 406–407
Employment laws, federal, 407–410
Endurance
    cardiovascular, 87–88, 88t
    muscular (See Muscular endurance)
Energy
    ATP production for, 62–64, 63f, 64f
    metabolic calculations for, 77–84, 219
Energy balance, 213–217
Energy drinks, 224–225
Energy equivalency chart, 77, 82f
Energy expenditure, 77–84, 213–216, 219, 220
    ACSM metabolic formula for, 82–84, 83t
    estimation, for common physical activities,
        83t
Energy intake, 213, 219, 220
Energy units, 77, 82f
Engagement, client, 358–359
Enjoyment, principle of, 113–114
Enthusiasm, 501
Environment
    in social cognitive theory, 328–329, 331f
    in social ecological model, 334–336, 335f
Environmental barriers, to physical activity,
        354–356, 367
Environmental reevaluation, 331t
ePARmed-X+ Physician Clearance Follow-Up
        Questionnaire, 32, 48
Ephedrine, 253
Epicondylitis, lateral, stretching exercise for,
        275f

Epidemiology, physical activity, 8–9, 8f
EPOC. *See* Excess postexercise oxygen consumption
Equal Employment Opportunity Commission (EEOC), 403, 409–410
Equal Pay Act of 1963, 409
Equipment maintenance, 412, 455, 456t
Equity, 457
Equity, owner's, 459
Ergonomics, 197
Errors and omissions (E&O), 402
Estradiol, and flexibility, 139
Ethics, 485, 489–495
    ACSM code of, 485, 489
    American Fitness Professionals & Associates code of, 499
    conflict of interest, 495
    definition of, 485
    scope of practice, 489–494
Ethics and Professional Conduct Committee, ACSM, 495
Eustress, 373
Eversion, foot, 167f, 167t, 268
Evidence-based clinical decision making (EBCD), 496–497
Evidence-based management, 418
Evidence-based practice
    behavior change, 348
    cardiorespiratory fitness, 61
    definition of, 495
    developing question in, 495, 498
    evaluating evidence in, 496, 498
    flexibility recommendations, 153t
    health behavior, 348
    incorporating evidence in, 496–498, 497f
    nutrition, 221–222
    physical activity as vital sign, 337
    providing information on, 495–498
    searching for evidence in, 496, 498
Excess postexercise oxygen consumption (EPOC), 65, 65f
Exculpatory clause, 401–402
Exempt employees, 441, 441t
Exercise. *See also specific exercises*
    abnormal responses to, 92
    acclimatization and, 96–97
    altitude and, 94–97
    chronic, by children and adolescents, 302–303
    chronic, by older adults, 313
    chronic, by pregnant women, 306–308
    cold stress and, 94–95
    definition of, 4
    for flexibility, 138
    graded intensity (*See* Graded intensity exercise)
    heat stress and, 94–95
    outcomes of, 4, 5f
    physical activity *versus*, 4
    resistance (*See* Resistance training)
    risks associated with, 19–21
    stress experience and, 376
    for stress management, 379–380
    for weight loss (obesity), 217–220, 236
        demonstrating exercises for, 218
        FITT recommendations for, 217–218, 218t
        training considerations in, 218–219
Exercise-induced muscle damage (EIMD), 267, 269
Exercise is Medicine (EIM) credential, 487–488
Exercise is Medicine (EIM) promotional strategy, 473

Exercise physiologist. *See* See ACSM Certified Exercise Physiologist®
Exercise physiology, history of, 7–12
Exercise prescription
    cardiorespiratory fitness, 84–94, 85t
    flexibility training, 153–154
    functional movement, 183–193
    goal setting in, 349
    guidelines on, 485
    history of, 7–8
    incorporating evidence in, 496–498, 497f
    for individuals with cardiovascular disease, 244
    for individuals with controlled diseases, 241–246
    for individuals with musculoskeletal limitations, 266
    interval training, 89
    Pollock and, 8
    for pregnant women, 308
    preventive *versus* rehabilitative, 493–494, 494t
    resistance training, 129
    weight loss, 218–219
Exercise testing
    abnormal responses in, 92
    cardiac events during, 20, 55
    cardiovascular fitness in, 9
    contraindications to, 51–53, 51b
    diagnostic, 48, 55
    exercise initiation in lieu of, 249
    guidelines on, 485
    informed consent for, 37, 38f
    nondiagnostic, 48
    for older adults, 313–314
    preparticipation, 48–49, 55
    stopping, signs for, 92
    submaximal, 48
    supervision criterion of, 49
Exercise Test Technician, 485
Exertion, perceived, 92, 257
    in children and adolescents, 302, 303
    in pregnant women, 308
    stress and, 380
Exertional dyspnea, abnormal, 47
Exhaustion, in stress response, 375–376
Exosystem, 335
Expectations
    affective, 339–340
    budget, 461
    job, 447
    outcome, 348
Expense forecast, 461
Expense management, 462–463
Expenses, 460–463, 460f
Experiential processes, of change, 331t
Extension PNF stretching, 141, 141f
External rotation, band, 191t, 193f
Extreme negligence, 400, 401
Extrinsic motivation, 338–339, 357

F

F as in Fat report, 213
Facebook Business, 464
Facility environment, as barrier to physical activity, 355
Facility management, 436–468, 453–457
Facility operations, 455
Facility policies and procedures, 410–412
Facility responsibilities, to membership, 406, 410–412
Facility settings, 453–454
Fainting (syncope), 47

Fair Credit Reporting Act (FCRA), 408–409
Falls
    aging and, 311
    fractures in, 266–267
    pregnancy and, 306
    prevention of, 290t, 291
Familiarization period, in strength assessment, 108–110
Fascia, 105
Fast-twitch (type II) muscle fibers, 105–106, 311
Fat, muscle *versus*, 219
Fatigue
    injury risk with, 271
    pregnancy and, 309
    as sign/symptom of CMR disease, 48
    stress and, 379
Fat percentage, body, 206–213
    bioelectrical impedance analysis of, 209–210
    in children and adolescents, 301
    laboratory measures of, 206, 211–213
    for men, 206, 207t
    myths about, 219–220
    in older adults, 311
    skinfold measurements of, 207–210, 209t, 211t, 212f
    stress associated with testing, 375
    in weight loss goals, 219
    for women, 206, 208t
Federal laws, 403–405
    employment, 407–410
    HIPAA, 404–405
    OSHA guidelines, 398, 404, 407, 450t
    sexual harassment, 403–404
Feedback, on programming, 467
Feelings (affect)
    expectations, 339–340
    regulation of, 352–353, 373–374
    self-efficacy and, 330–333, 332t, 353, 354t
Female athlete triad, 266, 285, 287
Females
    body fat percentage of, 206, 208t
    cardiorespiratory function in girls, 301
    CRF and maximal aerobic power in, 80t–81t
    flexibility of, 139, 301
    fractures in, 266
    growth of children and adolescents, 300–301
    musculoskeletal injuries in, 266
    osteoporosis in, 285, 286
    physical activity and energy expenditure in, 216
    pregnant (*See* Pregnant women)
    resistance training-related injuries in, 122, 122f
    social ecological model for adolescents, 336b
    waist-to-hip ratio norms for, 206t
Fibrates, 254t, 255
Fick equation, 66
Field tests, of cardiorespiratory fitness, 70t, 71
Fight-or-flight response, 372, 375, 379
Financial liability, 457, 459
Financial management, 457–463
    accounting terminology and principles in, 457–458
    accrual and cash accounting in, 458
    budgeting in, 461–462
    expense management in, 462–463
    financial statements in, 458–461, 459f, 460f
    income management in, 462
Financial statements, 458–461, 459f, 460f
Fingers, static stretches for, 161f, 161t
Fiscal year, 461

Fitbit, 351
Fitness director, 439t, 446t
Fitness instructor, 439t
Fitness Management (Tharrett), 438
Fitness-related income, 462
Fitness testing, stress in, 375
Fitness trends (2019), 471–472
FITT principle
    for cardiorespiratory fitness, 84–87, 85t
    in chronic diseases, 241–246, 242t, 243t, 257
    exercise for weight loss, 217–218, 218t
    in flexibility training, 153–154, 153t
    for interval training, 89
    in low back pain, 279t
    in overuse injuries, 272, 272t, 279t
    in pregnancy, 308–309
    in resistance training, 123–128, 124t
The Five Dysfunctions of a Team (Lencioni),
    437
Five Ps of marketing, 470
Five repetition maximum, 109
Fixed (long-term) assets, 458
Fixed costs, 462–463
Flexibility, 136–174
    activities of daily living, 137
    age and, 139, 311
    anatomical structures and, 138–139, 138f,
        144, 144f
    assessment of, 145–146
        goniometers for, 145–146, 146f,
            147t–152t
        sit-and-reach tests for, 145
    ballistic, 139, 140
    basic principles of, 137–139
    case study of, 170–171
    in children and adolescents, 301
    as component of health-related fitness, 137
    definition of, 137
    dynamic, 108, 137, 139, 142–143, 145,
        154–169
    factors affecting, 137–139
    gender and, 139
    joint specificity *versus* full-body, 137
    muscle properties and, 138
    in older adults, 311, 316
    physical activity/exercise and, 138
    progression in, 153–154
    recommendations/guidelines, 137, 153t,
        154–169
    static, 137, 139, 140f, 155t–168t
    yoga for, 143
Flexibility training
    antibiotics and injury risk in, 154
    for arthritis, 282–283
    ballistic, 139, 140
    dynamic, 108, 137, 139, 142–143, 154–169
    fitness/sports-specific, 154
    FITT principle in, 153–154, 153t
    health impact of, 154
    for low back pain, 279t
    modes of, 139–143, 154, 155t–168t
    for older adults, 316
    PNF, 137, 139, 140–143, 141f
    program design, 153–154
    progression in, 153–154
    recommendations, 153t, 154–169
    resistance, 138
    risks and injuries in, 154, 169
    static stretching, 139, 140f
    for tendinopathies and plantar fasciitis, 272t
    traditional, 139
Flexion PNF stretching, 141, 141f
Floor monitoring, 411

Foam rollers, 196, 196f, 197
Follet, Mary Parker, 430
Food
    dietary guidelines, 221–222, 221t, 222f
    thermic effect of, 214
Food and beverage, revenues from, 462
Foot, static stretches for, 166f, 166t–167t, 167f
Foot care, in diabetes, 245, 250
Foot injuries, 20
Force, muscular, 107, 108f
Force–velocity relationship, 107, 108f
Foresight, 426
Fracture Risk Assessment Tool (FRAX), 287
Fractures, 266–267
Fractures, osteoporotic, 285–291, 286t
Framingham Heart Study, 8
FRAX (Fracture Risk Assessment Tool), 287
Freely moveable (synovial) joints, 138–139,
    138f
Free weights, 116–117, 117f, 119–121, 456t
Frequency
    cardiorespiratory fitness, 84–85, 85t
    exercise for bone health, 288, 290t
    exercise for weight loss, 217–218, 218t
    exercise in chronic diseases, 241–246, 242t,
        243t, 257
    exercise in low back pain, 279t
    exercise in overuse injuries, 272, 272t, 279t
    exercise in pregnancy, 308, 309
    flexibility training, 153–154, 153t
    resistance exercise, 112, 123, 124t, 127–128
Frontal plane, 114–115, 114f
Full-time employees, 441–442, 441t
Functional movement, 175–199
    accommodations for, 176
    age and, 182
    alignment issues in, addressing, 191–193
    assessment and prescription, 183–193
    baseline for, establishing, 183
    capacity, physical activity and, 18
    in children and adolescents, 302
    inhibition of stabilizing muscles and, 180
    instability training for, 193, 194t, 195f
    integrative assessments and corrections in,
        185–193
    joint structure and, 181
    lifestyle recommendations for, 197
    mediators of, 180–182
    mobility in, 177–179
    motor learning in, 176
    neutral position and, 182–184
    in older adults, 182, 312, 314, 316
    overload and, 176, 182
    overweight/obesity and, 180
    physical inactivity and, 180
    posture and, 181
    previous injury/pain and, 180–181
    proprioception in, 176–177, 177f, 177t
    rolling patterns in, 187, 188t, 189f–190f
    sensorimotor control in, 176–180
    sensorimotor system in, 176–177, 178f
    specificity and, 182
    stability in, 177–180
    stretching and self-myofascial release for,
        194–196, 196f, 197t
Functional Movement Screen, 186

G

GAAP (Generally Accepted Accounting
    Principles), 457
Games, for children, 304
GAS. *See* General adaptation syndrome

Gas exchange, 61–62
Gastric ulcers, stress and, 376–377
Gastrocnemius
    eccentric loading of, 274f
    stretching exercise for, 276f
General adaptation syndrome (GAS), 128,
    374–376, 379
Generalized edema, 47
General liability insurance, 402, 452
Generally Accepted Accounting Principles
    (GAAP), 457
General manager, 439t, 446t
Gestational diabetes mellitus, 310, 317–318
GFR. *See* Glomerular filtration rate
Ghrelin, 213
Gleason, Benjamin, 130–131
Glenohumeral joint
    goniometry assessment of, 148f, 148t–149t,
        149f
    stretches for, 156f, 156t–158t, 157f
Glenohumeral stabilization, 178–179
Glomerular filtration rate (GFR), 238, 241
Glucose levels, 250–251. *See also* Diabetes
    mellitus
    exercise and, 240
    pregnancy and, 306, 310, 317–318
    stress and, 378
Glucose metabolism, 62–64
Glute bridge, 188t, 189f, 191t
Gluteus maximus, 106–107, 181
Glycolysis, 62–64, 64f
Goals
    employee, 447–448, 448t
    exercise, setting, 349
    SMART, 349, 429, 432, 432f, 448, 448t
    strategic planning, 431–432, 432f
    weight loss, 217, 219, 224
Golgi tendon organs (GTOs), 142, 143, 144f
Goniometers, 145–146
    components and use of, 146, 146f
    general guidelines for use, 146
    procedures for use, 147t–152t
Good cholesterol, 236
Good Samaritan law, 398
Good stress, 373
Google Ads, 464
Graded exercise test
    diagnostic, 48
    exercise initiation in lieu of, 249
    guidelines on, 485
    nondiagnostic, 48
    preparticipation, 48–49
Graded intensity exercise
    arteriovenous oxygen difference response
        to, 66
    blood pressure in, 67–69, 67f
    cardiac output in, 66–67, 67f
    cardiorespiratory responses to, 64–68
    heart rate in, 66–67, 67f, 68–69
    oxygen uptake kinetics in, 65–66, 66f
    pulmonary ventilation response to, 67
    rate pressure product in, 69
    stroke volume in, 66–67, 67f
"Great man (woman)" theory, 421
Greece, ancient, 7
Grip strength, 109
Gross negligence, 400, 401
Group exercise director, 439t
Group Exercise Instructor (GEI), 439t,
    486–487, 487t
Group mechanisms, in organizational
    behavior, 431
Growth, in children and adolescents, 300–301

GTOs. *See* Golgi tendon organs
Guidelines
  cardiorespiratory fitness, 85
  dietary, 221–222, 221*t*, 222*f*
  exercise in arthritis, 282*t*, 284–285
  exercise in children and adolescents,
    303–305
  exercise in chronic diseases, 242*t*, 243*t*
  exercise in low back pain, 279*t*, 281
  exercise in osteoporosis, 289–291, 290*t*
  exercise in overuse injuries, 272*t*, 279*t*,
    281
  exercise in pregnancy, 308, 309
  facility policies and procedures,
    410–412
  flexibility/ROM, 137, 153*t*, 154–169
  graded exercise testing, 485
  *Health/Fitness Facility Standards and
    Guidelines* (ACSM), 401, 404, 406,
    449, 450*t*–452*t*, 453
  OSHA, 398, 404, 407, 450*t*
  physical activity
    ACSM/AHA, 9–10
    ACSM/CDC, 9
    development of, 9–12
    USDHHS, 10–12
  preparticipation screening, 30, 31, 50–51,
    450*t*
  resistance training, 104, 124*t*
  risk management, 440–452
  weight loss, 217–218
*Guidelines for Graded Exercise Testing and
  Exercise Prescription* (ACSM), 485
Gynoid obesity, 204

H

Hand, static stretches for, 160*f*, 160*t*
Handgrip strength, 109
Harassment, sexual, 403–404, 407
Harris-Benedict equation, 215, 215*t*
Harvard Alumni Health Study, 8
Harvard Fatigue Laboratory, 7
Harvard Step Test, 70*t*
Headaches, stress and, 377–378, 384
Healing process and phases, 269, 270*t*
Health
  body composition and, 201
  flexibility training and, 154
  muscular fitness and, 104–105, 129
  physical activity and, 12–19
    in adults, 15–17, 17*t*
    case studies of, 22–24
    in children and adolescents, 13–15
    epidemiology of, 8–9, 8*f*
    heart/CVD, 8–9, 8*f*, 15–17
    in older adults, 18
  stress and, 372, 376–379, 377*t*
Health belief model, 348
2019 Health Club Consumer Report (IHRSA),
  466
*Health/Fitness Facility Standards and
  Guidelines* (ACSM), 401, 404, 406,
  449, 450*t*–452*t*, 453
Health fitness management, 436–468
  facility, 453–457
  financial, 457–463
  human resources, 437–449
  risk, 449–453
Health Fitness Specialist (HFS), 487
Health History Questionnaire (HHQ), 32, 39,
  40*f*–42*f*
Health information, protected, 404–405

Health Insurance Portability and
  Accountability Act (HIPAA) of 1996,
  404–405
Health-related barriers, to physical activity,
  355
Health-related fitness, 4, 5*f*
  body composition as component of, 201
  flexibility as component of, 137
  muscle fitness as component of, 104
Health risk appraisal, 411. *See also*
  Preparticipation physical activity
  screening
Healthy eating pattern, 221–222
Heart, anatomy and physiology of, 61–62
Heart disease
  cardiac rehabilitation in, 8, 238–241, 244
    concerns, precautions, and
      contraindications, 247–250, 248*t*
    Pollock and, 8
    risk stratification, 49, 50*t*
  economic costs of, 17
  events during exercise testing, 20, 55
  exercise concerns, precautions, and
    contraindications in, 247–250, 248*t*
  exercise prescription and programming
    in, 244
  exercise responses affected by, 246–247
  muscular fitness and, 104
  obesity and, 201, 202–203
  PA epidemiology in, 8–9, 8*f*
  pathophysiology of, 233–234
  physical activity and reduced risk of,
    15–17, 84
  preparticipation screening for, 37
  stress and, 376, 378
  sudden death in, 20, 55
Heart murmurs, 47–48
Heart rate (HR)
  altitude and, 96
  assessment before, during, and after
    exercise, 68–69
  blood pressure regulation in, 235
  in cardiorespiratory assessment, 71
  in children and adolescents, 301
  cold stress and, 95
  in Fick equation for $\dot{V}O_{2max}$, 66
  in graded intensity exercise, 66–67, 67*f*,
    68–69
  heat stress and, 95
  maximum, 90
  medications affecting, 93, 254*t*, 255–256
  in older adults, 312
  peak, 90
  in pregnant women, 305, 307, 308–309
  steady state, 71
  target, 90
Heart rate (HR) drift, 95
Heart rate (HR) monitor, 349
Heart rate reserve (HRR), 90
Heat, and flexibility, 138
Heat acclimatization, 96
Heat stress, 94–95
  in children and adolescents, 302
Hedonic principle, 339
Hedonic psychology, 339
Hedonic theory, 327, 339–340
Height, 202
  of children and adolescents, 300–301
Hematoma, 268–269
Hemoglobin, in children and adolescents, 301
Herbal medicine, 253
Herren, Joey, 402
Herzberg, Fredrick, 429

HHQ. *See* Health History Questionnaire
High altitude, 94–97
High-density lipoproteins (HDLs), 53, 236, 240
High-intensity interval training (HIIT), 89,
  241–242, 244–245, 466*t*, 467*t*
Hill, A. V., 7
Hi-Lo assessment, 186, 186*t*
Hindsight, 426
Hip, flexibility of
  assessment of, 150*f*, 150*t*–152*t*, 151*f*
  static stretches for, 163*f*, 163*t*–164*t*, 164*f*
HIPAA Privacy Rule, 404–405
Hippocrates, 7
Hiring, 442–446. *See also* Human resource
  management
Hiring statutes, 407–410
Hispanic Americans
  obesity in, 201
  participation in physical activity, 367
Historic trends, in physical activity, 7–12
HIV/AIDS, stress effects in, 378
Hold–relax, 142
Hold–relax with agonist contraction, 142
Hold–relax with antagonist contraction, 142
Homeostasis, stress and, 374–376, 379
Horizontal (transverse) plane, 114–115, 114*f*
Hormone replacement therapy (HRT),
  287–288, 289*t*
Hot yoga, avoidance in pregnancy, 306
Household physical activity, 3–4, 3*f*, 6*t*
HR. *See* Heart rate
HRR. *See* Heart rate reserve
Human resource management, 437–449
  compensation in, 445, 446*t*
  employee retention in, 449
  goal setting in, 447–448, 448*t*
  interview process in, 445
  organizational culture and, 437–438, 446
  orientation, development, and training in,
    446–447
  performance management and retention
    in, 447–449
  recruiting in, 442–444
  selection process in, 442, 444–445
  staffing in, 438–442
  teamwork in, 437–438
Hydrocodone + acetaminophen, 270*t*
Hydrostatic (underwater) weighing, 206, 211
Hygiene factors, in management, 429
Hygienic safety, 412
Hyperglycemia, 236, 237
Hyperkyphosis, thoracic, 291
Hypertension
  case study in, 258–259
  in chronic kidney disease, 238, 240
  definition of, 234–235
  economic costs of, 17
  exercise concerns, precautions, and
    contraindications in, 247–250, 248*t*
  exercise responses affected by, 246, 247
  exercise role in mediating, 239–240
  management of, 235
  medications for, exercise effects of, 253,
    255–256
  in metabolic syndrome, 237
  obesity and, 202–203
  in older adults, 311
  pathophysiology of, 234–235
  physical activity and reduced risk of,
    16–17, 17*t*
  in pregnancy, 307
  primary, 235
  risk factor assessment in, 52–53

Hypertension *(continued)*
  secondary, 235
  stress and, 378
Hypertonicity, muscle, 180, 181, 194
Hypertrophy, muscle, 220
Hyperventilation, 186
Hypotension, postural, in pregnancy, 307, 308
Hypothalamic–pituitary–adrenal (HPA) axis, 375
Hypothermia, 95

I

Ibuprofen, 253, 270*t*
IDEA method, 355
IHRSA. *See* International Health, Racquet & Sportsclub Association
Image marketing, 464
Immigration Reform and Control Act of 1986 (IRCA), 409
Immune suppression, stress and, 378
Improvised management, 427
Incentive program, 473
Inclinometers, 145–146, 146*f*
Inclusive Fitness Trainer, ACSM/NCHPAD Certified, 487
Income
  of fitness professionals, 474, 475*f*
  net, 457
Income management, 462
Income statement, 457, 460–461, 460*f*
In-demand programs, 466, 466*t*, 467*t*
Independent contractor, employee *versus*, 439, 440*t*
Indirect calorimetry, 215
Individual characteristics, in organizational behavior, 431
Individual factors
  in social cognitive theory, 328–329, 331*f*
  in social ecological model, 334–336, 335*f*
Individual mechanisms, in organizational behavior, 431
Individual outcomes, in organizational behavior, 431
Inflammation, musculoskeletal, 269–270
Inflammatory bowel disease, stress and, 376–377
Inflammatory phase, of healing, 269, 270*t*
Informational control, 383
Informational support, 351, 382
Informed consent, 37, 38*f*, 401
In-groups, 424
Inherent risk, 400–401
Inhibition
  reciprocal, 143
  stabilizing muscle, 180
Initiating structure, in leadership, 421
Injuries
  acute, 271
  antibiotic use and, 154
  in cardiorespiratory exercise, 93–94
  flexibility training and, 154, 169
  and functional movement, 180–181
  legal issues in, 397 (*See also* Law and legal system)
  limitations from, 266–281
  medications for, 269–270, 270*t*
  musculoskeletal, 20–21, 93–94, 121–123, 266–271
  overuse, 271–281
  resistance training, 121–123, 122*f*
  tissue repair of, 269, 270*t*
  traumatic movement-related, 266–271
Insight, 426

Instability training, 193, 194*t*, 195*f*
Instant Recess program, 330–332
Institute of Medicine (IOM), 215, 225, 306
Institutional factors, in social ecological model, 334–336, 335*f*
Instructor qualifications, 411
Instructor wages and benefits, 446*t*
Instrumental support, 351, 380–382
Insulin, 213, 236, 250–251, 256
Insurance coverage, liability, 402
Integrity, 501
Intelligence
  contextual, 425–426, 425*t*, 426*t*
  emotional, 424
Intensity
  brace, 185–186
  cardiorespiratory fitness, 84–85, 85*t*, 89–92
  determining, 89–92, 257
  exercise for bone health, 290*t*
  exercise for older adults, 315
  exercise for weight loss, 217–218, 218*t*
  exercise in chronic diseases, 241–246, 242*t*, 243*t*, 257
  exercise in low back pain, 279*t*
  exercise in overuse injuries, 272, 272*t*, 279*t*
  exercise in pregnancy, 308, 309
  flexibility training, 153–154, 153*t*
  interval training (HIIT), 89, 241–242, 244–245, 466*t*, 467*t*
  resistance exercise, 123, 124*t*, 125–126
Intentional misconduct, 399
Intentional tort, 399
Intermediate-density lipoprotein (IDL), 236
Intermittent claudication, 47, 235, 239, 250
2018 International Fitness Industry Trend Report—What's All the Rage (ClubIntel), 464, 466, 467*t*
International Health, Racquet & Sportsclub Association (IHRSA)
  on blood-borne pathogens, 404
  on business models, 453–454
  on fitness trends, 472
  2018 Profiles of Success, 438, 442, 462
  on program trends, 466, 466*t*
  Standards Facilitation Guide, 406
International Organization for Standardization (ISO), 488
Internet marketing, 464, 477
Internship programs, 442, 502
Interval training, 89, 241–242, 244–245, 466*t*, 467*t*
Interviewing
  job candidate, 408, 445
  motivational, 339, 359, 360–361
Intrinsic motivation, 338–339, 356, 357
Inversion, foot, 167*f*, 167*t*, 268
Irritable bowel syndrome, stress and, 376–377
Ischemia
  arterial (intermittent claudication), 47, 235, 239, 250
  myocardial, 233–234, 239, 244, 246–248
Ischemic threshold, 239, 244, 246–248
ISO (International Organization for Standardization), 488
Isokinetics, 117–118
Isometric muscle contractions, 107, 124
Isometric stretching, 139
Isotonic muscle contractions, 116

J

Janda, Vladimir, 180
Jerk lifts, 125

Jewish Community Center, 453
Job descriptions, 407, 442, 443–444
Job postings, 444
Job responsibilities, 447
Jobs, in fitness industry, 438, 439*t*
Jobs, Steve, 438
Job task analysis (JTA), 490–494
Jogging
  advantages and disadvantages of, 88*t*
  cardiorespiratory fitness in, 88
  MET values of, 6*t*
  musculoskeletal injuries in, 20–21
  weight loss in, 217
Joints
  freely moveable (synovial), 138–139, 138*f*
  goniometry assessment of, 145–146, 146*f*, 147*t*–152*t*
  inflammation of, 281–283
  pregnancy and, 306
  range of motion, 137–139
  structure of, and functional movement, 181
JTA. *See* Job task analysis
Jumping, plyometric training, 118–119, 118*f*

K

Kabat, Herman, 140
Karvonen method, 90
Kidney disease
  ACSM major signs or symptoms of, 46–48
  aerobic training guidelines in, 242*t*
  chronic, pathophysiology of, 238
  controlled, exercise for individuals with, 232–264
  exercise concerns, precautions, and contraindications in, 252–253
  exercise prescription and programming in, 246
  exercise role in mediating, 240–241
  FITT considerations in, 242*t*, 243*t*, 246
  known, 46
  medication effects on exercise in, 253–256
  preparticipation screening for, 29–47 (*See also* Preparticipation physical activity screening)
  resistance training guidelines in, 243*t*
  teaching and demonstrating exercises in, 256–257
Kilocalorie, 77, 219. *See also* Calories
Knee, static stretches for, 165*f*, 165*t*
Knee injuries, 20
Knott, Margaret, 140
Knowledge, research, 496
Knowledge and skill statements (KSs), 490–494
Krebs cycle, 63–64
KSs. *See* Knowledge and skill statements

L

Lactate/lactic acid, 63, 65, 312, 380, 385
Laissez-faire leadership, 423
Lateral band walks, 188*t*, 190*f*, 191*t*
Lateral epicondylitis, stretching exercise for, 275*f*
Lat pull-down, 119, 120*f*
Lat pull-up, 119, 120*f*
Lat stretch, 140*f*
Law and legal system, 396–414
  background checks, 408–409
  civil law, 398–399
  client responsibilities, 406
  client rights, 405

contract law, 406
criminal law, 398
drug testing, 408–409
employer and employee rights and
    responsibilities, 406–407
employment laws, 407–410
facility policies and procedures, 410–412
federal laws, 403–405
HIPAA Privacy Rule, 404–405
knowledge about, need for, 397
liability insurance, 402–403
negligence, 397, 399–402
OSHA guidelines, 398, 404, 407, 450t
primary sources of law, 397–403
risk management of liability, 400–403,
    449–453
sexual harassment, 403–404, 407
standard of care, 397, 398f, 399–400, 411
STEPS for avoiding liability, 397, 398f
tort law, 399
waiver/exculpatory clause, 400–402
LBP. *See* Low back pain
Leader–member exchange (LMX) theory, 424
Leadership, 415–426
    autocratic, 423, 428
    behaviors in, 421
    charismatic, 419–420
    classical model of, 419, 420
    competencies in, 416
    consideration in, 421
    construct of, 416
    contextual intelligence and, 425–426, 425t,
        426t
    democratic, 423
    emotional intelligence in, 424
    evolution and mixing of theories and
        models, 420–421
    as industry/professional standard, 416
    initiating structure in, 421
    intended outcome of, 417
    laissez-faire, 423
    Lewin's styles of, 423
    management integration with, 417, 417f
    management *versus*, 416–417, 418t
    operational definition of, 416–417
    organic model of, 420
    organizational behavior and, 431–432
    path–goal theory of, 422
    servant, 423
    situational, 421–422, 422f
    strategic planning in, 431–432, 432f
    theories of, 419–426
    trait theory of, 421
    transactional, 419, 422–423
    transformational, 419–420, 422–423
    visionary model of, 419–420
Leadership development, 420
Leads, in sales, 478–479
Legal system. *See* Law and legal system
Leg cycling, energy expenditure during,
    83t
Leg press, 110
Leisure-time physical activity, 6t, 9, 9f, 12–13,
    13f, 16f
Lencioni, Patrick, 437
Leptin, 213
Lewin, Kurt, 423
Liabilities, financial, 457, 459
Liability, legal, 397–403
    Good Samaritan law and, 398
    negligence and, 399–402
    risk management of, 400–403, 449–453
    STEPS for avoiding, 397, 398f

tort law on, 399
waiver/exculpatory clause and,
    400–402
Liability insurance, 402–403, 452–453
Lifespan. *See also* Adolescents; Children;
    Older adults
    exercise across, 299–323
    physical and physiological changes across,
        300
Lifestyle
    and diabetes mellitus, 252
    and functional movement, 197
    and health in older adults, 310–311
Ligament sprains. *See* Sprains
Light physical activity, 6t
Linear model of periodization, 128
Linear PNF stretching, 141f
Lipoprotein(a), 236
Lipoproteins, 53, 233, 236, 240, 378
Liquidity, 457
Listening, 359, 466
Lite, Randi, 502
LMX. *See* Leader–member exchange (LMX)
    theory
Load, in resistance training, 111–112, 115,
    125–126
Low back pain (LBP), 275–281
    assessment of, 276
    causes of, 275–276
    clinical presentation of, 276
    core musculature and, 276, 277t
    epidemiology of, 275
    exercise guidelines for, 279t, 281
    pregnancy and, 306, 307
    safe and effective exercises for, 276–281,
        278f, 280f
Low-density lipoproteins (LDLs), 53, 233,
    236, 240
Lower body
    goniometry assessment of, 150f, 150t–152t,
        151f
    static stretches for, 163t–168t
Low-volume interval training (LVIT), 89
Lumbar extension, goniometry assessment of,
    147f, 147t
Lumbar flexion, goniometry assessment of,
    147f, 147t
Lung disease. *See* Pulmonary disease
Lunge with hand weight, 280, 280f
Lung function. *See* Respiratory system
LVIT. *See* Low-volume interval training

M

Macrocycle, 128
Macronutrients, recommended proportions
    of, 221t
Macrotraumatic injuries, 266
Mail, promotion via, 464, 477
Maintenance, as stage of change, 327, 328t, 330b
Maintenance, equipment, 412, 455, 456t
Malcolm, Lydia, 388–389
Males
    body fat percentage of, 206, 207t
    CRF and maximal aerobic power in, 78t–79t
    flexibility of, 139
    fractures in, 266
    growth of children and adolescents, 300–301
    physical activity and energy expenditure
        in, 216
    resistance training-related injuries in, 122,
        122f
    waist-to-hip ratio norms for, 206t

Management, 415–418, 427–433
    authoritarian, 427
    behavioral model of, 430
    bureaucratic model of, 428
    case studies of, 433
    competencies in, 416
    country-club, 427
    evidence-based, 418
    facility, 453–457
    financial, 457–463
    health fitness, general, 436–468
    human resource, 437–449
    improvised, 427
    intended outcome of, 417
    leadership integration with, 417, 417f
    leadership *versus*, 416–417, 418t
    middle-of-the-road, 427
    motivator-hygiene theory of, 429
    operational definition of, 416–417
    organizational behavior and, 431–432
    performance, 447–449
    risk, 400–403, 449–453
    scientific, 427–428
    strategic planning in, 431–432, 432f
    team or democratic, 427
    techniques of, 427–430
    Theory X and Theory Y, 430
    total quality, 428–429
Management by objective (MBO), 429
Management grid, 427
Mantra meditation, 385
MAP (mean arterial pressure), 68
Marketing, 463–466, 469–483
    art of the deal in, 479
    call-to-action, 464
    content, 464
    Continuum Performance Center (CPC),
        481–482
    cost-benefit breakdown of tools, 478t
    five Ps of, 470
    image or brand, 464
    incentive program in, 473
    people (demographics) in, 470–472
    personal sales in, 478–479
    place in, 472–474
    price in, 474–475, 475f
    product in, 472
    promotion in, 464–465, 467, 475–480
    public relations in, 479–480
    tools for, 464–465
Market value, 474
Martial arts, for stress management, 386
Massage, 385
Master of Science in Applied Physiology,
    486
Master of Science in Clinical Exercise
    Physiology, 486
Mastery experience, and self-efficacy,
    330–333, 332t, 353, 354t
Maximal oxygen uptake ($\dot{V}O_{2max}$), 65–66,
    70–71, 70t, 78t–79t
MBO (management by objective), 429
McArdle Step Test, 70t
McClaran, Steve, 341–342
McGill, Stuart, 185
McGill Pain Scale, 276
McGregor, Douglas, 430
Mean arterial pressure (MAP), 68
Measurable goals, 349
Mechanoreceptors, 176
Medical emergencies, 412, 449–452
Medical examination/clearance,
    39, 48–49

Medications
 for arthritis, 284
 common, mechanics and rest/exercise
  response, 254*t*–255*t*
 effects on cardiorespiratory fitness, 93
 effects on exercise in chronic (controlled)
  diseases, 253–256
 interactions of, 253
 for musculoskeletal injuries, 269–270, 270*t*
 for osteoporosis, 287–288, 289*t*
Medicine balls, 116, 121, 121*f*
Meditation, 385
"Member down," 412
Membership dues, 462
Men. *See* Males
Menopause, and bone density, 286
Mental health
 exercise and, 380
 referral to psychologist, 386, 386*t*
 stress and, 376, 378–379
Mesocycle, 128
Mesosystem, 335
Metabolic calculations, 77–84
 ACSM metabolic formula for, 82–84, 83*t*,
  219
 energy units and conversion factors in,
  77, 82*f*
 for weight loss, 219
Metabolic disease
 ACSM major signs or symptoms of, 46–48
 aerobic training guidelines in, 242*t*
 controlled, exercise for individuals with,
  232–264
 exercise concerns, precautions, and
  contraindications in, 250–251
 exercise prescription and programming in,
  244–245
 exercise role in mediating, 240
 FITT considerations in, 242*t*, 243*t*,
  244–245
 known, 46
 medication effects on exercise in, 253–256
 pathophysiology of, 235–237
 preparticipation screening for, 29–47 (*See
  also* Preparticipation physical activity
  screening)
 resistance training guidelines in, 243*t*
 stress and, 378
 teaching and demonstrating exercises in,
  256–257
Metabolic equations, 6*t*, 219, 220
Metabolic equivalents (METs), 4, 77, 82*f*,
 83, 91
Metabolic pathways, for ATP production,
 62–64, 63*f*, 64*f*
Metabolic syndrome, 237, 240
Metabolism, 213–216
 in children and adolescents, 301
 in pregnant women, 306
METs. *See* Metabolic equivalents
Mexican Americans, obesity in, 201
MI. *See* Motivational interviewing;
 Myocardial infarction
Microcycle, 128
Microsystem, 335
Microtrauma, 267
Middle-of-the-road management, 427
Mifflin-St. Jeor equation, 215, 215*t*
Migraines, 377
Mind–body techniques, for stress reduction,
 383–386
Mindfulness, 385
Misconduct, intentional, 399

Mission statements, 432, 432*f*, 446
Mitochondria, 63
Mobility, 177–179. *See also* Functional
  movement
 age and, 182, 311
 assessment and prescription, 183–193
 lifestyle recommendations for, 197
 mediators of, 177, 180–182
 mobilizing muscles in, 179, 179*t*
 physical activity and, 137
Mobilizing muscles, 179, 179*t*
Model, 327. *See also specific models*
Moderate physical activity, 4, 6*t*, 9
 for older adults, 315
Modified cobra stretch, 188*t*, 189*f*
Monitors, physical activity, 349, 351
Morris, Jeremy, 84
Motivation. *See also* Behavior change
 client's engagement scale in, 358–359
 communication and, 359–360
 continuum of, 338–339, 357
 emotional regulation and, 352–353
 exercise physiologist and, 357–359
 extrinsic, 338–339, 357
 intrinsic, 338–339, 356, 357
 lack of, as barrier to physical activity, 354
 leadership and, 416
 in self-determination theory, 338–339
 in social ecological model, 335–336
 in theory of planned behavior, 337
 Theory X and Theory Y, 430
Motivational interviewing (MI), 339, 359,
 360–366
Motivator-hygiene theory, 429
Motor learning, 176
Motor skills, of children and adolescents, 302
Motor unit, 106, 106*f*
Movement, functional. *See* Functional
 movement
MTU (muscle-tendon unit), 267–268, 267*t*
Multiple-joint exercise, 119, 120*f*, 124
Multiple sclerosis, stress and, 378
Multipurpose facilities, 453
Muscle(s)
 aging and, 311
 agonist, 105, 181
 antagonist, 105, 143, 181
 contractions of, 3, 105, 106–107, 124, 137,
  142
 core, 124–125, 180, 276, 277*t*
 everyday posture and, 181
 fat *versus*, 219
 flexibility properties of, 138
 flexibility/stretching and performance of,
  137, 169, 194
 force produced by, 107, 108*f*
 force–velocity relationship, 107, 108*f*
 hypertonicity of, 180, 181, 194
 hypertrophy of, 220
 mobilizing, 179, 179*t*
 respiratory, 186–187
 stabilizing, 179–180, 179*t*, 191*t*, 276, 277*t*
  alignment faults and, 191–193, 191*t*
  corrective exercises for, 191–192, 191*t*,
   192*f*–193*f*
  propensity of inhibition, 180
 structure and function of, 105–107
 synergist, 105, 181
 types of action, 106–107
Muscle fibers, 105–106, 144, 144*f*, 311
Muscle mass, loss of, 201
Muscle relaxation, progressive, 384
Muscle soreness, delayed-onset, 218

Muscle spindles, 144, 144*f*
Muscle-tendon unit (MTU), 267–268, 267*t*
Muscular endurance
 aging and, 311
 assessment of, 110–111, 110*f*, 112
 development of, 104
Muscular fitness, 103–135. *See also* Resistance
  training
 anatomic considerations in, 105–107
 assessment of, 108–111
  absolute and relative values in, 108
  data from, 108
  endurance, 110–111, 110*f*, 112
  medical clearance for, 108
  specificity of tests, 108
  strength, 109–110
 as component of health-related fitness, 104
 guidelines on, 104
 health impact of, 104–105, 129
Muscular strength
 aging and, 311
 assessment of, 109–110
  familiarization period in, 108–110
  one repetition maximum (1-RM) in,
   109–110
 in children and adolescents, 301, 303–304
 development of, 104
 interventions for, 115–123
 in older adults, strengthening of, 315
Musculoskeletal injuries
 acute, 271
 antibiotic use and, 154
 in cardiorespiratory exercise, 93–94
 exercise to reduce risk of, 270–271
 flexibility training and, 154, 169
 healing process in, 269, 270*t*
 immediate care for, 269
 limitations from, 266–281
 medical referral for, 266
 medications for, 269–270, 270*t*
 overuse, 271–281
 prevention of, 21
 PRICE treatment for, 267*t*, 268*t*, 269
 in resistance training, 121–123, 122*f*
 risk of, 20–21, 93–94
 traumatic movement-related, 266–271
Musculoskeletal limitations
 case study of, 292–294
 chronic conditions and, 266, 281–294
 discharge considerations for, 266
 exercise for individuals with, 265–298
 exercise prescription and programming
  for, 266
 overuse injuries and, 271–281
 safety considerations for, 266
 traumatic movement-related injuries and,
  266–271
M$\dot{V}O_2$ (myocardial oxygen demand), 69
Myocardial infarction (MI). *See also*
 Cardiovascular disease
 exercise after, 238–239, 244, 247
 exercise responses affected by, 246–247
 medications for, exercise effects of, 255
 pathophysiology of, 234
 physical activity and reduced risk of, 18
 stress and, 376, 378
 sudden death in, 20
Myocardial ischemia, 233–234, 239, 244,
 246–248
Myocardial oxygen demand (M$\dot{V}O_2$), 69
Myofascia
 SMR for, 194–196, 196*f*, 197*t*
 triggers points within, 194–196

Myofibril, 105
Myotatic reflex, 143
MyPlate, 222, 222f
Myths, weight management, 219–220

N

Naproxen, 253, 270t
National Academy of Sciences, 495
National Center for Complementary and
    Alternative Medicine, 225
National Commission for Certifying Agencies
    (NCCA), 488–489
National Health and Nutrition Examination
    Survey (NHANES), 13, 14
National Institute of Mental Health (NIMH),
    387t
Natural killer cells, stress and, 378
Natural remedies, 253
NCCA. *See* National Commission for
    Certifying Agencies
Neck, static stretches for, 155f, 155t
Negative energy balance, 213
Negligence, 397, 399–402
    definition of, 397, 399, 400
    elements of, 397, 399–400, 400f
    extreme or gross, 400, 401
    liability insurance and, 402–403, 452–453
    risk management of liability, 400–403
    tort law on, 399
    waiver/exculpatory clause and, 400–402
Negligent conduct, 399
Net income, 457
Neuromotor exercises
    for arthritis, 284
    for older adults, 316
    for strains and sprains, 271
Neuropeptide Y, 213
Neutral position, 182–184
    definition of, 182
    progressive stages for, 183–184, 185t
    static, assessment of, 183–184, 184t
News releases, 480
NHANES. *See* National Health and Nutrition
    Examination Survey
Niacin, 255
NIMH (National Institute of Mental Health),
    387t
"No fault" conduct, 399
Nonclinical health/fitness facility settings,
    454–455
Noncurrent (long-term) liabilities, 459
Nondiagnostic exercise testing, 48
Nonexempt employees, 441, 441t
Nonexercise activity thermogenesis (NEAT),
    214
Nonlinear model of periodization, 128
Nonsteroidal anti-inflammatory drugs
    (NSAIDs)
    for arthritis, 284
    precautions in chronic diseases, 253, 255t
    for traumatic musculoskeletal injuries, 270t
Non–weight-bearing exercises, 88
Normative standards, 77, 78t, 78t–79t
Not-for-profit facilities, 453
NSAIDs. *See* Nonsteroidal anti-inflammatory
    drugs
Nutrition
    in adolescents, 221t
    for bone health, 287, 288t
    in children, 221t
    dietary guidelines on, 221–222, 221t, 222f
    EP role in, 491–492, 493t

obesity treatment through, 221–222
in pregnancy, 309

O

OA. *See* Osteoarthritis
Obesity
    adolescent, 14–15, 14f, 201, 203, 302–305
    behavioral strategies for, 224
    BMI classification of, 201, 202–203
    cardiovascular risk assessment in, 52–53
    case study, 226
    causes of, 213, 236
    central (abdominal), 204–205
    childhood, 14–15, 14f, 201, 203, 302–305
    definition of, 236
    and diabetes mellitus, 201
    exercise concerns, precautions, and
        contraindications in, 251
    exercise interventions for, 217–220, 236
        demonstrating exercises for, 218
        FITT recommendations for, 217–218,
            218t
        training considerations in, 218–219
    and functional movement, 180
    gynoid, 204
    inappropriate weight loss methods for,
        223, 223t
    increase in physical activity in, 16
    medical conditions associated with, 201,
        202–203, 236
    in metabolic syndrome, 237
    nutrition (diet) for, 221–222
    osteoarthritis with, 283
    pathophysiology of, 236
    pregnancy and, 310
    prevalence of, 201
    race and, 201
    surgery for, 223–224
    and thermoregulation, 302
    treatment of, 217–225
    weight management and, 213–225
Objective(s)
    in Exercise is Medicine, 473
    management by, 429
    strategic planning, 431–432, 432f
Occupational exposure, 404
Occupational physical activity, 3–4, 3f, 6t
Occupational Safety and Health
    Administration (OSHA), 398, 404,
        407, 450t
Occupational stress, exercise and, 380
Office for Civil Rights, 404–405
Office of Dietary Supplements, 224
Older adults, 310–316
    aerobic activity for, 315
    body composition of, 311
    cardiorespiratory fitness in, 312
    chronic exercise by, impact of, 313
    definition of, 300
    exercise programming for, 313–316
    exercise testing for, 313–314
    flexibility of, 311, 316
    functional movement of, 182
    lifestyle and healthy behaviors of,
        310–311
    moderate *versus* vigorous intensity for,
        315
    muscle-strengthening activity for, 315
    musculoskeletal function of, 311
    neuromotor exercises for, 316
    physical activity and health in, 18, 312,
        313, 366–367

physical activity guidelines for, 11t, 12
physical and physiological changes in,
    311–313
preparticipation screening of, 313
resistance training for, 315
thermoregulation in, 312–313, 316
working with, 366–367
OMNI scale, 302
1.5-mile run test, 70t, 78t–79t
One repetition maximum (1-RM), 109–110,
    126
Open-circuit spirometry, 70–71, 70t, 82
Open kinetic chain exercises, 124
Operating expenses, 462–463
Operations, facility, 455
Options, for physical activity, 356
Order of exercise, in resistance training, 125
Organic model, of leadership, 420
Organizational behavior, 431–432
Organizational culture, 437–438, 446
Organizational mechanisms, 431
Organizational structure, 446
Orientation
    employee, 446–447
    fitness facility, 411
Orthopnea, 47
OSHA. *See* Occupational Safety and Health
    Administration
Osteoarthritis (OA), 283–285
    assessment of, 283
    case study of, 292–294
    clinical presentation of, 283
    exercise guidelines for, 282t, 284–285
    medication effects for, 284
    obesity and, 283
    physical activity and, 17t, 18, 19
    safe and effective exercise in, 283, 284f
    yoga for, 143
Osteopenia, 285, 287
Osteoporosis, 285–291
    assessment of, 287
    clinical presentation of, 287
    epidemiology of, 285
    exercise guidelines for, 289–291, 290t
    in female athlete triad, 286, 287
    medications for, 287–288, 289t
    nutrition and, 287, 288t
    physical activity and, 18
    primary, 285
    resistance training and, 105, 289
    risk factors for, 285–287, 286t
    safe and effective exercise in, 288–291
    secondary, 285
    whole-body vibration for, 291
Oswestry Low Back Pain Scale, 276
Otto, Stephanie Marie, 170–171
Outcome expectations, 348
Out-groups, 424
Overload
    in cardiorespiratory fitness, 86
    context for principle of, 182
    in flexibility training, 153
    functional movement and, 176, 182
    in resistance training, 113, 182
Over-the-counter (OTC) drugs, 253
    for musculoskeletal injuries, 270, 270t
Overuse injuries, 271–281
    acute injuries *versus*, 271
    exercise guidelines for, 272t, 281
    medications for, 269–270, 270t
    prevention of, 271
    safe and effective exercises for, 272, 273,
        274–281, 274f–276f, 278f, 280f

Overweight, 201, 202–203. *See also* Obesity
  and functional movement, 180
Owner's equity, 459
Oxidative system, 62–64, 64*f*
Oxygen
  arteriovenous difference response to
      graded intensity exercise, 66
  gas exchange of, 61–62
  partial pressure of, 95–96
  supplemental, availability of, 412
  transport in blood, 61–62, 62*f*
  uptake kinetics
      during graded intensity exercise, 65–66,
          66*f*
      sex/age and, 78*t*–79*t*
      during submaximal single-intensity
          exercise, 64–65, 65*f*
Oxygenated blood, 61
Oxygen consumption (aerobic capacity),
      64–66
  in children and adolescents, 301
  cold stress and, 95
  excess postexercise, 65, 65*f*
  maximal ($\dot{V}O_{2max}$), 65–66, 70–71, 70*t*,
      78*t*–79*t*
  myocardial, 69
  in older adults, 312
  peak, 90–91
  in pregnant women, 306
  relative and absolute, 77
  reserve $\dot{V}O_2$, intensity measurement via, 91
  sex/age and, 78*t*–79*t*
  steady state, 64–65, 65*f*
  submaximal, 64–65, 65*f*, 70*t*, 71
Oxygen debt, 65, 66*f*
Oxygen deficit, 64–65, 65*f*, 66*f*

P

P(s), five, of marketing, 470
PA. *See* Physical activity
PAD. *See* Peripheral artery disease
*2018 PAG (Physical Activity Guidelines for
      Americans)*, 10–12, 11*t*–12*t*, 19*t*, 85,
      104
Pain
  calf (intermittent claudication), 47, 235,
      239, 250
  and functional movement, 180–181
  low back, 275–281, 306, 307
  musculoskeletal, medications for, 269–270,
      270*t*
  as sign/symptom of CMR disease, 46
Palpitations, 47
Panic disorder, exercise and, 380
Parathyroid hormone (PTH), 289*t*
PARmed-X, electronic (ePARmed-X+), 32,
      48
PARmed-X for Pregnancy, 308
Paroxysmal nocturnal dyspnea, 47
PAR-Q+ (Physical Activity Readiness
      Questionnaire for Everyone), 32,
      33*f*–36*f*, 71, 266, 411
Partial pressure of oxygen (PO$_2$), 95–96
Part-time employees, 441–442, 441*t*
Passive stretch, 139
Path–goal leadership theory, 422
Pathogens, blood-borne, 404
Peak heart rate, 90
Peak METs, 91
Peak $\dot{V}O_2$ method, 90–91
Pectoral wall stretch, 140*f*
Pederson, Gregory, 401

Pedometers, 349, 351
Pelvic floor muscles/training, 180, 279, 306,
      308
People, in marketing mix, 470–472
Peptide YY, 213
Perceived barriers, to physical activity, 354,
      356
Perceived exertion, 92, 257
  in children and adolescents, 302, 303
  in pregnant women, 308
  stress and, 380
Perceived Stress Scale (PSS-10), 381–382
Percentage body fat, 206–213
  bioelectrical impedance analysis of,
      209–210
  in children and adolescents, 301
  laboratory measures of, 206, 211–213
  for men, 206, 207*t*
  myths about, 219–220
  in older adults, 311
  skinfold measurements of, 207–210, 209*t*,
      211*t*, 212*f*
  stress associated with testing, 375
  in weight loss goals, 219
  for women, 206, 208*t*
Performance appraisals, 411, 448–449
Performance management, 447–449
Performance-related fitness, 4
Periodization, 106, 128, 271
Peripheral artery disease (PAD)
  aerobic training guidelines in, 242*t*
  exercise concerns, precautions, and
      contraindications in, 247–250, 248*t*
  exercise's effect on, 239
  pathophysiology of, 235
  resistance training guidelines in, 243*t*
Peripheral resistance, 67–68
Personal characteristics, of EP, 499–501
Personal contact, marketing via, 478*t*
Personal experience, as evidence, 496, 498
Personal sales, 478–479
  art of the deal, 479
  finding leads in, 478–479
  qualifying prospects in, 479
Personal Trainer®, ACSM Certified, 486–487,
      487*t*
Personal training director, 439*t*
Pew Health Professions Commission, 416
Physical activity (PA)
  adults reporting no leisure-time PA, 9, 9*f*
  aerobic, 3
  anaerobic, 3
  ancient times and teachings, 7
  and arthritis, 284–285
  barriers to, 4–5, 7*t*, 354–356, 366–367
  in children and adolescents, 302–305,
      303–305
      impact of chronic exercise, 302–303
      motor skills and, 302
  data on, 12–13, 13*f*, 470–471, 471*f*
  defining, 3–5
  epidemiology of, 8–9, 8*f*
  exercise *versus*, 4
  flexibility effects of, 138
  guidelines and recommendations
      ACSM/AHA, 9–10
      ACSM/CDC, 9
      development of, 9–12
      USDHHS, 10–12
  health impact of, 12–19
      in adults, 15–17, 17*t*
      case studies of, 22–24
      in children and adolescents, 13–15

heart/CVD, 8–9, 8*f*, 15–17, 84
  in older adults, 18
historic trends in, 7–12
history, in preparticipation screening, 46
household, 3–4, 3*f*, 6*t*
identifying benefits of, 348
leisure-time, 6*t*, 9, 9*f*, 12–13, 13*f*, 16*f*
light, moderate, and vigorous, 4, 6*t*
MET values of, 4, 6*t*
occupational, 3–4, 3*f*, 6*t*
outcomes of, 4, 5*f*
preparticipation screening for, 29–57, 108
promoting, 4
recreational, 3–4, 3*f*
risks associated with, 19–21, 19*t*
situational context of, 3–4, 3*f*
thermic effect of, 214
transportation-related, 3–4, 3*f*
as vital sign, 337
weight loss through, 217–220
Physical Activity and Health (U.S. Surgeon
      General), 9, 31
*Physical Activity Guidelines Advisory
      Committee Scientific Report* (2018),
      10
Physical Activity Guidelines for Americans,
      10–12, 11*t*–12*t*, 19*t*, 85, 104
Physical Activity in Public Health Specialist
      (PAPHS), 487
Physical activity level (PAL), 214–216
Physical activity monitors, 349, 351
Physical Activity Readiness Medical
      Examination, electronic
      (ePARmed-X+), 32, 48
Physical Activity Readiness Medical
      Examination for Pregnancy
      (PARmed-X for Pregnancy), 308
Physical Activity Readiness Questionnaire for
      Everyone (PAR-Q+), 32, 33*f*–36*f*, 71,
      266, 411
Physical fitness
  components of, 4, 5*f*
  definition of, 4
  as outcome, 4, 5*f*
Physical fitness movement, 7–8
Physical inactivity, 4
  data on, 12–13, 13*f*, 470–471, 471*f*
  and functional movement, 180
  health impact of, 15–16, 15*f*
  and obesity, 213
  and osteoporosis, 291
Physician Clearance Follow-Up
      Questionnaire, 32, 48
Physiological feedback, and self-efficacy,
      330–333, 332*t*, 353, 354*t*
Physique anxiety, 355
PICO format, for evidence, 497
Pilates, for pregnant women, 307–308
Place, in marketing mix, 472–474
Plaintiff, 399
Planks, 125
Planks, side, 185, 188*t*, 190*f*, 278*f*, 279–280
Planned behavior, theory of, 327, 337–338, 338*f*
Planning, strategic, 431–432, 432*f*
Plantar fasciitis, 273–274
  assessment of, 273
  clinical presentation of, 273
  exercise guidelines for, 272*t*
  management of, 273
  safe and effective exercises in, 274–275, 275*f*
  stretching exercise for, 275*f*
Play, for children, 304
Plethysmography, 206, 211–213

Plumb line assessment, 183, 184*t*
Plyometric training, 118–119, 118*f*, 303
PNF. *See* Proprioceptive neuromuscular facilitation
Policies and procedures
    emergency, 412, 449–452
    facility, 410–412
    human resource, 447
Pollock, Michael, 8
Positive energy balance, 213, 217
Posterior shoulder hyperextension, 140*f*
Postpartum period
    physical activity and health in, 18
    physical activity guidelines for, 12, 12*t*, 15, 305
Posttraumatic stress disorder (PTSD), exercise and, 380
Postural hypotension, in pregnancy, 307, 308
Posture
    awareness in, progressive approach to developing, 183–184
    and functional movement, 181
    integrative assessments and corrections for, 185–187
    neutral position in, 182–184
    plumb line assessment of, 183, 184*t*
    proprioceptive acuity and, 177*t*
    static, assessment of, 183–184, 184*t*
    stretching for deviations in, 184*t*
    verbal cues for correction, 183, 184*t*
    wall test of, 183
Power clean and snatch, 116, 117*f*, 125, 127
Powerlifting, resistance training *versus*, 105
PPIs. *See* Proton pump inhibitors
Prayer, 385
Precontemplation, as stage of change, 327, 328*t*, 330*b*
Predictive equations, of energy expenditure, 215, 215*t*
Pregnant women, 305–310
    cardiorespiratory fitness in, 305–306
    case study of, 317–318
    chronic exercise by, impact of, 306–308
    contraindications to exercise in, 309
    employee rights of, 409–410
    exercise guidelines for, 305, 308, 309
    exercise prescription for, 308
    exercise programming for, 308–310
    nutrition in, 309
    overweight or obese, 310
    physical activity and health in, 18, 305, 308, 309–310
    physical activity guidelines for, 12, 12*t*, 15, 305
    physical and physiological changes in, 305–306
    special considerations for, 310
    warning signs in exercise, 309
    weight and center of gravity, 306
    weight gain in, 306, 307, 317–318
Prehiring inquiries, 407–410
Preparation, as stage of change, 108, 327, 328*t*, 330*b*, 357–358
Preparticipation physical activity screening, 29–57
    algorithm for, 43*f*–44*f*
    assessment form for, 39, 45*f*
    case study, 54–55
    cautions in, 31
    challenges of, 49–51
    conservative approach in, 49
    contraindications to exercise testing, 51–53, 51*b*

decision tree for, 42*f*, 48
ePARmed-X + Physician Clearance Follow-Up Questionnaire, 32, 48
guidelines on, 30, 31, 50–51, 450*t*
Health History Questionnaire (HHQ), 32, 39, 40*f*–42*f*
history of, 31
importance of, 30
informed consent for, 37, 38*f*
known cardiovascular, metabolic, and/or renal disease in, 46
legal issues in, 411
levels of, 31–51
medical examination/clearance, 39
for older adults, 313
paradigm shift on, 48
PAR-Q +, 32, 33*f*–36*f*, 71, 266, 411
physical activity (or exercise) history in, 46
for pregnant women, 308
process of, 39–49
professionally supervised, 31, 37–49
recommendations *versus* requirements, 50–51
risk stratification/classification in, 30, 31, 48, 49, 50*t*
self-guided, 31–32
signs and symptoms of cardiovascular disease in, 46–48
Preschool-age children, physical activity guidelines for, 11*t*, 12, 14
Prescription drugs, for chronic disease, exercise effects of, 253, 255–256
President's Council on Physical Fitness and Sports, 7, 137
Preventive exercise prescription, 493–494, 494*t*
Price, in marketing mix, 474–475, 475*f*
PRICE treatment, 267*t*, 268*t*, 269
Primary appraisal, 372
The Principles of Scientific Management (Taylor), 427
Print advertisements, 464, 476
Privacy Rule, HIPAA, 404–405
Problem-focused coping, 373–374
Product, in marketing mix, 472
Professional behavior, 484–505. *See also* Ethics
Professional indemnity insurance (PII), 402
Professional liability insurance (PLI), 402, 453
Professionally supervised screening, 31, 37–49
    assessment form for, 39, 45*f*
    components of, 37
    decision tree for, 42*f*, 48
    informed consent for, 37, 38*f*
2018 Profiles of Success (IHRSA), 438, 442, 462
Profit and loss projections, 461
Profit and loss (income) statement, 460–461, 460*f*
Profit margin, acceptable, 474
Progesterone, and flexibility, 139
Programming, 466–467. *See also specific exercise types and conditions*
    in-demand programs, 466, 466*t*, 467*t*
    successful, steps to, 466–467
Progression
    accommodations for, 176
    in cardiorespiratory fitness, 86–87
    in core exercises, 277–281, 278*f*, 280*f*
    features optimizing, 176
    in flexibility training, 153–154
    functional movement and, 176
    in individuals with chronic diseases, 241
    in instability training, 193, 194*t*
    in resistance training, 111–112

Progressive muscle relaxation, 384
Progressive overload, 86
Promotion, 464–465, 467, 475–480
    advertising in, 464–465, 476, 478*t*
    art of the deal in, 479
    branding in, 464, 476
    business to business (B2B), 477, 478*t*
    cost/benefit breakdown of tools, 478*t*
    direct mail/e-mail in, 464, 477
    incentive program in, 473
    Internet in, 464, 477
    personal sales in, 478–479
    public relations in, 479–481
    referral in, 476
    sponsorship in, 477–478, 478*t*
Property insurance, 453
Proprioception, 176–177
    acuity in, salient features of, 176, 177*t*
    age and, 182
    arthritis and, 284
    assessment and prescription, 183–193
    definition of, 176
    feedback and feed-forward in, 177
    lifestyle recommendations for, 197
    mediators of, 180–182
    sensory input for, 176–177, 177*f*
Proprioceptive neuromuscular facilitation (PNF), 139, 140–143, 141*f*
    anatomical structures and, 144, 144*f*
    diagonal, 141, 141*f*
    hold–relax techniques in, 142
    muscle performance affected by, 137, 194
Proprioceptors, 143
Prospects, qualifying, 479
Prostate cancer, physical activity and reduced risk of, 17*t*
Protected health information, 404–405
Protective documents, legal, 400–402
Proton pump inhibitors (PPIs), 255*t*
Psychographics, 470
Psychological distress
    exercise and, 380
    referral for, 386, 386*t*
    stress and, 378–379
Psychological needs, and self-determination, 338–339
Psychologist, referral to, 386, 386*t*
Psychosocial barriers, to physical activity, 355
PTSD, exercise and, 380
Puberty, 300
Public Health Specialist, certified, 487
Public policy, 334–336, 335*f*
Public relations, 479–480
Pull-down, 119, 120*f*
Pull-up, 119–120, 120*f*, 138
Pulmonary circulation, 61–62
Pulmonary disease
    aerobic training guidelines in, 242*t*
    controlled, exercise for individuals with, 232–264
    exercise concerns, precautions, and contraindications in, 251–252
    exercise prescription and programming in, 245
    exercise role in mediating, 240
    FITT considerations in, 242*t*, 243*t*, 245
    medication effects on exercise in, 253–256
    pathophysiology of, 237–238
    resistance training guidelines in, 243*t*
    teaching and demonstrating exercises in, 256–257

Pulmonary ventilation
   altitude and, 94–97
   in children and adolescents, 301
   in graded intensity exercise, 67
   in older adults, 312
   in pregnant women, 305–306
Pulse palpitation, 68
Purpose
   in organizational culture, 437
   in programming, 467
Push-up, 120
Push-up tests, 104, 110–111, 110f, 112

Q

Qigong, 308
Qualifications
   employee, in job description, 444
   instructor, 411
Qualifying prospects, 479
Queens College/McArdle Step Test, 70t, 73

R

Race/ethnicity
   and BMI/waist circumference, 205
   discrimination prohibited on basis of,
      407–408
   and obesity, 201
   working with diverse populations, 367
Radial pulse, 68
Range of motion (ROM), 137–139.
      See also Flexibility
   activities of daily living, 137
   aging and, 311
   assessment of, 108, 145–146, 146f,
      147t–152t
   factors affecting, 137–139
   flexibility definition, 137
   functional movement and, 181
   joint specificity of, 137
   recommendations/guidelines, 137, 154–169
Rate pressure product (RPP), 69
Rating of perceived exertion. *See* Perceived
      exertion
Reactivity, in stress response, 376
Recertification, 498–499
Reciprocal determinism, 328–329, 331f
Reciprocal inhibition, 143
Recovery, in stress response, 376
Recreational activities, 3–4, 3f
Recruiting, 442–444
   definition of, 442
   strategies for, 442–444
Recruitment, of muscle fibers, 105–106, 106f
Red blood cells, in children and adolescents,
      301
REE. *See* Resting energy expenditure
Reengineering, 332
Referral
   business to business, 476, 478t
   client, 476
   employee, 442
   mental health, 386, 386t
Reflexes, myotatic or stretch, 143
Regression equations, for skinfold
      measurements, 208–210, 209t
Regularity, principle of, 112
Rehabilitative exercise prescription, 493–494,
      494t
Reinforcement management, 331t
Relapse prevention, 333, 356, 357b
Relatedness, as psychological need, 338–339

Relationships. *See also* Social support
   and change, 331t, 351–352
   and sales, 466
Relationship Selling (Cathcart), 465
Relative contraindications, 52
Relative oxygen consumption, 77
Relaxation, progressive muscle, 384
Releases, legal, 400–402
Relevant goals, 349
Remodeling phase, of healing, 269, 270t
Renal disease
   ACSM major signs or symptoms of, 46–48
   aerobic training guidelines in, 242t
   chronic, pathophysiology of, 238
   controlled, exercise for individuals with,
      232–264
   exercise concerns, precautions, and
      contraindications in, 252–253
   exercise role in mediating, 240–241
   FITT considerations in, 242t, 243t, 246
   known, 46
   medication effects on exercise in, 253–256
   preparticipation screening for, 29–47
      (*See also* Preparticipation physical
      activity screening)
   resistance training guidelines in, 243t
   teaching and demonstrating exercises in,
      256–257
Repair phase, of healing, 269, 270t
Repetition maximum (RM), 109–110, 126
Research knowledge, 496, 498
Resistance
   in motivational interviewing, 361
   in stress response, 375
Resistance training, 103–135
   anatomic considerations in, 105–107
   for arthritis, 282–283, 284f
   case study, 130–131
   for children and adolescents, 303–304
   choice of exercise, 124–125
   core, 124–125
   creativity in, 113
   definition of, 105
   dynamic constant external, 116–117, 117f
   enjoyment in, 113–114
   exercise prescription for, 129
   fitness trend in, 104
   for flexibility, 138
   frequency in, 112, 123, 124t, 127–128
   functional movement and, 182
   fundamental principles of, 111–115
   general recommendations on, 129
   guidelines for, 104, 124t
   health impact of, 104–105, 129
   injuries in, 121–123, 122f
   isokinetic, 117–118
   for low back pain, 279t
   modes of, 119–121
   muscle action in, 106–107
   muscle fiber recruitment in, 105–106, 106f
   for older adults, 315
   order of exercise, 125
   for osteoporosis, 105, 289, 290t
   overload in, 113, 182
   periodization in, 106, 128
   for persons with cardiovascular disease, 244
   for persons with chronic diseases, 243t,
      244, 245, 246, 257
   for persons with diabetes mellitus, 245
   for persons with kidney disease, 246
   plyometric, 118–119, 118f
   for pregnant women, 307–309
   program design considerations in, 115–123

   program variables in, 123–128
   progression in, 111–112
   for reducing risk of strains and sprains,
      270–271
   regularity in, 112
   repetition maximum in, 109–110, 126
   repetition velocity in, 127
   resistance load in, 111–112, 115, 125–126
   rest intervals between sets in, 127
   risk assessment for, 115
   safety concerns in, 121–123, 123t
   specificity in, 114–115
   stress experience and, 376
   supervision in, 115
   for tendinopathies and plantar fasciitis, 272t
   training intensity in, 123, 124t, 125–126
   training volume in, 123, 126–127
   2 + 2 rule in, 111–112
   types of, 116–119, 124–125, 124t
   weight loss in, 217
Respiratory muscles, 186–187
Respiratory system. *See also* Cardiorespiratory
      fitness
   altitude and, 94–97
   anatomy and physiology of, 61–64
   in children and adolescents, 301
   cold stress and, 95
   goal/function of, 61, 62f
   graded exercise responses of, 64–69
   heat stress and, 95
   in older adults, 312
   oxygen uptake kinetics in
      during graded intensity exercise, 65–66,
         66f
      sex/age and, 78t–79t
      during submaximal single-intensity
         exercise, 64–65, 65f
   in pregnant women, 305–306
Responsibilities
   client, 406
   employer and employee, 406–407
   facility, to membership, 406, 410–412
   job, 447
   supervisory, 400, 406, 410–411
Resting energy expenditure (REE), 213–215,
      215t
Rest intervals, in resistance training, 127
Retention, employee, 449
Revenues, 460–462, 460f
Reversibility
   in cardiorespiratory fitness, 86–87
   in resistance training, 112
Rhabdomyolysis, 255
Rheumatic cachexia, 281
Rheumatoid arthritis, 281–283
   assessment of, 281–282
   clinical presentation of, 281
   exercise guidelines for, 282t, 284–285
   medication effects for, 284
   safe and effective exercise in, 282–283, 284f
   yoga for, 143
Rights
   client, 405
   employer and employee, 406–407
Risk(s), 19–21
   assumption of, 401
   cardiac events during exercise testing,
      20, 55
   for children and adolescents, 303
   contraindications for, 51–53, 52b
   exercise, Thompson's study of, 55
   flexibility training, 154, 169
   inherent, 400–401

leadership *versus* management, 417
legal issues/liability in, 399–403
musculoskeletal injuries, 20–21, 93–94
musculoskeletal limitations and, 266
precautions against, 19, 19*t*, 49
preparticipation screening for, 29–57
resistance training, 115, 121–123, 123*t*
strain/sprain, exercise to reduce, 270–271
sudden cardiac death, 20
Risk classification, 30, 31, 48
Risk factor assessment and management, 52–53
Risk factor thresholds, 30, 31
Risk management, 400–403, 449–453
business liability insurance and, 452–453
standards and guidelines for, 449–452
Risk stratification, 30, 31, 48, 49, 50*t*
RM. *See* Repetition maximum
Rockport walking test, 70*t*, 72
Rogers, Renee J., 362–366
Roller massagers, 196
Rolling patterns
assessment of, 187, 188*t*
corrections for, 187, 188*t*, 189*f*–190*f*
verbal cues for, 187, 188*t*
ROM. *See* Range of motion
RPE. *See* Perceived exertion
RPP. *See* Rate pressure product
Running
advantages and disadvantages of, 88*t*
energy expenditure during, 83*t*
MET values of, 6*t*
musculoskeletal injuries in, 20–21
Running tests, for cardiorespiratory fitness, 70*t*, 78*t*–79*t*

S

Safe and effective exercise
in bursitis, 273
in low back pain, 276–281, 278*f*, 280*f*
in osteoarthritis, 283, 284*f*
in overuse injuries, 272, 273, 274–281, 274*f*–276*f*, 278*f*, 280*f*
in plantar fasciitis, 274–275, 275*f*
in rheumatoid arthritis, 282–283, 284*f*
in tendinopathy, 274–275
Safety
hygienic, 412
injury prevention, 21
musculoskeletal limitations and, 266
resistance training, 121–123, 123*t*
risks/risk reduction, 19–21, 19*t*
workplace, OSHA guidelines on, 398, 404, 407, 450*t*
Sagittal plane, 114–115, 114*f*
SAID principle, 87, 114
Sales, 466, 478–479
art of the deal, 479
finding leads in, 478–479
qualifying prospects in, 479
Sales manager, 439*t*, 446*t*
SAMHSA (Substance Abuse and Mental Health Services Administration), 387*t*
Sarcomere, 105, 181
Sarcopenia, 201
SBP. *See* Systolic blood pressure
Scales, for measuring weight, 202
Scapular retraction, 191*t*, 192*f*
Scientific management, 427–428
Scope of practice, 489–494
Capati v. Crunch Fitness, 492–493
decision tree, 490, 492*f*

definition of, 489
job task analysis in, 490–494
overlapping, 490, 490*f*, 491*f*
reviews of, 490
scenarios of, 491–494
Screen time, 303, 304–305
SCT. *See* Social cognitive theory
Scuba diving, avoidance in pregnancy, 309
SDT. *See* Self-determination theory
Sedentary behaviors, 4, 15–16, 15*f*, 53
and arthritis, 284–285
in children and adolescents, 303
and osteoporosis, 291
Selection process, for employees, 442, 444–445
Selective estrogen receptor modulators (SERM), 289*t*
Self-control, 382–383
Self-determination theory (SDT), 327, 338–339
Self-efficacy, 329–333
communication about, 359
definition of, 353
enhancing, 353
exercise physiologist and, 358
psychosocial barriers and, 355
and relapse prevention, 333
strategies for, 330–333, 332*t*, 353, 354*t*
and stress management, 382–383
supporting, in motivational interviewing, 361
Self-guided screening, 31–32
ePARmed-X+Physician Clearance Follow-Up Questionnaire, 32, 48
PAR-Q+, 32, 33*f*–36*f*, 71, 266, 411
Self-liberation, 331*t*
Self-monitoring, 349–351
consequences of, 350
facilitators of, 350
perceived barriers of, 350
perceived benefits of, 350
physical activity monitors for, 349, 351
recommendations for, 350
relapse prevention in, 356
Self-myofascial release (SMR), 194–196, 196*f*, 197*t*
Self-presentation, 355
Self-reevaluation, 331*t*
Self-stretching, 139
Selye, Hans, 128, 374–376
Senior Fitness Test, 314
Sensorimotor control, 176–180
Sensorimotor system, 176–177, 178*f*
Servant leadership, 423
Sets, in resistance training
periodization and, 128
rest intervals between, 127
volume of, 126–127
Settings, of health/fitness facilities, 453–455
Sex discrimination, 403, 407, 409
Sexual harassment, 403–404, 407
Shadowing, 447
Sheppard v. River Valley Fitness One, 403
Sherrington, Charles, 141, 176
Shortness of breath, 47, 245, 251–252
Short Physical Performance Battery, 314
Shoulder, flexibility of
assessment of, 148*f*, 148*t*–149*t*, 149*f*
static stretches for, 140*f*, 156*f*, 156*t*–158*t*, 157*f*
Shoulder external rotation, 191*t*, 193*f*
Shoulder hyperextension, posterior, 140*f*
Shoulder stabilization, 178–179

Side plank, 185, 188*t*, 190*f*, 191*t*, 278*f*, 279–280
Single-joint exercises, 119, 124
Siri equation, 209
SIT. *See* Sprint interval training
Sit-and-reach tests, 145
Situational context, of physical activity, 3–4, 3*f*
Situational leadership theory, 421–422, 422*f*
Size principle, of motor unit activation, 106
Skeletal muscle. *See also* Muscle(s)
agonist, 105, 181
antagonist, 105, 181
contractions of, 3, 105, 106–107, 124, 137, 142
fibers of, 105–106, 106*f*, 144, 144*f*
force produced by, 107, 108*f*
force–velocity relationship, 107, 108*f*
hypertonicity of, 180, 181, 194
hypertrophy of, 220
stretching/flexibility and, 137
structure and function of, 105–107
synergist, 105, 181
types of action, 106–107
Skill-related fitness, 4, 5*f*
Skinfold measurements, 207–210
assumptions and errors in, 207–208
equations for, 208–209, 209*t*
procedure for, 210
sites for, 211*t*, 212*f*
Slow-twitch (type I) muscle fibers, 105–106, 311
SMART goals, 349, 429, 432, 432*f*, 448, 448*t*
Smartphones
biofeedback apps on, 384
self-monitoring via, 351
Smartwatch, 349, 351
Smoking, risk factor assessment in, 53
SMS blasts, 465
Social cognitive theory, 327, 328–333, 331*f*, 348
Social ecological model, 327, 334–336, 335*f*, 336*b*
Social factors, in social ecological model, 334–336, 335*f*
Social liberation, 331*t*
Social media marketing, 465, 477
Social media presence, professional, 500–502
Social norms, of fitness facility, 355
Social support
for behavior change, 351–352
for older adults, 367
real-life example of, 383
for stress management, 380–382, 383
Society for Human Resources Management, 446
Soleus, stretching exercise for, 276*f*
Special populations. *See also specific populations*
children and adolescents, 300–305
individuals with controlled diseases, 232–264
individuals with musculoskeletal limitations, 265–298
older adults, 310–316
pregnant women, 305–310
Specialty credentials, 486–487
Specificity
in cardiorespiratory fitness, 87
context for principle of, 182
functional movement and, 182
in goal setting, 349, 429, 432, 432*f*, 448, 448*t*
in resistance training, 114–115

Spine
  goniometry assessment of, 147f, 147t
  neutral position of, 182–184
  pain, 275–281 (*See also* Low back pain)
Spirometry, 70–71, 70t, 82
Sponsorship, 477–478, 478t
Sports, MET values of, 6t
Sports conditioning, 303
Spot reducing, myth of, 220
Sprains, 268–271
  definition of, 267
  exercise to reduce risk of, 270–271
  medications for, 269–270, 270t
  pregnancy and, 306
  PRICE treatment for, 268t, 269
Sprint interval training (SIT), 89
Squat, muscle action in, 106–107, 107f
Stability, 177–180
  age and, 182
  assessment and prescription, 183–193
  core function in, 180
  definition of, 178
  instability training for, 193, 194t, 195f
  lifestyle recommendations for, 197
  mediators of, 177, 180–182
  muscles in (*See* Stabilizing muscles)
  optimal strategies for, 178
Stability balls, 121
Stabilizing muscles, 179–180, 179t, 191t, 276,
    277t
  alignment faults and, 191–193, 191t
  corrective exercises for, 191–192, 191t,
    192f–193f
  propensity of inhibition, 180
Stable ischemia, 234
Stadiometer, 202
Staffing, 438–442
  employee *versus* independent contractor,
    439, 440t
  exempt *versus* nonexempt employees, 441,
    441t
  full-time *versus* part-time employees,
    441–442, 441t
  job descriptions in, 407, 442, 443–444
  positions/jobs in fitness industry, 438,
    438t, 439t
  questions to consider in, 438
Stages of change, 327–328, 328t, 329, 330b,
    357–358
Stakeholders, 418, 431–432, 432f, 475
Standard of care, 397, 398f, 399–400, 411
Standards Facilitation Guide (IHRSA), 406
Static flexibility, 137, 139
Static flexibility testing, 145
Static muscle contractions, 3, 107
Static posture, assessment of, 183–184, 184t
Static stretching, 139, 140f
  ankle and foot, 166f, 166t–167t, 167f
  elbow, 158f, 158t–159t, 159f
  fingers, 161f, 161t
  hand and wrist, 160f, 160t
  hip, 163f, 163t–164t, 164f
  knee, 165f, 165t
  lower body, 163t–168t
  major muscle groups, 155t–168t
  muscle performance affected by, 137, 169,
    194
  neck, 155f, 155t
  recommendations, 154–169
  shoulder, 156f, 156t–158t, 157f
  toe, 168f, 168t
  trunk, 161f, 161t–162t, 162f
  upper body, 156t–162t

Statins, 254t, 255
Statutory law, 397–398
Steady state
  heart rate, 71
  oxygen consumption, 64–65, 65f
Steps (stepping)
  energy expenditure during, 83t
  pedometers for, 349, 351
STEPS, for avoiding liability, 397, 398f
Step tests, 70t, 71, 73
Stewardship, 501
"Sticking point" of exercise, 107
Stimulus control, 331t
Stogdill, Ralph, 421
Strain, as stress response, 374, 378, 382–383
Strains, 267–271
  definition of, 267
  exercise to reduce risk of, 270–271
  grading and characteristics of, 267t
  medications for, 269–270, 270t
  PRICE protocol for, 267t, 269
  treatment of, 267t
Strategic planning, 431–432, 432f
Strength. *See* Muscular strength; Resistance
    training
Stress, 371–394
  acute, 379
  allostatic load model of, 375–376
  appraisal of, 373
  as barrier to physical activity, 380
  chronic, 372–373, 375–376, 379
  coping with, 373–374
  cumulative, 373
  definition of, 372
  excessive, signs and symptoms of,
    376, 377t
  exercise and adaptation implications of,
    376
  fitness test–associated, 375
  general adaptation syndrome in,
    374–376
  good (eustress), 373
  health effects of, 372, 376–379, 377t
  perceived, assessment of, 381–382
  psychological functioning in, 378–379
  response to, 372–379
  sources of, 372–373
  transactional model of, 373
Stress in America report, 372, 374
Stress management, 379–389
  biofeedback for, 384
  case study of, 388–389
  diaphragmatic breathing and body scan
    for, 384
  exercise for, 379–380
  massage for, 385
  meditation and prayer for, 385
  mind–body techniques for, 383–386
  mindfulness for, 385
  personal (self-) control for, 382–383
  progressive muscle relaxation for, 384
  referral to psychologist for, 386, 386t
  resources for, 387t
  self-control/self-efficacy for, 382–383
  social support for, 380–382, 383
  yoga and martial arts for, 386
Stressors, 372–373
Stretching
  anatomical structures and, 144, 144f
  ankle and foot, 166f, 166t–167t, 167f
  antibiotics and injury risk in, 154
  ballistic, 139, 140
  dynamic, 108, 137, 139, 142–143, 154–169

elbow, 158f, 158t–159t, 159f
  fingers, 161f, 161t
  for functional movement, 194–196, 196f,
    197t
  hand and wrist, 160f, 160t
  health impact of, 154
  hip, 163f, 163t–164t, 164f
  knee, 165f, 165t
  for low back pain, 279t
  lower body, 163t–168t
  muscle performance affected by, 137, 169,
    194
  neck, 155f, 155t
  for overuse injuries, 274–275, 274f, 275f
  PNF, 137, 139, 140–143, 141f
  for postural deviations, 184t
  for pregnant women, 306, 307–308
  recommendations, 154–169
  for reducing risk of strain/sprain, 271
  shoulder, 156f, 156t–158t, 157f
  static, 137, 139, 140f, 154–169, 155t–168t,
    194
  for tendinopathies and plantar fasciitis,
    272t
  toe, 168f, 168t
  trunk, 161f, 161t–162t, 162f
  upper body, 156t–162t
Stretch (myotatic) reflexes, 143
Stroke volume (SV)
  blood pressure regulation in, 235
  in children and adolescents, 301
  in Fick equation for $\dot{V}O_{2max}$, 66
  in graded intensity exercise, 66–67, 67f
  heat stress and, 95
  in older adults, 312
  in pregnant women, 305
Strontium ranelate, 289t
Stults-Kolehmainen, Matthew, 388–389
Subcutaneous fat, skinfold measurement of,
    207–210, 209t, 211t, 212f
Submaximal exercise testing, 48, 64–65, 65f,
    70t, 71–72, 74
Submaximal oxygen uptake, 64–65, 65f, 70t,
    71
Substance Abuse and Mental Health Services
    Administration (SAMHSA), 387t
Sudden cardiac death, 20, 55
Sullivan, Geoff, 481–482
Summary judgment, 402
Supervision
  principle of, 115
  resistance training, 115
Supervisory responsibilities, 400, 406,
    410–411
Surgeon General's *Physical Activity and
    Health* report (1996), 9, 31
SV. *See* Stroke volume
Sweating, 95
  in children and adolescents, 302
  in older adults, 312–313
Swelling. *See* Edema
Swimming
  advantages and disadvantages of, 88t
  weight loss in, 217
SWOT analysis, 432
Syncope, 47
Synergist muscles, 105, 181
Synovial joints, 138–139, 138f
Systemic circulation, 61–62, 62f
Systems theory, 335
Systolic blood pressure (SBP), 67–68, 69,
    234–235
  in children and adolescents, 301

T

TAAG (trial of activity for adolescent girls), 336b
Tachycardia, 47
Talk test method, 91–92, 257, 308
Target body weight, 214
Target heart rate, 90
Taylor, Frederick W., 427–428
TDEE. See Total daily energy expenditure
Team management, 427
Teamwork, 437–438
Technology, for self-monitoring, 349, 351
TEE. See Total energy expenditure
TEF. See Thermic effect of food
Tendinitis, 271
Tendinopathy, 271–272
    assessment of, 271
    clinical presentation of, 271
    common sites for, 271
    definition of, 271
    exercise considerations for, 272, 272t, 274–275
    FITT principle in, 272
Tendinosis, 271, 272t
Tennis balls, for SMR, 196
Ten repetition maximum, 109
Tension headaches, 377–378, 384
Teser, Kaitlin, 22–23
Theory(ies). See also specific theories
    behavior change, 326–346
    definition of, 327
    importance of, 327
    interventions based on, 348
    leadership, 419–426
    translation to real world, 334
Theory of planned behavior (TPB), 327, 337–338, 338f
Theory X and Y, 430
Thermic effect of food (TEF), 214
Thermic effect of physical activity (TEPA), 214
Thermogenesis, nonexercise activity, 214
Thermoregulation
    acclimatization, 96
    in children and adolescents, 302
    cold stress, 94–95
    heat stress, 94–95, 302
    obesity and, 302
    in older adults, 312–313, 316
    in pregnant women, 306, 309
Thixotropism, 196
Thompson, Paul, 55
Thoracic hyperkyphosis, 291
Threat, stress appraisal in, 373
3D-thinking model, of contextual intelligence, 426
"Thrifty gene" hypothesis, 213
Time (duration)
    cardiorespiratory fitness, 84–85, 85t
    exercise for bone health, 290t
    exercise for weight loss, 217–218, 218t
    exercise in chronic diseases, 241–246, 242t, 243t, 257
    exercise in low back pain, 279t
    exercise in overuse injuries, 279t
    exercise in pregnancy, 308, 309
    exercise in tendinopathies, 272
    flexibility training, 153–154, 153t
    interval training, 89
    resistance exercise, 124t
Time, as barrier to physical activity, 354
Time-bound goals, 349

Tissue repair, 269, 270t
Title VII of the Civil Rights Act of 1964, 403
Toes, static stretches for, 168f, 168t
Tort, definition of, 399
Tortfeasor (defendant), 399
Tort law, 399
Total-body free weight exercises, 119–121
Total daily energy expenditure (TDEE), 213–215, 215t
Total energy expenditure (TEE), 215–216
Total peripheral resistance (TPR), 67–68, 235
Total quality management (TQM), 428–429
TPB. See Theory of planned behavior
TPR. See Total peripheral resistance
TQM. See Total quality management
Tracking/trackers, 349–351
Traditions, 437–438
Training, employee, 446–447
Trait theory, of leadership, 421
Transactional behaviors, 419
Transactional leadership, 419, 422–423
Transactional model of stress, 373
Transcendental meditation, 385
Transformational leadership, 419–420, 422–423
Transportation-related physical activity, 3–4, 3f
Transtheoretical model (TTM), 327–328, 328t, 329, 330b, 357–358
Transverse abdominis, isolation of, 278f, 279
Transverse plane, 114–115, 114f
Traumatic movement-related injuries, 266–271
    exercise to reduce risk of, 270–271
    healing process in, 269, 270t
    immediate care for, 269
    medical referral for, 266
    medications for, 269–270
    PRICE treatment for, 267t, 268t, 269
Treadmills, care of, 456t
Treadmill test, 9, 70t, 74, 78t–79t, 313
Trend-line budgeting, 461
Trends, fitness, 471–472
Trends, programming, 466, 466t, 467t
Trial of activity for adolescent girls (TAAG), 336b
Triceps brachii, 105, 159t
Trigger points, 194–196, 196f, 197t
Triglycerides, 53, 236, 378
Trunk flexibility, static stretches for, 161f, 161t–162t, 162f
Trust
    communication and, 359–360
    sales and, 466
TTM. See Transtheoretical model
12-minute walk/run test, 70t, 78t–79t
2 + 2 rule, 111–112
Type 1 diabetes mellitus, 236
Type 2 diabetes mellitus, 236, 244–245, 252, 378
Type I muscle fibers, 105–106, 311
Type II muscle fibers, 105–106, 311
Type of exercise (FITT)
    cardiorespiratory fitness, 84–86, 85t
    exercise for weight loss, 217–218, 218t
    exercise in chronic diseases, 241–246, 242t, 243t, 257
    exercise in low back pain, 279t
    exercise in overuse injuries, 272, 272t, 279t
    exercise in pregnancy, 308–309
    flexibility training, 154, 155t–168t
    resistance exercise, 124–125, 124t

U

Ulcers, stress and, 376–377
Underhand medicine ball toss, 121, 121f
Underwater weighing, 206, 211
Underweight, 202
Undistributed expenses, 462–463
Undulating model of periodization, 128
U.S. Department of Health and Human Services (USDHHS), 9, 10–12, 305, 387t
U.S. Department of Labor, 404
U.S. Diabetes Prevention Program (DPP), 252
U.S. Food and Drug Administration (FDA), on dietary supplements, 224, 253
Unstable ischemia, 234
Upper body
    endurance, assessment of, 110–111, 110f
    goniometry assessment of, 147f, 147t–149t
    static stretches for, 156t–162t
"Use it or lose it," 86–87

V

Value, market, 474
Values
    in organizational culture, 437
    professional, 485 (See also Ethics)
    in strategic planning, 432, 432f
Variable costs, 462–463
Variable resistance machines, 116–117
Variance, 457
Variation, in resistance training, 112, 127, 128
Vasculature, 61–62
Vastus lateralis, 106–107
Veins, 61–62
Velocity, muscular, 107, 108f
    in isokinetics, 117–118
    in resistance training, 127
Ventricles, of heart, 61–62
Venules, 61–62
Verbal persuasion, and self-efficacy, 330–333, 332t, 353, 354t
Very low-density lipoproteins (VLDLs), 236
Vicarious experience, and self-efficacy, 330–333, 332t, 353, 354t
Vigorous physical activity, 4, 6t, 10, 48
    for older adults, 315
Vision
    in leadership, 417, 419–420
    in organizational culture, 437
    in programming, 467
    in strategic planning, 432, 432f
Visionary model, of leadership, 419–420
Vital sign, physical activity as, 337
Vitamin D, 287, 288t, 289t
V̇O₂ (oxygen consumption), 64–66
    in children and adolescents, 301
    cold stress and, 95
    excess postexercise, 65, 65f
    maximal (V̇O₂max), 65–66, 70–71, 70t, 78t–79t
    myocardial, 69
    in older adults, 312
    peak, 90–91
    in pregnant women, 306
    relative and absolute, 77
    reserve, intensity measurement via, 91
    sex/age and, 78t–79t
    steady state, 64–65, 65f
    in submaximal exercise, 64–65, 65f, 70t, 71

Volume
    in cardiorespiratory fitness, 86
    in individuals with chronic diseases, 241,
        245
    in resistance training, 123, 126–127
Voluntary muscle contractions, 137

W

Wages, 445, 446*t*
Waist circumference, 203*t*, 204–206, 205*f*
Waist-to-height ratio (WHtR), 205
Waist-to-hip ratio (WHR), 205, 206*t*
Waivers, and liability, 400–402
Walking
    advantages and disadvantages of, 88*t*
    cardiorespiratory fitness in, 98
    energy expenditure during, 83, 83*t*
    injury risk in, 20
    MET values of, 6*t*
    pedometers for steps, 349, 351
    weight loss in, 217
Walking tests, for cardiorespiratory fitness,
    70*t*, 72, 74
Wall plank-and-roll (WPR), 185
Wall test, 183
Warm-up
    for children and adolescents, 303
    for flexibility/ROM, 138, 139, 143, 146,
        154, 169
    for injury prevention/management, 271,
        274
    for muscular strength assessment, 109
    for older adults, 316
    for pregnant women, 308
WBV. *See* Whole-body vibration
Weber, Max, 428
Weight (body weight), 202. *See also* Obesity;
        Weight gain; Weight loss; Weight
        management
    of children and adolescents, 300–301
    of pregnant women, 306
    self-monitoring of, 349

Weight-bearing exercises, 88
    for bone health, 290*t*, 291
    for low back pain, 279*t*
Weight gain
    exercise and, myth about, 220
    medications causing, 225
    in older adults, 311
    in pregnancy, 306, 307, 317–318
    preventing, 217
Weightlifting, 116–117, 119–121
    for children and adolescents,
        303–305
    DCER, 116–117, 117*f*
    power clean and snatch, 116, 117*f*, 125,
        127
Weight loss, 217–225
    appropriate methods of, 223
    behavioral strategies for, 224
    for diabetes mellitus, 245
    dieting for, 225
    exercise and, 217–220, 236
    FITT recommendations in, 217–218,
        218*t*
    goals for, 217, 219, 224
    inappropriate methods of, 223, 223*t*
    medications affecting, 225
    metabolic equations for, 220
    nutrition (diet) for, 221–222
    in older adults, 311
    rate of, 216, 219
    surgery for, 223–224
    training considerations for, 218–219
Weight loss supplements, 223*t*, 224–225
Weight machines, 116–117, 119–121, 120*f*
    for children and adolescents, 304–305
Weight management, 213–225
    case study, 226
    in children and adolescents, 304–305
    common activity factors in, 215, 215*t*
    energy balance in, 213–216
    estimating target body weight in, 214
    exercise and, 217–220
    medications affecting, 225

myths about, 219–220
    obesity treatment in, 217–225
    physical activity level in, 214–216
    weight loss goals in, 217
Wellness vision, 22–23
Western Ontario and McMaster Universities
        Osteoarthritis Index, 283
Whole-body vibration (WBV), 291
WHR. *See* Waist-to-hip ratio
Wisdom, 501
WISE (Wisdom, Integrity, Stewardship, and
        Enthusiasm), 501
WOM. *See* Word of mouth
Women. *See* Females
Word of mouth (WOM), 464, 476
Workers compensation insurance, 453
Workplace safety, OSHA guidelines on,
        398, 404, 407, 450*t*
Worrell, Chris, 481–482
WPR (wall plank-and-roll), 185
Wrist, static stretches for, 160*f*, 160*t*

Y

Yancey, Toni, 330–332
Yantra meditation, 385
YMCA Cycle Ergometer Test, 70*t*
YMCA/YWCA, 453
Yoga
    for arthritis, 143
    for flexibility, 143
    hot, avoidance in pregnancy, 306
    for pregnant women, 307–308
    program preferences/trends,
        466*t*, 467*t*
    for stress management, 386
*York Insurance Company v. Houston Wellness
        Center, Inc.*, 402–403

Z

Zero-based budgeting, 461